D1799128

# 1 MONTH OF
# FREE
# READING

## at

## www.ForgottenBooks.com

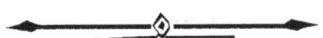

By purchasing this book you are eligible for one month membership to ForgottenBooks.com, giving you unlimited access to our entire collection of over 1,000,000 titles via our web site and mobile apps.

To claim your free month visit:

www.forgottenbooks.com/free1018860

* Offer is valid for 45 days from date of purchase. Terms and conditions apply.

ISBN 978-0-331-14324-9
PIBN 11018860

This book is a reproduction of an important historical work. Forgotten Books uses
state-of-the-art technology to digitally reconstruct the work, preserving the original format
whilst repairing imperfections present in the aged copy. In rare cases, an imperfection in
the original, such as a blemish or missing page, may be replicated in our edition. We do,
however, repair the vast majority of imperfections successfully; any imperfections that
remain are intentionally left to preserve the state of such historical works.

Forgotten Books is a registered trademark of FB &c Ltd.
Copyright © 2018 FB &c Ltd.
FB &c Ltd, Dalton House, 60 Windsor Avenue, London, SW19 2RR.
Company number 08720141. Registered in England and Wales.

For support please visit www.forgottenbooks.com

Dr. Jno. Wise.
— . —
— Third St. —
— . —
Dayton. O.

Dr. Jno. Wise,
Third St.
Dayton, O.

THE

# PRINCIPLES AND PRACTICE

OF

# MODERN SURGERY.

_Third St._
_Dayton. O._

THE

PRINCIPLES AND PRACTICE

Dr. Jn. Wise.
_Third St._
Dayton. O.

OF

# MODERN SURGERY.

## BY ROBERT DRUITT.

" Id potissimum agens, ut omissis hypothesibus, in praxi nihil adstruat quod multiplici experientia non sit roboratum."

ACT ERUD. LIPS , 1722.

FROM THE

## SECOND LONDON EDITION.

### Illustrated with Fifty Wood Engravings.

## WITH NOTES AND COMMENTS

BY

### JOSHUA B. FLINT, M.D.—M.M. S.S.

LECTURER ON THERAPEUTIC AND OPERATIVE SURGERY IN THE " LOUISVILLE
ACADEMY OF MEDICINE, AND LATE PROFESSOR OE SURGERY
IN THE MEDICAL INSTITUTE OF LOUISVILLE."

PHILADELPHIA:

## LEA & BLANCHARD.

WO
D794s
1842

Entered according to Act of Congress, in the year one thousand eight hundred and forty-two, by

**LEA &, BLANCHARD,**

in the Clerk's Office of the District Court of the Eastern District of Pennsylvania.

GRIGGS & CO., PRINTERS.

TO

# CHARLES MAYO, Esq.

SENIOR SURGEON TO THE WINCHESTER HOSPITAL.

IN ADMIRATION OF HIS SOUND JUDGMENT AND SKILL
IN SURGERY,

AND

IN GRATEFUL ACKNOWLEDGMENT OF EARLY KINDNESS,

# THIS WORK

IS DEDICATED BY HIS AFFECTIONATE NEPHEW

AND OBEDIENT SERVANT,

## ROBERT DRUITT.

*6, Bruton Street, Berkeley Square,*
*June 1st,* 1841.

# PREFACE

A LONG preface is not necessary to explain the purport of this work. Suffice it to say, that it is meant to afford a short but complete account of modern surgery; to contain every thing that is essential to the right understanding of its principles, and to embody the experience of the highest authorities as to the best rules for practice.

Short books have in general one of two faults. Either they are made short by the omission of much that is important, insomuch that they are very bad guides for the student, and utterly useless to the advanced practitioner; or they are made short by condensation, and are so crabbed and intricate in style, that some cannot understand them, and others will not take the trouble to read them. I cannot expect this work to be entirely free from both these faults; but yet the favourable reception which the former edition met with from readers and critics leads me to hope that it answered its intended purpose; and that by adhering to the most rigid method, and by making, where possible, a numerical division of the subjects, I succeeded in rendering it tolerably complete, readily comprehensible, and not difficult of retention by the memory. I have added a hundred pages to the practical department of the present edition, which I believe contains every novelty in surgery that deserves mention; but let me add, that in conformity with the motto on my title-page, I have carefully excluded all new-fangled modes of treatment that appeared to me to be contrary to the rules of sound English practice.

The arrangement of a work of this kind ought not, as I conceive, to be regarded as a matter of mere indifference, or at most of convenience, but it ought to embody in it something of a principle; and I believe that the arrangement of this work may be useful to the student, by showing him in what order he may best prosecute his researches into the principles of his profession.

Of the five parts into which it is divided, the first two are more especially devoted to the principles, and the three others to the practice of surgery. The first part treats of the disturbances of the constitution at large, that may be produced by injury or disease of a part; beginning with the simple faintness or collapse that follows a blow, and proceeding to consider the varieties of fever and tetanus.

The second part describes what may be called the elements of local disease; that is to say, those morbid changes of structure or function, which are produced either immediately by external causes, or secondarily, through some deviation from health. And this part includes not only the *common* changes of structure which may be produced, almost at will, in any constitution; but those diseases also, such as cancer and scrofula, which require some peculiarity of the system for their development, and which are consequently termed *specific*. Had my limits permitted, I would gladly have made this part of the work more complete, and have included in it an abstract of general pathology; speaking more fully both of local changes, and of the manners in which they are modified by different kinds of health. Let me observe here that the man who looks upon inflammation as a mere hydraulic derangement of the blood-vessels, or as something red, that must be bled and starved, may be what is vulgarly called simple and decisive in his practice, but is not very rational and cannot be very successful.

The third part treats of the various kinds of injuries, beginning with the simplest mechanical injuries; then proceeding to the effects of chemical agents, and lastly, considering the effects of animal poisons. With regard to the last-mentioned class of morbific agents, I may observe, that without a knowledge of hospital gangrene, dissection wounds, and glanders, no one can have very clear ideas on the subjects of infection and contagion, or of the action of those other morbid poisons, whose effects come within the so-called domain of physic.

The fourth part considers the various tissues, organs, and regions of the body in order, and describes the various accidents they are liable to, and such of their diseases as are commonly assigned to the care of the surgeon.

The fifth part describes such of the operations as were not included in the former parts. So much for the arrangement of the work; from which I have never hesitated to deviate in slight particluars, for the purpose of avoiding repetition, or of not separating subjects that might be better treated of in connexion.

To the whole is appended a collection of formulæ, the number of which is very much increased in this edition.

R. D.

6, *Bruton Street, Berkeley Square,*
*June* I, 1841.

# PREFACE TO THE AMERICAN EDITION.

The American Editor of the present volume can claim but little participation in the merits of it beyond what is due to an early appreciation of the excellencies of Mr. Druitt's book, and an earnest and successful effort to procure its republication. Upon a thorough examination of it with a view to this undertaking, it appeared that its author had been so eminently successful in collecting and arranging whatever could be introduced into such a work with advantage, as to forbid any aspirations for the honours of authorship to a revising Editor, even in the humble offices of annotation and commentary, and he engaged in the enterprize ambitious only to be instrumental in introducing to his profession in this country, and especially in the west, the best compend of the principles and practice of surgery extant.

The only work of the kind, to be compared with it, is the admirable Dictionary of Mr. Samuel Cooper, and though a high compliment, it is not an undeserved one to this volume, to say that, in view of its final purpose and uses, it is, in many respects, entitled to a preference. Mr. Cooper's disquisitions—historical and speculative—on various subjects, though always learned, ingenious and interesting, are frequently too elaborate and discursive for a book of practical reference, and the substance of them may generally be found in brief and comprehensive paragraphs, by Mr. Druitt, and accompanied by such ample biographical references as will enable the surgical student to prosecute his inquiries under the light of all the best guides and authorities which the science can supply. The systematic and methodical arrangement of topics in one volume, while it may be a little less convenient in a *manual* for the practitioner, than the alphabetical order of the "Dictionary," nevertheless contributes essentially to its excellencies as a *text-book* for the student. In this respect it will be found to answer an important desideratum in the apparatus of teaching, and cannot fail to become a favourite as well with Professors of Surgery as with their pupils.

A full course of surgical instruction, of which this should be an epitome or synopsis, would be as nearly a complete one, both in arrangement and matter, as the present state of the science and the didactic genius of the best teachers, could produce.

The extensive circulation which such claims cannot fail to secure to a work of this kind, among the teachers and practitioners of our art, in this

2

country, offered a tempting opportunity for the Editor to introduce to their notice such views and principles of practice, on the various surgical topics, as his own observation and reflection had contributed to establish and render favourite and important ones, in his own estimation. Among these results of his personal investigation are certain conclusions respecting the natural history of calculous affections, and the causes of their greater frequency on this than on the other side of the Alleghenies, which it would have been particularly agreeable to him to have communicated to the profession in this way, and which probably would have been interesting to most medical readers. But, a fear of rendering the book too voluminous for its peculiar uses, inability to find a single chapter or section in the original which could be dispensed with, and, especially, a reluctance to violate its rigid eclecticism determined him to abstain in the present reprint, from any such additions.

A few brief notes of a practical character, the transposition of two or three sections, and the *change of name*, from "'The Surgeons Vade Mecum" to the one now substituted—comprise the only material alterations on which he has ventured. The latter alteration was made partly as a matter of taste, but chiefly upon considerations of significancy and pertinence. "Vade Mecum" is a title by no means expressive of the true character of this work—it indicates indeed, the modesty of its author, but is far from comporting with the real dignity and merit of his production.

"THE PRINCIPLES AND PRACTICE OF MODERN SURGERY" is certainly a significant title for a book which, like the present, is a faithful codification of the opinions and practice of Hunter, Pott, B. Gooch, Abernethy, the Bells, Physick, Dupuytren, Hennen, Macartney, Larrey, the Coopers, Scarpa, Lawrence, Liston, Guthrie, Mayo, Brodie, Carmichael, Warren, Wardrop, Key, Travers, Dudley, Breschet, Tyrrell, Green, Dieffenbach, Civiale, Leroy, Arnott, Barton, Ricord, Colles, Stanley, and most of the other distinguished surgeons who have flourished since the commencement of the Hunterian epoch. Without any of the adventitious aids to which most publications of the present day owe their success—the previous heralding, and subsequent puffing which are usually in requisition at a literary début—without the prestige of rank or official distinction on the part of its author, the "Vade Mecum" has secured an extraordinary popularity in Great Britain, and the most flattering commendations of medical critics.

Such testimony to its intrinsic merits has encouraged its republication here, and will bespeak for it a favourable reception among the practitioners of our country, to whom it is respectfully commended, by

*Their Friend and Brother,*

J. B. F.

*Louisville, April 5th,* 1842

# CONTENTS.

## PART III.

### OF THE DIFFERENT SPECIES OF INJURIES.

## PART V.

### OF THE OPERATIONS OF SURGERY.

# PART I.

## OF THE CONSTITUTIONAL EFFECTS OF LOCAL INJURY AND DISEASE.

---

### CHAPTER I.

#### OF PROSTRATION OR COLLAPSE.*

DEFINITION.—We shall use the terms prostration, or collapse, in the present chapter to signify that general depression of the powers and actions of life, which immediately follows any severe injury.

SYMPTOMS.—The usual symptoms are, shivering; coldness of the surface and extremities; rapid, feeble, and tumultuous pulse; hurried and sighing respiration; dilated pupil, and oppression of the mental faculties. But these symptoms are liable to great variety; for they not only differ in degree, but the principal functions are unequally disordered in different cases. Sometimes depression of the vascular system predominates, and the patient lies in a state of perfect syncope, with the pulse and respiration imperceptible. Sometimes the nervous system is chiefly affected, the patient being bewildered and incoherent, as though intoxicated; or even comatose, as though he had taken a narcotic poison. Nausea and vomiting, hiccup, and suppression of urine; and in children, convulsions, are also extremely frequent symptoms.

TERMINATIONS.—The process of recovery from collapse is commonly called *reaction:* and the manner in which the case may terminate must depend on the nature and degree of that reaction. Thus,

*First,* if it is healthy and moderate, and especially if the collapse arise merely from *concussion* (or violent shaking) of an organ, without actual injury to its structure, it will lead to complete recovery. Thus it very often happens that a slight blow on the testicle, or particularly on the stomach or liver, causes an extreme degree of sickness and faint-

---

* The principal authorities to be consulted on the subject of the first two chapters, are Travers on Constitutional Irritation, third edition, and Hunter on the Blood, chap. ii.

3

ness, which, however, passes off gradually, and leaves no ill consequences.

*Secondly.* If reaction be excessive, the state of collapse will be gradually succeeded by *fever*, symptomatic of the inflammation to which the local injury has given origin.

*Thirdly.* If reaction be imperfectly developed, it will be converted into the state of *prostration with excitement*, of which we shall speak in the next chapter.

*Fourthly.* If reaction be altogether wanting, the collapse will terminate in *death*. And death may occur immediately on the receipt of the injury, if it be of extreme severity; or otherwise the patient may die more slowly, the pulse at the wrist becoming fainter, and finally ceasing; and the respiration more and more slow and oppressed, till life is gradually extinguished.

CAUSES.—These symptoms may be caused by every variety of injury to which the body is liable. Great and sudden extremes of grief, or joy, or fear, or cold;—large doses of any active poison, such as arsenic, or sulpheric acid, or tobacco;—the sudden impression of miasmata, or of morbid poisons, as the plague;—great loss of blood, and mechanical injuries. It is most important that the surgeon should know what injuries are most likely to be followed by fatal collapse, in order that he may have proper materials for giving his prognosis. They are,

*First,* those of organs that are necessary to life, as the stomach and brain; and it is well known that a severe concussion of either of these organs may extinguish life instantaneously.

*Secondly.* Injuries of organs which do not easily admit of reparation; as the joints.

*Thirdly.* Injuries that are severe in their nature; as punctured, lacerated, contused, and especially, gunshot wounds.

*Fourthly.* Injuries of great extent, although they may be trivial in degree;—as extensive burns.

*Lastly.* Injuries occurring to young infants or to the very aged; or to constitutions that are enfeebled by excess* and intemperance,† or by long standing bodily disease or mental depression. From this it will be learned, that the slightest injury, or surgical operation, the removal of a tumour for instance, may prove fatal to persons labouring under chronic organic disease, such as tubercles in the liver or lungs, or continued anxiety and despondency of mind; so that in almost any case, a firm persuasion that recovery is impossible, is almost sufficient to render it so.

---

\*———" Tibi quidnam accedet ad istam
Quam puer et validus præsumis mollitiem, seu
Dura valetudo inciderit, seu tarda senectus ?"

Hor. Sat. ii. 2, 86.

† Those who always live above par, says Hunter, are extremely liable to sink

TREATMENT.—The indication is to excite the vital organs to a moderate and healthy reaction. This is to be fulfilled by the use of diffusive stimulants, such as hot brandy and water, æther, and ammonia; and putting heated bricks or bottles of hot water under the axillæ and between the thighs, and covering the patient warmly till the circulation is restored, and the pulse has acquired permanent strength and firmness. *Vomiting* may be allayed by a large dose of solid opium (gr. ii.—iii.,) or by a large dose of calomel, (gr. v.) and opium (gr. ii.) or by an opiate enema (vide Formula 48) if the bowels are relaxed, or an aperient enema, especially of turpentine, (F. 49) if they are confined; or by effervescent draughts containing one or two minims of diluted hydrocyanic acid, with ten of Battley's sedative, every hour. Counter-irritation to the epigastrium, by means of very hot water or a mustard poultice, (F. 44) is also highly useful.—*Hiccup* may be relieved by a teaspoonful of sp. ætheris comp., or by sipping very frequently gruel, or some other bland fluid, and keeping very silent and quiet.—*Convulsions delirium* and *coma*, are to be treated according to the state of the circulation; by ammonia and stimulants whilst it is depressed, but by a very cautious bleeding, or leeching, or purging, or application of cold to the head, if they remain after the circulation is restored and the pulse has become firm.—One remedy that it might be well worth while to try in an extreme case, is the wrapping a patient in the skin of a sheep, or of any other animal, stripped off immediately after its death. Baron Larrey had seen this done by certain humane Esquimaux, with the greatest benefit, to some shipwrecked Frenchmen that were half dead with cold, fatigue, and hunger; and he put it in practice with equal success in the case of Marshal Lannes, Duc de Montebello, when he was dangerously bruised by a fall from his horse during one of Napoleon's Spanish campaigns.

CAUTIONS.—Care must be taken on the one hand to continue the use of stimulants long enough, and to desist from them gradually if there is any fear that the collapse may return; and, on the other, not to carry them too far—for if the action of the heart is excited beyond its powers it will be more liable to be permanently exhausted. Besides, if the patient be over stimulated, the succeeding fever and inflammation from the injury will be aggravated; and the danger of hæmorrhage will be increased from any blood-vessels that may have been ruptured. Finally, the vulgar and mischievous habit of bleeding patients immediately after an injury, before they have recovered from a state of faintness and depression, needs only to be mentioned to be condemned.

when attacked by disease or injury; for as they are habitually at the full stretch of living, their powers cannot be excited farther to meet any casual emergency.—On the blood, chap. ii. sect. 1.

# CHAPTER II.

## OF PROSTRATION WITH EXCITEMENT.

DEFINITION.—" Prostration with excitement, and excessive reaction," is the term used by Mr. Travers to signify a state which sometimes follows the collapse from a severe injury; in which there is a violent but transient excitement of the nervous and vascular systems, without the development of that more permanent and sthenic action which constitutes inflammatory fever.

SYMPTOMS.—The symptoms vary extremely in different cases, although they present the uniform character of extreme and exhausting excitement, without genuine febrile action. There is great anxiety about the region of the heart: the respiration is oppressed and sighing; the pulse exceedingly rapid and bounding, but soft and compressible; the face is flushed, and there is vomiting. But, in the majority of these cases, the principal feature is the excitement of the nervous system, which is manifested by a peculiar delirium (*delirium traumaticum*) precisely similar to the *delirium tremens*.* The tongue is moist and tremulous; there is a general tremor of the muscles; the patient is totally sleepless, irritable in his temper, answers questions in a snappish, or peevish, or incoherent manner; is often anxious to call himself perfectly well; and as the malady increases, he becomes restless, impatient, and talkative; wishes, perhaps, to get out of bed, and attempts to injure his attendants, and soon becomes most furiously maniacal. In some cases, however, the delirium is of a milder cast; the patient is haunted with extravagant ideas and spectral illusions; or fancies himself busied in his ordinary avocations, and talks perpetually about them.

TERMINATIONS.—The *prognosis* will be the more unfavourable, in proportion as the excitement is violent, as it cannot fail to lead to exhaustion, the pulse becoming irregular, the aspect livid and haggard, the extremities cold, and coma supervening, which is soon followed by death. There will be some hope, however, if the pulse becomes more tranquil and firm, and especially if the patient sleeps.

CAUSES.—The exciting causes of this state are (surgically considered) the various mechanical injuries before enumerated;—acting on constitutions that are weak, and consequently irritable;† that have " an increased

---

* Copland's Dict. Pract. Med. *Art.* Delirium with Tremor.
† Omne infirmum, naturâ querulum.

disposition to act, without the power to act with." Some examples of it occur in children, especially after burns; but they are most frequently met with in the case of persons of middle age and plethoric habit, who habitually indulge in excess of food and spirituous liquors, and who, as is well known, often die from many injuries and accidents which more temperate persons might have recovered from without difficulty.

TREATMENT.—The indications are to moderate the excitement, and support the strength. If there be violent delirium, with heat and dryness of skin, and the pulse very sharp, the scalp should be shaved and kept wet with evaporating lotions; the bowels should be evacuated with a dose of calomel combined with camphor, followed by an aperient draught, or by enemata if there be much vomiting; taking care, however, not to purge so freely as to reduce the strength. At the same time hyoscyamus should be given in moderate doses every hour or two; such as gr. v. of the extract or ℳ xxx. of the tincture—and if these means fail, one large dose (gr. ii.—iii.) of solid opium, or ℳ xl.—lx. of Battley's solution may be given after the bowels are opened. If, however, there be greater debility and restlessness, opium may be given in small doses, (gr. ¼—½ 2nda, vel 3tia, quâque horâ,) carefully watching its effects, and giving it up if it seem rather to augment cerebral excitement, or to induce coma. Enemata containing ʒß of laudanum may be preferable in some cases; or combinations of camphor and henbane with musk and anti-spasmodies. The strength should be carefully supported by beef-tea, arrowroot, &c.: and if the patient have been accustomed to ardent spirits or opium, they may be allowed with great advantage in considerable quantity. The patient must be confined, if necessary, in order to prevent injury to himself or others; and he should be treated with calmness and indulgence, but yet with firmness. In the last stage, when coma supervenes, counter-irritation by means of sinapisms or blisters to the scalp, or feet, or calves of the legs, may be tried, but scarcely any means will avail.

# CHAPTER III.

## OF FEVER.

### SECTION I.—OF FEVER GENERALLY.

GENERAL DESCRIPTION.—Fever may be described as a state in which all, or most of the functions of the body are deranged. The nervous system is shown to be deranged, by the headach, pain in the back, lassi-tude, muscular weakness, mental torpor, and confusion of the perceptive senses. Chilliness or burning heat, testify to disorder of the function by which animal heat is produced or regulated. Respiration and circula-tion are either slow and embarrassed, or performed with preternatural frequency and force. Digestion and nutrition are suspended, hence the rapid emaciation. The secretions are either deficient, or, if abundant, are depraved; hence the thirst, dry skin, scanty urine, and costiveness or diarrhœa. Moreover, the fluids have a tendency to be vitiated, and the solids to be diseased, as shown by congestion and effusion in either of the three great cavities.

Fevers are often divided into two grand families; the *idiopathic* and the *symptomatic*. The former arise from agents operating on the blood or nervous system; ague and typhus are examples. The latter are called *symptomatic*, because produced by disease or injury of some part. It is with these that the surgeon has to deal; and there are the following varieties, which we shall treat of successively.

(1.) If there be acute inflammation in a healthy system, the fever will be *inflammatory*, which is commonly called *symptomatic fever*. (2.) If there be acute inflammation in a weakened or cachectic system—or if the inflammation arises from certain specific causes of a depressing ten-dency, such as morbid poisons,—or if it attack certain structures, as the veins;—the fever is generally called *irritative*. (3.) If the inflammation have terminated in an exhausting suppuration, or if there be a permanent disease which the constitution has no power to vanquish, *hectic fever* will be established. (4.) When the vital powers are entirely exhausted, the fever assumes what is called a *typhoid* type; which, in the emphatic language of Hunter, is termed dissolution. (5.) Lastly, fever, even when arising from a local cause that is permanent, may be *intermittent;* that is, may occur in definite paroxysms, with intervals of health.—This is often the case in diseases of the urinary organs, such as strictures and fistulæ in perinæo: and sometimes in worms or other states of irritation of the intestinal tube.


SECTION II.—OF INFLAMMATORY FEVER.

*Syn.*—SYNOCHA, Cullen.

GENERAL DESCRIPTION.—This fever accompanies every acute inflam-mation which arises from a severe and considerable injury, or affects parts of great sensibility and importance in healthy subjects. And it is almost a natural and necessary concomitant. "Nature," says Hunter, "requires to feel the injury; for where after a considerable operation there is rather a weak quiet pulse, often with a nervous oppression, with a seeming difficulty of breathing and loathing of food, the patient is in a dangerous way. Fever shows powers of resistance; the other symptoms show weakness, sinking under the injury."*

SYMPTOMS.—Slight shivering; succeeded by increased heat of skin :† preternaturally frequent, hard, and vibratory pulse ;—pain and aching in the head, back, and limbs, with a sense of lassitude and muscular weakness;—general deficiency of the secretions; dry skin; dry and white tongue; thirst; nausea and loss of appetite; constipation; scanty and high-coloured urine;—the blood generally buffed and cupped;—slight aggravation of the symptoms in the evening, often delirium in the night, and slight remission in the morning.

TERMINATIONS.—(1.) If the patient recover, the urine becomes more copious, and deposites a lateritious sediment;‡ the tongue becomes moist and clean, the skin cool and perspiring; the local inflammation either is resolved, or proceeds to a healthy suppuration; and the return of the appetite and of the other natural functions 'indicate the patient's recovery. The formation of pus often appears to be a natural crisis.§ (2.) But if from the irreparable nature of the disease or injury, or from the irritability of the system, life is destined to be destroyed, the pulse becomes continually more frequent, and subsequently weak, irregular, and intermittent, the extremities cold, and life soon ceases with the failure of the circulation.

TREATMENT.—The treatment of this fever is included in that of acute inflammation, of which it is the shadow. But it must be observed in this place, that when it is symptomatic of an inflammation that is unavoidable, (as after a compound fracture, and most other severe injuries,) it cannot be cut short, although its undue violence may be abated;—and that great care should be taken not to weaken the patient too much by depletion, especially if the part injured be not of vital importance, and its reparation will require time and strength. The indications are, to allay vascular action and nervous irritation, and to restore the secretions. And the means are, rest, low diet, aperient and febrifuge medicines, anodynes at bed-time when the bowels have been cleared, and general or local bleeding if demanded by the exigencies of the case.

---

* On the blood. Chap. iv. sect. 6.

† From increased determination of blood to it, and deficiency of the secretion which naturally carries off the heat. In ordinary symptomatic fever, the real heat of the blood does not rise more than three or four degrees above the natural standard; but in scarlet fever it has risen as high as 1160.

‡ *Lateritious*, like brick-dust, from *later*, a brick.

§ Κρισις, any important phenomenon in a disease (mostly an evacuation of some sort) by which the patient's safety or danger may be judged of.

CAUTION.—Although it is always expedient to open the bowels, yet purging should be avoided when it is likely that the disturbance which it occasions may be detrimental to any diseased or injured part, as a compound fracture, or the like.

OF THE PULSE.—It may be convenient to say a few words in this place about the pulse. The *elements of the pulse* are three; namely, *first*, the contraction of the heart, which propels blood into the arteries;—*secondly*, the yielding and dilatation of the artery, which when felt constitutes the *pulse ;*\*—and, *thirdly*, the return of the artery to its former caliber. Now some of the properties of the pulse depend on the heart, and some on the arteries. Thus its *frequency* and *slowness* correspond to the number of the heart's contractions in a given time. Its *quickness* (or *sharpness*) depends on the velocity and impetus with which each individual contraetion is made. On the other hand, *hardness* of the pulse depends on the resistance offered to the ingress of the blood, by the constant tonic contraction of the contractile coat of the arteries; but if that contraction is trifling, so that the vessel yields readily to the impulse of the blood, or the pressure of the finger, the pulse will be *soft.* The *vibratory* feel, or *thrill*, or *jar*, is caused by an irregular dilatation of the artery, which dilates with an innumerable number of stops and interruptions. The *full* and *small* pulse depend in some measure on the quantity of blood in the system, but principally on the state of the vessel, for if that does not dilate freely, the pulse will be small. A small hard pulse is a much safer indication for bleeding than a full soft one.

In the fever accompanying acute inflammation of any *common* part, such as skin, cellular tissue, or muscle, or of the eye, dura mater, or pleura, the pulse is generally *frequent*, *hard*, and *full.*

During acute inflammation, however, of the brain and stomach—parts most essential to life—or of the peritoneum, testicle, and kidney, which are most intimately connected with the stomach by the sympathetic nerve, the vital powers seem to be more depressed, and the pulse is *frequent*, *hard*, and *small.*

Again, during acute inflammation in a very weak and irritable constitution, or after great loss of blood, the pulse may either be very *frequent, small*, and *soft*, or *frequent*, *large*, *soft*, and *jerking;* the soft jerking quality indicating an almost passive yielding to the heart's impulse, and being caused by an absence of that contractile tone which renders the pulse small and hard.†

---

\* If the artery is perfectly straight, and the circulation tranquil, the dilatations will not be so great as to be perceptible to the eye, and can only be appreciated by compressing the vessel slightly between the fingers; whereas if it is curved, each impulse of the blood will slightly straighten it, and cause a sensible motion.

† Wilson Philip. Experimental Inquiry into the Laws of the Vital Functions, p. 323, 3d edition. See also Hunter on the Blood, Chap. iii. sect. 8.

BUFFY BLOOD.—The reader need scarcely be reminded, that after healthy blood has coagulated, it divides into two portions, serum and crassamentum;—that the serum is a watery solution of the albumen and salts, whilst the crassamentum consists of the fibrine and red particles;—and that the fibrine, which by itself is yellowish white, derives a uniformly red tinge from the equal diffusion of these particles. But, on the other hand, the crassamentum of inflammatory blood has on its surface " *a buffy coat*," that is, a yellowish white layer of fibrine free from red particles;—which layer may vary from one line to one third of the clot in thickness, and is frequently so strongly contracted as to make its surface concave or *cupped*, and its edges fringed. We have therefore to inquire, first—what change in the blood causes this deviation from its ordinary appearance;—and secondly, what states of the system produce this change in the blood.

(1.) With regard to the first inquiry, there are four changes in the state of the blood which, together or singly, may be possibly concerned in the production of the buffy coat. First, a *slow coagulation*, so that the red particles have time to sink, and leave the upper surface of the clot colourless. Secondly, an *increased specific gravity of the red particles*, so that they have an unusual tendency to subside quickly. Thirdly, a *disposition of the fibrine to separate* itself from the mass of the blood. Fourthly, an *increase in the quantity* of the fibrine.

Now the *first* of these conditions, namely, the slow coagulation, generally exists in inflammatory fever, " when the powers of life are unimpaired, the circulation rapid, and the blood drawn in a full stream."[*] But still, as Hewson says, " something more than merely a lessened disposition to coagulate is necessary for forming the crust or size,"[†] because, in the first place, if blood be confined by ligatures in a vessel of a living animal, or if an animal die a sudden and violent death, although in both these cases the blood will coagulate very slowly, it still will be free from the buffy coat, and, in the second place, inflammatory blood sometimes coagulates very quickly. So that slow coagulation cannot be admitted as the essential cause.[‡]

The *second* condition, namely, increased gravity of the red globules, was supposed to be proved by an experiment of Hunter's;[§] but as it was soon after disproved by Hewson, who repeated Hunter's experiments with a totally opposite result, no great weight can be laid upon it.

The *third* alleged cause, the spontaneous separability of the fibrine, is

[*] Copland, Dict., *Art.* Blood.

[†] Hewson; Experimental Inquiry into the Blood. Lond. 1772. Chap. ii. pp. 34 *et seq.*

[‡] Muller's Physiology by Baly, 2d edition, vol. i. p. 129.

[§] Hunter says also that the serum is specifically lighter than usual.

established on better evidence. "The blood in inflammation," says Hunter, "more readily admits of a separation of its visible parts." In fact the fibrine (which was assumed by Hewson to be highly attenuated) may be seen to rise to the surface of inflammatory blood very soon after it is drawn, giving it a bluish appearance.

The *fourth* condition, the increased quantity of the fibrine, has been proved to exist, by the experiments of Thackrah,* Andral, and others. But whilst some authors assert that it is increased at the expense of the albumen of the serum, and that the serum of inflammatory blood contains less albumen than usual; others, as Gendrin, affirm that the serum is pre-ternaturally albuminous.†

From a due consideration of these circumstances, it appears most proba-ble that the buffy coat depends partly on some change in the vital properties of the blood, by which the fibrine is disposed to separate itself from the liquor sanguinis;—and partly, *perhaps*, on a diminished viscidity and slow coagulation, which permit the red particles to subside quickly.‡ The *cupping* is easily accounted for by the strong contraction of the buff; for the crassamentum of inflammatory blood is always extremely dense and firm, although there may be no buffy coat whatever.

(2.) In the second place, we have to consider by what states of the system these changes in the blood are produced. Hunter says that they are produced by an increase of the powers of life, and by an increase of the disposition to act with those powers. And we have both positive and negative evidence that this is correct. For the buffy coat is found on the blood of healthy pregnant women and animals, in whom the powers and actions of life are augmented without doubt; and it is always most conspicuous when the circulation is rapid, and when the blood is drawn in such a manner as to preserve its vital properties; that is, in a full rapid stream, into a deep vessel, the temperature of the apartment being high.

On the other hand, the buff will be deficient, when the blood is drawn in such a manner as to deprive it speedily of its life; that is, in a small slow stream, into a flat and shallow basin, the temperature being low. It is remarkable, that the buffy coat is occasionally absent at the com-mencement of some inflammations, especially of the lungs, whilst the circulation is slow and labouring and embarrassed, and whilst it may be

---

* Thackrah, C. T. on the Blood. Lond. 1834. Andral, in Dublin Med. Press, Oct. 28, 1840.

† Albumen and fibrine are almost identical in chemical composition; and the former, when coagulated, can scarcely be distinguished from the latter.

‡ Davy's Experimental Researches. Lond. 1839, vol. ii. This eminent physiolo-gist denies that the quantity of fibrine is increased, and advocates Hewson's doc-trine, that the fibrine is attenuated, and the blood less viscid, during inflammation.

supposed that the nervous system is oppressed by the intensity of the inflammation; and that it may make its appearance as soon as that oppression is removed by bleeding. Thus, during one venæsection, it has happened that the blood first drawn has not been buffed, owing, as we presume, to the embarrassed circulation;—the buff has appeared in a second portion when enough has been drawn to relieve that embarrassment;—and has again disappeared in a third, when the circulation has become languid at the approach of syncope.

Finally, the buffy coat, considered as an evidence of fever or inflammation, is, like every other symptom that our conjectural art presents us with, not to be depended on invariably. For, in the first place, it may be present when there is no inflammation;—as in pregnant women; in the plethoric; in persons accustomed to be periodically bled, or who are habitually exposed to the night air.* Again, its quantity is by no means proportioned to the intensity of inflammation; for it is constant to the last in rheumatism, even when subdued by bleeding. And there are certain inflammations of great intensity in which it does not exist at all; as in the commencement of sundry cases before mentioned;—in inflammations that have little of the adhesive tendency, as those of mucous membranes, or diffuse inflammation of the cellular tissue; and in the inflammations arising from certain morbid poisons, as glanders, or in the course of typhus fever,† when the blood, having lost its vital qualities, scarcely coagulates at all.

SECTION III.—OF IRRITATIVE FEVER.

GENERAL DESCRIPTION.—The term Irritative Fever seems to be conventionally assigned to a form of violent and dangerous constitutional disturbance, which apparently combines the characters of inflammatory fever and of prostration with excitement; and which is scarcely to be distinguished from the early stage of typhoid fever.‡ Or perhaps it may be more convenient to describe it as the set of constitutional symptoms which attend phlebitis, diffuse inflammation of the cellular tissue; the disease arising from glanders, and from wounds poisoned during dissection;—also severe phlegmonous erysipelas and inflammations in which there is great pain from the confinement of matter;—all of which cases

---

* Samuel Cooper. First lines of Surgery.

† Palmer's edition of Hunter. Vol. iii., p. 39, *note*.

‡ Some authors state that the blood is most buffed when there is an inflammation with considerable tendency to effusion of fibrine, as pleurisy or pericarditis; others state that it is most buffed when the inflammation has no adhesive tendency, as acute rheumatism, so that the fibrine cannot escape from the blood: a curious instance of contrary deductions from the self same facts, when partially viewed and hastily generalized.

exhibit a combination of violent local inflammation, great febrile commotion, and great depression of the vital powers.

The *Symptoms* and *Treatment* will be particularized under the head of the various local affections which this fever accompanies. The leading features are great restlessness and anxiety, debility, depression of spirits, weight at the præcordia, oppressed respiration; frequent rigors; rapid and sharp pulse, but variable in force; death, preceded by low delirium, and signs of great exhaustion. The treatment must, as a general rule, be directed to the invigoration of the vital powers by cordial stimulants and tonics, the evacuation of depraved secretions, and the removal of pain and irritation, and of local disease, by whatever measures are most appropriate.*

### SECTION IV.—OF HECTIC FEVER.†

DEFINITION.—Hetic fever is an habitual disorder of the system, when irritated by some long-standing disease, or source of weakness which it is unable to remove. It is a remittent fever, and is accompanied by a general tendency to increase of one or more secretions.

SYMPTOMS.—Emaciation and debility; tongue morbidly clean and red, especially at the tip and edges; appetite often inordinate; disposition alternately to diarrhœa and profuse perspiration;‡ pulse frequent and small;—a febrile exacerbation comes on every evening (or oftener, especially after meals) with slight chills, followed by heat of skin, burning of the soles of the feet and palms of the hands, and a circumscribed flush in the cheeks;—thirst and restlessness, preventing sleep till after the middle of the night, when the patient falls asleep, and suddenly wakes in a profuse perspiration;—often buoyancy of spirits and hope to the last.

TERMINATIONS.—(1.) If it be about to terminate fatally, the debility increases; the diarrhœa and perspirations become more profuse and exhausting; the legs become œdematous; aphthæ form; and great pain; griping and tenesmus attend the diarrhœa, owing to an inflammatory or ulcerated condition of the intestines. The patient may expire suddenly, the heart failing from mere debility; or death may be preceded by typhoid symptoms. And this fatal termination may be owing either to the continuance of the original disease, or to the induction of secondary disease in the lungs or mesenteric glands. (2.) Recovery from hectic is often remarkably rapid, if the causes be removed; provided that no secondary disease has commenced.

CAUSES.—Any chronic organic incurable disease;—whether incurable

---

* Vide part ii. chap. vii. sect. iv. on Diffuse Inflammation of the Cellular Tissue; and part iii. chap. ix. sect. ii. on Dissection Wounds.

† From ἕξις, ἑκτικος, habit, habitual.

‡ Called *colliquative*; (*liquo*, I melt ;) because they exhaust the system.

from its *nature*, as scirrhus, tubercle;—from its *seat*, as the lungs or mesentery;—from its *extent*:—or from *constitutional debility;* also exhaustion from profuse suppuration;—or from any other great and continned discharge;—as prolonged lactation, leucorrhœa, and so forth. Hectic is so frequently caused by profuse suppuration, that an absorption of pus was formerly deemed to be its invariable and efficient cause. Hunter denied this theory—1st, because hectic may arise from organic disease, or from excessive discharge of any secretion when there is no suppuration; 2ndly, because pus may be absorbed (as it often is from chronic abscesses and buboes, which are discussed without being opened) without the production of hectic.* It is certain, therefore, that absorption of pus is not the *only* cause of hectic. But it is equally certain that pus is absorbed from extensive suppurating surfaces; and it is probable that its presence in the blood adds to the hectic and constitutional debility; and that (especially if it be vitiated or decomposed) it tends greatly to the production of colliquative diarrhœa and ulceration of the intestines.† For the injection of pus or putrid matter into the blood almost invariably causes diarrhœa;‡—an effect also which is notoriously produced among students who absorb the putrid vapours of the dissecting-room.

TREATMENT.—The indications are (1) to remove the local cause; (2) or if that be impracticable, to enable the system to support it. The first indication may often be fulfilled by an amputation or other operation; and it is well known that hectic patients often bear operations extremely well, recovering from them rapidly, and making but one step as it were from death's door to perfect health.§ In cases not admitting or requiring an operation, local mischief must be remedied, and profuse discharges restrained as far as possible. As for the second indication, the strength must be maintained by a mild nutritious diet; that is, as much food may be given as the stomach can digest with comfort; and wine, porter, or beer, may be allowed in order to assist digestion; but the quantity of animal food and of spirituous liquors must be regulated, so that they may not add to the excitement, nor increase the heat of the skin, thirst, and perspirations. Arrowroot and other farinaceous preparations; jellies, Iceland and carragee moss, are useful as mild nutritives occasionally, when there is an excess of heat and feverishness; but these slops should not be given at such times or in such quantities as to interfere with the di-

* On the Blood. Ch. ix. sect. 1.
† Copland ; Dict. Prac. Med., Art. Hectic, p. 965.
‡ Vide part ii. ch. vii. of this work.
§ " The removal of a diseased part which the constitution has become accustomed to, and which is rather fretting the constitution, is adding less violence than the removal of a sound part in harmony with the whole." Hunter on the blood. Ch. ii. sect. 2.

gestion of more solid food, if there is an appetite for it. *Tonics* may be given to support the strength; such as bark, quinine, or cascarilla; or sometimes the preparations of iron; but if at any time, in the varying progress of the disease, excitement appear to prevail, the pulse being more accelerated, and pain aggravated, tonics and animal food must be for a time exchanged for saline medicines and farinaceous or milk diet. *Digitalis*, a remedy much used in hectic, may be of service at such times, if given in a few moderate doses, for not too long a time. Ten minims in a saline draught, at bed-time, are a proper dose. Sleep must be procured, and pain allayed, by sufficient doses of opium. Change of air is always advantageous. Profuse perspirations may be checked by dilute sulphuric or nitric acid, with tonics, as F. 1. As it will be recollected that the diarrhœa often depends on an inflamed or ulcerated condition of the intestinal mucous membrane, reason will suggest that attempts to stop it by port wine and large doses of catechu, or other stimulants and astringents, will often be not only unavailing, but irritating and mischievous;* although good enough in cases of mere debility. If, therefore, the diarrhœa is attended with tenderness, much pain, and tenesmus, the proper remedies are demulcents and anodynes; rest in bed; occasionally a poultice of bran with one fifth of mustard, applied to the abdomen, and suffered to remain till it causes slight smarting and redness;—the very mildest diet of milk, arrowroot, &c., enemata of starch, containing from twenty to sixty minims of laudanum (F. 48;)—Dover's powder at bed-time, and small doses of chalk mixture, with a few minims of laudanum, during the day; and one or two grains of blue pill, with three or four of rhubarb occasionally, if the liver is inactive. It may be added, that copious injec. tions of warm water give great relief in all cases of diarrhœa; soothing the irritating membrane, washing away acrid secretions, and enabling the patient to pass easily at once what otherwise would occasion several painful dejections.

### SECTION V.—OF TYPHOID FEVER.†

GENERAL DESCRIPTION.—This fever is an acute form of constitutional disturbance, occurring when the powers of life are much exhausted or depressed. It may be a sequel of the hectic; or of the state of pros_

---

* The author has known large doses of catechu purge violently, when administered to a young woman for passive menorrhagia.

† The pathological student, will not confound the affection spoken of here and else_ where, in the volume, as "typhoid fever," with the *dothinenteritis* of modern physicians. Mr. Druit and other surgeons still employ the term to indicate a sympathetic febrile affection, with adynamic symptoms, a Typhus-like condition or simulated synochus. F.

tration with excitement; or it may supervene very soon after an injury.

SYMPTOMS.—Pulse very frequent and weak, often quick and jerking in the early stages; skin hot and very dry: all the secretions deficient; tongue dry, brown, and tremulous; lips parched;—if there be a wound, it becomes dry, livid, and glassy, and ceases to suppurate.

TERMINATIONS.—(1.) If the patient is to die, the pulse becomes more rapid, thready, and tremulous, and at last is imperceptible at the wrist; the eyes look dull and glassy and sunken; the temples and nostrils are pinched from atony of their muscles;—the patient lies on his back, and sinks towards the foot of the bed;—there is frequent hiccough; the abdomen is tightly distended with flatus, and the sphincter is relaxed, so that stools are passed involuntarily; the patient dozes imperfectly, awaking with a start; he picks imaginary objects on the bed clothes, and mutters to himself;—there is starting or twitching of the tendons; at last the skin becomes cold and clammy, respiration slow and laborious, and coma supervenes, soon followed by death. (2.) If recovery occurs, the surest sign of amendment is a diminution of the frequency and increase of the firmness of the pulse, with sound sleep; the patient being sensible and composed, the eyes brighter, the tongue cleaning, and above all, suppuration returning, if there be a wound.

CAUSES.—Typhoid fever may be caused (1) by some circumstances producing immediate and direct depression of vital power; such as traumatic gangrene; a wound poisoned during dissection; or a severe injury or operation suffered by an habitual drunkard. (2.) It may be caused by some disease of long standing, which has completely exhausted the constitutional powers—as profuse suppuration with hectic. And both these conditions may be, and frequently are, combined with a third; (3) namely, contamination of the blood by putrid or other poisonous matter. Thus it is sure to supervene if putrid pus be confined in an abscess, or if putrid urine escape into the cellular tissue of the perinæum. M. Bonnet has proved incontestably that the hydrosulphate of ammonia, the product of putrefaction, is absorbed in these cases, and is one cause of the typhoid fever.*

PROGNOSIS.—The prognosis will of course be always doubtful; but there may be a chance of recovery, if the cause is of recent existence, and admits of removal by operation or otherwise; whilst there can be scarcely any, if the constitution has been exhausted by its long continuance. Thus, if this fever come on in erysipelas or small-pox, diseases of no long continuance, the constitution may rally;—or if it is caused by a recent injury, or by extravasation of urine, it may be removed perhaps by

* See part ii. ch. vii. sect. iii.

an amputation, or incisions in the perinæum: but it will scarcely be cured if caused by chronic abscess or disease of a joint, and preceded by hectic. And thus, if the hectic has been suffered to pass into the typhoid state, the season of amputation and hope of recovery are also past. " It is," says Hunter, " the more incurable, as it is more connected with the past than with the present."

TREATMENT.—The indications are to remove the cause; allay irrita-tion, and support the strength. If the removal of the cause by operation is likely to be successful, upon the principles just laid down, it should be done without delay; and even if not, it may be better to try a doubtful remedy than none at all.

As for the general treatment, opium or some of its preparations should be given in small doses, repeated frequently, or in a large dose at once, according to the judgment of the practitioner, for the relief of restlessness and delirium. The most potent tonics, especially quinine, should also be freely given. The author can particularly recommend F. 2. 3. 26. Moderate quantities of concentrated forms of nutriment, jellies, broths, beef-tea, arrowroot, &c., and wine or hot brandy-and-water, need not be spared, if the patient will take them. Hiccough is best relieved by a tea-spoonful of sp. æther, c.; and flatulence by an enema of turpentine. The catheter should be used if the patient cannot pass his water—a point that should always be most scrupulously inquired into.

## CHAPTER IV.

### OF TETANUS.

DEFINITION.—Tetanus is a disease manifested by tonic* spasm and rigidity of some, or many, of the muscles of voluntary motion.

DIVISIONS.—There are several varieties of tetanus. (1.) It is divided into the *idiopathic*, or that which arises solely from some disorder of the system, and the *traumatic*, or that which is caused by a wound. (2.) It may be *acute* or *chronic;* the former arising suddenly, and soon termi-nating, generally affecting the whole body, and often fatal; the chronic being of less intensity and of longer duration, usually partial in its extent, and mostly terminating in recovery. (3.) Tetanus may be *general* or

---

* Spasms are of two kinds; the *tonic* (τυνω, I*stretch*) in which the rigidity is per-manent, and the *clonic,* (κλονος, *commotion,*) in which contraction alternates quickly with relaxation, as in epilepsy and hysteria.

*partial;* and when partial it is mostly confined to the neck and jaws, constituting *trismus,* or locked jaw. (4.) It may be divided according to the set of muscles predominantly affected: being called *opisthotonos,* when the body is curved backwards so as to rest on the occiput and heels, which it most commonly is; *emprosthotonos,* when it is curved forward from a preponderance of the abdominal muscles;* and *pleurosthonotos,* when it is drawn to one side, this being the most uncommon.† (5.) The *trismus infantum,* or *neonatorum* which attacks children soon after birth, is usually made a distinct species. (6.) Tetanus may in its *type,* be *intermittent,* when it is caused by marshy miasmata, as it may be occasionally like almost every other nervous affection.

PREMONITORY SYMPTOMS.—(1.) In the true traumatic tetanus, there are seldom any premonitory symptoms, except sometimes severe shooting pains in the wound;—(2.) the genuine idiopathic is mostly preceded by foul tongue, loss of appetite, disturbed sleep, dejected spirits, and fugitive spasms in various parts;—(3.) and in one well-marked set of cases that will be more fully alluded to hereafter, the attack is preceded by shivering, pain in head, back, and limbs, and other symptoms of inflammatory fever.

SYMPTOMS.—The patient first complains of stiffness and pain of the neck and jaws, as from a cold; and his countenance is observed to have a peculiar expression, because the corners of the mouth and eyes are distorted and puckered by incipient spasm of the facial muscles. In the next place, the muscles of mastication and deglutition become fixed and rigid, with spasm, so that the mouth is permanently closed, and there is great difficulty of swallowing, especially liquids. To these symptoms succeed a fixed pain at the epigastrium, and convulsive difficulty of breathing, indicating that the diaphragm and muscles of the glottis are affected; and the spasm now extends to the other muscles of the trunk and limbs, rendering them completely fixed and rigid. The abdomen feels remarkably hard; there is obstinate constipation, and frequently difficult micturition from spasm of the perinæal muscles; the pupils are contracted, and the saliva flows from the mouth, because the patient is unable to swallow it. This spasm never ceases; but it has occasional remissions of violence, alternating with aggravated paroxysms, which are easily induced by the slightest irritation or disturbance. Meanwhile the in-

---

* Larrey conceived that the curvature of the body was determined by the situation of the wound; that if the wound was on the posterior surface, there would be opisthotonos, and so forth. But although this is sometimes the case, it is quite as frequently otherwise. (Clinique Chirurgicale, Paris, 1829, p. 85.)

† A case of acute tetanus, affecting one side only, is given in the Med. Gaz., May 12th, 1838. No mention is made of the pulse.

tellects are undisturbed, and the pulse may be natural, except during a severe paroxysm, which quickens it, and causes perspiration and thirst.

TERMINATIONS.—(1.) If the case is about to end *fatally*, the paroxysms become more frequent and violent, and the breathing more and more embarrassed by spasm of the diaphragm and of the muscles of the glottis; and at last the patient dies, either from exhaustion or from suffocation;— the nervous system being either worn out by the violence of the spasm, or the respiratory action being suspended long enough to cut off the necessary supply of arterial blood from the brain, and so induce insensi‐ bility. The most usual *period of death* is the third or fourth day; some‐ times it is postponed till the eighth or tenth, but rarely longer. On the other hand, there is the case* recorded of a negro who injured his hand, and died of tetanus in a quarter of an hour; and cases of death within twenty-four hours are by no means uncommon. (2.) When acute tetanus terminates favourably, still the patient's recovery is not complete for weeks or months—partly because of the strainings and lacerations which the muscles have suffered,—partly because of the remaining ten‐ dency to spasm, which very slowly yields, and is apt to be temporarily aggravated by very slight causes, especially cold and damp. But in some rare instances the disease has been removed almost instantaneously by the removal of its exciting cause.

PROGNOSIS.—The prognosis in acute tetanus is extremely unfavourable, especially if traumatic; it is more favourable in the idiopathic, and the chronic most generally gets well of itself. Death very seldom occurs after the twelfth day. Dr. Parry† attempted to found a prognosis on the state of the pulse, and thought that if on the fourth day it was under 100 or 110, the patient being an adult, the prognosis was favourable;—but if above 120, unfavourable. But although it is true that the pulse is in general accelerated towards the close of the malady, still some fatal cases have occurred in which it never rose above 80 or 90. As a general rule it may be said that the prognosis is *favourable* if the complaint be par. tial;—if it do not affect the muscles of the glottis;—if it has lasted some days without increasing materially in severity;—if it is sensibly mitigated by the remedies employed;—if the pulse is not much accelerated;—if the patient sleep; and if he have been subject to it before in an intermittent form. On the other hand, the prospect will be *unfavourable*, if the spasms continually increase in severity, and especially if they affect the muscles of the glottis.

DIAGNOSIS.—Tetanus resembles *hydrophobia* in the difficulty of swallowing and aggravation of the spasms by slight external irritants;

* Rees's Encyclopædia, *Art.* Tetanus.

† Caleb Hillier Parry, M. D. Cases of Tetanus and of Rabies Contagiosa. Bath, 1814.

but it may be distinguished by the spasms being *continuous*, and by the patient being sensible in general and calm to the last;—whereas in hydrophobia, there are fits of general convulsions with *perfect intermissions*, and the patient is mostly delirious, with a peculiarly wild haggard expression of countenance. *Inflammation of the spinal cord*, or its membranes, resembles tetanus in having opisthotonos and spasmodic difficulty of swallowing; but it may be distinguished by the pain in the back, and fever being more predominant than in any case of mere tetanus, and by the paraplegia and coma which supervene in most cases.

MORBID ANATOMY.—The morbid appearances that have been found in different cases are as follow. Increased vascularity of the membranes and substance of the *spinal cord*, with or without effusion of serum;— more rarely the same appearances have been found in the cranium; flakes of cartilage and spiculæ of bone deposited in the membranes of the spinal cord;*—vascularity of the nerves leading from the wounded part;—vascularity of the mucous membrane of the stomach;—of the sympathetic ganglia;—and congestion of the lungs. But there is not one of these morbid changes that is constantly, and, except the first, there is not one of them that is even frequently found. The muscles are extremely rigid after death, and ecchymosed or ruptured in many parts;—the blood is mostly coagulated.

PREDISPOSING CAUSES.—The best established predisposing causes are;—changes of temperature from warm to cold or damp;—a disordered state of the stomach and bowels;—the presence of worms, or of undigested food, or vitiated secretions in the intestines;—the existence of the above-named osseous or cartilaginous deposites, or of any other permanent cause of irritation near the spinal cord;—fear, anxiety, or fatigue, or any other circumstances that depress either mind or body. Tetanus is much more prevalent and fatal in warm than in cold or temperate climates; and men are much more frequently subject to it than women.

EXCITING CAUSES.—The *exciting causes* of tetanus may, for the sake of convenience, be arranged under three heads—the first two comprising the causes of the *idiopathic*, and the third, those of the *traumatic* variety.

The *first* consists of causes which operate on the nervous system generally, as cold and damp; the poisons of nux vomica, of the cicuta aquatica, and other narcotico-acrid poisons, especially a certain Javanese poison called *chetik*.

The *second* comprises causes which affect organs supplied with ganglionic nerves, especially the stomach or bowels; and there can be little doubt but that many of the cases which are styled traumatic, because there exists a wound, are in reality caused by visceral irritation, without which the tetantus could not have arisen. Thus in a case, which occurred

---

* Refer to the cases at p. 38.

in St. Bartholomew's Hospital, ten days after a wound on the toe, and
proved fatal in a fortnight, no morbid appearances, not even an increase
of vascularity, were found in the spinal cord; but almost all the intes
tinal canal was inflamed, and there were ulcers in the ilium and cœcum.*
Dr. Dickson† and Mr. M'Arthur‡ relate cases in which the intestines
were filled with a peculiar unhealthy yellow viscid secretion;—Mr. Aber
nethy§ commemorates the peculiarly unhealthy stools, like sloughs, in a
case which he observed;—Mr. Travers‖ strongly suspects that dysentery
and ulcers of the intestines may be coincident causes;—and some authors¶
have affirmed that intestinal worms are a strongly predisposing, if not
really efficient, cause. But besides, cases might be quoted, from various
authors, in which there was no wound at all,—gastro-intestinal irritation
was the only cause. Thus Andral relates a case produced by gastritis;
Lehman,** a case of partial tetanus by hernia; and another instance is
related,¶ in which it was caused by the irritation of an emetic on a sto
mach disordered by habitual drunkenness. But although irritation of the
stomach and bowels is the most frequent of this class of causes, still irri
tation of other organs may produce the disease. Begin†† states that it
has arisen from pericarditis; Gooch‡‡ gives a case produced by disease of
the breast; and Farr** knew it caused by pulmonary abscess. Uterine
irritation is by no means an uncommon cause. Whytt** gives the case
of a girl, aged twenty, who caught cold during the menstrual period, and
died of tetanus in eighteen hours; and the ease related in the adjoining
note gives a good example of fatal trismus from irritation of the womb.§§

* There were vascularity and serous effusion in the cranium, brought on most
likely by the large doses of opium which the patient took. Med. Gaz. vol. i. p. 646.
  † Med. Chir. Trans. vol. vii. p. 459.
  ‡ Ibid. vol. vii. p. 474 et seq.
  § Lectures on Surgery. Renshaw, London, 1835, p 23.
  ‖ Travers. Farther Inquiry concerning Constitutional Irritation. London, 1835,
p. 397.
  ¶ Laurent. Vide F. Pescay, Dict. de Sc. Med. Paris, 1821, vol. lv. p. 9.
  ** Quoted in Wenceslai Trnka de Ki'zowitz, Commentarius de Tetano, Vindo-
boniæ, 1777—the very best work on the subject extant.
  †† Dictionnaire de Médecine et Chirurgie Pratiques. Paris, 1836. Art. Tetanos.
  ‡‡ B. Gooch, Chirurgical Works. Lond. 1792. Vol. ii.
  §§ A young lady miscarried in the second month of pregnancy; but as the abdomen continued to enlarge, and the breasts to fill, and the menses to be absent, it
was surmised that one ovum only of a twin had been expelled, and that the other
was proceeding in the regular course of development. About the fifth month she
was seized with violent flooding, which yielded for a time to the ordinary remedies,
but recurred repeatedly. Soon after this she was suddenly attacked with stiffness
of the jaws, spasmodic difficulty of swallowing, and spasm of the glottis. A physi-
cian-accoucheur was now called in, who introduced bougies into the womb, with
the view, as he said, of inducing delivery; this manifestly aggravated all the symp-

The third class of causes are wounds and external injuries of every description, especially lacerated and punctured wounds of tendinous parts, as the hands and feet; gunshot wounds; compound fractures, compound dislocation of the thumb; wounds irritated by foreign matters,* or in which nerves are exposed. Tetanus has followed a blow with a pedagogue's ferrule;† but it is rarely if ever caused by clean simple incisions. There are three periods at which tetanus may be induced by wounds, viz. (1) it may supervene immediately, or very soon after the infliction,‡ if the patient be predisposed; (2) during the progress, when the wound is occasioning severe pain and irritation; (3) when it is nearly or quite cicatrised: and this is perhaps the most frequent period. Why it is so, is by no means clear; but some attribute it to the rapid stoppage of suppuration, and others (as Trnka and Travers) to an irritation of the nerves by the contraction of the cicatrix. Tetanus is sometimes induced very suddenly by cold, as well as by the poisons before mentioned.

PATHOLOGY, OR THEORY OF THE DISEASE.—In this part of the subject we must inquire, 1st, what is the seat of tetanus; 2ndly, what is its nature; and 3rdly, state whatever pathological deductions may fairly be established.

1. The *seat of tetanus* must evidently be some part capable of influencing all the voluntary muscles;—namely, the motor portion of the spinal cord, and medulla oblongata.

2. With regard to its *nature*, we may ask is it inflammatory? Now some authors§ hold, that it uniformly and essentially consists in inflammation of the spinal cord or its membranes, and they call it *tetanic mye-*

---

toms. The remedies used were calomel and opium ; she was not bled, as she had been much reduced by the flooding. She died in two days from the accession of trismus, having become comatose. On a post mortem examination, the womb was found swelled and congested, but containing no ovum; the other abdominal and thoracic viscera were healthy ; the base of the brain and cervical portion of the spinal cord immensely congested and loaded with serum. Similar cases are to be found in Trnka. See also Gooke's Morgagni, vol. i. p. 129; and the Lancet for June 2nd, 1838.

* The *Times* newspaper for September 17th, 1840, quotes the case of an American farmer who died of tetanus, after having been severely stung by bees.

† Morgan's Lecture on Tetanus ; a graphic portraiture of its horrors.

‡ Hunter says that small wounds may excite tetanus speedily, but that large ones only predispose. Small injuries will produce effects that larger ones will not;—thus a violent bruise will not excite laughter like a slight tickling. Lectures in Palmer's Ed. vol. i.

§ Especially Begin and Fournier-Pescay. As a curious instance of medical discrepancy, we may observe that the latter of these authors affirms that fever is invariably present, and that those who say otherwise cannot have seen the disease: whereas he himself in another place states that it may occur during the great collapse which immediately succeeds an injury ; a condition quite incompatible with fever.

*litis;*\* the arguments in favour of their doctrine being, *first*, that tetanic spasms do actually occur in genuine myelitis; and *secondly*, that congestion in the cord and its appendages are the most frequent morbid appearances observed. But, on the other hand, it may be urged that tetanus is *not always inflammatory; first*, because congestion of the cord is far from invariably found; and when it is, it may in some instances be considered rather an effect of the disease than its cause; *secondly*, because fever and inflammatory symptoms are by no means constantly present; *thirdly*, and most conclusively, because tetanus may co-exist with a state of depression and collapse, in which it would be impossible for inflammation to be established.† As, therefore, it certainly cannot be said that tetanus depends necessarily upon inflammation, it can only be said that it consists in some unknown change in the spinal cord, whereby it spontaneously excites contraction in the voluntary muscles—which contraction, in a healthy state, is only produced by the stimulus of the will, or by some impression on a sentient nerve.

Although, however, it is most certain that inflammation is not essential to the existence of tetanus, still it is equally certain that there is one class of tetanic cases which present a well-marked inflammatory character. They commence with shivering and pain, are attended with fever, and if fatal, display on inspection, congestion, serous effusion, softening or purulent deposite, in some part of the brain or spinal cord.‡ But if we

---

\* From μυελος *medulla*, and *itis* (ιενιι *ire*;) a termination signifying inflammation.

† " I have observed, sometimes after severe gun-shot wounds, attended with great disturbance and stunning, (*fracas et commotion*,) and after considerable hæmorrhages, a state of constant atony (*atonie*) during the course of tetanus. The pulse was slow, intermittent, small, and thready;—stupor and apparent insensibility preceded the spasms, and, so to say, announced them. The tetanus was universal, but the rigidity and tension of the muscles were moderate. This state was of but short duration; death occurred in fifteen or twenty hours."—Fournier-Pescay, Op. Cit.

‡ The following are examples. (1.) Case in which the disease was caused by a blow on the back of the neck—next day patient was seized with shivering and fixed pain at the injured part—pulse 130, and full—death in thirty-six hours. Head found loaded with blood, and cervical portion of the cord softened. Med. Gaz. vol. i. 645. (2.) A cavalier cut his hand, and applied cold—was immediately seized with shivering and fever and tetanus—was bled, but died in fourteen hours. Fournier-Pescay, Op. Cit. (3.) Patient was labouring under simple continued fever from cold and wet—tetanus came on after a week, with aggravation of fever and pain in the head and back; treated successfully by large bleedings, warm bath, purgatives, and mercury. Burmester in Med. Chir. Trans. vol. ii. (4.) A man after violent exercise was seized with rigors—fever—pain in forehead—emprosthotonos, and subsequently opisthotonos—was bled, but died comatose in five days—serum and blood found effused between the membranes of brain; cervical portion of cord softened. Francesco in Forbes's Review, Jan. 1838. (5.) A woman died of tetanus from cold, with decided inflammatory symptoms. The spinal canal contained much bloody serum; the pia mater was inflamed in the anterior columns, the white substance was con-

except this class, (which is by no means a majority,) and the very small class of cases in which there exists collapse, the remainder cannot be associated with any morbid condition of the circulating system.

3. It must be concluded, therefore, that tetanus is merely a manifestation of functional disorder in one department of the nervous system. In fact, that (like other spasms) it is to the motor system just what nervous pain is to the sentient, and delirium to the intellectual. For all these functional disorders of the nervous system have many points in common. They may all be symptomatic of the most varied states of local disease. They may all be accompanied with the most opposite states of vascular excitement and bodily strength. They may all be caused by the greatest conceivable variety of morbific agents ;—cold, mental anxiety, mechanical injury, sympathetic disorder, and poisons. And lastly, they all seem to be fatal in the same ratio in which they interfere with the actions of life, or exhaust its powers.

TREATMENT.—The treatment comprises both local and constitutional measures ; the indications are, to remove all sources of irritation, and diminish the spasm.

In the *local treatment*, the first points to be accomplished are,—to remove all extraneous bodies from the wound, if there be one ;—to make apertures for the free discharge of pus;—to make incisions for the relief of inflammatory swelling and tension;—and if any isolated portion of nerve or tendon happens to be on the stretch, to divide it. Then the part may be fomented with warm decoction of poppies; after which, a solution of a scruple of opium, or extract of belladonna in an ounce of water, may be applied on lint, and the whole part be enveloped in large soft poultices. Sundry other measures have been proposed, in order more effectually to remove local irritation: such as the division of the principal nerve leading from the wound; or, as Mr. Liston has proposed; the making an ∧ incision above so as to isolate it and cut off as much nervous communication as possible; or the destruction of a ragged, contused, ill-conditioned wound by *actual cautery*, as Larrey and others have practised with great benefit;—or the *excision of the wound* if cicatrized or nearly so. Sometimes, when the wound is nearly cicatrized, or has ceased to suppurate, the application of a blister or of strong stimulating ointments has been of service. But, as Mr. Curling* observes, it happens, unfortunately, that the tetanic condition of the spinal cord, when fully established, is mostly independent of its local exciting cause, and does not cease on

verted into a number of whitish yel'ow bodies, from the size of a millet to that of a lentil, very soft, with red spots; the posterior columns healthy.—Poggi, Lond. Med. and Phys. Jour. vol. lxi. p. 132.

* A Treatise on Tetanus, being the Jacksonian Prize Essay for 1834. By T. Blizard Curling. London 1836, p, 122.

its removal. Hence *amputation* of the injured part has very rarely been successful, and has even aggravated the mischief; so that, as a general rule, it ought not to be performed, unless desirable for some other reason besides the tetanus.

We must next review the *constitutional remedies* that have been employed in tetanus, stating their relative utility, and the cases in which they are most likely to be beneficial.

1. *Bleeding* has been employed with the most decided benefit in many cases, in which it may be presumed that there existed the inflammatory diathesis already spoken of. And in all cases attended with marked inflammatory symptoms, or if the habit be full, and the wound hot, swelled, and painful, bleeding from the arm, and cupping from the spine, are clearly indicated. And even if there should be no inflammatory diathesis, provided the patient be young, bleeding may be performed in *moderation;*\*—both to prevent congestion, and to faciliate the absorption and operation of remedies. But, in by far the majority of cases, it should not be employed at all; for its influence on the muscular system is but secondary; and though it may diminish spasm for a time, it consumes the materials of life, and hastens death from exhaustion.

2. *Purgatives* are always indicated, unless there is some known cause to the contrary;—both because there is always obstinate constipation, and because worms, or vitiated secretions in the digestive tube, may be among the exciting causes: and the most active ones must be chosen. Thus, at the outset of the malady, a scruple of calomel mixed with butter should be put at the back of the tongue for the patient to swallow, and should be followed in an hour with a draught containing $\mathfrak{Z}$j of turpentine and a similar quantity of castor oil, or by a drop or two of croton oil; and enemata of turpentine† should be frequently ministered till the bowels are completely unloaded. The circumstances which forbid this use of purgatives, are previous disease of the alimentary canal; dysentery, ulcers, &c.; but even then there would be no objection to unirritating enemata.

3. *Mercury*, given so as to induce ptyalism, has often cured tetanus; therefore two or three grains of calomel may be given every two or three hours; or large quantities of strong mercurial ointment may be rubbed into the thighs and legs.

4. *Tobacco* has certainly proved more efficacious than any other remedy in tetanus. An enema, therefore, of four ounces of the *enema tabaci*

---

\* Pelletier treated a case successfully after taking fourteen or fifteen pounds of blood; and Lisfranc in one case bled eight times, and applied seven hundred and ninety-two leeches: examples rather to be wondered at than imitated.

† A remarkable case of locked jaw, cured instantaneously by a turpentine clyster, is recorded in the Med. Chir. Trans., vol. vi., by that learned and excellent physician Dr. Phillips of Winchester.

(F. 50) should be given after the bowels are cleared, or without waiting for that, if the symptoms are urgent. It soon induces deadly sickness, cold perspiration, fainting, and relaxation of the muscles, followed perhaps by sleep. And the enema should be repeated twice or thrice a day, or just often enough to keep the muscles constantly relaxed. But care must be taken to keep up the strength, and to administer hot brandy and water, or other stimulants, if the heart's action appear enfeebled.

5. *Cold* is of eminent service to animals affected with tetanus; and a soldier was once most unexpectedly cured by exposure all night in severe weather. It may therefore do good in some instances to apply cold extensively to the surface by means of bladders filled with various frigorific mixtures; taking care to support the circulation by internal stimulants. But the cold bath, or cold affusion, although they are of great service in chronic tetanus, are most hazardous in the acute, and have more than once proved instantly fatal.

6. *Tonics*, especially the muriated tincture of iron, quinine, &c., are likely to be of great service in asthenic cases. They should be given in large doses every two hours; it being as important to support a right action as to diminish a wrong one.*

7. *Opium* is of most undoubted efficacy in some instances, probably those attended with a painful wound, and weakness. When it produces good effects, they are soon manifest. The best way of using it appears to be by frictions with liniments containing it; or by removing a small portion of cuticle over the spine with a blister, and sprinkling a grain of finely powdered acetate, or hydrochlorate of morphia, on the denued cutis. Very large doses may be given without any effect.

8. *Nutriment.*—It is in all cases necessary to keep up the strength by beef-tea, wine, arrowroot, &c., especially towards the close of the malady. Mr. Travers believes that more patients have been lost from want of nutriment than from want of medicine. But it is often by no means easy to administer food or medicine, in consequence of the closure of the jaws, and difficulty of deglutition. The former difficulty may sometimes be overcome by passing an elastic catheter through the nose, or behind the last molar teeth. But if the attempt at swallowing is attended with much spasm in the larynx, it must be abandoned, and our remedies be introduced solely through the skin, or by enema. It is both unneces-

---

* Travers, Second Inquiry concerning Constitutional Irritation. The subcarbonate of iron is well called by Mr. Travers a "most inconvenient form." It is difficult to conceive the use of giving it in such quantities that it passes unaltered through the intestines,—as was the case with Frazier, one of the tetanic patients treated with it by Dr. Elliotson. Moreover, it is doubtful whether this patient's recovery is to be ascribed to the iron, or to an evacuation of pus from the foot. Vido Elliotson, Med. Chir. Trans. vol. xv., and Tyrrell's Ed. of Sir A. Cooper's Lectures, vol. iii.

sary and barbarous to force the jaws asunder, or to extract any of the teeth.

9. The *resin of the Cannabis Indica,* or Indian hemp, a mild stimulant and narcotic, has been employed by Dr. O'Shaughnessy and others at Calcutta, in doses of gr. iij every half hour till the symptoms are mitigated. It cured eight out of twelve cases.

10. *Colchicum* has been much praised by Mr. Smith of Hayti, and appears likely to be of benefit in idiopathic cases brought on by cold.

11. *Antispasmodics.*—It is scarcely worth while to mention camphor, musk, æther, castor, the warm bath, assafœtida, nor yet antimony, stramonium belladonna, or digitalis. They may have done good in some isolated cases, but no reasonable person would trust in them, to the exclusion of more active and certain remedies.

12. *Wourali.*—It is well known that narcotics are of two kinds. Some of them, including opium, prussic acid, and alcohol, act on the brain, suspending sensibility and voluntary motion, and causing death by causing the breathing to cease. Others (as digitalis and tobacco) act immediately on the nerves of organic life, and cause death by stopping the motions of the heart. Now there is a poison belonging to the former class, called *wourali* or *woorara,* which was brought to England by Mr. Waterton from Guiana, where the natives use it to poison their arrows, and which, when introduced in inconceivably minute quantities into the circulation, instantly suspends the functions of the brain;—sensibility and consciousness are lost, and the movements of respiration cease. But the heart continues to beat for a little while after this apparent death, and if respiration be kept up artificially, so as to maintain the purity of the blood, the heart will continue to beat, and after a time the nervous system will recover its suspended faculties, and life will be restored.[*] Animals have been repeatedly subjected to the action of this poison, and have been restored to perfect health afterwards;[†] and Mr. Sewell has tried it in two instances on animals affected with tetanus, and with perfect success;[‡] for the nervous system, when it recovered from the poison, was perfectly free from the disease. The same practice has therefore been proposed by Mr. Morgan to be hazarded in the human subject when afflicted with hopeless tetanus;—the poison to be introduced into a small

---

[*] An ass that was experimented on in this manner in 1814, died in 1839 at Walton Hall. Vide Waterton's Wanderings; and Brodie's papers, Phil. Trans. 1811, p. 178, and 1812, p. 205.

[†] Human beings poisoned with opium or alcohol have often been saved by artificial respiration.

[‡] But unfortunately one of the animals, a horse, died subsequently of repletion, and the other, an ass, of inanition.

wound in the finger,—a ligature to be placed above, so as to regulate its admission into the system; (it acts in fifteen seconds:) —and as soon as apparent death has ensued, artificial respiration to be kept up assiduously till signs of reanimation appear. And in a hopeless case the experiment would certainly be justifiable.*

CHRONIC TETANUS is very seldom fatal, although in some rare instances the patient has died completely exhausted by its long continuance; for it sometimes lasts several weeks. The principal remedies are aperients, tonics, and the shower-bath. The bowels should be kept freely open, but the indiscriminate exhibition of drastics should be avoided. Electricity, in the form of sparks, or weak shocks down the spine, would probably be of service.†

TRISMUS INFANTUM is a form of tetanus which is almost unknown in England. It was formerly, however, exceedingly prevalent in Ireland,‡ and appears to be met with there occasionally even at present. It carries off a vast number of children in the West India islands; and we learn from Dr. Holland,§ that in the desolate rocky Vestmann islands, on the south coast of Iceland, one hundred and eighty-six infants perished of it in twenty-five years, although the population does not exceed one hundred and fifty souls. The causes appear to be, want of ventilation, and filth, or the innutritious and unwholesome diet of the parents, such as the fish and sea-bird eggs that form the only sustenance of the Vestmann islanders; and these causes probably co-operate with an unhealthy state of the wound left by the falling off of the navel-string. The time at which the disease appears is generally from the fifth to the tenth day after birth; hence the popular Irish term, *nine-day fits.*

The *symptoms* are, locked jaw, spasmodic difficulty of breathing and swallowing, and general convulsions. They are almost invariably attended with diarrhœa, and preceded by fretfulness, startings during sleep, and unusual greediness for the breast.

*Treatment* of any kind is seldom successful; but it may be presumed

---

* A most unique and preposterous remedy is recorded in Trnka, (Op. Cit. p. 444.) A ship was trading on the coast of Angola in 1763, and a native boy, who was ill with tetanus, had been treated for some days without benefit by the ship's Doctor. His case was considered hopeless, when one of the savages cured him in the following extraordinary manner. He made a small wound in the thigh, into which he inserted a pipe, and then blew with all his might, till the whole body was inflated with emphysema. Strange to say, the boy recovered from that mo rent.

† Holland, Med. Notes and Refl; and Addison on Electricity in Convulsive Diseases, Guy's Hosp. Rep. vol. ii.

‡ Clarke, Joseph. M.D., in Med. Facts and Observations. Vol. iii. Lond. 1792.

§ Medical Notes and Reflections, 2nd Ed. p. 29.

that free ventilation, the warm-bath, four or five doses of calomel (gr. i.—ii.) at intervals of four or five hours, a teaspoonful or two of castor oil to clear the bowels, and minute doses of laudanum (one-eighth of a minim cautiously increased) every two hours afterwards, are the measures most likely to be of service.*

* Maunsell and Evanson on Diseases of children, 3rd Ed. Dublin, 1840, p. 178.

# PART II.

## OF THE PRINCIPAL PROCESSES OF LOCAL DISEASE.

---

## CHAPTER I.

### OF THE GENERAL PHENOMENA OF INFLAMMATION.

DEFINITION.—Inflammation may be defined to be a state of increased vascularity and sensibility, with a tendency to morbid secretion and change of structure.*

SYMPTOMS.—The symptoms are redness, pain, heat, and swelling, with impaired function of the inflamed part;—and each of these symptoms requires a few observations in detail.

(1.) The *redness* is owing to the increased quantity of blood in the inflamed part; for all the vessels are dilated, and the red particles pass into capillaries that before conveyed only serum. When inflammation is acute, the redness is of the bright scarlet tint of arterial blood; when chronic, it is of a darker venous hue; and in certain specific inflammations it is purple or copper-coloured.† Again, in common inflammation, it is gradually diffused, and lost in the neighbouring parts, whilst it is abruptly circumscribed in some forms of specific inflammation.‡ There are several terms used by authors to express the varieties, degrees, and appearances of redness.§ Thus, 1. It is called *ramiform*, when seated in the small arteries and veins only, and not in the capillaries. 2. It is said to be *capilliform* when *some* of the capillaries are also distended. 3. It is

---

* P. H. Berard, Dict. de Med. vol. xvi. Paris, 1837.

† The dusky hue is probably caused by some effusion under the cuticle. which generally peels off afterwards. Macartney on Inflammation, Lond. 1838, p. 17.

‡ Hunter's Works by Palmer. Vol. iii. p. 330.

§ Carswell, Illustrations of the Elementary Forms of Disease. Lond. fol. 1837.

*uniform,* when *all* the capillaries are injected; as in erysipelas. 4. It is *punctiform* when occurring in minute dots; as when the villi of a mucous membrane are injected, but not the mucous tissue itself. 5. It is called *maculiform,* when the blood is either extremely accumulated, or else extravasated at certain points. This form of redness accompanies hæmorrhagic inflammation.

(2.) The *pain* of inflammation is sometimes attributed to a stretching of the nerves by the distended blood-vessels. But this is a very unworthy and mechanical explanation. It is more correct and philosophical to say that it is a disorder of sensation, accompanying the disorder of nutrition and function. There is good reason for believing that it occasionally is the first element of inflammation present; preceding the existence of vascular disturbance. It differs in its character and intensity according to several circumstances, but principally according to the part which is inflamed. Thus it is burning, or tingling in the skin; throbbing in the cellular tissue; sharp and lancinating in the pleura;—a mere sense of heat and soreness in the bronchial mucous membrane; and extremely dull and oppressing in a part largely supplied with ganglionic nerves;—as the stomach, kidneys, or testicles. It is always less severe if the fluid products of inflammation can readily escape, than if they are confined,—and comparatively slight if the part inflamed be yielding and extensile, but most severe if it be hard and dense, as bone or ligament; although these structures possess very little sensibility in health. It is also in general greater in common inflammation than in specific, with the exception of the gout. It is sometimes felt at a distance from the inflamed part; thus pain in the shoulder is often the first symptom of inflamed liver, and pain in the knee of diseased hip. Lastly, it may be entirely absent; as where inflammation occurs in a healthy constitution, and merely produces adhesion; thus adhesions are often found between the pleuræ after death, that never were suspected during life; or where inflammation, although disorganizing, is very insidious and indolent, as in scrofula;—or where the patient's mental and physical sensibilities have been benumbed by the habitual abuse of intoxicating liquors.*

(3.) The *heat* of inflammation was supposed by Hunter to be a mere effect of the increased afflux of blood. For it is most remarkable in inflammation of those parts which are farthest from the heart, and naturally the coldest; and in them it often does not rise so high as the mean temperature of the blood;—whilst in inflammation of internal parts, whose heat is uniform, and not depressed by external vicissitudes, it sometimes does not rise at all. But some modern authorities maintain that the heat of inflammation is owing not merely to the increased afflux of warm

---

* Latham, Lectures on Subjects connected with Clinical Medicine.—Lecture vi.

blood, but to a greater evolution of heat by the agency of the nerves; and it is said that more liquid will be evaporated by inflamed parts in a given time, than by healthy parts of equal temperature.*

(4.) The *swelling* is caused at first by the increased quantity of blood, and subsequently by the effusion of serum, blood, lymph, and pus. It is most remarkable in loose textures; also in the breast, testicle, and lymphatic glands.

(5.) The *impairment of function* which inflammation produces, consists at first in an increased irritability and morbid sensibility of external impression; but, subsequently, of an utter incapability of performing the usual offices, in consequence of structural change.

(6.) Inflammation may produce every possible *alteration of secretion. First*, in *quantity;* secretion is invariably diminished at the commencement of inflammation; but often increased at its close, as is the case with mucous membranes. *Secondly*, in *chemical composition;*—as the tears which in certain cases become hot and scalding, and excoriate the cheek. *Thirdly*, the secretions may be *mixed* with the products of inflammation; thus mucus is often mixed with blood, serum, lymph, and pus. *Fourthly*, gas is sometimes secreted in inflamed tissues.

(7.) ALTERATION IN STRUCTURE.—Inflammation is capable of altering all the mechanical qualities of parts. 1. The *weight* is always increased if the inflammation be recent, and if it have not existed long enough to induce atrophy. 2. *Cohesion* or *hardness* is always *diminished* in acute inflammation, although this is apt to be overlooked in consequence of the increased density. This softening arises partly from the serum which infiltrates the tissues; and is always most remarkable when there is the least cellular tissue to contain the serum; as in the brain. Hardness may be increased in chronic inflammation; sometimes because the whole bulk of the part is shrunken; sometimes because of the organization of lymph. Hardening from chronic inflammation was formerly termed *scirrhus.* (3.) *Transparency* and *polish* are always impaired.

MORBID ANATOMY.—The ordinary *post mortem* appearances of recent inflammation are, redness, softening, swelling, and infiltration with serum. It is necessary, however, to make a few observations respecting these phenomena, and especially concerning redness; because, in the *first* place, it may disappear altogether after death—*secondly*, it may be simulated by redness from congestion which existed during life—and *thirdly*, it may be simulated by certain appearances produced after death.

In the *first* place, then, redness, if very slight, may disappear from inflamed skin after death; but if the blood-vessels were injected, the vascularity would be found increased; besides that the part would be

---

* Berard, Op. Cit.; James on Inflammation, p. 239 ; Macartney, Op. Cit. p. 14 ; Latour, Revue Med., Jan. 1840.

softened, and slightly infiltrated with serum, and that the epidermis would peel off more readily than natural.

*Secondly.* Redness may have been caused during life, not by inflammation, but by congestion, from an obstacle to the return of blood; and congestion may also be attended with softening, and serous effusion, so that in some instances it cannot be distinguished at all from inflammation, and in others not with certainty. The general distinction is, that in congestion the larger veins are distended more than the capillaries, and previously to them; whereas it is the reverse in inflammation. The diagnosis will be aided by observing whether there is any cause of obstruction to the venous circulation.*

*Thirdly.* The redness of inflammation may require to be distinguished from certain appearances produced after death. And these may be produced, (1.) By the *action of the capillaries*, which persists after that of the heart has ceased: so that the arteries are emptied, and the blood accumulated in various internal organs, especially the lungs and spleen. (2.) By *gravitation*; by which the most depending parts of the body, and especially of the lungs, are always more or less congested. (3.) By *transudation* of the serum and colouring matter through the coats of the vessels in incipient putrefaction; which is a frequent cause of red spots and stains on internal surfaces, and of collections of bloody serum in the various cavities. But the author's space does not permit him to dilate upon these topics: they are merely adverted to for the purpose of showing, that redness, swelling, softening, and serous effusion, (unless accompanied by some more decided effect of inflammation, such as lymph or pus,) must not be hastily received as evidences of it; seeing that they may be produced by other causes, both before death and after it.

EFFECTS AND TERMINATIONS.—Inflammation has only one genuine *termination*; namely, *resolution*, or recovery; the inflammatory action subsiding, and the part returning to its former state;—but, beside resolution, it may have either of the following six terminations, or *effects*, or *consequences*, as they ought rather to be called. 1. *Hæmorrhage*; an escape of blood from the distended vessels. 2. *Effusion of serum.* 3. *Effusion of fibrine*, or of *coagulable lymph*, constituting *adhesion*. 4. *Suppuration*; the formation of a peculiar fluid called *pus*. 5. *Ulceration;* the disappearance or removal of the inflamed part. 6. *Mortification*, or its death. To each of these effects a chapter will be devoted.†

FORMS OF INFLAMMATION.—Inflammation may be divided—1. Into *healthy* and *unhealthy;*—the former being that which naturally ensues in

---

* Andral, Anatomie Pathologique, tom. i. p. 56.

† It must be understood that except suppuration, and perhaps adhesion, these effects may all be produced by other causes besides inflammation—congestion in particular may cause hæmorrhage, serous effusion, ulceration, and gangrene.

healthy constitutions, when a part of the organization is impaired;—being restorative in its tendencies, and injurious only if excessive or misplaced. Whereas, the unhealthy is essentially destructive, and has little or no spontaneous tendency to recovery. 2. Into *common* and *specific;* the common arising from ordinary causes acting on healthy constitutions;— the specific arising, either because the constitution is unsound, as in scrofula, so that (to use Hunter's words) it gives or reflects back upon the part inflamed a diseased disposition or action;—or because it is produced by a cause which is specific; as the poisons of small-pox or syphilis. 3. It may be divided into *acute* and *chronic;* the acute being sudden in its seizure, violent in its action, and rapid in its progress;—the chronic being less violent and more tardy. Acute inflammation is sometimes called *active;* and the term *passive* is applied to chronic inflammations in weak constitutions. 4. It may be classified according to its tendency to produce particular local effects ; thus we speak of adhesive, suppurative, hæmorrhagic, ulcerative, and gangrenous inflammation.

MODIFICATIONS.—Inflammation will always be modified by the *state of constitution* in which it occurs; being active and rapid in the young and healthy; but more indolent, and tending to destructive processes (such as ulceration and mortification) in the aged and debilitated. It will also present divers variations, according to the *cause* producing it; and will be greatly influenced by the *epidemic constitution* of the air. But its most important modications are derived from the *structure of the parts* which it invades; for it has a special tendency to a different termination in almost every different texture. Now all parts capable of being inflamed may be divided into two orders;—first, those which have no natural outlet, as the serous cavaties, and the cellular tissue of the body generally ; secondly, those which have; as the skin and mucous membranes. In the *first order*, inflammation is more disposed to produce adhesion than suppuration ; so as not only to render less likely the production of pus in a cavity from which it could not escape, but also if suppuration could occur, to limit the extent of suppurating surface, and circumscribe the fluid and prevent its diffusion. But the *second* order of parts is more liable to an inflammation that spreads ;—which has a tendency to produce suppuration before adhesion; because suppuration is but a trifling evil compared with the danger that would ensue if the mucous canals were closed by adhesive matter, from the slight inflammations to which they are perpetually subject. Yet if inflammation be of extreme *violence*, or if there be something particularly morbid in its *cause* or in the *constitution*, the natural precedence of these two effects will be inverted. Thus in violent inflammation of mucous membranes, as croup, lymph is poured out on the surface ;—and inflammation of the cellular tissue, arising in a vitiated habit, or from a morbid poison, (as after

7

dissection wounds,) may induce a diffused and widely spreading suppuration which is not limited by adhesion.

PREDISPOSING CAUSES.—The predisposing causes of inflammation may be connected with the constitution, or with the part. To the former belong plethora; the sanguine temperament, and excess in food and drink. The latter are chiefly over-stimulation, or exertion beyond power; besides previous disease, and original weakness of organization.

EXCITING CAUSES.—The exciting causes may be divided into two classes. 1. Those which act primarily on the *structure* of a part;—as mechanical and chemical injuries of all sorts. 2. Those which act primarily on its *functions* and *vital endowments;*—as over-exertion;—and the poisons, such as cantharides, which affect living matters only. The former class act *directly;* that is they inflame the part which they are applied to: the latter class may act *indirectly;* just as cold applied to the feet causes inflammation of the lungs. The former also act *immediately;* whilst some of the latter may take some time (which is called the stage of incubation) to produce their effects. Lastly, causes may be *common* or *specific;*—the former being those which are daily met with, and which can act on all constitutions;—the latter being unable to affect all constitutions, being peculiar in their origin, and producing a modified inflammation, with a specific train of consequences.

DIAGNOSIS.—It must be understood that both the blood-vessels and nerves are concerned in inflammation;—it must also be understood, that although either of these elements, if disordered, will tend to implicate the other, still that one of them may for a long time be deranged solely. Inflammation, therefore, requires to be distinguished from disordered action of the blood-vessels merely, or *hyperæmia*—in the forms of *congestion* and *determination of blood*—and from pain caused by disordered nervous influence.

(*a*) *Congestion* signifies an accumulation or stagnation of venous blood in a part which may be caused by some mechanical obstacle to its return; or by weakness and atony; it is a very frequent sequel of inflammation. It produces more or less weight and pain, with disturbance of function, especially of secretion; but it does not cause fever like acute inflammation, nor interstitial deposition like chronic;—although it may terminate in either.*

(*b*) *Active determination* of blood is produced by a dilatation and expansion of the arteries, whereby they convey more blood to a part. It is a process necessary to many natural actions; as, for instance, the en-

---

* The red noses of drunkards present instances of permanent congestion, distinct from inflammation.

largement of the womb during gestation, and the secretion of milk after delivery ;—blushing affords a very familiar example of it. When morbid, it causes excitement and functional derangement. Instances of it are seen in the injected capillaries of the intestines in cholera, and in headachs from excitement ;—in many cases it is the first stage of incipient inflammation.

(c) *Irritation* of the nerves, or *neuralgia*, is a peculiar state, attended with severe pain and tenderness. The irritable breast, irritable testicle, tic douloureux, neuralgic toothach and headach, and the mock inflammations which occur in weak, irritable, and hysteric subjects, (especially from abuse of blood-letting,) are examples. The pain of nervous irritation may in general be distinguished from that of inflammation, by its sudden accession and subsidence ;—by its being often relieved by measures that would aggravate inflammation, such as pressure, friction, &c.;—by the pain being severe out of all proportion to heat, redness, and swelling, even if they exist at all ;—and by the circumstance that although the pain may last for weeks or months, no local disorganization or suppuration follows.

THEORY OF INFLAMMATION.—It is not compatible with the scope of this work to give a detailed account of the various theories that have been invented respecting the *proximate cause* or *essential nature* of inflammation. Of the older writers, some attributed it to a *lentor* or viscidity of the blood ;—others to an *error loci*, that is, an obstruction of the capillaries by the entrance of globules too large to pass through them. Cullen supposed that it consisted in spasm of the extreme vessels. Hunter ascribed it to an increased action ;—Wilson, Philip, and Hastings, to a debility ;—and Mr. J. W. Earle to an obstruction of the capillaries.

But the theory that seems to be most reasonable and most useful, is that of Dr. Macartney ; who considers that the proximate cause of inflammation is a sense of injury felt by the organic (sympathetic or arterial) nerves ; and shows that inflammation after an injury may often be prevented by soothing and allaying this nervous irritation, and inducing a comfortable state of feeling.

With regard to the processes that actually occur in the inflamed part, many statements have been promulgated, that appear to be totally contrary to fact, and to have arisen from ill-devised microscopical experiments. Many authors, for instance, have described the phenomena that may be seen in the web of the frog's foot or fins of fishes, after the application of a red hot needle, or of acrid salts ; and having observed that after such applications the capillaries become dilated, the blood moves in them more slowly, and at last coagulates, and does not move at all, they have concluded that a retardation of the circulation is an essential element in inflammation. M. Latour, however, has shown satisfactorily, that this coagulation is merely the chemical effect of the heat, acids, or other

irritating matters employed to create the so-called inflammation; and both
Latour, Gulliver, Macartney, and other late authors of good credit, affirm
most positively that it is impossible to excite inflammation in cold-blooded
animals at all.

The facts that seem to be best established, are the following:—That
in the capillaries of every *acutely inflamed* part, and the larger vessels in
its vicinity, the blood is circulated with preternatural rapidity and abundance; that this vascular excitement is followed by effusions of serum,
lymph, and perhaps of blood into the interstices of the part, which effusions occur either by transudation through the parietes of the capillaries,
or by rupture of them. And that if the inflammation continue, the parts
thus softened and infiltrated lose their distinguishing characters, and pus
is formed;—or if the inflammation increases in severity, the blood coagulates in the vessels, the tissue becomes soft and flaccid, and in fact
mortifies.*

---

# CHAPTER II.

## OF ACUTE INFLAMMATION.

DEFINITION.—Acute inflammation is that which is sudden in its origin,
violent in its action, and rapid in terminating; and it is attended with
fever, either if it be considerable in its extent, or if it affect parts of great
sensibility and importance, or if the constitution be highly irritable.

TREATMENT.—In the *treatment* of acute inflammation and its attendant
fever, the *indications* are, to reduce the increased action of the heart and
arteries; to allay pain and nervous excitement, and to restore the secretions. The chief means are, evacuants, sedatives, and narcotics.

(1.) BLOOD-LETTING,† *Objects of.*—The first and most important mea-

---

* Vide Cullen's First Lines, book ii., chap. i. sect. 2. Hunter on the Blood;
Thompson's Lectures on Inflammation; Gendrin, Histoire Anatomique des Inflammations; Andral, Anatomie Pathologique: Wilson Philip's Treatise on Fevers, and
Experimental Inquiry into the Laws of the Vital Functions, 3rd ed.; Mayo's Outlines of Physiology, 5th ed.; the Papers by Mr. J. W. Earle in Lond. Med. Gaz. vol.
xvi; Latour op. cit.; Macartney op. cit.; Gulliver Phil. Mag. Sept. 1838. Kalten-
brunner de Statu Vasorum et Sanguinis in Inflammatione, 1826.

† On the subject of blood-letting, the surgical practitioner should always bear in
mind the difference between the *suppression* of inflammatory action and *the preven-*

sure is general blood-letting;—which, if carried far enough, induces a state of insensibility, and suspended circulation, to which the name *syncope*, or *fainting*, is given. Now it requires to be understood, that this suspension of the heart's action depends upon two causes; *first*, on the abstraction of its natural stimulus, the blood;—*secondly*, and principally, on a peculiar sedative influence transmitted to it from the brain, when the latter does not receive its due share of arterial blood. And although the mere loss of blood *per se* may be of service (when that fluid is morbidly abundant) by relieving the system from a source of excitement, still the principal good effects of bleeding in inflammation depend on its sedative effects on the brain, and through the brain on the heart. And as it is often absolutely necessary to bleed persons in acute diseases who are extremely debilitated, it is of importance to produce as much of that sedative effect with as little loss of blood as possible.

*Manner of Bleeding.*—For this purpose the blood should be drawn as quickly as possible*—from a large orifice; and, above all, the patient should sit or stand upright. For if the blood is drawn slowly, so that the vessels have time to adapt themselves to their diminished contents, or if the patient is in the recumbent posture, so as to assist the flow of blood to the brain, the bleeding may be continued almost to death without the occurrence of faintness.

*Quantity to be taken.*—As a general rule, the blood should be permitted to flow till paleness of the lips, lividity about the eyes, sighing, nausea, fluttering pulse, and relief of the pain, indicate the *approach* of syn-

---

tion of it, in determining the extent to which he may safely carry the means of depletion and depression.

In the case of a healthy man, for instance, who has received a wound involving either of the cavities of the trunk, where it is of the utmost importance to prevent inflammation, the lancet may be employed largely and frequently, the practitioner being careful only not to reduce the organic energies below the point at which immediate union of divided parts may be effected. But, violent reaction having taken place—inflammatory processes being fairly established, whether in spite of bloodletting, or by default of its more seasonable employment, the utmost discretion is necessary in the use of this potent means of subduing inordinate vascular action.

The circumspect practitioner will have in view the various consequences of inflammation which he cannot hope altogether to avert, and most of which require a good deal of constitutional vigour in the patient, to dissipate or render them harmless.

Of all therapeutical appliances there is none in which art ventures on such extreme liberties with nature as in this of blood-letting, and unfortunately there are few in regard to which the principles that are to regulate its administration are so unsettled and contradictory. Those which are briefly stated in the text, are the most approved and important the authorities furnish. F.

* About ℥viii. ought to flow in three minutes.

cope; but *full* syncope should always be avoided, for reasons that will presently appear. Then the patient may be suffered to lie down, and should be kept perfectly quiet, without any attempts to restore the circulation by stimulants;—that so the inflamed capillaries may resume their natural caliber, whilst relieved from the influx of the circulation.

*Tolerance.*—The tolerance, or power of bearing bleeding, without fainting, varies according to the age, sex, and temperament of the patient. It is less in the very young and old than in the middle-aged;—less in the female than in the male;—and less in the nervous and lymphatic temperament, than in the sanguine and phlegmatic. But the *tolerance* is besides affected most remarkably by the existing disease. Thus it has been ascertained by Dr. Marshall Hall, that 15 oz. is the average quantity that will produce syncope in an adult if healthy; but that in some diseases much more requires to be taken, and in others much less.

The diseases in which bleeding is best borne; are inflammations of the head, or of other vital parts. Those in which it is most injurious and worst borne, are putrid fevers and diseases of debility. And so, an observation of the tolerance is sometimes a very important aid to diagnosis. Supposing a woman to complain of violent pain in the head or abdomen, which is suspected to be inflammatory. If faintness occurs from the loss of a very small quantity of blood, it will be certain either that is not inflammatory, but nervous;—or that if inflammatory, it must be treated by other measures than blood-letting. But the junior practitioner must bear in mind that he may occasionally meet with some thin, bloodless patients, whom it would be very injurious to bleed, but who nevertheless, from some peculiarity of constitution, do not faint, even though bled to excess.

*Reaction.*—After the depressing effects of bleeding there naturally ensues a degree of reaction; the pulse rising in frequency, and the local pain returning; and this reaction will be the greater if the venesection has been carried to the extent of producing full syncope;—hence the importance of stopping short of this point. This reaction is, if possible, to be prevented by the sedatives, which we shall mention presently; but if, notwithstanding, well-marked inflammatory symptoms return, the bleeding must be repeated till the disease is permanently vanquished;—provided that the strength permit.

*Indications for Bleeding.*—But as general venesection is not to be resorted to indiscriminately in every case of acute inflammation, a few words must be said on the principles that regulate its employment. And there are three things to be considered; viz. 1st, the patient's strength, and state of his constitution; 2ndly, the part affected; 3rdly, the nature and amount of the injury or exciting cause which has produced the disease.

(1.) With regard to the state of the constitution, bleeding is most required, and best borne, when the *temperament* is sanguine, or that mixture of the sanguine and phlegmatic termed rustic;—when the *muscles* are large and firm;—when the blood-making powers are vigorous and the circulation strong, as indicated by redness of the face and lips, and by a full, hard, and frequent pulse. On the other hand, it will be borne *worse* when the muscles are large and flabby, and the pulse habitually open, soft, and full. And it will be borne worst of all, when the complexion is sickly and pale;—the pulse quick, small, and feeble;—the lips, conjunctiva, and tongue pale. And if there should happen to be a state of passive dilatation and weakness of the heart, syncope would most likely be instantly fatal;—and if there should be any organic disease which impedes the formation of blood, its loss is liable to be followed by irrecoverable sinking and exhaustion. *Fat people* generally bear bleeding worse, and in fact contain less blood, proportionably to their bulk, than those of a spare, lean habit and rigid fibre.

The propriety of a *second bleeding* must in a great measure be determined by the effect which the first has had on the pulse; for if that be more frequent and quick, or more sharp and jerking,\* instead of slower and softer, it would seem that the bleeding had diminished the strength more than it had reduced the disease. The state of the blood must also be regarded; for if the surface of the coagulum be flat, and its consistence loose, it is a sign that the vital powers are depressed, that farther bleeding will be injurious, and that the case must be committed to the other antiphlogistic powers.

(2.) Respecting the *part affected*, it may be observed that the necessity for venesection, and its beneficial effects, will be greater in proportion as the *tolerance* is greater ;—and that it would be indispensable where the organ affected is important to life, or to its enjoyment ; whilst it might not be so, if an equal degree of inflammation affected an unimportant part;—and that its good influence in inflammation of a vital organ will often be marked by a rise in the strength and fulness of the pulse.

(3.) With regard to the *nature of the cause*, bleeding is not well borne when that is such as to produce great depression of the vital powers, as in the case of dissection wounds;—nor when the inflammation itself causes great depression, as in phlebitis;—nor in the case of an injury requiring great constitutional efforts for its restoration, as a compound fracture;—nor if the disease be advanced towards suppuration or gangrene.

II. EVACUANT SEDATIVES.—Under this title may be included a number of antiphlogistic remedies, which reduce vascular excitement, either by increasing certain secretions, or by some specific lowering agency

---

\* Vide p. 24.

independent of any evacuation,—most of them being capable of acting
in both manners. (*a*) *Purgatives* are admissible at the commencement
of all cases, except when they would cause irritation or disturbance of
a diseased or injured part, as might be the case in wounds of the alimentary canal, and in compound fracture. Those should be selected which
excite free secretion from the liver and intestines, and evacuate them
rapidly : such as a good dose of calomel, followed by F. 4. (*b*) *Mercury**
reduces the heart's action, restores the secretions, and excites the absorption of diseased products; it is chiefly advantageous in inflammations of serous structures, with a tendency to adhesion. The best form
for its administration is calomel, of which from one to five grains may
be given, at intervals of from two to six hours, till a *slight* affection of
the mouth is manifested; which should be kept up by smaller doses if
necessary; but all violent salivation is an evil. The calomel should be
combined with opium or hyoscyamus, to prevent it from purging too
freely. (*c*) *Antimony* is another direct antiphlogistic; it may be administered in doses of $\frac{1}{8}$-$\frac{1}{2}$ grain, with each dose of calomel and opium; in
larger doses, such as gr. ii., it is a most potent remedy, especially in
pneumonia; it does not cause vomiting after the first few doses, but ex-
erts its sedative influence without producing any evacuation. (*d*) *Colchicum* is a remedy of precisely the same character; it is most useful in
gouty and rheumatic affections. It may and frequently does produce
bilious stools; but it is a vulgar error to suppose that they are indispensable to its good effects. (*e*) *Nitre* and the other salines, as in F. 5,
may also be given with great advantage; they abate heat and thirst,
purify the blood, and increase the secretion of urine.

III. SEDATIVES NOT EVACUANT.—These remedies reduce fever and inflammation, by acting on the nervous system without increasing the
secretions; they are hyoscyamus, conium, and digitalis, the first two of
which in particular are of eminent service, when combined with calomel
and antimony, (F. 6.) to prevent reaction, and soothe pain in inflammatory cases attended with great nervous irritability.

IV. NARCOTICS.—*Opium* primarily decreases the secretions, and increases vascular excitement; hence it must not be given in acute inflammation till after bleeding; but then a large dose (such as gr. ii.) may be
given in combination with five of calomel, to allay pain and prevent
reaction. But it is the *sine qua non*, and may be given without reserve

---

* I am disposed to think that very seldom if ever, shall we realize any advantage
from the administration of *mercurials* in inflammations occasioned by mechanical
injuries, involving only the textures, usually the subjects of such injuries.

I have long since ceased to use it myself in such cases, and generally when I
have seen it employed by others, it has proved to be any thing but antiphlogistic in
its effects.      F

in inflammations occurring in very debilitated habits, such as peritoneal inflammations from perforation of the intestine, or other cause, after fever, or after profuse hæmorrhage.

*The warm bath* acts in every way analogous to opium, and requires the same precautions; viz. as it stimulates before it soothes, it must be preceded by evacuations, if the habit be plethoric. The proper temperature is 97° Fahrenheit, and it should be continued long enough to induce complete relaxation.

V. DIET.—The *diet* in acute inflammation should, as a general rule, be of the least stimulating nature. But although water-gruel and tea might for many days suffice for the robust and plethoric, the starving system must not be indiscriminately applied to children, or the old or debilitated; on the contrary, their strength must be supported by mild fluid nutriment, arrowroot, beef-tea, &c., and even by wine if necessary.

VI. REGIMEN.—There must be a total avoidance of every thing that would irritate mind or body. Perfect rest in the recumbent posture, and in a position as easy as it can be made;—cool air;—free ventilation;—the exclusion of light and sound;—with mental consolation, to allay doubts and fears, and inspire resignation and cheerfulness, are most potent aids to medical treatment, which without them would often be utterly fruitless.

LOCAL TREATMENT.—In the local treatment of inflammation, the first thing to be done is to remove all exciting causes if possible, and to place the part at perfect rest, and in an elevated posture, so as to favour the return of blood from it;—and then the indications are, to diminish the morbid heat and afflux of blood; and to allay irritation and pain.

1. *The local means of abstracting bloo*d are leeches, cupping, and scarifications. In order to apply leeches, the part should first be washed, and if they will not stick, a little milk or blood should be smeared on it, or some small punctures should be made with the point of a lancet; and the leeches should be well dried in a cloth. The best plan of stopping hæmorrhage from leech-bites is to dip small pellets of lint in the tinct. ferri sesquichloridi, and press them on the holes for a few minutes, or to insert a finely-pointed pencil of lunar caustic into them. Sometimes it is expedient to touch them with a red hot knitting needle, or to stitch them up with a very fine needle and silk. But in order to prevent the very serious consequences that sometimes happen from this source to children and delicate persons, proper directions should always be given that the bleeding from leech-bites should be stopped before the patient is left for the night. Moreover, it will be prudent to apply them over some bone, so that pressure may be applied effectually. Again, leeches, if they stick too long, should be removed by touching them with salt, and should not be pulled off forcibly; nor should they be applied to the eyelids or prepuce, otherwise they will probably be followed by œdema-

8

tous swelling, or even erysipelas. *Cupping,* when it can be adopted, is a more active measure, and relieves pain sooner than leeches. *Scarifi- cations,* or *incisions,* are of use when inflamed parts are covered with a dense unyielding fascia, as in whitlow; or when there is great tension, as in phlegmonous erysipelas; or when the inflamed part is infiltrated with an irritating fluid, as in extravasation of urine, or with unhealthy matters, as in carbuncle.

2. *Cold applications* are of use to diminish heat, and cause contraction of the capillaries; but they should be applied continuously, otherwise the pain will be aggravated when the heat returns. The best lotion is one containing lead and spirit, as F. 11; it should be applied by means of a single piece of thin linen frequently changed; and care should be taken that the vapour may pass off freely, otherwise the cold lotion will soon be converted into a hot fomentation. In some severe cases, ice or frigorific mixtures (F. 12) may be applied in bladders. The following very ef- fectual means of applying a continuous degree of cold, is recommended by Dr. Macartney. The inflamed limb is to be placed in a trough or piece of oilcloth, with a piece of lint on the inflamed part. A large ves- sel full of cold water being then placed on a table by the bedside, one end of a broad strip of cloth should be dipped in the water, and the other end (which should be cut to a point) laid on the lint; and so the water will be carried in a constant gentle stream down the cloth to the inflamed part.

3. *Warmth.* Very often cold adds to irritation; and perhaps in most cases *tepid* applications (85° Fah.) are preferable; for they do not stimulate like heat, nor occasion painful reaction like cold, and are more directly sedative than either. *Warm* fomentations (92°—98° Fah.) are useful by relaxing the skin, soothing pain, and promoting perspiration, and are especially indicated in inflammations of dense tendinous parts. In every case the patient's feelings should be consulted, and the applica- tions be warm or cold according to his choice. Dr. Macartney very justly insists on the necessity of producing an agreeable state of feeling in inflamed parts, as a means of relieving that sense of irritation in the or- ganic nerves which he considers as the *point de depart* in inflammation. This gentleman has contrived an apparatus for conveying steam to any part of the body, which affords by far the best means of applying heat and moisture. It consists of a tube of woollen cloth, three feet long, twelve inches wide, and fitted with hoops of whalebone to keep it open; one end of it is applied to the part which it is desired to foment. the other is tied round the neck of a tin boiler in which the steam is generated.

4. *Stimulants,* and astringent solutions, are of great service in inflam- mation of mucous membranes, by decomposing and washing away their irritating secretions, and inducing contraction of the capillaries.

**5.** *Counter-irritants.*—When one part of a frog's foot has been irritated and caused to inflame, it is said that if a neighbouring part be likewise irritated, some blood may be seen under the microscope to rush to it from the former. On this principle one inflammation is relieved by establishing another near it. Blisters (or rather the strong acetum cantharidis) are the best form of counter-irritants; but they should never be applied too near the disease, and never till its activity has been subdued by previous antiphlogistic measures.

# CHAPTER III.

## OF CHRONIC INFLAMMATION.

DEFINITION.—Inflammation is said to be chronic when it is gradual in its origin, slow in its progress, and tending to last long, or even indefinitely. Its *consequences* may be, adhesion, thickening, induration, ulceration, or suppuration.

CAUSES.—Its causes may be local or constitutional. Thus it may in the healthiest subjects be caused by any slight and continued irritant;—or it may be the sequel of acute inflammation, the vessels being left dilated, weak, and irritable. But it is more frequently the local manifestation of some constitutional disorder, such as general debility, with a tendency to local congestion,—or over-stimulation and plethora,—or disorder of seme important organ, as of the stomach or liver.

TREATMENT.—The indications are, to remove all constitutional disorder, to allay local irritation, and restore the tone of the distended vessels.

1. In the first place, the patient's general appearance and condition must be examined. If he is bloated and plethoric, indulging freely in stimulating food and drink, and has unimpaired digestive organs, so that blood is constantly formed in too great abundance, the diet must be lowered and restricted principally to farinaceous articles;—free exercise must be taken in the air;—the bowels should be actively purged by a dose of calomel, followed by an aperient draught, and then a course of alterative medicine should be commenced, in order to regulate the circulation, increase the secretions, and relieve the system of its superabundant material. Plummer's Pill is an excellent form; it acts on skin, liver, and bowels; F. 6, 7, 10, have similar effects. Aperients should be administered occasionally, so as to carry off the mercury; such as seidlitz powders, or F. 8, 9, 42; but in severe and obstinate cases, it may be necessary to bring the constitution under the influence of that mineral,

taking care, however, to desist at the least appearance of ptyalism, and maintain a gentle and continued, but not violent action.

2. But if the chronic inflammation occur in an enfeebled and irritable constitution, (as when it succeeds an acute attack that has been too actively treated by bleeding and mercury,) a nutritious and liberal diet must be adopted, wine and tonics (F. 26, 1, 2, 3, 28) should be administered, in order to improve the digestion and vigour of the circulation; irritation and pain must be allayed by sedatives and opiates; the secretions of the bowels must be maintained by the gentlest laxatives; and if mercury is required to keep up the biliary secretion, it must be given in small doses of the mildest forms, (F. 10, 52,) and at intervals.

3. Any marked disorder must be carefully sought for and rectified. If the tongue is furred and red at its tip and edges, and there are acid eructations, flatulence, and other signs of irritation of the stomach, the diet should consist principally of boiled mutton, or chicken, rice-pudding, boiled milk and bread, and similar unirritating and easily digestible articles; and small doses of alkalies (F. 54) may be given after meals; with a mild mercurial (F. 7, 10, 52) occasionally at bedtime, and an aperient (F. 8, 9, 55) in the morning. If the complexion is sallow, and the stools clay-coloured, a few doses of calomel or blue pill, with morning aperients, are indicated. When steel or bark is administered, it is always necessary to have a proper action of the liver and bowels, otherwise headach and feverishness will ensue. If the skin is dry and harsh, it should be stimulated by exercise, by warm clothing, especially flannel, by the flesh-brush or horse-hair gloves, and by an occasional ten minutes' immersion in the hot bath; 92°—102° Fah. In females the uterine system must be regulated by the exhibition of steel, aloes, or other emmenagogues, if necessary. There are some remedies that seem to possess peculiar powers in chronic inflammation, by supporting the strength and dispelling congestion: such as serpentaria and ammonia in combination with bitter infusions;—very small doses of corrosive sublimate in combination with tincture of bark (F. 48;) sasaparilla (F. 56, 57) and the liq. arsenicalis, which is eminently serviceable in dry, scaly eruptions of the skin.

The *local treatment* of chronic inflammation has for its objects, to remove exciting causes, to unload the distended vessels and make them contract to their natural caliber, and to exercise the part in its proper functions, so that it may gradually resume the actions and sensations of health.

*Local bleeding* must be employed at intervals to unload the vessels, whilst they must be excited to contract by various stimulants and astringents; such as the sulphates of zinc, copper, and alumina, nitrate of silver, salts of mercury, &c. The application of cold by pumping is often highly serviceable. These or any other measures will be known to do good if they make the part feel stronger and more comfortable, although their first application may have been painful; but if they render it hotter and more vascular it is a sign that they stimulate too highly, and may thus endanger the production of acute inflammation.

*Counter-irritants* are more useful in chronic inflammation than in the acute, especially those which establish a permanent suppurative discharge.

# CHAPTER IV.

## OF EFFUSION OF SERUM.

GENERAL DESCRIPTION.—Effusion of serum, as a local disease, is generally produced either by obstruction to the return of venous blood, or by inflammation. It is the earliest and most constant effect of inflammation occurring equally into the interstitial cellular tissue,—into the parenchyma of organs,—from mucous and serous surfaces, and from the skin. If it is followed by any of the other effects of inflammation, it is always more widely extended than them all. But it may be the chief or only effect of inflammation, as in acute dropsy, which, whether it affect the cellular tissue or serous cavities, is an example of an inflammatory state rapidly producing serous effusion. The serum in these cases is always of greater specific gravity, and contains more albumen, than in dropsy from debility. In patients of a lax, flabby habit of body, and in parts of loose cellular structure, inflammation always produces more of this effect than in those of a firmer texture.

ŒDEMATOUS INFLAMMATION.—Under this term Hunter describes a peculiar form of inflammation terminating rapidly in serous effusion, which occurs in those who are affected with dropsy, or disposed to it. It mostly attacks the lower extremities; the swelling is bright red, much diffused, very sore, but not throbbing. It is very apt to terminate in sloughing or suppuration, but not adhesion, and is the frequent cause of large ulcers on the legs of the dropsical. *Treatment.*—The bowels must be well cleared; but other constitutional measures (whether antiphlogistic or tonic) must depend on the state of the system. The best local application is a tepid spirituous lotion (F. 13;) leeches should be avoided, as they may cause ulceration and sloughing.

After inflammation in any part, some degree of œdema is apt to remain in consequence of the distention and weakened tone of the capillaries; and if the habit be weak, great œdema may arise from a very slight cause, as a blister. It must be treated by flannel or other bandages, gentle friction, cold affusion, and attention to the general health.

When any parts, especially the legs, are very much distended with serum, it may be necessary to evacuate some of it, in order to prevent the sloughing of large patches of skin. But instead of making scarfications, as was formerly recommended (which are almost certain to degenerate into ulcers) numerous punctures should be made with a grooved, or acupuncture needle; and they should always be made as near the heart as possible.*

---

# CHAPTER V..

## OF ADHESION, OR THE PRODUCTION OF NEW TISSUES.

DEFINITION.—Adhesion may be defined to be the effusion and organization of the fibrine of coagulable lymph of the blood,—a process which occurs under an infinity of circumstances, healthy and morbid, restorative and destructive.

Two FORMS.—This effusion may occur under either of the two following forms: (1) the fibrine may be poured out by itself, as in iritis; or (2) it may be effused together with serum, as they naturally co-exist in the *liquor sanguinis;* and in this case the fibrine soon coagulates,—either forming a layer on the inflamed surface, or diffused in shreds and flakes through the serum.

THREE STAGES.—In the process of adhesion three stages are observable; in the *first*, the lymph or fibrine is recently effused, and as yet unorganized; in the *second*, it becomes vascular and organized; in the *third*, it assumes the nature of the definite textures of the body.

*First Stage.*—In the first stage, the fibrine, if examined, appears a soft and gelatinous mass. Originally diffluent, like thin mucus or cream, it gradually increases in consistence, and becomes a reticular or cellular substance, containing serum in its meshes; and if that fluid be squeezed out, it seems like a mass of cobwebs moistened with water.† Its colour is yellowish white,—or pinkish if blood have been effused with it.

*Second Stage.*—In this stage the fibrine becomes permeated with blood-vessels, which are often numerous enough to make it intensely red.

* Mayo, H., Outlines of Pathology, p. 428; Copland, Dict. of Pract. Med. *Art.* Dropsy; Andral, Anatomie Pathologique, vol. i. p. 320; Hunter on the Blood, Palmer's Ed. vol. iii. pp. 314, 331.

† Carswell, op. cit.

Respecting the mode in which this process is accomplished, two opinions are entertained. Some suppose that the vessels are prolonged into the fibrine from the inflamed and softened surface to which it is attached;—or, to speak more correctly, that blood-globules shoot into it in a continuous stream, and that the vessels are formed by a solidification of the fibrine around their track. Others conceive that the fibrine, like the vitellary membrane of the egg, has the power of forming blood within its substance; and that the blood so formed is endowed with a spontaneous motion, and forms channels through the plastic mass; which extend themselves and join the general circulation. But this latter opinion is not at present held by the best pathologists.* The *time* within which recently effused fibrine may acquire vascularity, varies according to the vigour of the constitution; it has been completed in man within twenty-nine hours;† but in feeble habits it may require some days. It scarcely needs to be added, that lymph causes the adhesion of two serous surfaces, by its blood-vessels communicating with both. It is not necessary for the union of two serous surfaces, that both should be originally inflamed; for the contact of one inflamed surface will produce enough of inflammation in adjacent sound one to make it participate in the effusion and organization of lymph.

During this second stage, the fibrine may be the seat of various phenomena;—it may be pushed off and broken up by fresh effusions;— or it may secrete blood, or pus, or tubercle.

*Third Stage.*— In the third stage, the fibrine becomes completely organized, and assumes the character of some of the standard tissues of the body. And it is capable of being converted into almost any of them; the conversion in any particular case being determined by the surface from which the fibrine was effused, or by the function which it is made to perform. Thus, if a bone be broken or inflamed, the effused fibrine will be converted into bone. If a bone die, or is abstracted, still the lymph effused from the surrounding parts—from bone, muscle, fascia, cellular tissue, indiscriminately will become bone. If (as in the case of unreduced dislocation) the lymph is subject to frequent motion, part of it will be converted into bone, part into cartilage, part into ligament, so as to form a new joint. But there are some tissues which cannot be replaced; and

* Some interesting observations on this subject were published by Sir A. Carlisle, in the *Guy's Hosp. Rep.* May 1840. He shows that when blood, or any fluid holding an essential oil in suspension, are dropped on the buffy coat of a coagulum, or on any similar soft substance—chalk made into a paste with water, for instance; they have a power of dispersing themselves through the soft mass, in channels which have an arborescent shape precisely like newly-formed blood-vessels.

† Sir E. Home. Practical Observations on the Treatment of Ulcers. London,. 1801, and Phil. Trans. 1818.

then the lymph which they secrete is transformed into some other tissue, which occupies a similar place in other animals. Thus, muscle cannot be formed anew ; but if divided, the uniting lymph will become ligament, or dense fascia-like cellular tissue, which occupy the place of many mus-cles in animals of inferior development.

It appears that almost all the simple *tissues* are capable, if divided, of being thus united by a tissue similar to themselves, and of being to a certain extent restored, if partially abstracted. But complex *organs*, such as muscle or gland, do not enjoy this faculty.

All newly-formed tissues possess certain common properties. They are less vascular, and less endowed with vitality than the original ;—they are more prone to run into disease during states of constitutional cachexy ;[*] and they are liable (especially new cellular tissue) to shrink and become atrophied, or even (as in the case of pleuritic and peritonæal adhesions) to disappear altogether.[†]

The *parts most disposed* to the adhesive inflammation are the serous membranes, and shut cavities generally—those least disposed to it are the mucous membranes. In the latter, suppuration is the result of a less degree of inflammation than adhesion ; in the former, the reverse. But although the layers of lymph formed on mucous surfaces, when violently inflamed, (as in croup,) never become organized, but are detached by subsequent secretions of mucus or pus, still if two abraded or inflamed mucous surfaces are placed in opposition and left undisturbed, they may adhere ;—as sometimes happens in the vaginæ of female children ;—in the os uteri and Fallopian tubes of prostitutes, and in the ureters and biliary ducts when abraded by the passage of calculi.

The *uses* of adhesion are infinite. It unites wounds ;— it circum-scribes inflammation in serous cavities, and in the cellular tissue, by prevent-ing the diffusion of irritant fluids, whether the products of inflammation, (as pus,) or introduced by accident or injury ;—thus it forms cysts for ab-scesses, and for foreign bodies ;—and the readiness with which it occurs, is an excellent measure of the integrity of the constitution.

*Is adhesion inflammatory?*—Adhesion, when it occurs favourably after injuries, is produced by a very low degree of inflammation ; in fact, if there be more than a certain degree of inflammatory action, the lymph effused will be broken up by fresh exudations, pus will be formed, and

---

[*] Thus in the scurvy, old cicatrices have been known to break out afresh into ulcers, and old fractures to become disunited.

[†] In examining the body of a madman who had stabbed himself in the abdomen fifteen different times during his life, the parts near the *most recent* wounds were found united by considerable false membranes :—at the situation of some that were older, there were only a few thin cellular adhesions ; whilst, at the oldest, there was no trace of adhesion or false membrane whatever. Andral, Anat, Path., vol. i. 486.

the process of reparation must be commenced anew by means of granulations, as will be described hereafter.*

*Is blood organizable?*—It has been a matter of dispute, whether coagulated blood, like pure fibrine, is capable of becoming organized. Hunter believed that it was capable of being so, and in his work on Inflammation he adduced two cases in which he thought to afford examples of it. The first is the coagulum in an artery that had been tied, in which he had been able to inject what he thought was an incipient vascular formation ;— the second is a piece of coagulum adhering to a testicle, which he had certainly injected. Some succeeding pathologists, however, have denied that coagulated blood can ever become organized ; and affirm, that whenever it is effused into the substance of a part, it is either absorbed or removed by suppuration as an extraneous body. They allege in support of their objections, that in the above-mentioned injection of the coagulum in the artery, the coloured material was merely mechanically forced into its substance, and not distributed through any blood-vessels ;—and that the supposed coagulum on the testis was merely effused fibrine. And they farther allege, that well-authenticated instances of organized coagula are extremely rare, or rather altogether wanting ; whereas they ought to be common enough, because coagula are frequently placed under circumstances favourable for their organization, if they were capable of it :—as for instance in the sacs of aneurisms ; in sanguineous apoplexy, and in ecchymoses generally.

A reference, however, to facts can scarcely fail to show that Hunter's opinion was correct. For not only have coagula been distinctly injected by Home and Macartney, but it may be seen that coagulated blood, whether contained in a tied artery, or in a serous cavity, or in an apoplectic cyst, first loses its colour,—then assumes a fibrous or laminated structure—adheres to the surrounding parts—is converted gradually into a cellular or cellulo-fibrous texture—and is in most cases, like lymph, ultimately absorbed. Although, however, it is incontestable that blood is capable of becoming organized, still it must be admitted that effused lymph is much more so;—and that lymph, and not blood, is the material employed by nature in the production of new tissues, and the reparation of injuries.†

* We have not space to enter into a full discussion of this question. The arguments used by Macartney and others against the inflammatory nature of adhesion are, that if a wound presents any sensible degree of inflammation, it will suppurate and not adhere ;—and that the lowest divisions of the animal kingdom have the greatest powers of reparation, although they are least subject to inflammation, even if they are subject to it at all. But after all, the dispute is merely about words ; and any one who attends to the directions under the head of treatment, will practise very safely, let him adopt what theory he may.

† Vide Palmer's Ed. of Hunter, vol. iii. Catalogue of the Huntarian Museum, vol. i., Carswell, op. cit. ; Macartney, op. cit., p. 51, and Home, Phil. Trans., 1818.

TREATMENT.—If it be the object to promote adhesion, the general principles of treatment are, to maintain the most peifect rest and apposition, and to use such local and constitutional measures as will prevent heat, pain, and throbbing; in other words, to prevent the inflammation from proceeding to a grade of greater intensity than the adhesive. In a few cases (as after the operation for harelip, in a languid scrofulous habit) it may be necessary to excite vascular action by wine, to render it sufficient for the production and organization of lymph.

If it be wished to counteiact the adhesive inflammation, then use must be made of the antiphlogistic treatment generally, and of calomel in particular.

If it be wished to remove adhesions, or thickening; the results of previous acute or existing chronic inflammation, the rules must be attended to which were laid down for the treatment of chronic inflammation. Plethora, or debility, or any other existing disorder, must be removed by appropriate remedies. Absorption is to be excited by the administration of mercury, with which it is often necessary to affect the system. Such local means should also be used, if possible, as will make the circulation vigorous and promote absorption; such as friction with the hand, or with the flesh-brush; aided by stimulating liniments, (F. 14,) or by ointments containing iodyne, F. 25, 75; gentle exercise; passive motion, shampooing, pressure, by bandages or otherwise; cold affusion; electricity and galvanism; discutient lotions, especially those of zinc, F. 15, or muriate of ammonia, F. 16; blisters, or other counter-irritants—taking care not to reproduce active inflammation by too violent stimulation.

# CHAPTER VI.

## OF HÆMORRHAGE.

HÆMORRHAGE, like serous effusion, may be a consequence, 1st, of inflammation or excitement; 2ndly, of obstruction to the return of venous blood; and 3dly, of atony of the blood-vessels and thinness of the blood, as in scurvy and putrid fevers. The first form is called *active*, the last two *passive.*

(1) *Active hæmorrhage* consists in the exhalation of arterial blood from the capillaries. In almost every instance of violent inflammation, it is probable that some blood escapes either by rupture of the capillaries, or by exudation through their parietes. It occurs during the formation of abscess in the cellular tissue and in the liver. But the most common

seat of inflammatory hæmorrhage is mucous membrane, especially that of the lungs, and it often appears accidental whether irritation of that membrane shall produce secretion of blood or of mucus. The principal instances of it which fall under the surgeon's care, are epistaxis or hæmorrhage from the nose; hæmorrhois or hæmorrhage from the rectum; hæmorrhage from the urethra during gonorrhœa; and from granulating wounds. It has also been known to occur from the conjunctiva; and more rarely from the pleura, pericardium, and peritonæum.

*Diagnosis.*—Inflammatory or active hæmorrhage is distinguished from that which is the result of congestion or debility, by the presence of local pain, heat, and throbbing, and of a febrile state of the pulse and system generally.

*Treatment.*—This form of hæmorrhage is to be treated by bleeding, if it can be borne; and it may be observed, that it is less debilitating to employ one full venesection, so that the cause may be at once removed, than to let the blood dribble perpetually away from the part in small quantities. Purgatives and sedatives, especially lead, (F. 60, 61,) are also useful. Cold, if it can be applied, perfect rest, and an elevated position, are the local measures.

(2) In *passive hæmorrhage* the blood which escapes is venous. The principal instances of it are hæmorrhage from the nose in old subjects with diseased liver, melæna, or hæmorrhage from the liver, and passive menorrhagia and hæmorrhois. The chief remedies are, dilute sulphuric acid, sulphate of alumina, catechu, and ergot of rye.

---

# CHAPTER VII.

## OF SUPPURATION AND ABSCESS.

### SECT. I.—OF THE THEORY OF SUPPURATION, AND PROPERTIES OF PUS.

PROPERTIES OF HEALTHY PUS.—Pus is a yellowish white, opaque fluid, of the consistence of cream; free from smell, neither acid nor alkaline, said to have a sweetish, mawkish taste, insoluble in water, although freely miscible with it, and very slow to putrefy. Like many other animal fluids, it consists of a thin serum, holding a vast number of solid particles in suspension, from which it derives its colour and opacity.

PUS GLOBULES.—When these solid particles are examined under the microscope, they are found to be opaque spherical globules, somewhat granulated like mulberries. They measure from 1-5000th to 1-2000th

of an inch in diameter; some even are much larger; especially if they proceed from a surface that is actively inflamed.* If mingled with water
they soon appear plumper, more regular in shape, and more transparent;
but after a time become ragged and flabby, as if torn, or partially dissolved. If acetic acid is added, they undergo a still greater change.
They then seem as if composed of two distinct substances,—of an exterior capsule, which the acid acts upon and renders clear and transparent;
and of two or three central opaque granules;† and after a little while the

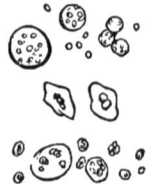

acid completely dissolves the capsule, and sets the granules at liberty.
Besides the globules, other smaller granular bodies are also found in
pus.‡

Many of the properties of pus depend on these globules. Its specific
gravity, for instance, (which varies from 1.021 to 1.040,) and its density,
depend on the number of them. Moreover, pus is coagulated by a strong
solution of hydrochlorate of ammonia. But this coagulation is not produced by the solidification of matters previously fluid, like the coagulation of blood or milk; neither is it caused by the salt merely abstracting
the water of the pus, as Pearson supposed; but it depends on a change in
the globules, which become more transparent, elongated, and adherent.
Freezing also renders pus viscid, and has a similar effect on the globules.
A heat of 165°, however, coagulates it by coagulating the albumen of the
serous portion.

CHEMICAL ANALYSIS.—The most recent analyses, especially those of
Bonnet of Lyons,§ Gueterbock,‖ and Davy, show that pus contains all
the proximate elements of blood, except the colouring matter. Thus it
contains, according to Gueterbock, water, (86.1 per cent.,) fat soluble in
hot alcohol (1.6,) fat and osmazome soluble in cold alcohol, (4.3,) and
albumen and the matter of the globules, soluble neither in hot nor cold
alcohol, (7.4.) The substance of which the globules are composed has

* Mayo, Med. Gaz., Oct. 19th, 1839.

† The uppermost group gives a pretty accurate idea of the appearance of pus
globules, under the microscope. The middle figures represent globules ragged after
maceration in water. The lowest group shows, very imperfectly, the action of
acetic acid.

‡ Vogel, über Eiter und Eiterung, p. 35 ; Davy, op. cit., vol. ii. p. 468.

§ Bonnet, Med. Gaz., vol. xxi.

‖ Gueterbock de Pure et Granulatione, Berol, 1837.

received the name of *pyine;* but it seems to differ very little from fibrine. Pus also contains about 0.8 per cent. of salts; chiefly common salt, and muriate of ammonia.

PRODUCTION OF PUS.—We shall give as brief an outline as possible of the most prevalent opinions and best ascertained facts relating to this most interesting pathological problem.

(1) It was for some time supposed that pus was merely blood modified by stagnation in its vessels, and that the pus globules were blood globules enlarged and decolourized.* But this opinion now seems to be abandoned, because the mamillated pus globules have no sort of resemblance to the smooth cup-like discoid blood globules, and because animals such as the paco, llama, and dromedary, which have elliptical blood globules, have their pus globules round notwithstanding.†

Yet as the blood globules are said by Barry and others to undergo very important changes of form during the process of development and of determination of blood, and even to expand themselves into cells, it seems premature to deny that they may occasionally form pus globules.‡

(2) Another opinion has prevailed, that pus might be formed by a softening down of coagulated blood or fibrine. This was supposed to be proved by the phenomena of phlebitis. For when a vein is highly inflamed, the blood in it coagulates and softens down into a whitish fluid which resembles pus;§ and Gendrin found that the same change might be effected by confining blood in an artery or vein, or in the cellular tissue, if previously inflamed by irritating injections.

Mr. Gulliver, however, has proved that the fluid produced in these cases, as well as the pus-like matter occasionally found in the centre of clots and fibrinous concretions in the heart, is not real pus, although it may resemble it in some of its external qualities. For it contains very many irregular particles, but no real pus globules; and its particles are all easily dissolved by the acetic and other acids, while real pus globules are not. Dr. Davy, moreover, has shown that the softened lymph of pneumonia is equally different from real pus; and Mr. Gulliver‖ has produced a similar fluid by subjecting fibrine mingled with water to a heat of 96—104° for about three days.

(3) A third opinion is, that pus globules are produced by a peculiar concretion of particles of fibrine. The facts which bear upon this view of the question are as follows:—

---

* Gendrin, (Hist. Anat. des Inflam.) describes this process as he saw it in frogs; but all recent writers say it is impossible to excite inflammation in cold-blooded animals.

† Gulliver, Med. Gaz., 1839, p. 415.

‡ Barry Martin, Phil. Mag., Oct. 1840.     § Carswell, op. cit.

‖ Med. Chir. Trans., vol. xxii., and Phil. Mag., Sept. 1838.

Sir E. Home having wiped a healthy ulcer quite dry, collected the colourless fluid, that soon afterwards exuded, upon a piece of talc. This he examined, and found that it contained no globules. He next covered it with another piece of talc, and placed it upon the ulcer again, that it might be under natural conditions of temperature, and then he found that after ten minutes pus globules had formed in it. This experiment has often been repeated with similar results.*

Again, it is well known that globules which cannot be distinguished from pus globules are formed in the blood of all animals when it has ceased to circulate: they are also to be found in almost every tissue of the body. The same globules are also found in the fibrinous concretion that exudes on vesicated skin; and according to Mandl,† they may be seen to form in the serum of frogs' blood, when its red particles have been separated by filtration.

Hence it has been concluded that pus globules are not elaborated by a peculiar secretion, but merely formed by the concretion of fibrine. But this explanation is too easy and mechanical.‡

(4) A fourth series of observations is highly interesting as explaining the relation of pus to mucus. It appears from the investigation of Henlé§ and others, that the cutis vera and mucous membranes are covered with regular layers of flattened cells, with central nuclei, which constitute the cuticle of the former, and the epithelium of the latter. Now healthy mucus is composed almost entirely of abraded epithelium, swollen with water, and mingled with very many granular globules, and a few bodies like pus globules. But during inflammation the secretion is altered; and the adjoining diagram after Vogel shows more clearly than

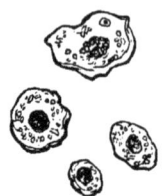

any words the transition of the flattened epithelium cells with their central granules, into the spherical pus globule.‖ From this it will] be evident, that although healthy mucus may be easily distinguished from pure

---

* Home on Ulcers, Lond. 1801, p. 35.

† Mandl, Louis, l'Experience, Aout 15, 1838, and Jan. 1839.

‡ Vide Babington, Med. Chir. Trans., vol. xiv. ; Raspail, Organic Chemistry.

§ Henlé, Lancet, May 18, 1839; also Symonds, in Provincial Med. Trans. for 1840.

‖ The uppermost figure is an epithelium cell—flat, irregularly five-sided, with a central nucleus. The others show the transition into pus globules by a diminution of the flat transparent portion.

pus, the former having many epithelium flakes and few globules,—the latter being crowded with globules, and having little, if any, epithelium,—still that the two fluids pass into each other by intermediate stages, in which distinction is impossible. Any chemical test is of course out of the question, although the older authors abound in them.

(5) There is lastly, another idea closely connected with the theory of the conversion of epithelium cells into pus. It is, that pus globules are *organic cells*, and that they are developed from nuclei in the same manner that those cells are in the embryo, from which the various tissues are formed. But it will be more convenient to explain this in the introductory section to the chapter on malignant disease.

Such are the chief facts known and opinions entertained respecting *pyogenesis*. To adopt any exclusive theory, and draw definite conclusions from them, would in the present state of our knowledge be presumptuous.

*Suppuration in the Cellular Tissue.*—The successive steps in the formation of pus in this tissue are as follows. First, there is a general softeuing and effusion of serum;—next an effusion of fibrine, known by its faculty of coagulating spontaneously; and this fibrine may be combined with more or less blood;—or pure blood may even be effused with it at the spots where the inflammation is most intense. These effusions increase; the tissues become distended and broken down, and at last pus appears in the thin reddish mixture of serum and lymph with which they were infiltrated. It is at first dispersed in minute collections; but these soon communicate by the solution of the intervening parts, and form a cavity termed an *abscess*. Meanwhile (in healthy inflammation) the lymph which is effused into the parts around the pus, becomes organized and converted into a *cyst* or *sac;*—which circumscribes the pus already formed, and may secrete fresh quantities of it, or absorb some of it, according to circumstances.

*Mucous Membrane and Skin.*—The mucous membranes, and the cutis deprived of its cuticle, readily produce pus by a process of secretion. They at first exude a thin serous fluid, which gradually becomes thick and opaque, and perfectly purulent.

*Serous Membranes.*—The suppuration of serous membranes is preceded by an effusion of serum and lymph; and the pus may be secreted, —either from the surface of lymph which has become vascular and organized;—or from the surface of the serous membrane itself;—the layer of lymph having been disintegrated and detached.

VARIETIES OF PUS.—1. *Healthy Pus* (called also *creamy* or *laudable*) is that which has already been described, and is the product of healthy inflammation in healthy parts. It is album, læve, liquidum, et laudabile.

2. *Serous Pus* is thin, almost transparent, and yellowish or reddish. It differs from the last in containing very little fatty matter or fibrine,

and in being the product of a low degree of inflammation in weak consti‑
tutions.

3. *Clotty or Curdy Pus* resembles the serous, but has numerous
white clots and flocculi of coagulated fibrine floating in it. Under the
microscope it displays the globules of healthy pus, and numerous other
particles of irregular shape. It contains very little fatty matter, and is
commonly found in scrofulous abscesses.

4. *Mucous Pus.*—When a mucous membrane is inflamed, the thin
serous fluid;—the ropy, viscid mucus,—and the muco-purulent matter
that are successively secreted, are, as has been shown, various transition-
steps between mucus and pus. Muco-purulent matter, when examined
under the miscroscope, displays both globular particles, leafy masses, and
numerous particles of irregular form. It is occasionally found in chronic
abscesses. It contains a large quantity of hydrochlorate of ammonia,—
a salt which abounds in unhealthy pus.*

5. *Concrete or Lardaceous Pus* may either consist of common pus,
thickened by the absorption if its watery parts, in consequence of having
remained for a long time in a chronic abscess, or bony cavity†—as the
antrum and nasal sinuses:—or it may originally be secreted in a thick
condition; and in this latter case differs little or nothing from the meli-
cerous or ætheromatous matter found in wens or other encysted tumours.

6. *Putrid Pus* has a fœtid smell, and alkaline reaction, in consequence
of the presence of hydrosulphate of ammonia;‡ which is formed by the
decomposition of albumen, when pus is exposed long enough to air and
heat.

7. *Specific Pus,* capable of producing the venereal disease or the small-
pox, may not differ in its sensible qualities from the healthiest.

8. The pus from spreading ulcers and cancers almost always contains
some debris of the ulcerating tissue. It is said to be *ichorous* when thin
and acrid; *sanious* when thin and bloody; and *grumous* when mingled
with dark half-curdled blood.

PUS IN THE BLOOD.—The effects of pus in the blood demand a few
observations, on account of the doctrines which have been promulgated
on the subject by some modern pathologists.

Mr. Gulliver, for instance, having found in the blood of persons who
had died of small-pox or fever, those white pus-like globules which other
investigators have shown to be present in all dead blood, was led some.
what prematurely to announce the existence or formation of pus in the
blood, as the proximate cause of most fevers.

* Pearson, Phil. Trans. 1810. Mucus gives out more ammonia, when treated by
lime or potass, than pus does.

† Mayo, Pathology, p. 159.

‡ A compound of sulphuretted hydrogen and ammonia. Albumen contains sulphur, hydrogen and nitrogen;—all the elements of this salt.

Other pathologists, moreover, have conceived, that in phlebitis, glanders, puerperal fever, and other cases in which there is great suppuration, and great vitiation of the blood, pus is absorbed from the seat of disease, and is deposited in the liver, lungs, joints, or other parts, and is the cause of the abscesses which so frequently form there, and which have been called *consecutive abscesses.*

Now, although it is probable that pus may be formed in the blood, and although it is certain that it may be absorbed into it, still these premises do not warrant all the conclusions that have been drawn from them.

For, in the first place, pus often finds its way into the blood in vast quantities after abscess of the liver, and is copiously excreted by stool, urine, and vomit. But no consecutive abscesses occur. So that, at all events, healthy pus may pass through the blood without occasioning any severe derangement.* But yet if pus be vitiated or putrid, it is very certain that its absorption will cause fever and diarrhœa—as will be shown in the Section on Chronic Abscess.

Again, although it is very possible that pus, if present in the blood, might be deposited in the lungs or liver, (because we know that quicksilver, when injected into the blood, is quickly found in those parts,) still it is very certain that consecutive abscesses are not universally caused by a deposite of pus into an uninflamed part. For abscesses in the liver often follow injuries of the head; and other consecutive abscesses sometimes follow other injuries, which have not given rise to any suppuration, and from which consequently there was no pus to be absorbed.†

SECTION II.—OF ACUTE ABSCESS.

DEFINITION.—An *abscess* may be defined to be a collection of pus in the substance of any part, or in any cavity. There are three kinds; 1. The *acute or phlegmonous;* 2. The *chronic* or *cold;* 3. The *diffused.*

SYMPTOMS.—Acute abscess (which, when occurring in the subcutaneous cellular tissue, is called *phlegmon*) commences with all the ordinary signs of acute inflammation, namely, inflammatory fever; severe throbbing pain; bright redness; and much swelling;—firm in the centre, and œdematous around. The occurrence of suppuration is indicated by severe rigors, by an abatement of the fever, and a change in the pain,—which is converted into a sense of weight and tension, with a pulsatory feel at each beat of the arteries. Then the tumour becomes softer, and

* Malcolmson on Abscess of the Liver, Med. Chir. Trans. vol. xxi.

† Vide Copland, Dict. Pract. Med., *Art.* Abscess; Carswell, op. cit.; Ferguson on Puerperal Fever, Lond. 1839; Ancell, case of purulent deposite into all the joints after small-pox; Med. Chir. Trans. vol. xxi. The author has also borrowed from a lecture on Phlebitis delivered by Sir B. C. Brodie at St. George's Hospital, in Nov. 1839.

loses its bright arterial colour; and as the quantity of matter increases, its centre begins to *point*, that is, to project in a pyramidal form, and *fluctuation* can be felt by alternate pressure with the fingers.

PATHOLOGY.—The successive steps in the formation of an abscess in the cellular tissue have already been described.

PROGRESS.—The pus having been formed, the next step is its evacuation, which is effected either by what Hunter called *progressive absorption;* that is, the successive absorption of all the parts intervening between the abscess and the surface;—or just as probably by their successive softening and disintegration.   Be this however as it may, the tumour becomes more and more prominent and soft; the surrounding inflammation and tumefaction subside; the centre becomes of a dusky red or bluish tint, the cutis is removed, the cuticle bursts, and the pus escapes.

Although abscesses may burst into serous cavities, or mucous canals if they happen to be near, still their general course is that which is least prejudicial;—namely, towards the skin.   The cause of this happy provision has much engaged the attention of pathologists.   It has been partially explained by supposing that in proportion as the quantity of pus increases, it advances towards the skin, because in that direction it is opposed by the least pressure.   But in many instances where the pressure on both sides is equal, as in abscesses of the alveoli of the teeth, and fistula lachrymalis, the matter tends to the outer side notwithstanding.   Hunter said that inflammation is always more violent on the side nearest the skin;—and that superficial parts are more disposed to suppuration than the deep-seated.   But these are mere enunciations of a fact, of which, as of the upward growth of a plant, we can appreciate the advantage better than we can assign the cause.

GRANULATION.—The matter having been discharged, the cavity of the. abscess contracts, the pellicle of lymph which lines it is cast off, and its surface becomes covered with numerous, small, red, vascular eminences called *granulations*.   These are formed by the effusion of lymph in successive layers;—each of which soon becomes vascular and organized, and secretes pus.   The reason why the lymph is effused in the form of these little eminences is supposed to be, that each of them is formed by one minute artery, which runs through its centre, and then divides into numberless ramifications on its surface.   So that if the restorative actions are vigorous, and the blood-vessels numerous, the granulations will also be numerous, but small and florid;—whilst in the opposite state they will be large, pale, an flabby.   And the pus from healthy granulations will be laudable and creamy,—from the other, thin and flaky.*

CICATRIZATION.—When the cavity has become filled up by the growth

---

* Granulations are often extremely sensible, and of course supplied with nerves; perhaps also with absorbents.

and union of granulations, the red inflamed skin around its orifice is
removed by ulceration, so that the margin of the sore becomes adherent
and fixed;—and then *cicatrization* begins. A white pellicle extends
from the circumference, gradually covers the whole surface, and becomes
organized into a new cutis and cuticle, called a *cicatrix*. The cicatrix
is at first thin and red, but soon becomes denser and paler than the original skin, and, like all new textures, is less vascular and less vital. The
colouring matter between the cutis and cuticle is later in appearing. But
this process is accompanied by two others, namely, the contraction of
the surrounding skin, so that the surface to be healed is very much diminished before cicatrization commences, and the contraction of the cicatrix
subsequently. The preliminary contraction of the skin appears intended
to diminish the labour of an extensive reparation;—the subsequent contraction of the cicatrix is in conformity with a law mentioned in the
Chapter on Adhesion, and depends on the absorption of the newly-formed
subcutaneous cellular tissue. It is always greatest where the preceding
granulations have been pale, flabby, and exuberant, as in burns.

But it is to be remarked, that the filling up of a vacancy in the tissues,
whether in consequence of accident, abscess, or ulceration, need not necessarily be attended with suppuration, nor with the peculiar appearance
of granulations. On the contrary, if all inflammation be subdued, and
all irritation excluded, the chasm may fill up with red lymph, which
speedily cicatrizes. This is constantly observed after trifling injuries;
they speedily become covered with a *scab* formed of dried blood, or
lymph, under the protection of which they soon cicatrize; and when it
can be effected, larger wounds should be made to heal in the same way.

CAUSES. Acute abscess is mostly *idiopathic,* that is, depends on constitutional causes, and is a frequent sequel of fevers;—it may, however,
be caused by blows, ecchymoses, or by foreign bodies introduced into
the skin or flesh.

TREATMENT.—The *indications,* in the first stage, are, to procure
resolution of the inflammation, and prevent the formation of matter.
After it has formed the indications are, to cause its evacuation and induce granulation and cicatrization.

In the *first stage,* therefore, the patient should be purged, or perhaps
bled; his diet should be low, and leeches should be applied to the part.
But when the cold applications feel chilly and uncomfortable, (as they
will when suppuration begins,) they should be exchanged for warm
poultices;—and when fever abates, the diet should be increased.

*Poultices* are admirable remedies;—they relax the skin, promote perspiration, soothe pain, encourage the formation of pus, and expedite its
progress to the surface. They should be large,—so as not soon to become cold or dry; they should be soft, that they may not irritate,—light,
that they may not fatigue, and they should be renewed frequently,

They may be made of bread and water, or of oatmeal boiled till it is soft, or of linseed meal, F. 45, 47. Some modern surgeons, who affect to despise poultices, (probably because they have only seen them in hospitals where they are seldom well made, and are often suffered to remain till they become sour and stinking,) recommend the *water dressing* instead,—that is, a piece of soft lint or folded linen dipped in warm water, and covered with oil silk to prevent evaporation; but this is a very inadequate substitute for the luxurious softness of a well-made poultice.

If, after the formation of matter, the inflammation does not subside, but swelling, hardness, and pain remain, then the application of leeches may be repeated; but in other cases the continuance of depleting measures after matter has formed, or when its formation is inevitable, will only weaken the patient, and delay the cure.

Respecting the *opening of abscesses*, it may be laid down as a general rule, that if they point and become pyramidal, without enlarging in circumference, they may be left to burst of themselves; but that if they enlarge in breadth and circumference, without tending to the surface, they should be opened. In the following eight cases, however, the surgeon's aid is imperatively demanded.

1. When matter forms beneath fasciæ and other dense ligamentous textures, such as the sheaths of tendons, or under the thick cuticle of the fingers. Because, as these are absorbed or softened with the utmost difficulty, the pus, instead of coming to the surface, will burrow amongst muscles and tendons, extending the abscess to great distance;—producing extreme pain and constitutional disturbance, by its tension of the fasciæ which cover it, and pressure on the parts beneath,—endangering extensive sloughing, and impairing the future motions of the part. Hence, as a general rule, all abscesses beneath fasciæ, or among tendons, or under the thick cuticle of the fingers, should be freely opened, as soon as the existence of matter is suspected.

2. When the abscess is covered by a thick layer of fat; this tissue being indolent, and not readily absorbed.

3. When matter forms near a bone, whether under or over the periosteum, lest exfoliation or necrosis ensue from the contiguous irritation.

4. When an abscess is formed in loose cellular tissue, (as around the anus,) which would readily admit of great distention and enlargement of the sac, and more especially if the cellular tissue is partially covered with muscles, (as in the axilla,) under which the matter might burrow.

5. When abscess is caused by the extravasation of urine, or other irritant fluids.

6. In suppuration of very sensitive organs, as the eye or testis.

7. In suppuration near a joint or great serous cavity, or the trachea, lest the abscess burst into them, which might be fatal.

8. When it is desirable to avoid the scar which always will ensue when an abscess ulcerates spontaneously.

And in the first five of these cases it is much better to make an opening before matter has formed, than to delay it for one moment afterwards.

The best *instrument for puncturing abscesses* is a straight-pointed, double-edged bistoüry. It should be plunged in at right angles to the surface, till it has entered the cavity, which may be known by a diminution of the feeling of resistance, or by slightly withdrawing the instrument, so that a drop of pus may exude by its side. Then the aperture may be enlarged sufficiently as the instrument is being withdrawn. A trocar may be used if the pus is covered by several loose unconnected layers of fasciæ. The puncture should be made at the most depending part of the abscess; and if it seems likely to close, its edges may be separated for the first forty-eight hours by a piece of oiled lint, formerly called a *tent.* After the opening, no rude attempts should be made to squeeze out the matter, as they might induce inflammation; but it should be allowed gradually to exude into a poultice or fomentation, which may be changed as often as necessary.

The poultices may be continued till all pain has subsided, and the cavity has begun to granulate;—but not too long, lest the granulations become weak and flabby. And then the best plan is to apply a compress of linen, and a bandage. If the cavity does not contract speedily, it must be treated as a *weak ulcer* or *fistula.* If the suppuration continues profuse, tonics, change of air, and a good diet, are advisible, in order to prevent hectic, and enable the constitution to repair the local mischief.

It occasionally happens that acute abscesses (especially those occurring in glandular textures and venereal cases) are cured by the absorption of their pus. This is likely to happen when, after acute inflammation, the matter remains without tending to come to the surface, and without pain.

The means best adapted to promote it are leeches and cold mercurial ointment worn as a plaster,—purgatives and remedies adapted to increase the secretions generally,—and above all things a sea voyage, so as to cause considerable sickness.

### SECTION III.—CHRONIC ABSCESS.

GENERAL DESCRIPTION.—Chronic abscesses are the result of a low degree of inflammation ; so slight indeed, that their existence is often unsuspected for a long time. They are mostly lined with a thin, reddish-gray, distinctly-organized cyst;—there is little or no vascularity in the parts adjoining ;—and the pus usually is *serous* or *curdy.* But sometimes the cyst is thick and cellulo-fibrous, and the matter *concrete*, so as hardly to differ from an encysted tumour. Chronic abscesses are often deep-seated, whilst the acute are mostly superficial.

CAUSES.—The causes are a weakened and scrofulous habit, chronic disease of bone, or other source of slow irritation.

SYMPTOMS.—When first detected, a chronic abscess appears as an obscure tumour, with a fluctuation more or less distinct according to its distance from the surface; it is free from pain, tenderness, swelling, or redness, unless far advanced or accidentally inflamed.

PROGRESS.—These abscesses may attain an enormous magnitude, partly because the sac being thin is readily extensible, and partly because of the atonic and indolent grade of the inflammation, which is insufficient to implicate the adjoining textures, and make the coverings ulcerate. When, however, from the increasing distention, or from some accidental irritation, this does happen, the skin reddens, inflames, and ulcerates, and so the matter is discharged.

TERMINATIONS.—(1.) In slight cases the stimulus of the air causes the interior of the sac to pour out granulations;—the reddened skin around the orifice ulcerates;—and the sore so formed may heal. (2.) If the restorative powers are weak, and the parietes of the sac have been unequally pressed together, one or more *sinuses* may remain. (3.) If, on the other hand, the abscess is very large, or if it is connected with a permanent cause of irritation, (as diseased vertebræ,) or if, after the admission of air, the pus have not a free exit, a most serious train of consequences will ensue. The pus, exposed to the atmosphere, putrefies;—the hydrosulphate of ammonia (the product of putrefaction) is absorbed into the blood;*—the interior of the sac inflames, partly from the irritation of the air, but chiefly from that of the putrid pus;—and then the grave and irreparable local disease, together with the contamination of the blood induces typhoid fever, under which the patient sinks.

PROGNOSIS.—Hence the danger of these abscesses will be great; (1.) If they are connected with a source of permanent irritation, which, by continuing the production of matter, prevents the sac from closing. (2.) If the sac has attained a large size;—and (3.) If under these circumstances it has advanced so far towards ulceration, that a spontaneous and permanent aperture is inevitable.

TREATMENT.—There are three *indications*; (1.) To amend the general health and remove all causes; (2.) To procure absorption of the matter; (3.) If that be impracticable, to open the abscess with such precautions as may induce a speedy contraction and obliteration of the sac.

(1.) In order to fulfil the first indication, the necessity of wholesome and sufficient food, pure air, warm clothing, and freedom from avocations that fatigue the body or harass the mind, need scarcely be adverted to;

---

* It may be detected in the blood and urine. The blood in these cases is black, and refuses to coagulate;—which is precisely the effect produced by adding the hydrosulphate of ammonia to healthy blood. Vide M. Bonnet's Papers in the Med. Gaz. vol. xxi.

whilst the appetite, digestion, strength, and secretions of the skin, liver, and bowels, must be improved after the manner detailed in the Chapter on Chronic Inflammation. If (as in the case of psoas and lumbar abscess) the abscess has been caused by some local disease, the latter must if pos. sible be ascertained, and removed by proper measures.

(2.) The best local means for causing absorption of the matter are stimulants and counter-irritants applied to the tumour or its vicinity. Plasters of Empl. Galbani c., or Emp. Thuris c., or Emp. Hydrargyri, or Emp. Ammoniaci cum Hydrarg.; or of F. 25; or an issue, or blister kept open in the vicinity; or a succession of blisters, when one is nearly healed, another being placed beside it; or friction with Ung. Iodin.; electric sparks; and cold affusion, are the most useful remedies; but they do harm if they cause heat or pain. Leeches, cold lotions, and purgatives must be employed if the tumour should inflame from any constitutional or local cause of irritation.

(3.) But if notwithstanding these efforts, the tumour continues to en-large, it cannot be opened too soon;—especially if there is any incipient redness of the skin. And a different proceeding is requisite in different cases.

*If the abscess is superficial and small,* without a hardened base, and freely fluctuating, a grooved needle may be passed into it, twice or three times a week, so as to cause a little matter to exude ;—moderate pressure being used in the intervals by means of a compress and bandage wetted with cold lotion. If this does not shortly succeed, and the abscess is small, a pretty free aperture may be made into its most depending part, so as to empty it completely. It is a great object to evacuate all flakes of unhealthy lymph, which if retained would be sure to prevent adhesion, and cause an open sore to be formed; but no violent pressure or squeez-ing must be employed. After the opening the patient should observe quietude, and a bandage, or adhesive plaster and compresses, should be passed round the part, so as to keep the sides of the sac in apposition with a moderate degree of pressure; and thus a free exit being provided for the pus, the opposing surfaces will often granulate and adhere;—then the external aperture heals, and the case is cured. If from deficiency of action this adhesion will not take place, weak stimulating injections may be used (such as Zinc. Sulph. gr. j, ad Aquæ ʒi.) Or another aperture may be made, and a seton be passed through the sac;—or if it be long and fistulous, it may be slit up, and made to heal from the bottom.

If the abscess is seated in the neck or other exposed part of a female, it is of the greatest consequence to make an early opening, so that all scars and deformities may be avoided. The instrument recommended by Sir A. Cooper for this purpose is a very fine lancet, only one-eighth of an inch broad. The puncture should be large enough to extract all flakes, but no larger; and it should be made transversely, so that its minute cicatrix may be hidden by the folds of the neck. Adhesive plaster should then be applied with moderate pressure;—and weak injections, especially F. 76, may be used, if the sac does not become obliterated in the course of a few days.

In some cases, when a considerable portion of skin has become thin and red—evincing that it will certainly ulcerate and form a large aperture, it will be advisable to apply the caustic potass, so as to destroy it, and avoid the more painful and tedious process of ulceration.

*Large Chronic Abscesses.*—If the abscess is so large that the exposure of its cavity would lead to the evil consequences that have been enumerated;—or if it is connected with disease of the spine, or other bone, (as in the case of psoas abscess,) the following plan should be resorted to, with a view of inducing a contraction of the sac, and of diminishing the danger from a permanent opening, should one be established subsequently. A *small puncture* should be made with a lancet at the most depending part of the tumour. It may be made *valvular*, by drawing the skin a little to one side before introducing the instrument, but this is not of much consequence. As much matter as flows spontaneously should be permitted to escape, and then the puncture should be carefully closed by lint and plaster, and the patient be kept at rest till it is healed. During the flow of the matter, the greatest care ought to be taken to prevent the admission of air into the sac. At the expiration of ten days or a fortnight, when it is nearly refilled a second puncture should be made (but not too near to the former) and should be healed again in like manner. This operation should be repeated at proper intervals, taking care never to let the abscess become so distended as it was before the previous puncture,— and using *moderate* support by bandages in the intervals. Thus, in fortunate cases, these repeated partial evacuations, combined with proper constitutional measures, will cause the abscess gradually to contract;—so that it either becomes completely obliterated or degenerates into an insignificant fistula.

The credit of discovering this method of treatment is due to the late Mr. Abernethy. He, however, recommended as *much as possible* of the matter to be evacuated at each operation, instead of allowing it to run spontaneously;—which latter method is much better calculated to preclude the admission of air, and avoids all irritation of the cyst by rough handling or squeezing.

But if air have gained admission into the cavity of the abscess, and the pus has become putrid, and prostration of strength and dry brown tongue show its influence on the system, then the indications plainly are, to make free openings and counter openings, so as to prevent all lodgment of the putrid pus;—and to wash out the sac occasionally with injections of warm water, containing a very little of the solution of chloride of soda. At the same time the general treatment of typhoid fever must be adopted, and the strength supported, in order that the absorption of noxious matter may be prevented, and its elimination be facilitated. The sedulous administration of wine, nourishment, opium, quinine, camphor, &c. as in Formulæ 1, 2, 3, may in fortunate cases enable the patient to recover, and at all events will retard his passage to the tomb.

M. Bonnet has suggested an expedient in these cases, that might often be worth the trouble of adopting. He proposes to immerse under water the part in which the abscess is situated, at the time it is punctured. This would, of course, render the ingress of air impossible;—an occurrence which, in the ordinary way of operating, will often happen in spite of every precaution.

SECTION IV.—DIFFUSED ABSCESS, OR DIFFUSED INFLAMMATION OF THE CELLULAR TISSUE.

GENERAL ·DESCRIPTION.—This is an inflammation, characterized by an absence of the disposition or of the power to form healthy adhesive lymph. It consequently spreads rapidly and widely, and is attended with constitutional symptoms of the gravest character.

SYMPTOMS.—An extensive and rapidly increasing swelling appears on one of the limbs, or on some part of the trunk. Its surface is tense, shining, and usually pale. When pressed upon, it feels in some cases hard and resisting, but more frequently it yields that peculiar, semi-elastic sensation described by the terms *boggy*, or *quaggy*. There is always most excruciating pain;—which in some cases is burning and throbbing, in others heavy and tensive. The disease is invariably attended with fever of an irritative or typhoid character. The pulse is always frequent; —it may be sharp and jerking, but it is without strength and steadiness. The countenance is anxious and haggard;—the mind irritable and desponding, and delirious at intervals. Respiration is quick and laborious,— more especially if the disease be seated on the chest, as it frequently is;—because the pleura is affected through contiguous sympathy. In unfavourable cases, low muttering delirium, subsultus tendinum, copious offensive perspiration, and jaundiced skin, usher in the fatal termination.

CAUSES.—The *predisposing* causes of this disease comprise all the agents capable of lowering the vital energies. Unwholesome food; confined air; disorder of the secretions of the alimentary canal and its attendant glands; exhaustion of the mind from excessive study;—the depressing passions;—and certain epidemic noxious states of air;—to which last must be attributed the extraordinary prevalence of this disease in the Plymouth dockyards in the year 1824.

The *exciting causes* may be of the most trivial nature, if the patient

11

be predisposed; such as very slight punctures or abrasions. This is the disease which is excited by the bites of venomous serpents;—and by inoculation with septic animal poisons;—especially by that which is generated in bodies recently dead;—it also occasionally follows certain surgical operations, as lithotomy and venæsection.

MORBID ANATOMY.—On examination of the parts affected, (at an early period of the disease,) the cellular tissue is found loaded with a limpid reddish serum. In a more advanced stage, this fluid becomes thicker, and less highly coloured. Subsequently, the cellular tissue is found to be gorged, partly with white semi-fluid matter, partly with a brownish purulent sanies, which is mingled with detached flakes of the sphacelated tissue. The muscles, and other structures in the vicinity, are discoloured and softened;—and the larger veins which permeate the diseased part, have their coats inflamed, and often in a state of suppuration.

DIAGNOSIS.—This disease is to be distinguished from the common phlegmonous abscess, by its having a smooth and level surface, without any tendency to point;—also by the asthenic nature of the accompanying fever. It presents many points of resemblance to *phlegmonous erysipelas;*—and, in fact, is not unfrequently combined with it;—but it is to be distinguished from it by the circumstance, that in phlegmonous erysipelas the skin is inflamed from the first;—whereas in diffuse cellular inflammation it is only affected secondarily, and after the disease has lasted for some days.

TREATMENT.—This will be more fully discussed in the Chapter on Dissection Wounds, (Part iii. ch. 9.) It may, however, be summarily observed, that leeches, hot fomentations, and free incisions;—emetics purgatives, and enemata, followed by ammonia, bark, opium, and wine, are the measures that are sanctioned by the most authoritative and experienced writers.*

## OF THE DISEASES OF THE SKIN.

### SECTION V.—ERYSIPELAS.

DEFINITION.—A diffused inflammation of the skin, with a tendency to spread.

VARIETIES.—1. Erysipelas is called *simple* when the skin is solely or principally affected; there being only more or less œdema of the subcutaneous cellular tissue. 2. *Plegmonous* erysipelas is complicated with an unhealthy inflammation of the cellular tissue, of that kind which is called *diffuse inflammation.*† 3. Erysipelas of the *head* is often compli-

---

* Vide two papers in the Edinburgh Medical and Surgical Journal for 1825, vol. xxv. Copland's Dict., Art. Cellular Tissue. James on Inflammation. Travers on Constitutional Irritation, and Butter on Irritative Fever, Devonport, 1825.

† Vide Part II., chap. vii., sect. iv., p. 81.

cated with delirium in the early stages, and coma in the latter—owing to inflammatory excitement of the cerebral membranes, with tendency to serous effusion.   4. *Gastric* or *Bilious* erysipelas is complicated with bilious vomiting, tender and puffed abdomen, red tongue, and perhaps diarrhœa.   5. *Erratic* erysipelas wanders progressively; some parts being attacked, whilst others are recovering.   6. *Metastatic* erysipelas ceases suddenly at one part of the skin, and flies to another.   7. *Recurrent* erysipelas suddenly leaves the skin, and then some internal organ is attacked with inflammation.

SYMPTOMS.—*Simple* erysipelas is known by redness of the skin, which *disappears momentarily on pressure*; considerable swelling, owing to serous effusion into the cellular tissue;—and severe stinging, burning, or smarting pain.   The redness is generally of a vivid scarlet hue; but it may be faint and yellowish if the disease is attended with much debility, or if it affect the eyelids, scrotum, or other loose cellular parts, and is consequently accompanied with a good deal of serous effusion.

In the *phlegmonous* erysipelas, the redness is deeper, and in some cases dusky or purple, and it is *scarcely*, if it all, *dispelled by pressure* —the swelling is much greater, and is hard, brawny, and tense;—and the pain is not only burning but throbbing.

Both varieties are ushered in by shivering, headach, pain in the back, and nausea;—and both are attended with fever;—which in the young, robust, and plethoric, will be of an ardent inflammatory character;—but in the aged and debilitated, or after the occurrence of sloughing, may rapidly become low and typhoid.

TERMINATIONS.—*Simple* erysipelas may terminate, 1. in *resolution*, leaving nothing but desquamation of the cuticle, and slight œdema; 2. but more frequently it produces large vesicles, from effusion of serum under the cuticle;—and these dry into scabs, which peel off, and leave the cutis either healed or superficially ulcerated.—3. Sometimes, however, it is followed by small *abscesses*.

*Phlegmonous* erysipelas *may* terminate as favourably;—but it more generally leads to unhealthy suppuration and sloughing of the cellular tissue:—in which case the swelling becomes flaccid and *quaggy:*— patches of the skin become purple and covered with livid vesications, and these patches slough, giving exit to a thin sanious pus, and to flakes of disorganized cellular tissue.   And not only the subcutaneous, but the intermuscular tissue and fasciæ may slough, rendering the limb useless, even if the patient escape with his life.

PROGNOSIS.—This must be *guarded* if the patient is old, enfeebled, and habitually intemperate;—if the constitutional affection is low and typhoid;—if the malady is situated on the head or throat, and there is coma or great dyspnœa;—or if the erysipelas is of the phlegmonous variety, and a large portion of the cellular tissue and skin is on the point of sloughing.

PATHOLOGY.—Erysipelas is one of a class of diseases, of which inflammation is a principal, but not the only element. For it needs scarcely be said that every inflammation of the skin is not erysipelas. In fact, it requires a peculiar state of constitution to give rise to it;—which state of constitution is remarkably analogous (if not identical) with that which accompanies puerperal fever, phlebitis, and the *suppurative diathesis*;—that is to say, the state in which abscesses form all over the body, and especially in the lungs, liver, and joints. Thus erysipelas and puerperal fever are often epidemic together;—the mothers perishing of one, and the infants of the other.* And in the London hospitals, during the prevalence of erysipelas, phlebitis and consecutive abscesses are often prevalent likewise.

CAUSES.—The causes which produce this state of the system are threefold. *First*, intemperance, fatigue, close confinement in foul air, and whatever other causes are capable of irritating the digestive organs, exhausting the nervous system, or vitiating the blood. The origin of erysipelas in the close air of hospitals is unhappily too notorious to need mention. *Secondly*, the disease may be *epidemic;* that is, may be produced by certain states of the atmosphere at large, affecting several people in the same district simultaneously. *Thirdly*, it may be propagated by *contagion* or *infection*, by means of the emanations from patients affected with it.

These causes may be sufficient of themselves to produce the disease (which then is said to be *idiopathic;*) or they may be *predisposing* merely, and require the addition of some *exciting cause*. Any injury of the skin may be an exciting cause of erysipelas;—especially leech-bites, caustic, and burns. Idiopathic erysipelas generally attacks the head.

TREATMENT.—The indications are, to diminish inflammatory action and febrile excitement,—to support the strength,—to correct the secretions,—and *locally*, to allay irritation,—to arrest the extension of the disease, —and to give free exit to sloughs and discharge.

*Emetics and Purgatives.*—In the first place an *emetic* may be given, composed of a scruple of ipecacuanha with a grain of tartar emetic. It should be followed by a good dose of calomel, and by black draughts (F. 4) containing a few grains of soda, every six or eight hours, as long as they bring away hardened lumps of fæces, or as long as the secretions continue to amend under their use. If, however, the patient be weak, an emetic of ipecacuanha and ammonia (F. 94) may be substituted for the tartar emetic. If the constitution is very much broken down, or if there are symptoms of early coma or typhoid debility, Copland recom-

* Vide Ferguson on Puerperal Fever, p. 28.

mends the calomel to be combined with camphor, and to be followed by the turpentine draught (F. 18) or turpentine enemata.

*Antiphlogistic measures.*—*Bleeding* will be required if the patient is young and vigorous, the pulse full and strong, the face flushed, and delirium violent;—and if the inflamed part is full, tense, and vividly red, and especially is seated on the head or throat. In similar active inflammatory cases, *calomel* may be given in doses of two grains every six hours with antimony (F. 6;) or *colchicum*, in doses of ♏ xx of the wine; and *saline draughts* with excess of alkali, (such as F. 5, or liq. am. acet. &c.) in the intervals;—but, in most cases of *simple* erysipelas a dose of mercury at night, and purges and salines during the day, will suffice. For it must be recollected that as the disease is not purely inflammatory, it can very rarely be cut short by mere antiphlogistic measures; and that debility is much to be dreaded; especially in cases occurring in the crowded habitations of London.

*Tonics and stimulants.*—*Bark* should be given in all cases as soon as the tongue becomes clean and the skin moist; or if the pulse is soft, tremulous, or very rapid, the heat moderate, and the delirium low and muttering;—or if the patient is naturally delicate, and subject to periodic or recurrent attacks;—or if antiphlogistic measures do not arrest the disease, or if suppuration or sloughing have commenced. If there be any doubt of its propriety, it should be given in small doses;—but, in decided cases of debility, a strong decoction should be administered, with the acids or ammonia,—and with wine or gin, if the patient is used to it.

*Opium* may be given in full doses at bed-time in the later stages, to allay restlessness, provided there is no cerebral congestion nor coma.

In the *gastric variety*, small repeated doses of hydr. c. creta et pulv. ipec. c. should be given with effervescing draughts; and fomentations or rubefacients be applied to the abdomen.

And in what may be called *chronic* or *habitual erysipelas*, when it comes on at intervals, when the stomach is disordered or the general health deranged, a course of aperients, alteratives, or tonics, (especially sarsaparilla and alkalis,) should be administered according to the principles laid down in the Chapter on Chronic Inflammation, page 59.

Local Measures.—*Leeches* are useful in the early stages, provided the patient can bear the loss of blood. *Minute punctures* about one-eighth of an inch deep, made with the point of a lancet, have been recommended as substitutes; but they are very inefficient as a means of abstracting blood, and cause considerable pain.

*Cold Lotions* may be used when the heat is great and the pulse good, and especially in erysipelas of the head. But they must be avoided if the circulation is languid, or if the erysipelas is *recurrent*, or is manifestly connected with gastric irritation, or any other internal disorder.

*Warm* or *tepid* fomentations of dec. papav. vel cydonii should be pre‐
ferred in cases arising from local irritation; and perhaps are safest at all
times, but the patient's feelings are the best criterion.

*Flour,* dusted on the inflamed part, is a very soothing application; and
is well calculated to allay the heat and itching of simple erysipelas, and
to absorb the acrid serum that escapes from the vesications.

*Pressure* by bandages is serviceable in the latter stage of most cases:—
and *from the very first,* if the inflammation be atonic and œdematous.

*Mercurial ointment* smeared on the part, or applied as a plaster, has
been much praised by some people, but its efficacy is questionable.

*Stimulants.*—The *nitrate of silver* in substance or solution;—or *blisters,* or fomentation of dec. cydonii oj. cum liq. am. sesquicaib. 3j, are of
great use in putting a stop to tedious cases of simple erysipelas, after pro‐
per constitutional remedies have been used. When there is a tendency
to sinking, warm cloths moistened with turpentine or sp. camp. may be
applied externally, whilst diffusive stimulants are administered inter‐
nally.

The *extension of the disease may sometimes be arrested* by applying
a strip of blistering plaster, or still better the nitrate of silver, so as com‐
pletely to encircle the inflamed part. The skin should be well washed
first, and care should be taken to leave no interstices through which the
disease might creep and extend itself. But of course, proper constitu‐
tional remedies must not be neglected for these local means.

*Incisions* are, to use a French expression, the *heroic* remedy in phleg‐
monons erysipelas. When the swelling is great and increases rapidly;—
when it is hard, tense, and resisting, not soft and œdematous as in simple
erysipelas;—when the pain is severe, and throbbing, and not relieved by
leeches;—when there is the least sensation of fluctuation or *quaggi-
ness;*—or when the skin is becoming livid or dusky, or covered with livid
vesicles, they are imperatively demanded. They are absolutely neces‐
sary for the discharge of pus and sloughs;—for, as James observes, these
matters are neither brought to the surface by pointing, nor walled in by
adhesion. But it must be recollected, that they are not to be considered
merely in the light of apertures for the discharge of matter; but as the
most effectual means of cutting short the inflammation, by relieving the
tension, and by emptying the distended blood-vessels. They are also
requisite in erysipelas of the throat, when great swelling threatens suffo‐
cation by pressure on the trachea. They should be made of sufficient
length,—in as many places as required;—they should be carried quite
deeply through the diseased tissues, and should be repeated as often as
necessary. Three, four, or five inches will be of sufficient length in
most cases; but no precise rule can be laid down on this subject. At
all events they should be made long enough, but not wantonly long from
adherence to any system. They should not be permitted to bleed longer

than the strength permits;—and hæmorrhage, if profuse, is best stopped by continued pressure with the fingers on the bleeding points. The subsequent measures are poultices, followed by stimulating dressings (as in carbuncle) and bandages to prevent lodgment of matter and sinuses.*

# CHAPTER VIII.

## OF ULCERATION.

### SECT. 1.—OF THE PATHOLOGY OF ULCERATION.

PATHOLOGY.—The observations of the most recent pathologists have shown that ulceration is a mere variety of mortification; in fact, that it consists in the progressive softening, death, and disintegration of successive layers of the ulcerating tissue; hence the term *molecular gangrene.*

Now ulceration, like mortification, may occur through two opposite precesses. *First,* from inflammation; and *secondly,* from congestion; that is, from a stagnation of venous blood in the capillaries.

(1) *Inflammatory Ulceration.*—The formation of an ulcer through inflammation is precisely similar to the formation of an abscess; the only difference being that the former commences on the surface, the latter in the substance of a part. Supposing the skin to ulcerate from the application of venereal poison, for instance. In the first place, its surface inflames, and secretes some unhealthy pus, which elevates the cuticle into a pimple or pustule. When the pustule is opened, there appears a little hollow, filled with a whitish or grayish tenacious mattei consisting of the skin which has already perished, and of unhealthy flaky pus. If this is wiped off the surface underneath is seen to be red, and it easily bleeds. Supposing the case to proceed, there is formed a chasm, eaten into irregular hollows, with intervening red eminences, which easily bleed if touched; its edges are ragged, loose, and undermined; the surrounding skin red, hot, and swollen; there is a thin serous, or bloody discharge, and a constant severe gnawing pain. An ulcer having these characters may always be considered as extending itself.

An *excoriation* is sometimes the first stage of this ulcer; that is to say,

* Vide James, op. cit.; Copland, Dict.; Higgingbottom on Nitrate of Silver: Copland, Hutchinson's Surgical Observations; the Lectures of Abernethy, Cooper, and Lawrence; and two Lectures, by Velpeau, Med. Gaz., August 14 and 21, 1840.

a portion of skin inflames, discharges matter, and loses its cuticle, and
the excoriated portion may either heal, or, as we have just observed, may
ulcerate.

Of course, ulcers spread with varying degrees of rapidity. An attack
of violent inflammation may cause the death of a considerable portion in a
very short time; this is said to be a *sloughing ulcer.* When an ulcer
spreads very rapidly, but regularly and without sloughing of any great
portion at one time, it is called *phagedenic.* And when it spreads more
rapidly still, not by one fit of sloughing, but by the constant reiterated
mortification of considerable layers, it receives the name of *sloughing
phagedæna.*

(2) *Conjestive Ulceration.*—This may be very briefly described as it
occurs on the legs of old dropsical people. A small portion of skin has
its capillaries distended with venous blood, whose return is nearly or quite
suspended. Some of the serum (with which the cellular tissue is already
distended) exudes under the cuticle, raising it into a blister. When this
is removed, there is seen a darkish layer of sloughing skin. This, like
the last, may spread with every degree of rapidity; but whether a large
tract of skin mortifies at once, or whether the smallest portion ulcerates the
process is one and the same.

(3) *Combination of the two Forms.*—But it most generally happens
that ulceration consists in a combination of inflammation and congestion;
that is, in the inflammation of a part already congested, or incapable,
through weakness, of supporting inflammation without loss of life. It
may be observed also, that ulcers which have commenced through congestion may be extended by inflammation.

As this account which we have given of the ulcerative process differs
very materially from the doctrines of Hunter, which are still adhered to
by many people, it is necessary to say a few words in proof of its cor-
rectness.

Now Hunter taught that ulcers are formed by a variety of absorption,
which he denominated ulcerative; that is, that the ulcerating tissue, feeling
its incapability of performing its functions, is absorbed by the agency of
its own lymphatics.

But to this doctrine it must be objected, first of all, because it is void of
all proof. Hunter says that it is so, and that he was the first to show it;
but nowhere does he attempt to prove it.

In the second place, it is opposed by the following undoubted facts.
(1) Ulcers often spread rapidly when inflamed; but absorption is always
diminished during inflammation; so that a quantity of nux vomica which
would prove fatal if applied to a recent wound, or to a healthy mucous
membrane, may be applied with impunity if these parts are inflamed. (2)
The tissues best supplied with absorbents, do not ulcerate so readily as
others (cartilage, for instance) which are very imperfectly supplied. (3)

Parts (such as bone) which are very quickly absorbed before the progress of an aneurism, do not ulcerate so readily as cartilage, which is absorbed before an aneurism very slowly, if at all. (4) The state which favours ulceration in the legs, is one adverse to the action of absorption either by lymphatics or veins. (5) Absorption is a very slow process; ulceration often very rapid. (6) Granulations ulcerate more readily than cicatrices; although they cannot be presumed to be better supplied with lymphatics.

(7) A surface to be absorbed by the minute lymphatics must necessarily become fluid; but if so, what is to hinder it from passing off, at least in part, with the discharge? (8) Injections demonstrate that old ulcers are always attended by a dilated state of the surrounding veins, but show no development of the lymphatics.*

PREDISPOSING CAUSES.—The *Tissues* most disposed to ulceration are the skin, mucous and synovial membranes. From these it may spread to other subjacent tissues, which yield to it with varying degrees of rapidity. The cellular tissue ulcerates very easily; but mueles, blood-vessels, and nerves very slowly; so that they often appear to be as it were dissected out in spreading sores by the destruction of the cellular tissue around them. Tendons and ligaments are also very slow to ulcerate; but cartilage, bone, and the cornea, are in certain constitutions extremely liable to it.

The *Constitutions* most liable to ulceration, are those which are debilitated by intemperance or privations; tainted with syphilis or scrofula;—or broken down by the excessive use of mercury.

The *parts* most disposed to it are those whose circulation is most weak and languid; such as the lower extremities; and more especially if the return of their venous blood be in any way impeded by a varicose state of the veins. On this account tall persons are much more frequently affected with ulcers of the legs than the short. Sir. E. Home shows, on the authority of Dr. Young, that twenty-two out of one hundred and forty-five tall men, and only twenty-three out of two hundred and seventy-six short men, were discharged from a regiment in the West Indies in four years, on account of ulcers.

*Parts newly formed* are, as has been before said, more liable to ulce-

---

* The authorities to whom I am indebted for these arguments are. J. W. Earle, *Med. Gaz.* for 1835. C. Aston Key, *Med. Chir. Trans.*, vol. xviii. and xix. Copland, *Dict. Pract. Med. Art. Inflammation;* and particularly Wallace *on the Venereal Disease,* Lon. 1838, p. 47; and S. Gaskell, *Jacksonian Prize Essay on Ulceration* MS. in the Library of the College of Surgeons in London. An inspection of the preparations accompanying Mr. Gaskell's Essay ,would convince the most skeptical. It is maintained that cartilage ulcerates through absorption, because large patches of it sometimes ulcerate without any pus or debris being found in the joint. But although this may be true, it does not alter the above mentioned facts relating to the skin. Vide Brodie, Lancet, Feb. 15, 1840.

rate than those of original formation. And this is equally true, whether they have been produced, *first*, in consequence of injury, as cicatrices and callus; or, *secondly*, whether they are developed from hypertrophy of a standard structure; as cutaneous tumours which often remain stationary for years, and then, from some slight irritation, will give rise to the most destructive and spreading ulceration; or, *thirdly*, whether they consist in the deposite of a texture alien to the normal organization. Thus cancerous diseases appear to depend mainly on the deposite of a new texture, which from its low powers of vitality, yields after a time to disorganization.

EXCITING CAUSES.—In constitutions or parts predisposed to it, the slightest irritation may be sufficient to excite ulceration. In the healthy it may be produced by the continuous application of some irritant so as gradually to exhaust the vital powers of the part;—such as continued pressure; the presence of irritating fluids; or depraved secretions. But it is not easy to excite genuine spreading ulceration in the healthy, unless by some specific cause, such as the venereal poison.

### SECTION II.—OF THE VARIETIES OF ULCERS.

I. THE HEALTHY ULCER is nothing more than a healthy granulating and cicatrizing surface. The granulations are small, numerous, florid, and pointed, and yield a moderate secretion of healthy pus. The edges are smooth, and covered with a white semi-transparent pellicle, which is gradually lost on the margin of the granulations. It will be recollected that a healthy sore of this description will be greatly diminished by the contraction of the surrounding skin, before any cicatrization has actually occurred.

*Treatment.*—The only treatment required will be a little dry lint, if there be much discharge,—or the water-dressing, or simple ointment, if there be not. If there be not much discharge, the dressings should not be changed more frequently than every second or third day. If the granulations are too luxuriant, they may be touched with lunar caustic, and dressed with dry lint;—or the sore may be exposed to the air for some hours. If the granulating surface is very extensive, or if all applications disagree with it, as sometimes happens, it will be expedient to form a *scab* on it surface. This may be done by allowing the pus to dry, or by sprinkling a little flour, or calamine, or chalk to absorb it. But the best plan in these cases is to pass a stick of lunar caustic over the surface of the sore, as recommended by Mr. Higginbottom. This salt instantly coagulates the fluids on the sore, and forms a white pellicle, which soon becomes dry and black, and is much less irritating than an ordinary scab. If the scab act favourably, suppuration ceases, and cicatrization will be found complete when it is detached. No other dressing is required, except, perhaps, a piece of goldbeater's skin, or a slight fillet to prevent injury. If pus continue to be formed, a small hole should be made in the middle of the scab to let it out.

II. THE INFLAMED ULCER has already been described.

*Causes.*—Ulcers (though not originally formed by inflammation) are liable to inflame from any of the ordinary local or constitutional causes, especially errors in diet. Sores situated over projecting parts of bones or ligaments, as the outer ankle, or over the bellies of muscles, are apt to assume this character; hence care should be taken to avoid making issues in such situations.

*Treatment.*—In a few instances, when the patient is very plethoric and strong, it may be expedient to bleed, and to administer calomel and opium till the mouth is slightly affected. In all cases the bowels should be cleared, the secretions kept up, and the diet be regulated. The patient should keep at rest, with the affected member in an elevated posture. Leeches may be applied in the vicinity of the sore; but not too near it, and not to any place where the skin is much thickened and congested, lest the leech-bites themselves take on ulceration. The part should be fomented night and morning for half an hour with poppy fomentations, and then a poultice or the water-dressing be applied, or the steam-bath described at p. 58 may be tried;—and if the pain be very severe, the poultice may be medicated with opium, F. 63, or conium. If the ulcer diminish under these applications, but yet its surface remain foul, they may be continued till it is healed; but if the surface become healthy, it may be treated as an ordinary ulcer.—If warm applications aggravate the pain, cold, evaporating, or saturine lotions (F. 11) should be used, the sore being protected by a piece of oiled silk or simple dressing.

If all these soothing measures prove ineffectual, as they occasionally will, even though aided by the most judicious constitutional treatment, recourse must be had to the measures directed for irritable ulcers.

III. THE IRRITABLE ULCER is a variety of the inflamed. It is defined by Mr. Skey* as having an excess of *organizing action*, with a deficiency of *organizable material*; so that the granulations are too small, and are morbidly sensitive and vascular.

*Treatment.*—In the first place, the constitution, which is generally out of order, must be corrected by alteratives and tonics. Plummer's pill, or F. 6, 7, 10, 52, at bed-time; and sarsaparilla, soda, and hyoscyamus, F. 56, 57, during the day; or the extract of conium in doses of gr. v., ter die, will be of great service.

In the local treatment, all sources of irritation must be removed, and

* F. C. Skey, F.R.S. A new mode of treatment employed in the cure of various forms of ulcer. London, 1837.

the soothing applications directed for the inflamed ulcer may be tried
first.   But the most successful plan, generally speaking, is the application of a succession of mild stimulants, so as to alter the actions and exhaust the irritability of the part.   Weak lotions of nitric acid, (F. 17,) of
nitrate of silver (gr. i. ad ℥j.,) of arsenic, (F. 68,) of sulphate of zinc (gr.
i.—v. ad. ℥j.,) of sulphate of copper (gr. i.—ii. ad. ℥j.,) of acetate of
zinc (F. 21,) of corrosive sublimate (F. 37,) of chloride of soda (F. 39,)
of iodine (F, 76,) the linimentum æruginis, black wash (F. 70, yellow
wash (F. 71,) lime water, solution of sulphate of iron (gr. i. ad ℥j.,) *forge
water,* that is water in which red hot iron has been extinguished, strong
green tea, powdered chalk or charcoal mixed with cream, ointments of
Peruvian balsam, of oxide of xine, chalk, lead, and calamine; weak mercurial ointment, liniment of ung. hydr. nitratis (73;) moderated pressure
with strips of soap plaster, or of linen spread with sop cerate, or with a
smooth piece of sheet lead; all of these measures will occasionally be of
service in the cure of obstinate and irritable ulcers.   For it very often
happens that an application which at first soothes the pain will soon lose
its good effects, and then become positively hurtful.

IV.   THE WEAK ULCER is the direct reverse of the preceding.   Its
powers of organization are deficient.   The granulations are large, pale,
flabby, and insensible, rising above the margin of the skin, and showing
no disposition to cicatrize.

*Causes.*—This state of ulcer may be owing to debility of the system;
but the healthiest granulations, if their healing be delayed, become
weak;—and conversely, if any granulations do not cicatrize, they should
be considered as weak, and treated accordingly.

*Treatment.*—The indications are to augment the vital forces of the .
granulations, and to retain their exuberant growth.   The diet should be
liberal, and should include a moderate quantity of wine, or beer.   If there
is much debility, some preparation of bark or steel should be exhibited.
If the granulations are extremely exuberant, they may be destroyed by
escharotics, such as cupri sulphas;—or sometimes may be shaved off
with a thin knife;—but it is better to cause their removal by over-stimulation than by actual destruction.   So that the best applications are, fine
dry lint, which by itself is an excellent stimulant; or lint dipped in a
lotion of sulphate of zinc, or of sulphate of copper, or of nitrate of silver,
or the ung. hydr. nit.   The formation of a crust or scab with the lunar
caustic, on Mr. Higginbottom's plan, may be often resorted to with advantage.   At the same time, pressure by means of strips of plaster, or
compress, and bandages, are necessary to prevent languor of the circulation;—especially if the muscles are wasted and flabby.   In some cases a
scab may be formed by covering the sore with powdered rhubarb, taking
care to oil the edges, so that they may not be irritated by it.   If the
patient is young and weakly, with great coldness and blueness, and ten.

dency to œdema in the extremities, the limb may be immersed in tepid salt water for fifteen minutes twice a day; to which an equal part of decoction of poppies may be added if pimples are produced.

V. The Indolent Ulcer is characterized by a deficiency of *action* as well as of *power*. Its surface is smooth and glassy, and of a pale ashy colour, like a mucous membrane. Sometimes, however, it displays a crop of weak fungous granulations. The edges are raised, thick, white, and sensible; the discharge scanty and thin. The most frequent *situation* of these ulcers is the small of the leg, and they are almost exclusively met with amongst the lower orders. They are often stationary for a great length of time; but, from any slight cause of irritation, may enlarge rapidly by ulceration or sloughing; and even when they have made considerable progress in healing, the granulations and cicatrices that have been months in forming may perish in a few hours from some constitutional disturbance or local injury.

*Treatment.*—The general rules are, to promote constitutional vigour by good diet and tonics, and to excite the local actions by various stimulants. The patient should take moderate exercise; but when he is at rest, the affected limb should not be permitted to hang down. In treating these cases, we must endeavour not only to effect a cure, but to make it permanent; and this can only be ensured by attending to the growth of the granulations, and rendering them as healthy and firm as possible.

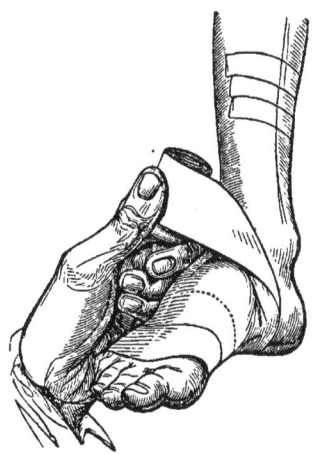

The following is perhaps the best plan of curing these ulcers. A number of pieces of lint, thoroughly soaked in the nitric acid lotion, should be laid in the sore, and be covered with a warm soft poultice. These applications should be changed twice a day, and be continued till the discharge becomes healthy, and granulations begin to arise. If there is any degree of inflammation about the parts, (which often happens when these ulcers first come under treatment,) the patient must be confined to bed and be purged. Afterwards, when the surface is clean, the following mode of dressing should be adopted. First, some pieces of lint, saturated with the nitric acid lotion, or zinc lotion, (F. 15,) or with some other stimulating substance, should be laid on the sores. Then strips of adhesive plaster, about 1½ inch wide, should be applied *two-thirds round the limb*, from an inch below the ulcer to an inch above it; and in applying each strip, the edges of the sore should be drawn together with a moderate degree of force. Next, a compress of soft linen must be placed over the plaster, and finally, the limb must be well and evenly bandaged from the toes to the knee; observing that the bandage is to be applied most tightly below, and more loosely by degrees as it ascends.

*Baynton's Plan.*—If, however, the whole limb is very much thickened, and the edges of the ulcers are very callous, it will be better to follow Mr. Baynton's method;*—that is, to encircle the *whole circumference* of the limb with strips of plaster, from an inch below to an inch above the ulcers. Each strip is to be first applied by its middle to that part of the limb which is opposite the ulcer, and then the two ends are to be brought forwards over it, and they should be long enough to overlap about two inches. A compress and bandage are to be applied afterwards. These modes of dressing almost always cause severe pain;—but it ought soon to subside, and the part to feel stronger and more comfortable afterwards. If, however, it continue to be painful and hot, some pure water should be poured on the bandage from a watering-pot or teapot.

If the adhesive plaster irritate the skin, it may be diluted with soap-plaster;—or the isinglass-plaster may be substituted. Mr. Baynton employed a combination of 4 oz. of common lead-plaster with ʒß of resin. The isinglass-plaster is made by dissolving isinglass in spirits of wine, and spreading the solution on silk. It readily adheres, if moistened with a warm sponge.

But although the plastering and bandaging are adapted for most cases, the immediate application to the ulcer will require to be frequently varied. Sometimes the strapping may be applied without any thing else; or dry lint may be placed under it; or lint imbued with lotions of sulphate of copper, or alum; or with lotions made by adding half an ounce of the tincture of myrrh, or of benzoin (comp.,) or aloes (comp.,) to four ounces of water; or the balsams of copaiba or Peru; but metallic preparations agree better in general than the vegetable. Ointments agree better with the indolent than with the other varieties of ulcer, because they do no harm if rancid. The ung. hyd. nitric. oxyd. is very useful;—and the ung. hydrarg. intrate. dilut. is praised for its efficacy in reducing thick callous edges.

---

* Baynton, T., Descriptive Account of a New Method of Treating old Ulcers of the Legs. Bristol, 1797.

If a crop of granulations threaten to slough, they should be fomented with hot decoction of poppies, to which a little spirit of wine has been added. The gastric juice of animals is said to be a specific for certain sloughing ulcers occurring in persons debilitated by the use of ardent spirits and salt provisions, and by residence in hot climates. During any febrile disturbance of the system, the local applications must be mild.

*Mr. Skey's Plan.*—Mr. Skey conceiving that the chief obstacle in the cure of these ulcers is the want of a vigorous capillary circulation:—and seeing that opium produces a uniform warmth of skin, and excites the circulation in the remotest parts, proposes to employ it in the treatment of these cases. He recommends it to be given in doses of half a grain night and morning, which may be increased gradually, according to its effects. He says that this treatment, without any local applications, will suffice for the cure of all weak and indolent ulcers, especially if the patient be old, and reduced by intemperance or starvation. He observes that in general the opium proves rather laxative than otherwise; and that it will have no ill effect in any case, whilst artificial support is needed;— or whilst the natural powers are languid;—or "so long as there remains a drain on the circulation." Mr. Skey also recommends the employment of opium with a similar view in other cases of deficient circulation, or passive congestion,—as in chronic catarrh, and the red noses of drunkards; and in phagedæna after the active symptoms have been combated.

*Should old ulcers be healed?*—The propriety of healing old ulcers will sometimes be made a question, in as much as certain diseases, and especially apoplexy and palsy, are apt to supervene on their suppression. Sir E. Home has specified the following cases in which a cure ought not to be attempted. 1. If the ulcer be "evidently affected with the gout, having regular attacks of pain, returning at stated periods; and those attacks similar to what the patient has experienced from gout in other parts." 2. If an ulcer habitually occur whenever the constitution is disordered. 3. If the patient be very infirm and old; for under these circumstances the removal of an habitual source of irritation, or the diversion of habitual afflux of blood, may prove fatal;—more especially as very old ulcers have been known to heal spontaneously a short time before death. In the first two cases, however, an issue placed in a convenient situation might be substituted for an ulcer in an inconvenient one. But in other cases, where the ulcer has not displayed any connexion with constitutional disorder, there need be no reluctance to heal it, provided that the secretions are properly maintained during the cure and for some time afterwards. And if any symptoms of congestion in the head or other organ should arise, an issue may be inserted in the arm.

Whately* mentions a case in which an ulcer was healed, but some time afterwards it reappeared of itself, and soon after that the patient died suddenly; and he observes that his death would infallibly have been attributed to the healing of the sore, if it had occurred before its second outbreak.

VI. THE FISTULOUS ULCER (Fistula or Sinus) is a variety of the indolent, and consists of a narrow channel lined by a pale pseudo-mucous membrane, which may or may not lead to a suppurating cavity. In old cases the parietes of the tube are often dense and semi-cartilaginous.

*Causes.*—Fistulæ are produced when abscesses are not thoroughly healed from the bottom, and when their sides have been too hastily approximated, or when there is some standing cause of irritation, as a ligature, or a piece of dead bone, which keeps up a discharge of pus.

*Treatment.*—The first indication is to prevent the lodgment of matter; for which purpose it may perhaps be necessary to make another opening. The second indication is to produce the adhesive inflammation;—to which the mucous lining of the fistula is naturally indisposed. The means to be adopted are, stimulating injections, (F. 17,) tents smeared with irritating ointments; the caustic bougie; or a seton consisting of a few threads of silk, which may be passed through the fistula, and may be gradually diminished as the passage contracts. When granulations have been created by these means, graduated pressure should be made, that the sides may coalesce. If these means fail, the fistula should be slit up with a bistoury; and then a thin piece of lint be introduced in order to prevent premature union of the cut edges, and make it heal from the bottom.

If there have been a succession of small unhealthy abscesses in a part;—or if ulceration have spread irregularly in the cellular tissue, so as to leave the skin ragged, and extensively undermined with tortuous sinuses, it will be advisable to destroy the whole of the parts so diseased by the potassa fusa; and this will stimulate the neighbouring sound parts, so that when the slough separates, a healthy surface will be left, which may be healed by the ordinary means.†

VII. THE VARICOSE ULCER occurs in consequence of a varicose state of the veins of the lower extremity. This greatly impedes the return of blood, and, by producing habitual venous congestion, weakens the parts, and renders them prone to ulceration. The ulcers are usually three or four in number; situated above the ankle. They are oval in shape, indolent in their progress, and neither extensive nor deep:—but they are

* Whately, T., Practical Observations on the Cure of Wounds and ulcers. Lond. 1816, p 144.

† Liston, Elements of Surgery.

attended with considerable pain, which is of a deep-seated, aching character, and not sore like that of ordinary ulcers.

The *Treatment* must be directed principally to the veins, and may either be palliative or radical; but for this we must refer to the chapter on that subject. We will merely observe here, that the applications to the ulcers must be suited to their condition, whether irritable or indolent;—and that great relief to the pain is frequently obtained by opening one of the enlarged vessels, and abstracting a moderate quantity of blood. The advantages of proper support by bandages or laced stocking needs scarcely to be noticed. Sometimes there is a constant desquamation of the cuticle, with serous discharge, for which the best remedies are equal parts of lime water and milk, or the ointment of oxyde of zinc.

VIII. The SLOUGHING ULCER is formed whenever either of the other varieties of ulcer is attacked with sloughing;—which is particularly liable to occur to the *indolent*, when subjected to undue irritation. Or, this name may be given to ulcers originally produced by a sloughing of the skin;—as on the legs of the dropsical.

*Treatment.*—The best applications are warm spirituous fomentations and stimulating poultices of yeast or carrots; or the nitric acid lotion on lint, with a warm poultice over it.

IX. PHAGEDÆNA is a peculiar variety of ulceration, extremely rapid in its progress. The surface of the sore is irregular, generally whitish or yellowish; the matter scanty and bloody; and the pain extreme. Some cases are attended with fever and acute inflammation, the margin of the sore being highly painful, swelled, and red;—others with atony and debility, the margin being pale, dusky, or livid.

*Causes.*—This disease may be induced either by extraordinary local irritation, or by some peculiar constitutional disorder. It may attack primary or secondary venereal sores in consequence of filth, intemperance, the abuse of mercury; or of a weakened and vitiated, or scrofulous habit. Sometimes it appears in the throat after scarlatina;—it may attack a blistered surface when the constitution has greatly suffered from an acute and exhausting disease, as measles, &c.;—in many instances it affects the mouth or genitals of children, constituting *cancer oris; phagedæna of the mouth; noma, &c.*

*Treatment.*—If the habit is inflammatory and the pulse full and strong, bleeding and the antiphlogistic regimen should be employed, and opiate lotion be applied to the sore. If the condition of the system is the reverse, tonics and narcotics, (FF. 1, 2, 3,) should be administered, and the diseased surface should be destroyed by nitric acid in the manner to be presently described.

X. SLOUGHING PHAGEDÆNA seems, says Mr. Lawrence, to be the state of phagedæna carried to its fullest extent;—or, as was explained at the commencement of this chapter, it may be described as a process interme-

13

diate between common ulceration and gangrene. Its causes are, either
local irritation, acting on a vitiated state of the constitution, or infection,
or exposure to foul air. We shall show presently that these causes operate in various proportions in different instances; and that infection, for
example, sometimes acts immediately on the wound; and sometimes
through the constitution. We shall first treat of it as it occurs sporadically in civil practice, where it bears the name of *sloughing phagedæna;*
and next, of those more serious visitations that decimate the patients in
crowded naval or military hospitals, whence it derives its other name,
*hospital gangrene.*

In the cases seen in civil practice, the disease is mostly seated in or
near the genital organs; in the cleft of the nates, in the groin, or at the
upper and inner part of the thigh. It often, but far from invariably,
supervenes on syphilitic ulcers; especially in young prostitutes who have
been exposed to cold and wet, and privation of solid food, and the abuse
of ardent spirits. It is especially liable to be induced by the too free
administration of mercury, or by intemperance and exposure to wet during a mercurial course. The worst cases, however, appear to arise from
neglected local irritation, without any specific virus; as from acrid discharges and defective cleanliness. Mr. Lawrence mentions the case of
a young woman who had suffered from severe small-pox, and from diarrhœa after it. The continual moisture from the rectum, with a mucous
discharge from the vagina, irritated and inflamed the skin of the nates,
and caused a large sloughing phagedænic excavation on both sides.

*Symptoms.*—"It usually commences as a highly irritable and painful
boil, surrounded by a halo of dusky red inflammation, and much elevated;
the patient also in general having mucous discharges from the vagina,
and a diffused redness of integument in the vicinity of the pudenda."
There are severe darting and stinging pains; which are at first intermittent, but gradually establish themselves as a constant symptom, with
occasional exacerbations. When the pustule is ruptured, the exposed
surface of the ulcer displays a stratum of adherent straw-coloured flocculi, mottled with darker points of reddish brown and gray. The sore
thus formed soon enlarges in breadth and depth;—the edges become
everted and attended with a circumscribed thickening, which is surrounded by dusky inflammation and diffused puffy swelling. The surface
is composed of gray or ash-coloured sloughs, which may become brown,
or resemble coagula of blood. The discharge is reddish-brown and
peculiarly fetid, and there is occasionally severe hæmorrhage. Meanwhile the agonizing pain, the hæmorrhage, and the absorption of putrid
matters, soon induce severe irritative fever;—ushered in by loss of sleep,
anxiety, restlessness, and thirst; which, with an exhausting diarrhœa,
produce death in about three weeks; and as delirium is rare, the patient
retains a miserable consciousness of severe suffering till the end. This

disease is *highly contagious,* but it appears to be a *local* disease, and both the constitutional and local symptoms may be removed by measures which destroy the acrid secretions of the ulcer.*

Hospital Gangrene is the name given to this affection when occurring in military and naval practice.

*Causes.*—Like other putrid maladies, it is engendered by crowding together a number of sick and wounded men;—and by inattention to cleanliness and comfort, and to free ventilation, which is so necessary for carrying off the noxious miasmata always generated under those circumstances. It frequently is a concomitant of dysentery or typhus, originating in the same sources. It may affect any kind of wound, or even a bruise, unaccompanied with external solution of continuity.

*Propagation.*—This disease, when once generated, may either spread by *contagion*; that is, may be propagated by the contact of its morbid secretions;—or may be *infectious;* that is, propagated through the medium of its vapour or effluvium. It may, although rarely, occur *sporadically;* that is, may be induced in isolated cases by improper and irritating local and constitutional treatment of the wounded.

*Symptoms.*—According to Mr. Blackadder, it begins in the form of a livid vesicle at the edge of a wound or sore, accompanied with an occasional painful sensation like the sting of a gnat. Sometimes it first appears as a small livid spot on the sore, and near its circumference. In either case the disease soon spreads, and converts the whole surface of the ulcer into an ash-coloured or blackish slough. The discharge, if previously healthy, is at first diminished in quantity, and sanious;—but soon becomes profuse, and dirty yellowish or brown. According to this gentleman, the hospital gangrene is at first a purely *local* affection, like the sloughing phagedæna;—and he says that the constitutional symptoms (typhoid fever, &c.) do not make their appearance before the third or fourth, sometimes not till the the twentieth day.†

*Dr. Hennen's Account.*—The following quotations, however, from Dr. Hennen, display a slight variation from Mr. Blackadder's account. "Let us suppose," says Dr. H., "that our wounded have all been going on well for several days, when suddenly one of our most promising patients complains of severe pain in his head and eyes, a particular tightness about the forehead, loss of sleep, and want of appetite; and that these feelings are accompanied with quickness of pulse and other symptoms of fever; his wound, which had been healthy and granulating, at once becomes tumid, dry, and painful, losing its florid colour, and assuming a dry and glossy coat. This is a description of the first stage of our Bilbao hospital gangrene, and if a brisk emetic were now exhibited, a sur-

---

* Welbank, Med. Chir. Trans. vol. xi.; Lawrence, Lectures in Med. Gaz., vol. v.

† Observations on Phagedæna Gangrenosa. By H. Home Blackadder, Edinburgh, 1818.

geon, not aware of the disease that was about to form, would be aston-
ished at the amelioration of the sore, and the unusual quantity of bile and
of indigested matter evacuated by vomiting."—" If this incipient stage
was overlooked, the febrile symptoms soon became aggravated; the skin
around the sore assumed a higher floiid colour, which shortly became
darker, then bluish, and at last black, with a disposition to vesicate;
whilst the rest of the limb betrayed a tendency to œdema. All these
threatening appearances occurred within twenty-four hours;—and at
this period the wound, *whatever might have been its original shape,
soon assumed the circular form.* The sore now acquired hard prominent ragged edges, giving it a cup-like appearance, with particular
points of the lip of a dirt-yellow hue; while the bottom of the cavity was
lined with a flabby, blackish slough. The rapid progress and circular
form were highly characteristic of hospital gangrene."—" The discharge
in this second stage became dark-coloured and fetid, and the pain extremely poignant."—" The face of the sufferer assumed a ghastly, anxious appearance; his eyes became haggard, and deeply tinged with bile;
his tongue loaded with a brown or blackish fur; his appetite entirely failed
him, and his pulse was considerably sunk in strength, and proportionably
accelerated."—" The third and last stage was now fast approaching.
The surface of the sore was constantly covered with a bloody oozing;
and on lifting up the edge of the flabby slough, the probe was tinged with
dark-coloured grumous blood, with which also its track became immediately filled; repeated and copious venous bleedings now came on;"—" at
length an artery sprung, which, in the attempt to secure it, most probably burst under the ligature."—" Incessant retchings soon came on,
and, with coma, involuntary stools, and hiccough, closed the scene."*

It thus appears, by collating the observations of these two military authorities, that the hospital gangrene may either be a *local disease ;* being produced by local contamination of a wound, and existing for some days before
the system at large is effected by it ;—or it may be *constitutional* from the
first ;—that is, may be induced by the absorption of poisonous miasmata
into the blood; in which latter case the constitutional symptoms precede the
local mischief. In fact, the ordinary constitutional symptoms of hospital
gangrene might be induced in the nurses and attendants on the sick, from
washing the bandages, and from general exposure to noisome effluvia,
without being followed by any local affection whatever.

*Treatment.*—The indications in the treatment of all the forms of
sloughing phagedæna are, 1, to destroy the diseased surface and its secretions;—and, 2, to correct the concomitant contamination of the system.

The first indication is to be carried into effect by means of caustics.
The French use the actual cautery; Mr. Blackadder recomends the liq.

---

* Principles of Military Surgery. By John Hennen, M. D., F. R. S. E., 3rd ed.
London, 1829, pp. 217 *et seq.*

arsenicalis;—but the following mode of using the concentrated nitric acid, as directed by Mr. Welbank, is preferable to either. In the first place, the sore must be thoroughly cleansed, and all its moisture be absorbed by lint or tow. If the sloughs are very thick, they may be removed by means of forceps and scissors. The surrounding parts must next be defended with a thick layer of ointment; then a thick pledget of lint, which may be conveniently fastened to the end of a stick, is to be imbued with the acid, and to be pressed steadily on every part of the diseased surface till the latter is converted into a dry, firm, and insensible mass. This application of course causes more or less pain for the moment, but when that subsides, the patient expresses himself free from his previous severer sufferings. The part may then be covered with simple dressings, and cloths wet with cold water. " It is always prudent, often necessary," says Mr. Welbank, " to remove the eschar at the end of sixteen or twenty hours; and then, if the patient be free from pain, and the ulcer healthy and florid, it is to be treated with common stimulating dressings;—such as cerat. calaminæ, or solution of argenti nitras; or a cerate of turpentine, which may be melted and poured in warm.'' If, however, there be any recurrence of pain, or the least reappearance of the disease, the acid is again and again to be applied till a healthy action is restored.

As for the general treatment;—if the constitution is not affected, opium may be given to allay the pain caused by the disease, and by the application of the escharotic; the bowels should be opened, and the diet regulated so as to support the strength without exciting feverishness.

If the disease, as observed by Hennen, begin with fever of an inflammatory type, and the patient be robust, and the local inflammation intense, a moderate blood-letting may be performed with advantage; with an emetic, purgatives, and the antiphlogistic regimen generally. Mercury is for the most part highly pernicious,[*] (although Mr. Babington says that it may be employed with advantage, if the surrounding inflammation be vivid and intense.)

If, however, the constitutional affection assume a low or typhoid type, either from the beginning or subsequently, the principal dependence is to be placed on opiates and tonics, in order to allay irritation and support the strength, (having first used emetics and cordial laxatives.) If there be much diarrhœa, bark will be hurtful.

*Prevention.*—It will be most necessary to prevent the spreading of this dreadful affection by the freest ventilation, by frequent ablution of the bodies of the sick and wounded, and changes of their bedclothes and linen;—by the instant removal of all excrements or filth;—and by the most scrupulous care in washing the bandages in boiling water, if they

---

[*] Babington on Sloughing Sores. Lond. Med. Journ., vol. lvii. p. 204, and vol. lviii. p. 288.

are to be used again, and in destroying them immediately if they are not. The walls also should be daily whitewashed, and the floor perpetually sprinkled with a solution of the chlorides. All the affected patients should be instantly removed to the greatest possible distance from the others; every thing connected with them should be thoroughly cleansed, and the utmost care to be taken not to convey the infection by means of sponges or dressings, or even by the fingers or instruments of the surgeon; in fact, tow or lint might well supersede sponges, as they might be destroyed after using.

XI. MALIGNANT PUSTULE (Charbon) is a contagious and very fatal disease common in France, but almost unknown in England. It commenees as a little dark red spot, with a stinging or pricking pain; on which there soon appears a pustule or vesicle seated on a hard inflamed base. When this is opened, it is found to contain a slough; black as charcoal; and the sloughing rapidly spreads, involving skin and cellular tissue, and sometimes the muscles beneath.

The account given of this malady by the continental writers is exceedingly confused; but it appears pretty certain, that it is caused by infection or contagion from horned cattle, who at certain seasons are affected with a precisely similar disease; and it further appears that, like hospital gangrene, it may commence in two ways:—

1st. By general infection of the system, from respiring air loaded with miasmata from diseased animals; or from eating their flesh. In this case it commences with constitutional symptoms; and it is this form which is more particularly styled *charbon*.

2ndly. By inoculation of the diseased fluids; and in this case the local symptoms begin before the constitutional. Mr. Lawrence gives an account of a man in Leadenhall Market, who accidentally smeared his face with some stinking hides from South America. The part touched by the putrid matter very soon became red, and swelled, and mortified, and the mortification spread over half the cheek. It is believed that flies which have alighted on the ulcers of the diseased animals, convey the virus, and infect other animals and human beings.

The constitutional symptoms and morbid appearances are those of putrid typhus; the treatment, both constitutional and local, is the same that we have directed for hospital gangrene.*

XII.—MORBID ULCERS.—Under this term Sir E. Home includes a variety of ulcers connected with a disordered state of the constitution, and capable of being removed by particular remedies. Arsenic is said by Mr. Eccles† to be highly useful in sores which are dry and little inflamed,

---

* Lawrence, Med. Gaz. vol. v. p. 392; Dict. de Med. *Art. Charbon, pustule maligne;* Schwabe, Brit. and For. Rev. vol. vii. p. 550.

† Eccles on the Ulcerative Process and its Treatment. Lond. 1834.

and surrounded by much scabbing and exfoliation of the cuticle. Ulcers about the instep and foot, with their edges and the surrounding skin much and extensively thickened like elephantiasis; and often occurring in the lazy and over-fed servants of the opulent;—sometimes yield to mercurial fumigations, or the application of mercurial ointment with camphor.

XIII. THE CUTANEOUS ULCER spreads widely but superficially over the skin, and often heals in one part whilst it spreads to another.

*Treatment.*—Any constitutional disorder must be ascertained and remedied. The best local applications are stimulants, especially the arg. nit., employed in solution, or rather on Mr. Higginbottom's plan.

XIV. THE ULCER OF THE CELLULAR MEMBRANE;—which destroys that tissue more widely than the skin, must be treated as the fistulous or weak, according to circumstances.

XV. MENSTRUAL ULCER.—This name is given to ulcers occurring in chlorotic young women, and exuding a sanguineous fluid at the time of their monthly discharge, if that be absent. Wounds made in operating will frequently do the same.

*Treatment.*—The constitutional disorder must be remedied by proper emmenagogues, and the ulcer be treated on general principles.

XVI. ULCERS ABOUT THE NAILS.—1. A very common and troublesome affection is that which is popularly termed "*the growth of the nail into the flesh,*" and which most usually occurs by the side of the great toe. It does not, however, arise from any alteration in the nail as its name would imply, but the contiguous soft parts are first swelled and inflamed by constant pressure against its edge from the use of tight shoes. If this state be permitted to increase, suppuration occurs, and an ulcer is formed with fungous and exquisitely sensible granulations, in which the edge of the nail is embedded, and which often produces so much pain as totally to prevent walking.

*Treatment.*—The objects are, to remove the irritation caused by the nail, and reduce the swelling of the soft parts. In most cases, if the nail, having been well softened by soaking in warm water, is shaved as thin as possible with a knife or file or bit of glass, the pain and irritation may easily be allayed by rest for a day or two, with leeches and poultices; and then any ulcer that has formed will soon heal. But if the case is more obstinate, the edge of the nail must be removed. This may either be done in the frightfully painful way laid down by Sir A. Cooper and Dupuytren; that is, by passing the sharp blade of a pair of scissors under the nail, cutting it through, and then tearing away the offending portion with forceps;—or it may be effected after a milder fashion, by cutting through the nail with a penknife, just down to the thick layer of cuticle intervening between it and the quick, (as it is called,) and then turning it back.* If the complaint return after this, the whole nail had better be

* Lawrence, Lectures in Med. Gaz.

removed by the application of a blister; or by dissecting it out, together with the gland that secretes it. Persons disposed to this affection should always wear loose shoes, and cut their nails square without removing the corners.

2. ONYCHIA MALIGNA *is a peculiar unhealthy ulcer occurring at the root of the nail, either of the fingers or toes, but more frequently the lat-ter. It commences with a deep red swelling, and an oozing of a thin ichor from under the fold of skin at the root of the nail; and lastly, an ulcer is formed, with a smooth tawny or brown surface, a very fetid sanious discharge, and swelled jagged edges of a peculiar livid dusky hue. It is in general extremely painful, especially at night.

*Treatment.*—Mr. Wardrop recommends mercury to be employed, so as to affect the gums in about a fortnight; and says that then the swell-ing will generally subside, and the ulcer become clean. The mercurial effect should be continued gently till the sore is healed, and for a short time afterwards. The best local applications are, solution of arsenic, (lip. arsen. 3ij. ad aq. ℥ij.) as recommended by Mr. Abernethy, which will generally be found to succeed; solution of corrosive sublimate, (P. L.,) of nitrate of silver, black and yellow wash, and other compounds of the same description.

---

# CHAPTER IX.

## OF MORTIFICATION.

### SECTION I.—OF THE PATHOLOGY OF MORTIFICATION.

DEFINITION.—Mortification signifies the death of any part of the body, in consequence of disease, and a distinction must be made between the mere *death* of a part, immediately following a violent injury, and *morti-fication*, which is preceded by some process of disease.

VARIETIES.—Some persons use the terms *mortification, gangrene,* and *sphacelus,* indiscriminately; but the majority signify by *sphacelus* an utter and irrecoverable loss of life;—and restrict the term *gangrene* to the state which precedes, and commonly (but not inevitably) terminates in sphacelus;—a state in which, as Thompson says, " there is a diminu-tion, but not a total destruction, of the powers of life;—in which the

---

* James Wardrop, F.R.S.E., on Diseases of the Toes and Fingers. Med. Chir. Trans., vol. v.

blood appears to circulate through the larger vessels; in which the nerves still retain a portion of their sensibility, and in which perhaps the part may still be supposed to be capable of recovery."

Another distinction is made between *humid* and *dry* gangrene. The *humid* is often the consequence of inflammation, and the mortified part being loaded with fluid effusions soon undergoes decomposition;—whilst the *dry gangrene* is either preceded by no inflammation at all, or by one so rapid that there is no time for interstitial effusions to occur, and the · mortified part becomes dry and hard;—in the first case being called a *slough*, in the latter an *eschar*.

Another and a most important division is into constitutional and local. By *constitutional* mortification is meant that which primarily originates in constitutional disorder;—or that which, having begun from a local injury, is propagated and maintained by constitutional disorder. By *local mortification* is understood that by which the system is not implicated, and with which it does not sympathize in a violent or dangerous degree.*

CAUSES.—The *local predisposing* causes, are the same as those of ulceration;—namely, congestion, or structural weakness. The constitutional causes of mortification are,—debility from old age, poverty, starvation, hæmorrhage, scurvy, or long-continued disease of any kind;—disease of the heart with contraction of the aortic orifice, so as to impede the arterial circulation;—and the peculiar state induced by the use of diseased grain, especially by the ergot of rye.† These causes are in

* Guthrie, G. J. F.R.S. A Treatise on Gunshot wounds, p. 116. 3rd ed. Lond. 1827.

† A very extraordinary instance of mortification resulting from constitutional disturbance, came under my observation last autumn, in the case of a little girl about six years old, living in Indiana. The child was well nourished and developed, and in good health, until about the middle of September, when an intelligent practitioner of the neighbourhood, visiting another member of her family, was requested to prescribe for her, as she appeared to be slightly indisposed. He examined her, and perceiving no symptoms of serious illness, ordered some gentle cathartic medicine and departed. During his visit the next day, he was summoned from the room of his patient, to another apartment, where the little girl had been amusing herself, as usual, in the morning, and found her prostrate, unconscious, almost pulseless, and somewhat convulsed. The symptoms of sinking became more and more urgent, and, while the surface of the whole body was rapidly losing its temperature, that of the left half—trunk and extremities—became also uniformly livid. She was placed in the warm bath, frictions employed, and, as soon as the power of deglutition was restored, diffusible stimuli were carefully administered. Consciousness and sensibility were restored in about three quarters of an hour, and after the operation of some cathartic medicine, the next morning, she seemed to be as well as ever, with the exception of the left foot and ankle, which continued to be cold, livid and insensible, notwithstanding the most diligent and assiduous employment of the proper means of restoration. No considerable constitutional reaction attended her recovery from the

general *predisposing* merely; but sometimes they are sufficient of themselves to induce mortification, which is then mostly seated in the lower extremities. The *exciting causes* may be divided into—*First, mechanical and chemical injuries*, violent in their degree, but still insufficient'to cause death immediately;—especially gunshot wounds, and compound fractures;—the injection of urine or other stimulant fluids into the cellular tissue;—the application of irritants to constitutions weakened by previous disease; as the application of blisters to children after measles or scarlatina;—long-continued pressure under the same circumstances; hence the sloughing of the skin over the sacrum or trochanters of patients confined to bed with some exhausting disease;—or the application of heat after exposure to cold.

*Secondly*, an *insufficient supply of arterial blood;* whether from ligature of a main artery;—from thickening of its parietes so as to contract its caliber;—from coagulation of the blood within it, or effusion of fibrine into it, as in arteritis;—or from ossification of the artery, and its conversion into a ligamentous cord, which is the cause of *senile gangrene.*

*Thirdly, impediments to the return of venous blood;* whether from ligature of a venous trunk ;—from coagulation of the blood in it;—from tumours (diseased liver for instance) compressing it, or from disease of the heart.

*Fourthly, injury or division of nerves.*—Thus the cornea has been known to slough after division of the fifth nerve. But, in general, deficient nervous influence operates merely as a predisposing cause.

The tissue most disposed to mortification is the cellular; and next to it, tendinous and ligamentous structures, if the cellular tissue surrounding them have been destroyed; then bone, if deprived of its periosteum;— next the skin, especially if the subjacent cellular tissue have mortified, or have become infiltrated with fluid; and lastly, parts of higher organization, as muscles, blood-vessels, and nerves, resist it most.

SECTION II.—OF THE SYMPTOMS AND TREATMENT.

Like ulceration, mortification may either be preceded by inflammation

sudden prostration, and, neither about the foot nor elsewhere were there pain nor any of the usual phenomena of inflammation. About the seventh day from the attack, a circle of demarcation began to form between the dead and living parts, about two inches above the ankle. It was thought best to accelerate the separation by artificial section, and I amputated at the usual point below the knee. The vessels and other textures at the point of division appeared to be sound—the wound healed kindly, and the patient made a good recovery. The foot was black, dry, and wrinkled—no dissection of the wounded part was permitted. The patient resided in a neighbourhood subject to epidemics of what is called bilious fever, and where, during this season, adynamic symptoms were more or less urgent in most of the cases. F.

or not. On the one hand, a part weakened by disease or injury may mortify, because it has not strength to support the inflammation which ensues;—or, on the other hand, it may mortify slowly, and the mortification may spread slowly, without there being energy enough in the system to set up inflammation;—which in its adhesive form is necessary to check the mortification and repair its ravages.

*Symptoms.*—When inflammation is about to terminate in mortification, its redness gradually assumes a darker tint, and becomes purple or blue; the heat, sensibility, and pain diminish; but the swelling often increases in consequence of the continued effusion of sanguinolent serum, which not unfrequently exudes through the skin, and elevates the cuticle into blisters. If the *gangrene* proceed to *sphacelus*, the colour becomes dirty brown or black; the parts become soft, flaccid, and cold, and they crepitate when pressed, and emit a cadaverous odour from the gases that are evolved by incipient putrefaction. Whilst gangrene is spreading, the dark colour is diffused, and insensibly lost in the surrounding skin; but when its progress is arrested, a healthy circulation is re-established up to the very margin of the sphacelated portion, and a bright red line of adhesive inflammation (called the *line of demarcation*) separates the living parts from the dead. And the appearance of this line is most important as a means of *prognosis*, because it shows that the mischief has ceased, and that there is a disposition to repair its ravages.

*Separation of the Mortified Part.*—It is at this line that the dead part is separated, which separation is said, according to Hunter's theory, to be produced by ulcerative absorption; although according to J. W. Earle, it is more probably the mere result of the softening and suppuration of that layer of the living parts which is contiguous to the dead. Be this, however, as it may, a narrow white line, consisting of a narrow circular vesicle, and formed by a separation of the cuticle, first appears on the bright line of adhesive inflammation before mentioned;—and when this is broken, a chain of minute ulcers are seen under it. These gradually unite and form a chink;—which widens and deepens till the slough is entirely detached;—and then a granulating and suppurating surface remains. In this manner the whole of a mortified limb has been spontaneously amputated;—the bone and tendons separating higher up, and being more slowly detached than the skin, muscles, blood-vessels. When the adhesive inflammation has duly occurred, this process of separation is unattended with hæmorrhage; the smaller vessels being, as Dr. Carswell thinks, obliterated by the effusion of lymph, and the larger ones by the coagulation and organization of the blood within them. And this coagulation extends some distance from the mortified part, so that a limb has been amputated in the thigh for mortification of the leg, without the loss of any blood from the femoral artery. Sometimes, however, as in hospital gangrene, these vital processes of adhesion are deficient, and the blood is found fluid in the vessels, so that the separation of the slough is attended with severe hæmorrhage.

*Constitutional Symptoms.*—The constitutional symptoms of mortification vary with its cause. If it arise, in a healthy subject, from acute inflammation which is still progressing, there will be healthy inflammatory fever;—but, on the other hand, if the mortification be very extensive;—if the inflammation of the adjacent parts be unhealthy, with no disposition to form the line of demarcation, but, on the contrary, with a greater tendency to serous effusion;—or if the mortified part be of great importance, as intestine or lung, the constitutional symptoms will be of a low typhoid cast;—there will be great anxiety, hiccough, a jaundiced skin, a soft or rapid, thready, and jerking pulse; and frequently profuse perspiration of a cadaverous odour.

*Diagnosis.*—It is important not to mistake the lividity and vesication of bruises, especially when they accompany fractures, for gangrene. They may easily be distinguished by their sensibility and temperature; and by the fact, that in gangrene the whole cuticle has lost its adhesion to the cutis; so that pressure will cause the vesicle to shift its place.

*Treatment.*—The general indications are, to allay inflammation if excessive:—to support the strength; and to cause the formation of a line of a healthy adhesion, by which the mortification may be arrested.

If there be an acute inflammation which threatens to terminate in gangrene;—or if gangrene have actually occurred in a healthy, young, robust subject, with great pain, and a full, hard, strong pulse; and if it appear likely to spread from the violence of inflammation;—it will be necessary to prevent its occurrence or extension, by bleeding, purging, and the general antiphlogistic treatment; whilst leeches, poultices, or lotions may be applied locally. But care must always be taken to reduce the strength as little as possible, whenever a part is so injured that its death is probable.

But an opposite treatment must be pursued if the pulse is quick and feeble, and there are the other signs of deficient vital power that have been before mentioned. The principal remedies for this state are bark, opium, and wine;—whose united effect should be to render the pulse slower and firmer and to induce a warm, gentle perspiration, and sleep;— whilst it will be a sign that they are injudiciously administered, if they induce or aggravate delirium and restlessness. The best form of administering the bark is a good decoction of *cinchona lancifolia*, to which opium, acids, ammonia or other stimulants, may be added; as in F. 1, 2, 3, 26. If the decoction disagree with the stomach, quinine may be given by itself in doses of three grains. *Opium* is of prodigious utility from its power of allaying irritability; so that it renders the constitution insensible as it were to the local mischief;—or, in Hunter's language, " It does good by not letting the disease do harm to the constitution." At the same time, by supporting the capillary circulation, as justly insisted on by Mr. Skey, it favours the production of the much desired boundary line of adhesive inflammation. It may in general be combined with the bark, in the dose of from seven to fifteen minims of the tincture every four hours; but if there be at any time very great restlessness, especially towards night, it will be better to give a full dose at once;—such as fifty or sixty minims of the tincture, or two or three grains of the solid opium, which will not be too much, if the patient have been taking it liberally before. Vomiting, and hiccup are to be treated as directed in Part I., chap. i. Wine—especially port—and nutriment, in the shape of arrow-root, beef-tea, gruel, &c. should be administered at moderate intervals.

*Local Measures.*—If a part be gangrenous, but not quite dead, its temperature must be carefully maintained, and its actions supported by warm poultices and fomentations.

If sphacelus has actually occurred, and the powers of the system are languid, and there is little disposition to form the line of demarcation, or throw off the dead parts, stimulating applications are necessary, especially the nitric acid lotion, F. 17, which may be liberally poured on the parts, and afterwards applied on lint under the poultice;—the ung. resinæ, thinned with turpentine;—the balsam of Peru;—tincture of myrrh, or of benzoin;—solution of the chlorides probably diluted, (F. 39;)—or poultices of yeast, (F. 46,) or of stale beer grounds. Any loose portions of slough may be cut away by scissors, taking care not to tear them away violently.

*Incisions* are of great service in spreading inflammatory mortification, attended with extensive effusion of serous or purulent fluids; which not only contaminate the blood, and depress the nervous system by their absorption, but also propagate the disease by diffusing themselves into parts that are still sound, and rendering them incapable of healthy inflammation.

*Question of Amputation.*—When a portion of an entire limb has mortified, it will be expedient to perform amputation, in order to avoid the delay and annoyance of a spontaneous separation. And the operation may in any case be performed as soon as the disease is arrested, and the line of demarcation is established;—provided always that the patient has vigour enough to bear the loss of blood which must in some degree necessarily ensue. Sir A. Cooper mentions a case in which a mortified leg was separating favourably through the calf, when the projecting bones were sawn off, with the view of expediting the process. A few granulations were accidentally wounded, and the trivial hæmorrhage that ensued was fatal.* But the rule generally given is to wait till the disease is arrested by a line of healthy inflammation, otherwise the stump may become gangrenous.

* Lectures by Tyrrell, vol. i. p. 237.

But still it will be proper to *amputate, without waiting for the line of separation*, if the mortification be strictly local as to its cause, and if it have not yet affected the constitution; as, for instance, in mortification of a limb from injury or aneurism of the large arterial trunks; or from severe compound fracture.    And as far as can be gathered from the works of Guthrie, Larrey, and James, it is justifiable as a last resource whenever there appears little or no disposition to limit gangrene, and whenever it spreads rapidly.  " Where gangrene," says Mr. Guthrie, " is rapidly extending towards the trunk of the body, without any hope of its cessation, the operation is to be tried; for it has certainly succeeded, where death would in a few hours have ensued."*

### MORTIFICATION FROM OBSTACLE TO THE RETURN OF VENOUS BLOOD.

This form of mortification mostly effects the lower extremities, and is always preceded by great œdema.   It may occur *before* inflammation, or may be a *consequence* of inflammation, which in œdematous parts is always liable to terminate in gangrene.  In the former case, the skin of the œdematous limb having become pale, smooth, glossy, and tense, assumes a mottled aspect of a dull red or purple colour from distention of the subcutaneous veins.  " Then, at some part where the conjestion is greatest, or where the skin is less yielding, as over the tibia, or above the malleoli, phlyctenæ, or large bullæ, are formed by the effusion of serosity, either alone or mixed with blood, under the cuticle.  When these burst, the cutis beneath presents a dark red or brown colour, and very soon is converted into a dirty-yellow or ash-gray slough."†   After the spread of the mortification to a given extent, inflammation occurs; and the slough, which is mostly an oval patch of skin and cellular tissue, separates.—This form of mortification, and the ulcer that is caused by it, are to be treated by warm fomentatious ; poultices of yeast, carrots, or stale beer grounds, and stimulating dressings, of which the nitric acid lotion is the best.

### MORTIFICATION FROM PRESSURE.

When a patient is confined to bed with some very tedious and dehilitating malady, as a fever ;—and especially if he has not strength to shift his posture occasionally, the skin covering various projecting bony points, (as the sacrum, brim of the illium, or great trochanter,) is apt to inflame and rapidly ulcerate or slough; and more particularly if irritated by negleet of cleanliness, or by the contact of urine.  The first thing often complained of by the patient is a sense of pricking, as though there were crumbs or salt in the bed.  The part, if examined at first, looks red and

* Op. cit. p. 132.                              † Carswell, op. cit.

rough; then becomes excoriated and ulcerates, or turns black, and mortifies.

*Treatment.*—If detected before actual sloughing, the best plan is to apply the admirable soft poultice described under F. 47, in the Appendix;—if, however, the sloughing has begun, a stimulating or fermenting poultice should be applied; and in either case it is indispensable to arrange small pillows or cushions, so as to take off all weight from the part affected.

### SENILE GANGRENE.

*Symptoms.*—This affection commences by a purple or black spot on the inner sides or extremity of one of the smaller toes; from which spot "the cuticle," says Pott, "is always found to be detached, and the skin under it to be of a dark red colour." "In some few instances, there is little or no pain; but in by far the majority, the patients feel great uneasiness through the whole foot or joint of the ankle, particularly in the night, even before these parts show any mark of distemper, or before there is any other than a small discoloured spot at the end of one of the little toes."* Its progress in some cases is slow, in others rapid and horribly painful. After its first appearance, the actual gangrene will generally be preceded by a dark red conjestive inflammation. The dead parts become shrunk, dry, and hard; and when the disease makes a temporary pause, which it frequently does, they slowly slough away; but a fresh accession of gangrene mostly supervenes before any progress has been made towards cicatrization. In this way the patient may live several winters, but generally sinks exhausted with the nocturnal pain before the whole foot is destroyed.

*Pathology.*—This disease is supposed by Andral to be the result of debility of the capillaries, with coagulation of the blood in them; but the more prevalent opinion is that it is caused by the ossification of the arteries, and obliteration of the smaller trunks, which are converted into ligamentous cords by a fibrous tissue generated in their cavities or between their walls.

This affection mostly happens to old persons, especially if they have been great eaters. They are generally found to have lost their hair and teeth, and their face and hands betray a languid circulation. It mostly attacks men. Mr. James,† however, relates a case in which it happened to a woman at forty-two; but she had disease of the heart.

*Treatment.*—The chief reliance is to be placed on opium, both in order to soothe the pain and support the capillary circulation. The solid form is best, and should be given in sufficient quantity to procure

* Pott's Chirurgical Works. 8 vo. Lond. 1771.
† James on Inflammation, pp. 545 and 552.

ease and sleep.  Stimulating poultices of beer grounds, port wine, and oatmeal, the chloride of soda.  F. 39, 17, &c. are the best local applications.  Amputation may perhaps be justified in very few cases.  Pott mentions the curious fact, that the ligaments by which the dead loose bones may be retained, often preserve their sensibility, and cause intense pain if cut through.

---

# CHAPTER X.

## OF SCROFULA.

*Syn.—Struma, King's Evil.*

DEFINITION.—Scrofula is a state of constitutional debility, with a tendeney to indolent inflammatory diseases.

GENERAL DESCRIPTION.—There are two varieties of scrofulous habits, which, although they agree in the main essential of constitutional debility, are yet totally opposite in many respects.  In the *first*, (or *sanguine variety*,) the skin is remarkably fair and thin, showing the blue veins through it, and presenting the most brilliant contrasts of red and white;—the eyes are light blue;—the hair light or reddish, the forehead ample, and the intellect lively and precocious.  Sometimes, however, as Mayo observes, the skin is *dark* and transparent, and the eyes dark, although there is the same general characteristic of delicacy and vivacity.*

In the *second* (or *phlegmatic*) *variety*, the whole aspect is dull and unpromising;—the skin thick and muddy; the hair dark and coarse;—the eyes greenish or hazel, with dilated pupils—the belly tumid—the disposition dull, heavy, and listless to outward appearance; although persons of this conformation will very generally be found to possess a clear and vigorous intellect, and powers of application far above the average.  The great Dr. Johnson is an example.†

In both varieties the natural functions are liable to be performed irregularly.  Digestion is weak, the tongue often furred, and red on its tip and edges;—the upper lip swelled;—the appetite sometimes deficient, but more usually excessive, and attended with a craving for indigestible sub-

---

* Philosophy of Living, 2nd edit. 1838, p. 24.

† Of seventy two scrofulous children, Mr. Carmichael found that forty-four had blue eyes, and twenty-eight hazel or black eyes.  Of the forty-four with blue eyes, twenty one had fair delicate skins and light hair;—and twenty-three had sallow or brown skins and dark hair  An Essay on Scrofula, by Richard Carmichael, Lond. 1810.

stances;—the bowels torpid;—the blood thin and watery;—the muscles pale and flabby;—and the heart and arteries, as well as the intestines, thin and weak.

In the sanguine variety, the growth is generally rapid, and the bodily conformation good, as far as outward form is concerned;—the limbs well made, the stature tall, and the chest broad.  Puberty also is early, and sexual passion is often strongly manifested before the degree of bodily strength permits it to be indulged in with impunity.  This is peculiarly the case with the females; who are usually remarkable for that early and evanescent beauty which arises from a great development of the adipose tissue.  In the phlegmatic variety, on the other hand, the growth is often stunted, the chest narrow, and the limbs deformed with rickets, and puberty retarded, especially in the females, who are liable to prolonged chlorosis.

CAUSES.—Scrofula being thus defined to be a peculiar state of the constitution, it may be shown, first, that it may be *congenital* and *hereditary;* that is to say, that scrofulous parents may transmit their peculiar organization, and predisposition to disease, to their children.  Not that it follows (as some foolishly quibble) that all the offspring of all scrofulous parents will necessarily have scrofulous disease; nor yet does it follow that the parents must necessarily be scrofulous, although the children are so born.  For parents may beget scrofulous children, if debilitated by privation or disease;—if either of them is very old or very young; and probably if either of them labours under a venereal tint, or has been profusely treated with mercury, or has a decided tendency to gout.

2ndly.  The scrofulous habit, if not congenital, may probably be created by any circumstance capable directly or indirectly, of lowering the vital energies, especially poverty and wretchedness; meager, watery, and insufficient food;—neglect of exercise;—confinement in close, foul apartments;—insufficient clothing;—and habitual exposure to damp and cold. It is exceedingly common in the insular and variable climate of England, and still more so in Scotland;—and it is well known that monkeys and parrots, as well as human beings, brought to this country, from the tropics, not unfrequently die of consumption or other scrofulous disease.

3rdly.  The scrofulous habit may be so intense, that the child is attacked with some of the diseases that we shall presently describe, in spite of all care.  Or, on the other hand, actual disease may not appear unless the health is first depressed by want of the necessaries of life, or by some other disease.  Thus scrofulous disease is exceedingly apt to follow scarlatina, measles, the small-pox, or any other acute malady, especially if treated by too much bleeding and mercury.  Moreover, every thing that disorders the digestive organs may bring it into action.  Hence it may be excited in the rich by gross, stimulating, irregular diet, as well as the poor by their flatulent fare of potatoes or oatmeal.  It rarely breaks

15

out before two or after thirty years of age;—although it may be called
into active operation at any age by circumstances which lower the health.

PATHOLOGY OF TUBERCLE.—The most characteristic element of scrofulous disease is the deposite of a peculiar kind of unhealthy lymph,
generally found in round masses, whence it derives the name of *tubercle.*
Like the unhealthy formations that will be spoken of in the next chapter, it may be deposited in three forms; viz.—1st. In distinct masses,
rounded or irregular. 2ndly. It may be infiltrated generally through the
tissues of an organ. Or, 3rdly. It may entirely usurp the place and
form of some tissue; which is then said to be converted into it. In the
first form it is most frequently found in the lungs, (where it gives rise
to pulmonary consumption,) in the follicles of the intestines in the cancelli of bones, in the pleura or peritonæum, and in the cellular tissue. In
the second and third forms, it is found in the lymphatic vessels and
glands, and in the breast, testis, liver, and kidneys; although it is also
frequently deposited in these glands or in their tubes, in distinct nodules.
But wherever it may be, its course is the same. In its *first stage* it is
deposited slowly and insidiously;—causing no pain or other symptom,
unless it mechanically interfere with some function. In this quiescent
state it may remain for an indefinite period, till at length the *second stage*
arrives. Then the surrounding tissue inflame, and form an abscess,
which contains the tubercle, softened and brokened down by the effusion
of serum and pus. In the *third stage* the abscess bursts, allows the
tubercle to escape, and then in favourable cases may contract and heal.
Sometimes the tubercle undergoes a natural cure by being converted into
a chalky or earthy substance, which may be quiescent for years.

Tubercle is generally considered to be unorganized, and destitute of
vitality. In its first stage, however, it is of a lightish gray colour, semi-
transparent, and commonly called *crude, miliary,* or *unripe;* and in this
stage Mr. Grant Calder thinks it alive and organized; and that it only
excites suppuration in its second stage, because it dies and becomes a
foreign substance. In this stage it becomes yellow, opaque, and curdy,
and is said to be *ripe;* moreover, its softening is by some supposed to be
an organic process.*

Besides tubercular disease, scrofulous patients are liable to a variety of
insidious, lingering, and obstinate inflammations. The lymph effused is
often frail and curdy;—the pus serous and flaky;—and scrofulous ulcers,
weak, with pink surface, flabby granulations, and loose edges.

GENERAL TREATMENT.—The indications are to strengthen the system
and prevent local disease by rendering the blood pure and the circulation
vigorous, and by keeping up the secretions. The means are both *regi-*

---

* Vide Latham's *Lectures*, xii.; Carswell, *op. cit.* Fasciculous *Tubercle;* Grant
Calder, *Med. Gaz.*, vol. xxii. p. 286.

*menial* and *medicinal.* The former, which are infinitely the more important, are food, air, exercise, and bathing.

(1) The *diet* of the scrofulous should be nutritious, digestible, and abundant, consisting of meat, bread, and farinaceous substances generally, with a sufficient quantity of beer or wine to promote digestion, without creating drowsiness or feverishness. The greatest attention should be paid to the quality of the milk of the mother or nurse; and to feed the child judiciously during the second year.

(2) The *clothing* should be warm, especially for the neck, chest, and feet;—so as to keep up the cutaneous circulation, and prevent congestion in the chest or abdomen. Flannel should be worn nearest the skin both in winter and summer;—in the former, for direct warmth; in the latter, to neutralize any accidental changes of temperature.

(3) Free *exercise* of the muscles and lungs in pure open air is indispensable. The accelerated venous circulation which it causes, and the compression of the abdominal viscera by the contraction of its muscles, are, as Mr. Carmichael has justly shown, the best means of promoting the action of the liver, and of preventing costiveness with its attendant evils. But exercise should be *voluntary,*—because then it will not be likely to be carried to the pitch of *fatigue,* than which nothing can be more injurious. *Gymnastic exercises* should be used with the utmost cantion.

(4) The best *residence* for the scrofulous is one that is warm, without being damp in the winter, and cool and bracing in the summer. The high lands of the interior, Malvern, for instance, or Clifton, in the summer;—" in the late autumn, when the air loses its freshness, and is tainted with the falling leaf and decaying vegetation, the sea side;"*—in the winter and spring, the mild climate of the Isle of Wight or coast of Devon, or a town residence, are alternations that are advisable for those that can afford them. But if the habit be extremely delicate, and disposed to phthisis, nothing can be better than a removal to Madeira;—provided that it be adopted in time;—and the sufferer be not expatriated (as is too often the case) merely to die.

(5) Daily *washing and friction* of the skin are as beneficial to the scrofulous as they are to every one else; and if the patient be precluded from taking exercise, friction is indispensable. Cold *sea-bathing* is in general so advantageous, that it has been deemed a specific. An aperient dose should be given before commencing it, if the habit be gross; and it is a good plan to use a tepid bath or two (90°—80°) first. The object in using the cold bath is to produce a *vigorous reaction;*—consequently, before taking it, the nervous and circulating systems should be in some degree of excitement; and the skin should be warm although not per-

* Mayo, Philosophy of Living.

spiring.  If the bather be strong, he may plunge into the open sea early
in the morning on an empty stomach, not only with impunity but with
advantage; but the forenoon is the best time for a weakly child, when the
air has become warm, and the system is invigorated with a breakfast.
If after bathing the surface is cold, numb, and pinched, (immersion not
having been protracted,) it is injurious.  In many cases, especially of
scrofulous ulcers, *river bathing* will be found more efficacious.

MEDICINAL TREATMENT.—The medicines of use in scrofula are, first,
*aperients*, to restore and maintain a proper action of the liver and bowels;
—secondly, *antacids;*—and thirdly, medicines capable of promoting digestion, and rendering the flesh and blood more sound and healthy.

(1) If at any time the bowels are much confined, or if there is a state of
feverishness, or if there is any scrofulous disease going on that is attended
with pain and inflammation, it will be advisable to give an active dose of
calomel, jalap, or scammony.  And the bowels should to kept always
regular by some mild aperient, such as rhubarb, magnesia, or castor oil;
with a little aloes, blue-pill, or hyd. c. creta occasionally, if the stools
are not properly tinged with bile.  But the patient must not be weakened
by unlimited purging, nor must calomel be used without consideration.

(2) *Alkalis* are of great service in scrofula, not only by neutralizing
acrid secretion in the stomach and bowels, but (as we may suppose) by
altering the constitution of the blood.  They are especially indicated if
the patient complains of heartburn, or great thirst, or if the tongue is
very red, or if there is a sinking and craving for food soon after meals.
Carmichael recommends a combination of chalk and sesquicarbonate of
soda, (gr. x. of the former, gr. v. of the latter,) thrice a day after meals;
F. 27 will answer the same purpose.  The liq. potassæ is more useful
for adults.

(3) Before reviewing the remedies that come under our third head, we
must warn our junior readers not to be too credulous when they hear of
a new *specific* for scrofula.  Common sense ought to teach, that diseases depending on an original vice of constitution are not in every instance to be cured by one remedy, still less that an organization feeble
in every tissue, and low in vitality, is infallibly to be renewed and per-
fected by any remedy.  If a medicine improves the appetite and flesh
and strength, it may be persevered in; but if it causes feverishness, emaciation, or debility, no vague idea of its specific virtues ought to induce
the practitioner to continue it.

*Bark* is of immense service when there is great exhaustion from suppuration, or when ulcers spread rapidly.  The decoction with quinine, or
liq. cinchonæ flavæ (F. 26.) are the best forms.

*Iron* is better adapted for permanent administration than bark; especially for thin, pale, flabby children, whose liver and bowels are kept in
proper action.  The *muriated tincture*, F. 63; the *ammonio-chloride,*

F. 62, (whose advantage is that it can be combined with alkalis, although it is often too stimulating for children;) the *sesquioxyde*, F. 82; and a combination of the protoxyde, with aloes and an alkali, will all be found useful.—(F. 28.)

*Sarsaparilla* often produces the most unlooked for benefit, especially the alkaline infusions, F. 56, 57, or the compound decoction (without mezereon and guiacum) given in a concentrated form, so that the stomach may not be offended by the bulk of fluid in which it is too much the fashion to prescribe it. As we cannot explain its operation, the existence of the disease is the only indication for its administration. It may always be given in cachectic diseases, when there is no palpable cause; in fact, when we are at a loss what to prescribe. But it is of most peculiar service when there is great weakness with great irritability; when tonics and nutriment cause feverishness, when the tongue is flabby, coated and rather sore, and nothing seems to agree.

*Iodine* should always be administered in combination with a metal, or alkali, or salt that renders it soluble—not in the form of simple tincture dropped on water. It should, moreover, be given in small doses for a long period; half a grain per diem, gradually increased to a grain, is quite enough for an adult. A slight action on the bowels and increase of the urine may be expected; but it should not be permitted to cause emaciation. The iodide of iron in doses of gr. ¼ *ter die;* or a combination of tinct. ferri. mur. ℥ xv. with the tinct. iodin. comp. (P. L.) ℥ v. *ter die;* the iodide of potassium in doses of not more than gr. iii.-v. *ter die*, with decoction of sarsaparilla; and F. 74; are convenient forms of administration. *Burnt sponge* in doses of ʒss *ter die*; and the oil of the cod's liver, of which two drachms may be given daily to a child, and four to an adult, are said to have similar virtues. The latter is said to relax the bowels gently, and promote nutrition, and contains a little iodine.*

The *sulphates of zinc and copper* in small doses are sometimes serviceable as tonics. The *chlorides of calcium* and *barium* were formerly much praised, but seem to have fallen into merited oblivion.

Pain, when violent, must be relieved with opium or other anodynes; and the extracts of conium and aconite in regular doses thrice a day, are often of great service when there are intractable ulcers. The aconite requires caution in its use.

We may add, that F. 26, 28, 52, 54, 58, 80, are combinations of various tonics, aperients, and alteratives, that will occasionally be found serviceable.†

* Taufflied, Lond. Med. Gaz. Feb. 28, 1840.

† Dr. Negrier of Angers has for some years past been trying the effects of an infusion of the leaves of the walnut-tree, in a variety of forms of scrofulous disease, with very favourable effects. A handful of fresh or slightly dried leaves may be

## PARTICULAR SCROFULOUS DISEASES.

(1.) OF THE SKIN.—Scrofulous children are extremely subject to eruptions of small flat pustules about the ears and mouth and other parts, and with excoriations of the skin, and exudation of thin acrid matter which dries into scabs;—to be *treated* by attention to the health;—the frequent use of soap and water, and the application of mild and stimulating ointments of oxyde of zinc, white and red percipitates, or nitrate of mercury, or of lead. This description and treatment may include almost all the multifarious forms of impetigo and porrigo.

(2.) CHRONIC ABSCESSES (independent of those which are caused by diseased glands or bone) may occur under three forms.—1st. They may commence imperceptibly in the cellular tissue. 2ndly. A circular piece of skin, of the size of a shilling or half-crown, with the tissue immediately beneath, may slowly inflame and swell, forming a hard red painless tumour, like a carbuncle. After a time it suppurates imperfectly, and it does not get well till the whole of the diseased part is destroyed by ulceration. 3dly. A small hard tumour of unhealthy lymph may form in the cellular tissue, which after a time inflames, causes abscess, and then sloughs out.

The *treatment* of the first variety is the same as that of chronic abscess generally. The two others should be left to themselves till they suppurate;—then it may be expedient, if there is a great piece of thin purple skin, to destroy it by potassa fusa; and the case afterwards comes under the head of scrofulous ulcer.

(3.) DISEASE OF THE LYMPHATIC GLANDS, especially in the neck is the commonest of scrofulous maladies, and depends on a deposite of tubercle into them or their vessels adjoining. One or more glands enlarge, and form tumours that are perfectly indolent and painless. Thus they may remain for years, stationary or slowly enlarging, till at length, from local irritation or disorder of the health, they inflame, and chronic abscesses form between them and the skin. In some few cases after the abscess is opened, the cyst contracts and heals, the glands remaining nearly as before. But more generally, all the skin covering the abscess becomes red and thin, and ulcerates; and the ulcer heals with an ugly puckered cicatrix, but not till the whole gland has wasted with suppuration. These swellings have been known to destroy life by compressing the trachea

boiled in a pint of water, and a small cup full taken twice a day. An extract may also be used in pills or thick sirup. A strong decoction is also applied to scrofulous ulcers with excellent effects.

The Editor of the Medica Chirug. expresses a favourable opinion of the remedy, and remarks respecting it what all observing practitioners have noticed, " that scrofu. lous diseases are on the whole much more benefited by vegetable remedies than those of a metallic nature," with the exception perhaps of Iron.        F.

or cervical vessels, or by bursting into them. Sometimes they undergo a cure by the chalky transformation before spoken of.*

*Treatment.*—The health must be amended by the measures before detailed;—and an endeavour must be made to cause absorption, by fomentation with hot salt water, or the zinc lotion, or cold poultices made with sea-weed;—by an occasional leech when irritated;—and by ointments of iodine when indolent. It may sometimes be expedient to extirpate one or more glands. But if suppuration occurs, and *if the skin begins to redden;* an opening should be made in the manner, and with the precautions, laid down in the section on *chronic abscess* (p. 80.)

TABES MESENTERICA, or MARASMUS, consists in a tubercular disease of the mesenteric glands, and of the follicles of the intestines, precisely similar in its course and phenomena to the same disease in the cervical glands. The numerous abscesses that form in the mesentery burst into the intestines, or into the abdominal cavity; and on examination the peritonæum is found as thick as leather, and the intestines resembling a collection of cells rather than a simple tube.

*Symptoms.*—Emaciation and voracity, owing to the obstructed course of the chyle;—the belly swelled and hard;—the skin dry and harsh;—the eyes red;—the tòngue strawberry-coloured;—the breath foul;—the stools clay-coloured and offensive, sometimes costive, sometimes extremely relaxed. The patient of course dies hectic, although he often lasts wonderfully long.

*Treatment.*—Animal food and other nutriment given in small quantities at short intervals;—mild mercurials to amend the intestinal secretions, especially the combination of hydr. bichlorid. with tinct. cinchonæ; —tepid bathing;—stimulating liniments to the abdomen;—change of air; and the cautious administration of the antiscrofulous remedies before mentioned.

(4.) SCROFULOUS ULCERS may be a result of the pustules and excoriations of the skin that have been spoken of;—or they may be formed by the ulceration of chronic abscesses; in which case they sometimes destroy extensive tracts of skin and cellular tissue, and may kill the patient by exhaustion, or render a limb rigid and useless if he recover. Or they may be attended with a hardened base, thick everted edges, a copious formation of pale granulations, and deposite of unhealthy lymph into the adjoining cellular tissue, which, with the granulations, is liable to fits of sloughing, preceded by severe pain.

* Ulceration of the tonsils and chronic disease of the mucous membrane of the fauces, whether of a specific character or not, are often exciting causes of these engorgements of the cervical lymphatics, and the surgeon should always examine the throat in such cases, with a view to this connexion. The use of stimulating gargles or the application of nitrate of silver will generally relieve the throat, and the glandular enlargements on the outside will often disappear immediately, unless they have already proceeded to suppuration. F.

*Treatment.*—We have nothing to add to the treatment of the *weak* and *irritable ulcer*, to which classes these must be referred. The preparations of iodine, F. 75 *et seq.* should have a fair trial.

Scrofulous diseases of the *bones, joints,* and *eye,* will be described under the head of their respective tissue.

### NOTE.

Genuine tuberculous scrofula is less common in the Valley of the Mississippi than on the Eastern coast of the Union. But a very large portion of what is regarded and treated as scrofulous disease in this part of the country appears to me to be merely the result of indiscreet mercurialization. Under the prevalent idea that biliary derangements either constitute, or co-exist with, every departure from health, some form of mercury is administered, in almost every prescription, and the whole capillary system of persons, who happen to be occasionally unwell, soon becomes impregnated and poisoned by this subtile mineral.

So too, if an alterative impression be desired, under any morbid condition, whatever, instead of employing regimen, diet and more harmless medicaments, it is common to resort indiscriminately to mercurial agents. The consequences of such reckless medication present themselves to the physician in dyspeptic affections, chronic headachs, pains in the limbs called rheumatic, &c. and to the surgeon in the more striking forms of alveolar absorption and adhesions, inveterate ulcerations of the fauces and nostrils where no specific taint has been suspected, and in various degenerations, malignant or semi-malignant, of glandular organs.

Moreover, the evil does not stop with the individual,—for where important elementary tissues are so deteriorated in the parents, a constitutional infirmity will be impressed on the offspring, while, if it may not properly be called scrofulous from birth, is the most favourable condition possible, for the development of the phenomena of that diathesis, whenever co-operating influences shall assail the unfortunate subject.

The interests of humanity, no less than the honour of medicine demand that those who observe and understand these things, should utter, on all proper occasions, the most unqualified protestations against such abuses of a medicinal agent whose timely and judicious use is so important to the healing art, and thus prevent it from becoming so detestable, that its employment will not be tolerated at all. F.

---

# CHAPTER XI.

## ON MALIGNANT DISEASES.

### SECTION I.—INTRODUCTORY.

DEFINITION.—Malignant diseases consist in the deposite and ulterior changes of a substance altogether alien to healthy structure. They possess the following characteristics. (1.) They terminate in the gradual destruction or transformation of the tissues which they affect. (2.) They progressively invade and destroy the tissues in their vicinity.

(3.) They travel in the course of the lymphatics, and attack the nearest glands. (4.) They generally affect several organs in the same individual; and (5.) If mechanically removed from any part, they mostly reappear in or near the cicatrix.*

It will be manifest from this definition that malignant diseases are essentially *constitutional;* and that many ulcerations (such as *lupus,*) although destructive, and perhaps incurable, are yet not truly malignant, because they are purely *local;*—because they do not attack several organs in the same individual, and because if they are removed thoroughly they do not return.†

FORMATION.—According to Carswell, malignant diseases may either be formed by *secretion;*—that is, may be deposited into the interstices, or upon the surface of tissues;—or they may be formed in the way of *nutrition* or *formation;*—that is, may be deposited as part of the molecular texture of organs; the normal tissue being gradually replaced by one composed of the malignant growth.

ANATOMICAL CHARACTERS.—It appears from the researches of Müller, that malignant tissues are developed in the same manner that Schwann has shown the earliest normal tissues of the embryo both of animals and plants to be. The earliest organic formation in the structureless jelly of the embryo is a little granule, called a nucleus or *cytoblast,‡* which has other minuter granules or nucleoli adhering to it. The nucleus, imbibing nutriment from the fluids around it, throws out a delicate vesicle which projects from it as a watch-glass from a watch. This vesicle enlarging, becomes a cell, with the nucleus imbedded in its parietes. The cell thus developed may undergo an infinity of transformations. It may become elongated or *caudate,* and form a fibre. The apposition of cells so elongated may form a fibrous tissue. Lastly, a cell-formed tissue may increase, by the formation of new nuclei and cells either within the old ones, or exterior to them and in their interstices.

Now Müller describes all malignant growths as being composed of

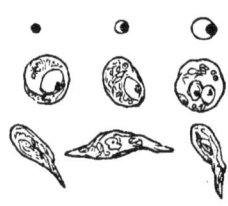

two parts. 1st, of granules, cytoblasts, and cells of different kinds; whose formation may be understood from the rough sketch we have given of Schwann's opinions aided by the diagram;§—and, 2ndly, of a cellular tissue, in which the former parts are imbedded; which cellular tissue is perhaps formed sometimes of adherent caudate cells,

* Carswell's Pathology.

† C. Hawkins on Malignant Disease of the Face. Med. Chir. Trans. vol. xxi.

‡ From κυτος, cells, and βλατος, germ.

§ The upper three figures of the cut are intended to illustrate the development of cells. The others represent the nucleated cells both round and caudate, of cancer and medullary sarcoma.

sometimes of the distended parietes of old cells which have become filled by the growth of new ones in their cavity. It must be added, that malignant growths are almost entirely composed of albumen;—that they are all supplied with ordinary blood-vessels, some more and some less;— and that they scarcely differ from some innocent albuminous growths in their chemical composition and microscopic elements.*

VARIETIES.—There are four varieties of malignant disease, viz. seirrhus; medullary sarcoma; gelatiniform cancer, and melanosis. That they are very nearly allied to each other is shown by the circumstance that two or more of them may affect different organs in the same individual; or may even exist together in one tumour; and that if one variety be extirpated, another may make its appearance in the cicatrix. But it does not seem probable that they are *identical*, or that one can be transformed into another by any process of development.

### SECTION II.—OF SCIRRHUS, OR CARCINOMA SIMPLEX.

SYMPTOMS.—Scirrhus begins usually as a rounded and peculiarly hard tumour, subject to occasional fits of severe lancinating pain.

ANATOMICAL CHARACTERS.—When examined, it is found to be hard, heavy, and nearly of the consistence of cartilage. It cuts with crispness like a potato or unripe pear. On a section, it appears to be composed of numerous dense white bands, intersecting each other irregularly, and having their interstices filled with a bluish, yellow, or reddish granular substance.

A thin slice examined under the microscope appears to be composed of a cellular tissue filled with globules, granules, and cells. One variety, called by Müller *carcinoma reticulare*, contains a network composed of opaque granular bodies, three or four times the size of blood-globules.

SEAT.—Scirrhus may occur in any organ or any texture; but by far the most frequently in the glands, especially the female breast, and the lymphatic glands in the vicinity.

PROGRESS AND TERMINATION.—The progress of this disease is two-fold. On the one hand, it spreads and successively invades all the adjoining tissues;—and at the same time the older portions of the morbid growth perish by ulceration or sloughing. At first the tumour is indolent and painless, so that the patient may be for a long time ignorant of its existence; it is also circumscribed and freely moveable. After a time it is affected with fits of severe lancinating pain, which gradually increase in frequency and severity. Then it slowly enlarges;—loses its

---

† *Vide* Müller on Cancer and Morbid Growths, translated by C. West, M.D., Lond. 1840. Review of Schwann on the Identical Development of Animals and Plants. Forbes's Rev. vol. ix. p. 495.

distinctness, becomes blended with the adjacent parts, and adheres to the skin and to the parts beneath it. At last the *destructive stage* commences. Portions of the tumour soften down, and form irregular abscesses; the skin ulcerates or sloughs,—and thus an open sore or *cancer* is formed. This ulcer enlarges in every direction; its edges are thick and jagged;—sometimes undermined and inverted;—sometimes swelled and everted. The surface is tawny or ash-coloured, and eaten into irregular hollows. The discharge is thin, sanious, fetid, and irritating,— and there is an almost constant burning pain. Sometimes a feeble attempt is made towards reparation;—pale, flabby granulations are thrown out, and a portion of the sore cicatrises for a time. In some few cases, the whole of the diseased growth has sloughed out, and a permanent cure has followed.* But in general the ulceration spreads, the neighbouring glands or viscera become contaminated, and the patient sinks from the constant pain and irritation.

CONSTITUTIONAL SYMPTOMS.—From the first there is a state of ill-health which cannot be solely attributed to the local disease, and which is denominated the *cancerous cachexia.* The patient is lanquid, depressed, and emaciated;—the complexion is leaden and sallow, the appetite bad, and digestion imperfect. As the disease advances, hectic is induced by the pain and exhaustion,—the vital energies are farther lowered by the absorption of deleterious secretions; and the patient suffers perhaps from the co-existence of the disease in other organs. An extraordinary *fragility of the bones*, so that the femur might be broken by turning in bed, is by no means an uncommon phenomenon;—partly arising from atrophy, partly from schirrous disease.†

DIAGNOSIS.—The diagnosis of scirrhus from other chronic tumours is at times most uncertain. Its principal characteristics are, *hardness, lancinating pain*, the co-existence of the *cancerous cachexia*, the patient's *age*, and the *situation* of the tumour. But as none of these characteristics may be well marked; and as tumours which have been harmless for years may ultimately assume a malignant aspect, the diagnosis must often be *guarded;*—that is, hedged in with intimations of its fallibility.

PROGNOSIS.—Although the destiny of a scirrhous tumour and of the patient are pretty certain, still the time in which the disease may prove destructive is most uncertain. So that if the patient is old;—if the disease has lasted long, and has been slow in its progress;—if the health is tolerable, and the cachexia not well marked;—much comfort may be derived from the assurance, that although the disease is incurable, yet life may be prolonged for many years, and may perhaps at last be terminated by some other malady.

---

* Travers on Malignant Diseases, Med. Chir. Trans., vol. xv. p. 213.
† S..lter in Med. Chir. Trans., vol. xv.

CAUSES.—The genuine cause of cancer is some unknown bodily conformation, which may be congenital and inherited, or may be engendered
by some causes equally unknown. Grief and the depressing passions,
and whatever tends to impair digestion and nutrition, are the best-esta-
blished *predisposing causes*. Females are more liable to it than males;—
and persons above forty than those under it;—and persons of spare,
bilious temperament and dark complexion, than those who are light, fat,
and ruddy. But it has occurred in girls under twenty. Some authors
think it most liable to attack the unmarried or barren; others state the
direct reverse. Blows or other injuries may act as *exciting causes,* and
produce it in a particular pait;—but they are insufficient unless the constitutional tendency exists.*

TREATMENT.—If no circumstance forbid, a scirrhus should be extirpated with the knife, care being taken to remove every particle that
appears unsound. Extirpation, however, will not effect a cure. In
ninety-nine cases out of a hundred the disease returns. But (to use the
words of an accomplished author†) "the period of the return of scirrhus
varies from six months to two or three years, or even longer. The interval may be one of health and hope; and even when the disease reappears, it does not in general return in a character of such formidable
suffering as in its ordinary course it presents." The operation may be
performed with some confidence if the disease is recent, moveable, circumscribed, and indolent. If, however, the skin is extensively tuberculated and adherent to the scirrhus;—if the surrounding fat and cellular
tissue are implicated;—if the diseased part is firmly adherent;—if it is
extensively ulcerated;—or if the original disease is much less in degree
than co-existent scirrhus of the adjoining lymphatic glands;—or if the
patient's health is fast sinking;—or if there is any palpable internal disease, the operation should not be attempted. Yet, although there be
*extensive ulceration*, it may be justifiable occasionally, in order to afford
even a month's respite from agonizing pain. Before operating, the health
should always be regulated by a course of alteratives and tonics.

Sundry *caustics* have been proposed, in order to cause sloughing of
the diseased growth. But they are on the whole more painful and dan-
gerons than the knife, and infinitely less effectual.

*Arsenic* and the *chloride of zinc* are the most useful, and may occasionally be resorted to in the case of flat superficial cancerous affections
of the skin; but the use of either of them in glandular scirrhus is much
to be reprehended.‡

The general *indications* in the treatment of scirrhus and cancer are, to

---

* Dr. Walshe's Paper on Cancer in the Cyclopædia of Practical Surgery, contains
the best account of the ætiology of malignant disease.

† Mayo, Pathology, p. 573.          ‡ Vide *Lupus*, in Part IV. Chap. II.

amend the general health;—to restore the secretions;—to diminish irritability;—to support the strength;—to counteract any accidental inflammation;—and to allay pain.

If the patient is young and plethoric;—and the fits of pain are frequent, and accompanied with heat and throbbing;—the diet should be reduced, the bowels be freely opened, and leeches be applied. In fact, frequent leeching is almost always of service in the early stages of any form of malignant disease; retarding its progress, and relieving the *common* inflammation with more or less of which it is always accompanied. As a general rule, Sir A. Cooper recommends the administration of five grains of Plummer's Pill at bed-time, and a draught containing *ammon. sesquicarb.* gr. v., *sodæ sesquicarb.* $3\beta$; *tinct. calumbæ* $3j$; *inf. gentianæ* $\overline{3}\beta$, twice in the day. But mercury, although highly useful as an *alterative*, must never be given so as to affect the system, or the ravages of the disease will be hastened.

The preparations of *iron* have been highly extolled, especially the carbonate and the ammonio-chloride. Either may be given with benefit when the lips are pale, the pulse weak, and the patient low and emaciated. The *ammonio-chloride* in pills, in doses of gr. ii. ter die, was a favourite medicine of the late Mr. Cline, and often effected the dispersion of chronic indolent tumours not really scirrhus.

*Narcotics* of all descriptions are necessary to relieve the pain. They are most advantageously given in combination, and require to be frequently changed and varied.

*Vegetable diet*, or low diet approaching starvation, has been much recommended. But by weakening the system, and increasing the irritability of the heart and nervous system, it cannot fail to be mischievous.

In fine, the treatment may be thus briefly summed up. The health must be improved by alteratives and tonics, by change of air, freedom from anxiety, and a diet that will support the strength, without heating the system. Wine may be allowed in moderation, if the patient is weak and is accustomed to it; narcotics must be given according as they are demanded. The *local treatment*, during the scirrhous stage, consists in occasional leeching, and the application of any mild plaster, (*E. saponis, plumbi, belladonnæ vel opii*,) to preserve the part from mechanical injury, and from changes of temperature. Fine flax is often used for the same purpose. It is sometimes useful to make an issue in the vicinity.

In the ulcerated or *cancerous stage*, the objects of local treatment are to allay pain, and to correct the fœtor and acrimony of the discharge. A copious list of applications for this purpose will be found in the remarks on irritable ulcers. Poultices made of the pulps of carrots;—or with the leaves of conium, hyoscyamus or belladonna;—poultices medicated with the extracts of those plants, or with opium, or the extract of poppies;—

ointments or lotions containing the same narcotics, or the salts of morphia, may be tried in succession. Sometimes relief is afforded by alternation with mild stimulants; as weak lotions of the chlorides of lime and soda;—or of the nitric or nitro-muriatic acid;—or nitrate of silver. Affusion with very cold or iced water is sometimes of use. *Carbonic acid,* a powerful narcotic and allayer of irritability, may be often advantageously applied by means of fermenting poultices; or by generating the gas in a bottle, and directing the stream on the surface of the sore through a tube.

Although, in the present state of our knowledge, it is utterly impossible to procure the absorption of a scirrhous tumour, still, if there be any doubt as to its nature, it may be advisable to employ iodine, or the iodides of potassium, iron, arsenic, or lead, externally and internally;—by which means some suspicious tumours have been dispersed.

SECTION III.—OF MEDULLARY SARCOMA, AND FUNGUS HŒMATODES.

Syn.—*Carcinoma medullary; encephaloid disease; soft cancer; spongy inflammation.*

Symptoms.—Medullary sarcoma usually commences as a soft, rounded, elastic tumour, growing rapidly, generally free from pain or tenderness, and not circumscribed or moveable, but blended with the surrounding tissues.

Anatomical Characters.—On a section this tumour appears to be composed of a white opaque substance of the colour and consistence of brain, streaked with numerous blood-vessels. But its appearance varies very much according to certain pathological conditions. Thus it very often happens that its delicate blood-vessels are ruptured, and the tumour becoming infiltrated with blood resembles a coagulum: in this state it is called *fungus hæmatodes.* Sometimes after rupture of a vessel the effused blood is absorbed, as after apoplexy of the brain, and there is left in its place a cyst containing a clear or coffee-coloured serum. Sometimes large masses of it are softened and sloughy, and of the consistence of thick cream or putrid brain. Under the microscope this form of malignant disease is seen to be composed of a delicate fibrous tissue, filled with rounded and caudate nucliferous cells.

Progress and Termination.—This tumour enlarges rapidly; and its arterial circulation is sometimes so vigorous as to cause pulsation like an aneurism. The skin covering it soon becomes purple or livid ; and the subcutaneous veins enlarged and tortuous. It is now subject to fits of aching or throbbing pain, but by no means so severe as that of scirrhus. At length one of the most projecting points ulcerates, and discharges a grumous fluid,—and a rapidly increasing fungus grows from the aperture.

Sometimes this fungus exudes an enormous quantity of a thin, colourless serum;—sometimes it is covered with a slight crust of coagulum;—sometimes its blood-vessels give way, and there is a profuse hæmorrhage;—and sometimes large portions of it soften down or slough. The constitution suffers in the same manner as in scirrhus, but much more early and severely; and the patient expires after a few months, worn out by the irritation of the external malady, and by its invasion of the viscera.

DIAGNOSIS.—This disease is to be distinguished from scirrhus by the absence of hardness and lancinating pain;—by the greater rapidity of its growth:—by the earlier and more decided cachexia;—by its attacking persons of every age, and being more frequent in the young; whereas scirrhus is exceedingly rare under thirty;—and by its disposition to fungate rather than to ulcerate.

PROGNOSIS.—This of course will be highly unfavourable, the patient sinking much sooner than in scirrhus.

CAUSES.—Some unknown constitutional peculiarity.

TREATMENT.—The constitutional treatment is the same as directed for scirrhus. *Leeches* frequently applied at the earliest appearance of the disease will somewhat retard its progress. *Cold* or *iced* applications, and the ligature of the principal arteries supplying the tumour have been recommended for the same purpose, but are not worth trying. Early *extirpation* of the whole of the diseased growth is the surest method of prolonging the patient's life, because it gets rid of, at once, what otherwise would cause protracted sloughing. But the disease is sure to return, and if the operation is delayed, it may return before the wound has healed.* *Hæmorrhage* in this disease, or in cancer, may be restrained by pressure with a piece of lint.

* Exceptions to this discouraging fact are nevertheless occasionally observed, and justify the attempt to rescue the sufferer from impending death, by the removal of the local disease, when it is so situated that the whole of it can be excised, when the neighbouring glands and lymphatics appear to be unaffected, and when no suspicious tumours or induration can be detected in the abdomen.

I frequently meet with a gentleman of this city, from whom I removed the left testis, affected with decided fungoid degeneration, between two and three years ago. In his case the cord was sound, and the original glands were unaffected at the time of the operation, although they had been enlarged, at a previous period of the disease. On the other hand, I performed a similar operation for another gentleman just two months since, in whose case the appearances were still more promising than in the former one; but last week I received information that although the wound had healed perfectly and the cicatrix remained sound, the disease had manifested its wonted inveteracy by symptoms which boded certain and speedy destruction to the patient. F.

SECTION IV.—OF GELATINIFORM CANCER, MELANOSIS, AND OTHER RARER VARIETIES
OF MALIGNANT DISEASE.

GELATINIFORM CANCER.—(SYN. *Tumeur Colloid, carcinoma alveolare.*)

This remarkable growth is seen, on a section, to be composed of innumerable white interlacing fibres, containing cells in their interstices.
The cells vary from the size of a grain of sand to that of a pea, and are
filled with a soft, viscous jelly, which generally is clear and transparent,
but occasionally turbid and opaque.  This jelly-like matter is composed
entirely of albumen, and retains its transparency in alcohol.  Its structure
differs from that of the other species of carcinoma in the greater size and
continued growth of the cells.

MELANOSIS is a disease consisting in the deposite of a brown or black
substance like the pigment of the choroid.  There is some difference of
opinion respecting its nature.  Carswell considers it an unorganized
substance, and not injurious except when its presence mechanically interferes with some function, or when it is deposited into some organ essential to life.  Müller, on the other hand, describes it as composed of organized cells and granules like the other malignant growths, but differing
from them in containing a black pigment.  In the human subject, it is
generally found in combination with medullary carcinoma.*

The *mammary* and *pancreatic sarcoma* are tumours which were so
designated by Mr. Abernethy, from there resemblance in structure to
those glands.  They appear to be varieties of scirrhus or medullary sarcoma; and to form, as it were, transition-stages between them and the
ordinary fleshy sarcoma: being not so certain as the former to lead to
destructive changes, but more so than the latter.

* Carswell, op. cit.  Fawdington on Melanosis, Lond. 1826 ; Mackenzie on the
Eye, p. 553.

# PART III.

## OF THE DIFFERENT SPECIES OF INJURIES.

---

## CHAPTER I.

### OF INCISED WOUNDS.

DEFINITION.—These are wounds made with clean-cutting instruments; they generally bleed more at first than the other kinds of wounds.

TREATMENT.—There are four indications:—1, To arrest hæmorrhage; 2, to remove foreign bodies; 3, to bring the divided parts into apposition, and keep them in union; 4, to promote adhesion.

(1) To arrest hæmorrhage, moderate pressure, a raised position, and the application of cold, will be sufficient in most cases;—but if an artery have been wounded, or the bleeding prove obstinate, the measures must be adopted which will be indicated in the Chapter on Wounds of Arteries.

(2) The removal of foreign bodies will be much more easy both for surgeon and patient if done at once, than if delayed till inflammation supervene. The best instruments for this and every other surgical purpose which they can perform, are the fingers;—but they may be aided by probes and forceps, if necessary. Dirt, gravel, &c., are best got rid of by affusion with water. All clots of blood must likewise be removed, or they will act as foreign bodies and prevent adhesion.

(3) In order to bring the sides of the wound into apposition, the part must be placed in such a position as will relax any muscular fibres that may have been divided, or that may be subjacent to the divided parts. Then the edges must be made to meet as nicely as they can without undue straining, and must be retained by cross strips of adhesive or isinglass-plaster, one end of the plaster being first applied to that side of the wound which is loosest, and the other being brought across with a mild degree of traction. If the wound, from its severity or situation, compel the patient to keep his bed, no farther application will be needed save a

17

cloth dipped in cold water;—otherwise a light compress and bandage may be applied to keep on the dressings, and protect the parts from injury. If the wound is so situated that the plasters cannot be applied smoothly, a slip of lint may be laid on it first. The surgeon should not be in too great haste to close deep and extensive wounds, lest they begin to bleed again when the patient becomes warm in bed. It is better to put the patient to bed with merely a piece of linen dipped in cold water on the wound; and to approximate it accurately after two or three hours, when all fear of hæmorrhage is over, and the cut surface is beginning to be glazed with lymph.

*Sutures.*—In some cases it is requisite to have recourse to sutures; although from the pain occasioned by their application, and their tendency to produce suppuration, they should never be used if they can be avoided. *Five species* are enumerated in the older authors.

1. The *Interrupted Suture* is thus made. A needle armed with

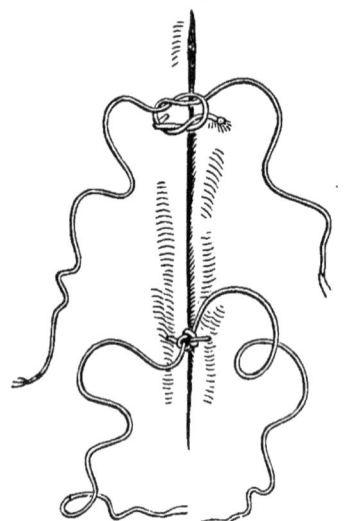

a single ligature is passed through one lip of the wound *from without*, inwards;—then at a corresponding part through the other lip *from within*, outwards. Then the ends of the ligature (which should be made of good stay-silk, well waxed and flattened, that it may lie easily in the wound) are to be drawn together, without, however, any great straining, and are to be tied tightly in a double reef knot, as represented in the adjoining figure.

The needle should be carried deeply enough to obtain a firm hold, but should not include any tendinous part. As many of these stitches are to be made as are necessary; half or three quarters of an inch is a proper interval.

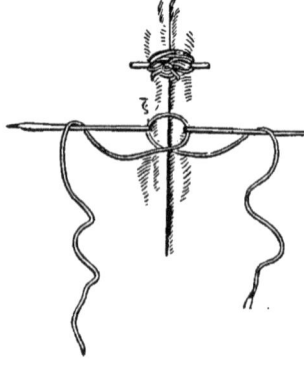

2. The *Twisted Suture* is made thus. The edges of the wound having been placed accurately in contact, a sufficient number of pins are to be passed through both of them at convenient distances. The first pin should be placed at any loose angle which there may happen to be. When all the pins have been introduced, and the parts are accurately adjusted, the middle of a long piece of silk is to be twisted around the uppermost, in the form

of a figure of 8. Then the two ends are to be brought down and twisted round each of the other pins successively in like manner;—and lastly, are to be secured by a knot.

The pins are usually made of silver, with steel points, that may be removed after they have been inserted. The fine pins used by entomologists for fixing insects, or the fine steel needles with lancet points, recommended by Mr. Liston, and depicted in the adjoining cut, are excellent substitutes. They are so small that they excite little irritation; and a great number of them may be employed, so as to ensure as nice an adaptation as possible. But after they are inserted, their points must either be cut off, or else be guarded with a lump of wax, in order that they may do no mischief.

3. The *Glovers* or *Continuous Suture* is nothing more than the ordinary way of sewing things together practised by seamstresses and housewives. It is sometimes employed in wounds of the intestines.

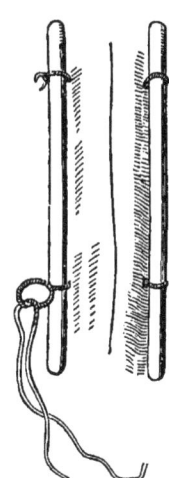

4. The *Quilled Suture* is performed by passing a sufficient number of ligatures, as in the interrupted suture. But instead of being tied to their opposite neighbours, all the threads on each side of the wound are fastened to a quill, or bougie, or roll of plaster. This suture is now nearly or quite obsolete; it was formerly supposed to be very advantageous in pressing the deep parts of a wound together.

5. The *Dry Suture* was made by sticking a strip of adhesive plaster, or (before that was invented) a strip of linen smeared with white of egg and flour, to the skin on each side of the wound. The adjacent margins of the plaster or linen were then sewed together.

*Rules for the use of Sutures.*—1. They are not to be used with the view of exerting great *force* in drawing the edges of the wound together, but simply with a view of obtaining a better *purchase.* 2. They are to be employed upon parts that are naturally loose and unattached, or that are very moveable, or that have no firm part under them against which they can be fixed. Thus the *twisted* suture is used in wounds of the lips; and the *interrupted* in those of the scrotum—of the abdominal parietes—of the female perineum, or where a portion of the nose or ear has been detached; in fact, in those cases, and those only, where sticking-plaster would be insufficient. 3. Sticking-plaster may, if possible, be used as an auxiliary, to prevent only strain upon the pins or stitches. 4. They are to be removed about the fourth or fifth day, before they begin to ulcerate—sooner, if violent inflammation and suppuration come on; but not so soon, if there be no great action,—in order that adhesion may be more perfect.

(4) The fourth indication is to keep down inflammation; that is, to prevent it from surpassing the degree necessary for adhesion. This is to be effected by opening the bowels, lowering the diet, enjoining rest, avoiding tight bandages, and every other source of irritation and constriction, and maintaining the injured part in as comfortable a state of feeling as possible; which, as was before observed, is the surest means of preventing inflammation. If, however, much pain and swelling supervene, leeches and cold applications (or warm if the patient prefers them) must be resorted to, and plasters, bandages, and sutures be abandoned till granulation commences. Then the parts may be again. gently aproximated, that they may heal by the *second intention;* that is, by the inosculation of their granulations.

CASES OF COMPLETE DISUNION.—If any small portion of the body (a finger or part of the nose for instance) has been completely cut off, if it be reapplied as soon as possible, and retained by plasters or sutures, and wrapped up so as to preserve its temperature, it will very probably unite again. And even if such a part have been separated for a considerable time, the attempt should not be given up:—but it should be well washed in warm water to free it from dirt, and the stump should also be bathed, so as to remove any dry coagulated blood, before they are reapplied to each other. Part of the left forefinger, an inch and a half long, after having been cut off for twenty minutes, was replaced and united perfectly in four days. The case is related by Dr. Balfour of Edinburgh, and is quoted in Sir A. Cooper.

### CURE OF OPEN WOUNDS.

If a part has been abstracted which cannot be restored; or if any kind of wound cannot be covered by skin, there are two ways in which it may heal—either with suppuration, or without it.

According to the first process, it inflames and suppurates, then granulates and heals like an ordinary ulcer.

There are two ways in which open wounds may heal without suppuration; viz, by scabbing; the surface being dry;—or by the modelling process, if the surface is kept moist.

The ordinary form of the second method of cure is that by *scabbing;*— the natural and simple way in which most slight accidents heal when not interfered with by art. It may be effected by permitting the blood to dry on the surface of the wound;—or perhaps in some few cases a crust may be formed with the nitrate of silver, on Mr. Higginbottom's plan. Under this protection the wound heals without suppuration.—Mr. Wardrop has seen the large surface exposed by the removal of a diseased breast heal completely under a crust of blood in thirty days, without suppuration. Common experience shows that it is better to leave slight scratches and abrasions to heal by themselves in this natural manner, than to interfere with them by plasters or ointments.

The second form of healing without suppuration, is that first described by Macartney, under the term *modelling process*. When the water-dressing is applied, and the part is kept under the most favourable conditions of rest and temperature, the wound fills up by a process of growth as it were; its surface being pale and moist, without the least sign of suppuration, till, having attained its natural level, it forms a small pliant cicatrix.

In the following cases no attempt should be made to bring the divided parts together, or to procure adhesion. (1.) When the skin cannot be brought into contact with the parts beneath it;—as after castration, and the removal of certain tumours; because the closure of the wound, by confining matter and causing sinuses, only protracts the cure. (2.) When the divided parts are thickened and inflamed. (3.) When the wound is complicated by the introduction of a poison, or of some foreign body that cannot be removed.*

# CHAPTER II.

## OF PUNCTURED WOUNDS.

GENERAL DESCRIPTION.—These are justly esteemed the most dangerous of all wounds. (1.) Because from their depth they are liable to implicate blood-vessels, nerves, viscera, and other deep-seated parts of importance. (2.) Because the parts which they traverse are stretched and torn, and consequently are disposed to inflame and suppurate. (3.) Because matter when formed has no free exit, and is liable to burrow extensively. (4.) Because foreign bodies may be carried in to great depths without being suspected, and create long-continued irritation. (5.) Because they are most liable to be followed by tetanus.

TREATMENT.—The first point usually mooted in discussing the treatment of these wounds is the propriety of dilating them, and converting them into simple incisions, in order to avert the deep-seated suppuration and confinement of matter. But as those evils are incident on the inflammation that supervenes, and as they by no means follow of necessity, an

---

* Palmer, note on Hunter, vol. iii. p. 259.

endeavour should be made to prevent or mitigate inflammation, so that there may be no necessity for such a severe measure.

In the first place, therefore, rest, low diet, purgatives, cold lotions,* and leeches, must be sedulously employed, to counteract all excess of inflammation, and to cause the absorption of any blood that may be effused in the course of the wound;—and perhaps of pus, if formed in very small quantity. But if, notwithstanding, there should be severe pain, and swelling, and fever, a free incision must be made for the relief of tension and the discharge of matter;—and the case must be treated in the same manner as a deep-seated abscess.

Diagnosis.—If the instrument with which a puncture is made be angular, the shape of the wound will in general be the same. But it is a remarkable fact that a punctured wound made with a *circular conical weapon* is not *round* but *linear*, as though it had been made with a narrow, flat instrument. And the direction of the wound varies in different situations;—thus in the neck, in the axilla, and near the linea alba, it is vertical; and on the sides of the abdomen, oblique.

# CHAPTER III.

## OF LACERATIONS AND CONTUSIONS.

### SECTION I.—OF CONTUSION AND ECCHYMOSIS.

Definition.—A contusion signifies an injury inflicted by some obtuse, blunt object, without perforation of the skin.

Consequences.—The consequences of contusion are, (1) a degree of *concussion*, or benumbing, which may be pretty severe, without much farther mischief; (2) some *structural injury*, which will be followed by inflammation. The degrees of this structural injury are three.

1. There may be *rupture of the smaller vessels*, the blood from which infiltrates the cellular tissue, and causes an ordinary *ecchymosis*.

2. A *large vessel* may be ruptured, so that blood is effused in consi. derable quantity, and tears up the cellular tissue forming a cavity.

3. The tissues may be irretrievably pulpified and *disorganized*.

Ecchymosis.—When ecchymosis has been produced in the skin or

---

* The *warm* water or vapour bath sedulously employed, will be much more likely to relieve the pain of such injuries at first, and to prevent serious consequences, than any cold applications.     F.

immediately beneath it, there appears a swelling of a reddish colour, which speedily becomes black. On the' third day it is violet, and the margin which was at first well defined, is found to be faint and diffused. About the fifth or sixth day the colour becomes green; on the seventh or eighth, yellow; and it gradually disappears about the tenth or twelfth;—sooner or later, according to the vigour of the individual and the quantity of the blood effused.

If an ecchymosis be formed in the cellular tissue without injury of the skin, no discolouration may appear for twenty-four hours;—and if it be more deeply seated among the muscles, it will not affect the skin for some days, and may then appear at a part quite remote from the seat of the injury;—and in this last case will usually be in the form of irregular yellow spots, marbled with green and blue.*

CAUSES.—Ecchymosis may be produced by many other causes besides contusions. It is a symptom of certain disease, as scurvy, purpura, and the last stage of fevers. It may be a consequence of oblique wounds, which do not permit the blood to flow freely out;—of spasms, and other violent contractions of the muscles;—it may also be caused by suction, (as after leech-bites,) especially in a part where the skin is thin. It may farther be simulated by the application of colouring matters to the skin. Lastly, ecchymosis produced during life may require to be distinguished from various appearances arising after death.

DIAGNOSIS.—*Ecchymosis produced by suction* may be distinguished from that which is the result of injury, by being generally in the form of small round spots, and situated on the inside of the arms, or female breasts; and the surgeon required to decide on the cause of such marks should consider whether they correspond in their appearance to the date which is assigned to them.

*Artificial discolouration of the skin* may be distinguished from ecchymosis by its being generally in round or irregular spots, fringed at the edges.†

Ecchymosis produced during life may be distinguished from the livid discolouration of *incipient putrefaction*, or that which is' caused by the gravitation of blood in a dead body, by noticing that in the first case, blood is effused into the cellular tissue, and is incorporated with the cutis, which is thickened; whereas in the latter two cases, the blackness will be confined to the surface of the cutis, and if blood is effused into the cellular tissue, it will be only at some depending part, and it will be fluid, and ·not coagulated.‡

TREATMENT.—The indications are (1) to check extravasation of blood;

---

* Devergie, Medicine Legale. Paris, 1836, tome ii. p. 57.

† Fallot de la Simulation et de la Dissimulation des Maladies. Bruxelles, 1836, p. 67.

‡ Beck's Medical Jurisprudence.

(2) to prevent inflammation; (3) to produce absorption of the fluids, and restore the use of the parts.

If the patient be robust, and the bruise seated on the head or trunk;— or if it be extensive elsewhere; and the swelling increase rapidly, and become very tense, it will be expedient to bleed. The bruised part should, if possible, be elevated;—and cold water or the white of an egg curdled with alum, or evaporating lotions, or a bladder filled with water, in which an ounce or two of nitre or common salt has been dissolved to render it cold, should be applied at once;—and a sufficient number of leeches, as soon as there are any signs of inflammatory pain and swelling, but not before. These measures, together with purgatives and low diet, will suffice for the first two indications;—whilst the third will be fulfilled by friction with stimulating liniments; by cold or hot affusion; and passive motion after inflammation has subsided.

Sometimes, however, the effusion of blood increases very fast, and the tumour becomes tense and shining, so as to threaten rupture of the skin. It will be well in this case to imitate the practice of prize-fighters, and make a very small aperture with the point of a lancet, and let as much blood be sucked out as can be without difficulty; although this should not be done unless absolutely necessary, because the pressure of the blood already effused tends to prevent the escape of more. If, however, this cannot be done, because the blood has coagulated,—and if the skin is so tense that it will inevitably either burst or slough,—and if the pain and tension are not adequately relieved by the free employment of antiphlogistic measures, so that the clot, instead of being absorbed, will be removed by suppuration, an incision of sufficient length should be made into the swelling, and a poultice be applied. Then the clot will most likely be gradually extruded by the contraction of the cavity, and a simple granulating wound will be left. But it is very bad practice to squeeze or scoop out the coagulum, as the bleeding might be brought on afresh, and severe inflammation be excited.* ˌ

If an artery of considerable size is lacerated, which will be known by the situation of the contusion, and the great and rapid swelling, the case becomes a *diffused aneurism*, and must be treated accordingly.

If the skin is so much injured as to endanger sloughing, tepid applications are to be preferred, especially the water-dressing, the steam-bath, or poppy fomentation and spirit of wine.

If the fingers or toes have been severely bruised, so that it may seem impossible to save them, they should not be too hastily amputated, as they often recover under unfavourable circumstances.

If any superficial part have been killed by injury, the water-dressing or a poultice will be the best and most convenient application till the

---

* Hunter on the Blood, part ii. chap. ii. sect. i.

slough separates. But should violent inflammation or gangrene come on they must be treated as has already been directed.

If any bruise be attended with severe collapse, the measures described in Part I., Chap. I., must be adopted. In no case should cold be applied extensively to the trunk; extensive superficial extravasation (to counteract which it was recommended above) rarely occurs there :—and if there be extravasation into the cavities, it must be combated by bleeding.

SECTION II.—OF LACERATED AND CONTUSED WOUNDS.

GENERAL DESCRIPTION.—These wounds are attended with less hæmorrhage than the incised;—both because their surface, being irregular, renders it easy for the blood to adhere and coagulate;—and because arteries, when torn, do not bleed so much as when cut. But in all other respects they are infinitely more serious. (1) They are liable to inflame violently and slough ; (2) they are often complicated with foreign bodies; and (3) they are more liable than simple wounds to occasion severe constitutional disturbance and tetanus.

TREATMENT.—In the first place, bleeding must be restrained;—secondly, foreign bodies must be removed ; thirdly, the divided parts must be brought into opposition, in case the whole or any part of them may be inclined to unite by adhesion. But as this is not very likely to occur, and as the wound mostly inflames highly and suppurates, there should be no straining with plasters or tight bandages. Then the patient must observe rest and low diet, and be purged;—and a cloth dipped in cold water;—or a soft poultice ;—or the water-dressing, or a poppy fomentation, or the steam-bath; may be applied locally, according to his feelings. Cold must not be applied too extensively, especially if the injury is seated on the trunk, or is very severe, or if much blood has been lost, or the patient is very old, or young, or feeble.

When pain and inflammation appear, bleeding may be performed, if the injury is important enough to require it, and the patient's strength can bear it; otherwise leeches should be applied. But the patient must not be reduced too much, or tetanus will be more liable to come on. Openings are to be made if necessary, in order to prevent the lodgment of putrid blood in the early stages, and of matter subsequently. When sloughs have separated, and suppuration is kindly established, the parts should be brought into apposition as much as can be done without leaving sinuses, and the case must then be treated as an ordinary sore.

18

# CHAPTER IV.

## OF GUNSHOT WOUNDS.

DEFINITION.—Under the term *gunshot wounds* are included all the injuries caused by the discharge or bursting of firearms. They consist of "severe contusions, with or without solution of continuity."

SYMPTOMS.—When a musket or pistol-ball has penetrated an ordinary fleshy part, there is seen a hole, perhaps rather smaller than the ball itself, with its margin livid and *inverted*,—and if the ball have passed completely through, there will be another larger and more ragged orifice, with its edge *everted*. The wound will, besides, be attended with more or less *pain, hæmorrhage,* and *constitutional disturbance.*

(*a*) The *pain* in these cases is said, by most authors to be inconsiderable at the moment of infliction. Mr. Guthrie, however, both from observation and personal experience, affirms that this is by no means the case, and says that in general the pain is severe;—that it is a dead, heavy, painful blow;—although still the injury may not be felt at the moment, if it is inflicted while the patient's whole attention is absorbed by other objects.

(*b*) Most authors state that gunshot wounds are attended with very little *hæmorrhage,* unless some considerable blood-vessel has been divided. But Mr. Guthrie asserts that this is equally erroneous; that there is in general considerable hæmorrhage of an arterial colour; but that a wound of a large artery is only to be feared if the blood continue to be poured out in great quantity and *per saltum,* in spite of pressure.

(*c*) The *constitutional disturbance* accompanying these wounds is severe and peculiar. The surface is pale, and bedewed with cold perspiration; every limb trembles; the patient cannot stand without support; and suffers from vomiting, faintness, and peculiar alarm, anxiety, and confusion of the mind. The severity of these symptoms will, in general, be proportionate to the extent of the injury, the importance of the part wounded, and the habitual fortitude of the sufferer; but the anecdote related in the subjoined note will show that they may be most severe under circumstances the most trivial.*

---

* During a rapid advance of part of the British army in Portugal, "one of the skirmishers suddenly came upon his adversary, with only a small bank between them;

COURSE OF BALLS.—A remarkable circumstance connected with gunshot wounds is the facility with which the ball may be diverted from its course by the slightest obstacles. Any trifling obliquity of surface, or difference of density in the parts which it traverses, may cause it to take a most circuitous route. Thus a ball may enter on one side of the head, chest, or abdomen, and may pass out at a point exactly opposite, just as if it had gone entirely through the cavity, whereas it may be found to have travelled round beneath the skin. Sometimes it will make a complete circuit, as in the case of a friend of Dr. Hennen, who was struck about the *pomum Adami* by a bullet, which passed completely round the neck, and was found lying in the very orifice by which it entered. The track of the ball in these cases will often be indicated by a blush, or dusky red line, or wheal on the skin, or sometimes by a peculiar emphysematous crackling;—and the diagnosis will of course be aided by the presence or absence of the symptoms of wounds of the great cavities. In a similar manner balls will run along concave surfaces. Thus a soldier may be struck on the wrist when the arm is bent in the act of firing, and the ball may graze along the arm, and fly off at the shoulder; or a ball may strike the outside of the calf of a mounted officer, and be thrown up into the popliteal space; or one may enter the thorax or abdomen, glide along the inner surface of the peritonæum or pleura, and pass out or be lodged near the spine.

LODGMENT OF BALLS.—It is always important to ascertain whether the shot have passed out of the body, or whether it is lodged;—and supposing that there are two holes, it must be considered whether they are produced by the *entrance* and *exit of one* or by the *entrance of two* distinct balls. If there are two holes, and they are distant from each other, some light may be thrown on the question by ascertaining the position of the patient at the time he was wounded, and the posture of his assailant. Thus a soldier has presented himself with two shot-holes, one on the outside of the ankle, the other near the trochanter; but they were both caused by the same ball, which entered at the ankle when the foot was raised in the act of running.*   In another instance, a soldier, who was ascending a scaling-

both parties presented, the muzzles of the pieces nearly touching ; both fired, and both fell. The British soldier, after a minute or two, thinking himself hit, but still finding himself capable of moving, got up, and found his adversary dead on the other side of the bank. " I saw him," says Mr. Guthrie, " immediately afterwards in considerable alarm, being conscious of a blow somewhere, but which, after a diligent search proved to be only a graze from a ball on the ulnar side of the arm; yet the certainty he was in of being killed, from the respective positions of the parties, had such an effect upon him at the moment of receiving this trifling injury, as nearly to deprive him for a short time of his powers of volition: whereas, had the wound been received from a concealed or distant enemy, it would in all probability have been little noticed."—Guthrie, op. cit. p. 11.

* Guthrie, op. cit., p. 17.

ladder, was wounded in the right arm, and the ball was found under the skin of the opposite thigh.* But even though there may be only one opening, it by no means follows that the ball has lodged; for it may have escaped by the very hole at which it entered, after having made the circuit of the body, as in the case of Dr. Hennen's friend just mentioned.

Or it may have impinged against some part, such as the cartilage of a rib, which has caused it to recoil; and a ball has been known to drive a piece of bone into the brain, and fall out of the wound afterwards. In some instances a ball has been unable to perforate a fold of linen, but has carried it for the distance of one, or even three or four inches into the wound; and on drawing this out, the ball of course comes out with it.†

Again, it is very possible that two balls may enter by the same aperture, one of which may pass out, and the other diverge and wound some important organ. So that, in many cases, the prognosis should be guarded, especially if the state of constitutional alarm and depression, instead of diminishing, increase considerably, and disproportionately to the apparent extent of the injury. Sometimes it will happen that a ball splits, either from a defect in the casting, or from its striking against some sharp bony ridge, as the vomer or shin.‡

But it frequently happens that large masses of metal are impacted in the substance of a part without much external indication of their presence, it appearing as though they made room for themselves by compressing the surrounding soft parts.§

FOREIGN BODIES.—Gunshot wounds may be complicated by the pre-

* Hennen, op. cit., p. 35.

† A silk handkerchief sometimes saves life in the same way ; and Mr. Home, in his Report on Gunshot Wounds in Canada, in 1838, speaks of the great power which the canvass lining of soldiers' stocks has in resisting the passage of balls.— Edinburgh Med. and Surg. Journ., July, 1840.

‡ A Brunswick soldier at Waterloo " was struck by a musket ball on the tip of the nose, which split upon the bony edge where joined by the cartilage. A piece of of the ball was extracted on the spot, and it was supposed that the ball itself had been purposely cut into pieces, as is sometimes done by foreign riflemen. The cure went on without accident until the tenth day, when the man was seized with a vio. lent hæmorrhage from the nose and mouth, which came on suddenly, and carried him off in the course of the night. On dissection, it appeared that a very minute portion of the ball had penetrated along the basis of the skull, lodged in the sinus of the left internal jugular vein, forming a sort of sac for itself close upon the vein, and which having inflamed the coats of the vessel, they at last ulcerated and burst."— Hennen, op. cit., p. 91.

§ Hennen relates the case of a young officer who was killed at the siege of Serin. gapatam by a cannon-ball of thirty-two pounds, which completely buried itself in the muscles of his hip. A mass of grape-shot, the size of the closed fist, has been extracted from under the plantar aponeurosis. Guthrie gives a case in which a ball of eight pounds weight lodged in the thigh without making a large opening, and was not discovered till it accidentally rolled out on amputating the limb.

sence of other foreign bodies besides the ball: and these are divided by Dr. Hennen into two classes; namely, 1st, pieces of the clothing, or of matters contained in the pockets, or portions of the body of some unfortunate comrade;* 2ndly, pieces of bone or muscle belonging to the individual, but which have become virtually extraneous, in consequence of being dead and detached. These are infinitely more mischievous than the former.

SPENT BALLS.—Injuries from spent balls have at all times attracted great attention from the extreme violence of the injury inflicted, with very little external appearance of it. In some rare cases a cannon-ball has passed close to the head, and has caused death, either immediately or within a few hours, without leaving any morbid appearance that could be detected by dissection.† But in the majority of instances it is found, that although the skin may be intact, or but trivially grazed, still that the parts beneath have been irreparably disorganized;—the muscles pulpified, the bones comminuted, and large vessels and nerves torn across. The patient is severely stunned; and the part injured is motionless, and senseless, and benumbed for some distance. Swelling soon comes on, but more from extravasation than from inflammation, which, although attempted to be set up, never attains any height. Gangrene occurs speedily, and is propagated to the neighbouring parts, weakened as they are by participation in the injury, and by their contact with tissues that have ceased to live.

These cases were formerly called *wind contusions*, being ascribed to a compression and displacement of the air by the ball. Some later theorists have conceived that they are produced by a current of electricity, which it generates in its passage through the atmosphere;—and others have

---

* A pocket of course linen, containing two five franc pieces and two copper coins, have been extracted after some days from the vastus externus muscle, in which they were deeply imbedded. Three pieces of coin were extracted on the fifth day after the battle of Waterloo, from a wound in the thigh of a poor Hanoverian soldier. As he possessed neither money nor pocket to put it into, they evidently came from a comrade who stood before him, and who was killed by the same shot. Part of the cranium has been found imbedded in the thigh;—a tooth in the temporal muscle,—and the olecranon of one man in the bend of another man's elbow.

† A lad was carrying a sand-bag on his head, when it was struck by a twenty-four pound shot from a distant battery. He immediately fell, senseless and comatose, with a slow, weak pulse, labouring respiration without stertor, and incessant attempts to vomit. The pupil of one eye was dilated and motionless, that of the other natural; the hair along the sagittal suture was erect, resembling that of a person placed on the insulating stool and electrified. In this state he remained for twenty-four hours, and then expired in convulsions. No cause of death was discovered on a minute examination, so that it must be attributed to a violent concussion; but it is remarkable that the ball should cause such a concussion, without also causing some more palpable lesion.—Hennen, p. 96.

imagined that a vacuum is formed behind it, and that the dreadful consequences we have enumerated arise from the eagerness of the living
tissues to start from their places to fill up this vacuum. If, however,
as these theorists assume, a ball can produce such effects merely by
passing *near* the body, and without actually *touching*, it must, *à for-
tiori*, produce them, when it indubitably touches;—as when a leg is
knocked off;—but this is not the case. The subjoined quotation from
Baron Larrey offers the most probable explanation of the phenomenon.*

PROGRESS AND CONSEQUENCES.—*In favourable cases,*—Inflammation
generally comes on from twelve to twenty-four hours after a gunshot
wound of some common part. The wound becomes swelled, stiff, and
painful, and exudes a little reddish serum. On the third or fourth day pus
begins to be formed; but the suppuration is limited by the effusion of
lymph around the wound. About the fifth day the parts in the immediate track of the ball, which have been killed by the violence of the contusion, begin to separate, and change from a blackish red to a brownish
yellow colour;—and on the tenth or fifteenth day, sooner or later, according to the vigour of the constitution, the slough is thrown off.† In the
mean time granulations form, the wound contracts and becomes impervious at its centre, and generally heals with a depressed cicatrix by the
end of six weeks or two months,—the lower aperture always healing
first. These are the symptoms observed in healthy constitutions, and
they will be attended with little constitutional disturbance, and that of no
long duration.

*Inflammatory Complication.*—But if the patient, previously to the
receipt of his wound, or after it, has committed excesses, or has been
exposed to vicissitudes of temperature;—or if the wound has been irritated
by want of rest, or improper applications, the local and constitutional

---

* "A cannon-ball is propelled at first with a rectilinear movement; and if, during
this part of its course, it strikes against any part of the human body, it carries it
away ; but the ball, after having traversed a certain distance, undergoes some change
in motion, in consequence of the resistance of the atmosphere and the attraction of
the earth, and turns on its own axis, in addition to the direct impulse received from
the explosion of the powder. If it should strike any part of the body when the
velocity with which the ball is passing is greatly diminished, it does not carry it
away, as in the preceding case; but in consequence of its curvilinear or rolling motion, it turns round the part, in the same manner as a wheel passes over a limb,
instead of forcing a passage through it. The soft elastic parts, such as the skin and
cellular membrane, yield, whilst the bones, muscles, tendons, arteries, &c., offering
a greater degree of resistance, are either bruised or ruptured. If the ball should
strike one of the cavities of the body, the viscera suffer in like manner."—Mem. de
Chir. Mil. quoted by Guthrie.

† It is by no means true, as is generally stated, that the whole track of the ball
must slough, for the separated parts are never equal in extent to the depth of the
wound.—Guthrie.

affections will be much more formidable. The pain will be more severe, the redness and swelling more extensive, the wound dry, and fever violent. When suppuration is established, instead of being confined to the track of the ball, it is diffused amongst the neighbouring muscles and under fasciæ, forming numerous and irregular sinuses;—so that the treatment is protracted for many months; and even after the cure is completed the limb remains disabled by contractions and adhesions of the muscles, and is liable to œdematous swellings from the structural and vital weakness which a continuance of inflammation always induces.

*Lodgment of Foreign Bodies.*—If the ball or any other foreign bodies remain lodged, the present inflammation and constitutional disturbance will be proportionably more severe, and the resulting suppuration more profuse and exhausting; and it will besides be accompanied with more or less pain, till the exciting cause is got rid of. But if the constitution or parts do not possess much irritability; if the ball be small and polished, and if it press against no nerves, or vessels, or other sensitive parts, it may, and often does, remain for years without creating any disturbance —a cyst being formed for it in the belly of a muscle, or in the interstitial cellular tissue. And this is much more likely to happen if the force with which it was propelled was *not very great*;—because, in that case, the wound is formed rather by *penetration* than by *contusion*,—it is a *slit*, rather than a *hole*,—and it may close by adhesion, with very little suppuration or separation of sloughs.

*Rare Complications.*—Mr. Guthrie has described two rare and peculiarly fatal forms of inflammation occasionally supervening on gunshot wounds. The *first* is a most acute inflammation, attacking the muscles and other deep-seated parts, with very little affection of the skin. In the instance related, the wounds were apparently going on well, when they became extremely painful towards evening; the pain increased during the night, and death occurred before morning. On dissection, says the learned author, the whole limb " seemed so stuffed or gorged with blood, that the texture of the parts, muscular as well as cellular, was soft, and readily giving way to a moderate pressure with the fingers. I can only compare it to the appearance of a part just falling into a state of gangrene."

The *second* variety made its appearance after the first two days, and in every case which Mr. G. saw, the wound was in the upper extremity. The part swelled, and was rather œdematous, and affected with a burning pain: the skin was bright and glossy. In fatal cases, the swelling rapidly extended up to the axilla, and then difficulty of breathing came on, and was soon followed by death. One patient only, out of six, was saved, by the most vigorous antiphlogistic treatment. The first three cases were not inspected p, m.; in the fourth, the great veins were inflamed, and in the fifth there was effusion into the chest.

*Mortification* supervening on gunshot wounds may occur under the
following conditions:—(1) When the injured parts are irrecoverably
disorganized, so that they immediately cease to live, which happens to
the tissues in the immediate track of a musket-ball, or to a whole limb
struck by a spent shot. (2) From excess of inflammation following a
wound;—either because the action induced is too great to be borne by
the weakened powers of the part;—or because the excess of inflammation
is due to a disordered state of the constitution. (3) From division of the
great arterial and venous trunks. This is indicated by its commencing
in the extremity of the limb; the foot or the hand for instance; and it
presents a combination of the two forms of dry and humid gangrene.
The most distant parts become cold, pale, and insensible; this state
spreads up the limb; then the patient complains of pain and numbness;
and the parts above those which are actually dead become slightly tumefied and discoloured. In the course of three or four days heat and redness supervene, and the swelling greatly increases. The constitution
now becomes affected with restlessness, anxiety, and fever;—the swelling rapidly increases, with great pain, the skin being yellowish and
streaked with bluish lines. The patient mostly sinks;—there being but
few cases in which, if the first stage has passed by, and the constitution
has become affected, (as indicatad by the rapid extension of the gangrenous swelling,) there will be power to arrest the disease, and form a line
of separation.

*Secondary Hæmorrhage.*—This is the last complication of gunshot
wounds that will here require notice. It may be caused, *first*, in consequence of excessive arterial action, by which the coagula in the mouths
of the divided vessels are displaced. This may occur at any time from
the first day till the fifth. *Secondly*, by the separation of a slough from
a large artery. This may occur from the fifth till the twentieth day;
and it is this peculiar variety of secondary hæmorrhage which is generally thought to be so frequent in its occurrence, but which Mr. Guthrie
asserts not to happen in more than three or four out of a thousand cases.
*Thirdly*, from ulceratian of the coats of an artery; and this may happen
at any time until the wound is healed. The *fourth* and most common
variety is a real *inflammatory hæmorrhage*; the blood not being poured
out from any particular trunk, but exuding from the general surface of a
granulating wound. This kind of hæmorrhage may be caused by every
thing capable of exciting the circulation;—by excess in food, drink, or
muscular exertion, and particularly by venery;* and the same causes will,

---

* The tendency of the great excitement produced by the venereal orgasm to cause
hæmorrhage is well known. Hennen (p. 189) enumerates three cases; in the first
of which, fatal hæmorrhage from the lungs took place from this cause; in the second,
"an officer died of uncontrollable bleeding from an amputated arm, from the same;"
in the third, "a young officer with an amputated thigh, which was healed within half

of course, tend greatly to induce either of the other varieties.—It is most liable to occur in persons of a sanguine temperament;—and especially if they have been exposed to the close air of a crowded hospital. The hæmorrhage is preceded in these cases (and in the other varieties also, if partially induced by the same causes) by pain, heat, and throbbing of the wound..

*Of Simple Cases.*—When a ball has passed completely through some common fleshy part, such as the thigh or buttock, the wound should be sponged clean;—and when the ordinary hæmorrhage is arrested, the best application is a piece of lint, (which may or may not be dipped in oil,) and which should be secured by two or three cross strips of plaster. Tremour and mental confusion may be allayed by a mouthful of wine or spirits, and by a few consolatory words from the surgeon;—or, if severe, by an opiate. When they have subsided, a compress wetted with cold water, or with some innocent lotion, will be the only other application needed. If the patient can be kept at rest in bed, all bandages, at this stage, will be unnecessary and injurious. In military practice, one or two turns of a roller may be necessary to keep on the dressings, but they should not be applied with any degree of tightness;—and as a general rule, their application on the field of battle should be as limited as possible, lest there be a deficiency of them in the later stages of treatment, when they can scarcely be dispensed with.

These primary dressings need not be removed for the first three or four days; and if they have become dry and stiff, they should be well moistened with warm water previous to their removal. During the succeeding inflammatory stage, there is the choice of hot or cold applications, each of which has its advocates. Mr. Guthrie greatly prefers the use of cold water;—but if it make the patient feel chilly or uncomfortable, or if it augment stiffness and pain, warm poultices, or the water-dressing, should be substituted. But it is found that the too frequent use of poultices weakens parts, and renders them incapable of the necessary restorative actions; whilst they too often serve as a cloak for negligence, and prevent the adoption of more active measures;—in fact, the experienced military surgeon just quoted considers a poultice applied to a compound fracture, or wounded joint, as the sure precursor of amputation.* When suppuration is well established, the cure is to be completed by mild stimulating lotions, and bandages. Particular care must be taken to prevent sinuses, by pressing out all stagnant matter, and pre-

---

an inch, had, seven weeks after the amputation, an hæmorrhage so violent from an excess of this nature, and a subsequent opening up of the stump to such an extent, as detained him under cure for three months longer." Instances of death in coitu are mostly to be assigned to a like cause.

* They were recommended by Hunter, on the plea that it is expedient to promote suppuration; whereas it is a great object to have as little suppuration as possible.

venting its accumulation by compresses; or by free openings if requisite, to ensure its discharge.   Gentle friction and passive motion, are the best means for preventing or removing subsequent stiffness.   The *constitu- tional treatment* must be antiphlogistic.   If inflammation be slight, purging, low diet, and rest may suffice;—but if it be severe, and the patient robust, bleeding may be employed freely.*   A combination of sulphate of magnesia and tartar emetic, F. 59, is a most convenient form for the military surgeon.   *Leeches* may be applied to allay inflammation. *Opiates* should be given at bed-time, if there be much spasmodic twitch- ing and pain.

Superficial wounds, made by musket or cannon-balls, are to be treated in the same way.   It must be recollected that cold lotions are never to be extensively applied to the trunk.

*Dilatation.*—The same observations are to be made concerning the dilatation of gunshot as of punctured wounds.   Scarifications or in- cisions are never to be made from routine, nor without some definite object.†   But if there be great swelling of muscular parts confined by fasciæ, or if matter form in the same, there can be no doubt of the pro- priety of a sufficiently long and deep incision to relieve the tension and discharge the matter.   Dilatation may also be required in compound gunshot fracture, to remove splinters of bone.

The two peculiarly fatal forms of inflammation specified by Mr. Guthrie are to be combated by vigorous antiphlogistic measures and in- cisions.

FOREIGN BODIES.—In *every case* the surgeon should ascertain whether foreign bodies are lodged in the wound; for even although it may be satis- factorily demonstrated that the *ball* has passed out,—or although there may be a mere laceration from grapeshot or shell, still pieces of the clothing or other matters may remain in the wound.   If there is only one open- ing, such an examination is indispensable.   The parts should be put as much as possible into the posture they were in when the injury was received; and the finger should be passed in as far as it will reach, counter-pressure being at the same time made on the opposite side of the limb.   In unimportant parts, the finger may be aided by a long probe or bougie, or a deeply-seated ball may sometimes be detected by a long, fine acupuncture needle.

If the foreign body is found lying under the skin, it should be immedi- ately removed by an incision, which will require to be larger than at first

* Soldiers, from their generous diet, active exercise, and regular discipline, bear depletions of every kind much better than rustic labourers or mechanics, although, perhaps, more ruddy and healthful in appearance.

† Yet we read of the orifices of these wounds being scored in a radiated manner by foreign surgeons, as though in compliance with some religious ordinance.   Sir C. Bell's Dissertation of Gunshot Wounds, p. 459.

would be imagined.  Pressure should be made to prevent the ball shifting its place during the incision, otherwise the operation will be long and vexatious.  If the foreign body is near the wound, it should be removed by forceps, the simpler the better.  The orifice will mostly require to be dilated for this purpose, because from the natural elasticity of the skin, and the ensuing tumefaction, it will be too much contracted to allow it to repass.

It is a well-established rule, that on no account are incisions to be made for the removal of foreign bodies, unless they are certain of being successful; both because of the fruitless pain created, and because of the depressing effects of a failure on the patient's mind.  If a ball is lodged in the middle of the thigh or other thick fleshy part, and from the direction of the wound it cannot be extracted without a very considerable incision, it should be left to itself; and it will probably be either brought within reach by the natural contraction of the parts, and by the flow of matter—or it may become encysted, and give no farther trouble.  Bullets that have become encysted, are to be cut out, if they come near the skin. or if, during any of their extraordinary changes of position, they impede the functions of any important part, otherwise they are to be left to themselves.  The cyst that envelopes them is frequently so dense, and adheres so firmly, that a portion of it must be removed at the same time.

If a ball has lodged in the substance of a bone, it should be removed by a chisel, or trephine; otherwise caries, or necrosis, and so much mischief as to necessitate amputation, may follow.  In a few rare cases, however, balls have remained imbedded in bone, without mischief.

SECONDARY HÆMORRHAGE.—The *fourth* of the varieties of secondary hæmorrhage is to be treated by rest; by the application of cold or iced water, or ice itself;—by pressure on the bleeding surface, or on the arterial trunks above;—and if the blood seem to ooze from any particular spot, it may be touched with nitrate of silver.  If there be fever and plethora, bleeding and purging;—if weakness and irritability, tonics, opiates, and the mineral acids;—and, in all cases, removal from a crowded hospital will be expedient.

NECESSITY OF AMPUTATION.—It will not be wondered at, that this operation will be frequently required in gunshot injuries of the limbs, on account of the fracture and comminution of bones, the exposure of joints, the division of blood-vessels, and the irreparable violence inflicted on the skin and soft parts.

The points for consideration in determining its necessity are twofold;— viz. 1st, would the preservation of the limb endanger the patient's life? —and 2ndly, supposing that it would not, would the limb be of use, if saved?  In deciding on the first point, we must be guided by the patient's *age;*—for an old person would succumb to an injury that a young one might recover from;—by his *habits;*—for temperance, sobriety, and a

well-disciplined mind, will be greatly in his favour;—by *previous dis-*
*ease;*—for (as has already been insisted on\*) if there be organic disease
of any viscus, the patient will be infinitely more liable to sink;—lastly,
by the *supply of necessaries*, and extent of accommodation;—hence, in
compound fractures, and other cases demanding perfect quiescence, many
more limbs may be saved in civil practice than in the accidents of naval
and military warfare.

PRIMARY OR SECONDARY?—But supposing amputation to be decidedly
required;—that the limb, if preserved, could be but a burden to the patient;—and that the attempt to preserve it would endanger his life;—the
question next arises, whether amputation ought to be *primary;*—that is,
performed within the first forty-eight hours, before fever and inflammation have set in;—or whether it ought to be *secondary;*—that is, delayed
till inflammation has subsided, and suppuration is established—which is
not generally the case in less than from three to six weeks.

Now this question is one which cannot be decided by argument, but by
experience; and the general experience of modern military surgeons has
decided that amputation when necessary ought to be primary. We may
gather from Mr. Guthrie's† works, that the loss after secondary operations
is at least three times as great as that after primary.

Hunter, however, and other surgeons before his time, advocated secondary amputations; the arguments in favour of their practice being, that
persons in a rude state of health do not bear operations so well as those
who have been labouring under some chronic suppurating complaint of
the part to be removed;—and that if the patient is not able to support the
inflammation arising from the accident it is more than probable that he
would not be able to support the amputation and its consequences;‡ and
farther, that the patient is liable to sink sooner or later from the shock of
the amputation speedily succeeding that of the injury. Moreover, Mr.
Alcock, surgeon to the Anglo-Spanish legion, found in his§ practice that
secondary was less fatal than primary amputation.

But it may be seen at a glance, that there is not one reason in favour
of secondary amputation that is worth much. For, in the first place, it
must be evident that many will die of the inflammation of an extensive lacerated and contused wound, who would not die of the minor inflammation arising from a clean incision; and that many will die of secondary
amputation, when exhausted by suffering, and weakened by confinement
in a hospital, who might have survived a primary operation. In the
second place, Mr. Alcock's experience in Spain is neutralized by another

---

\* Part I. chap. i.                         † Guthrie, op. cit. p. 224.
‡ Hunter on Gunshot Wounds.
§ Notes on the Medical History of the British Legion in Spain, by Rutherford Al.
cock, K. T. S. Lond. 1838.

isolated set of cases, viz. the secondary amputations after the battle of Navarino, all of which proved fatal.* And lastly, it must be recollected that the question is,—not whether a hundred men just wounded and requiring amputation are more likely to survive it than a hundred who have gone through the ordeal of six weeks in a hospital;—but whether the first hundred would live to that period; which most probably they would not.

When amputation is decided upon, it should then be primary. But there are two errors as to time, that even here must be avoided. The first is, that of *amputating too soon*, before the patient is in any measure recovered from the immediate shock and collapse; the second is, that of *waiting too long*, so that he becomes exhausted by pain. Therefore, when the patient is brought to the surgeon with a limb knocked off, and with a low pulse, cold skin, hiccup, fainting, or other symptoms of extreme collapse, the first endeavour should be to comfort him; to explain the nature of his loss; to assure him of his safety, and to administer small quantities of wine or cordials, and apply warmth; at the same time providing by the tourniquet against immediate peril from bleeding. And in this way, by waiting an hour or two, the agitation of mind and body will be appeased, and the operation may be performed without farther delay. But if the pain be so intolerable that the patient eagerly demands to be relieved from his sufferings, the request should be immediately complied with; for the shock of the operation will be infinitely less detrimental than the endurance of such torments.

Care should always be taken, before amputating, to *ascertain the whole amount of injury;* for it would be of little use to cut off a leg, if the patient were shot through the liver.

If, from any unavoidable circumstances, the favourable period has elapsed, and violent fever and inflammation have set in, still the operation must be done without delay in some few cases, to give the patient a chance of surviving. But, in the majority, free antiphlogistic measures should be first employed; and then "On the very day," says Hennen, "that a subsidence of fever is effectually announced by a free and healthy suppuration, by the abatement of local inflammation; by a restoration of the skin to its functions, demonstrated by returning coolness and elasticity, particularly on the affected limb; we should proceed to perform our amputation on those patients in whom no hope of an ultimate recovery without it can be entertained."†

RULES FOR AMPUTATION.—1. When a limb has been completely knocked off by a cannon-ball, the stump must be amputated; and if the bones be splintered and shattered up to the next joint, or if the wound be so near the

---

* Lizars' Practical Surgery.
† Hennen, op. cit. p. 256; Guthrie, Clin. Lect. Med. Gaz., March 10th, 1838.

joint that mischief is to be apprehended, the operation must be performed above it.

2. Gunshot fracture of the femur always requires amputation, and so does division of both femoral artery and vein, or of the sciatic nerve. But it is not necessary for considerable destruction of the soft parts, provided the bone, vessels, and nerves are intact, and that there are conveniences for the cure.

3. Injuries of the knee, or ankle-joints, or extensive fracture of the tibia with division of the arteries, require it, but not mere laceration of the calf.

4. The arm should not be amputated for almost any *musket-shot* injury. If the head of the humerus is shattered, it should if possible be sawu off;—if the elbow is shot through, it may be cut out;—and the fore-arm will bear so much fracturing and cutting, that it should not be con-demned without very great injury both to bones and arteries. But exten-sive injury of the wrist-joint, or of the humerus, with division of the vessels, generally requires the operation.

5. When a main artery is wounded, and gangrene is commencing, and spreading beyond the toes or fingers, amputation should be performed just above the level of the wound.

# CHAPTER V.

## OF THE EFFECTS OF HEAT, BURNS, AND SCALDS.

GENERAL DESCRIPTION.—The distinction between scalds and burns refers only to the difference in the agent through which the heat was applied; although, by some, the term *scald* is used to signify any minor degree of burn that has not produced disorganization. When the injury has been inflicted through the medium of a fluid, it is generally diffused in its extent, and equable in its severity. It is also generally superfi-cial;—for the heat of boiling-water is not sufficient to cause the death of the cutis, unless immersed in it for some time;—although that effect may be readily produced by boiling soap or oil, or other liquids whose point of ebullition is high.

The degree of heat which may be borne without inconvenience or injury, depends on the manner in which it is applied. The body may be exposed to *air* of a temperature of nearly 300° F. without injury, whereas the contact of a *solid* or *fluid* of the same heat would instantly cause burning. Again, some parts of the body will from habit tolerate a degree of heat that would be extremely painful to others.*

DIAGNOSIS.—It is sometimes important in medico-legal investigations, to determine exactly the medium by which a burn has been inflicted. Those caused by some sudden and intense heat of short duration,—as by the ignition of turpentine or gunpowder, or the inflammable gases, are more diffused, uniform and regular than those occasioned by the contact of heated substances;—and all the hair is burned off smoothly.

After burns from the explosion of gunpowder, the injured parts are said to be of a peculiar bluish white. The irritation of these injuries is often aggravated by the numerous grains of gunpowder that escape combustion, and are projected with such force as to stick into the skin. In many cases caused by the explosion of gas in coal mines, particles of the coal dust adhere to the skin in the same manner.

DIVISION.—The most useful division of burns, for practical purposes, is the three fold one which has existed from time immemorial, into, 1st, burns producing *mere redness*; 2ndly, those causing *vesication*; 3rdly, those causing *death of the part burned.*

1. The first class are attended with mere superficial inflammation, terminating in resolution, with or without desquamation of the cuticle. The pain is philosophically said to consist of a perpetuation of the original sense of burning.

2. In the second class, there is a higher degree of inflammation, causing the cutis to exude serum and form vesicles. These in trivial cases dry up and heal; but if the injury to the cutis have been sufficient to cause it to suppurate, they will be succeeded by obstinate ulcers. The pain of these burns is much more severe than in the former class, especially if the vesicles have been torn, and the surface of the true skin exposed to the air and the contact of foreign bodies. The formation and increase of vesicles may often be prevented. They generally appear immediately after the accident, although cases are recorded in which they did not rise for three days.

(3) The third class of burns are attended with mortification;—either *primarily*, from disorganization of structure;—or *secondarily*, from excessive inflammation. These are, for obvious reasons, not attended with so much pain as the last class; but in every other respect they are infinitely more serious, and the sores which remain after the separation of the sloughs, are often months or years in healing.

* " Those smiths who are daily employed in making of anchors, have the palms of their hands extremely hard and insensible like horn, insomuch that they are capable of holding burning coals, or even hot iron from the furnace, without danger ; but the same smiths, when they lie sleeping by the fireside after they have been tired by their day's labour, have the skin of their legs often burnt and raised into a blister by a small particle of such fire."—Van Swieten Comment. quoted in Kentish's First Essay on Burns.

CONSTITUTIONAL SYMPTOMS.—The constitutional symptoms of severe burns are those of great collapse. The surface is pale, the extremities cold, the pulse quick and feeble;—there are violent and repeated shiverings, and the patient often complains most urgently of cold. In some fatal cases these symptoms are soon succeeded by laborious breathing, coma, and death;—in others, dissolution is preceded by a period of imperfect reaction, with delirium, sharp jerking pulse, and the other symptoms indicative of *prostration with excitement.*

PROGNOSIS.—The danger of burns must be estimated by their extent, their severity, their situation, the age and constitution of the patient, and by the symptoms actually present. *Extensive* burns, even of small severity, are always dangerous; and especially if vesication has occurred early, and the cuticle has been stripped off. *Burns on the trunk* are always more dangerous than those of an equal extent on the extremities; and it need not be said that *infancy* and *old age* will be alike unfavourable. With regard to the *symptoms actually present,* it may be noticed, that although the severe pain, such as is common in burns of the second class, is in itself a source of great danger, from its tendency to exhaust the vital powers, still that it is on the whole a favourable symptom, if the injury is extensive; and that the want of it indicates urgent peril. " The early subsidence of complaint," observes Mr. Travers, " unwillingness to be disturbed, apathy approaching to stupor, as if the scale of sensibility had shrunk below the point of pain, is invariably a fatal symptom. Constant shivering is an ill omen. The failure of the pulse and consequent coldness of the extremities, with a livid hue of the transparent skin of the cheeks and lips from congestion in the capillaries, drowsiness, with occasional muscular twitchings, are sure prognostics of death." Subsidence of swelling is an equally ominous symptom.

The *periods of danger* in burns are three; 1st during the first three to five days; from collapse or imperfect reaction; 2ndly, during the sympathetic fever which follows, in which the patient may sink with an affection of the head or chest; 3rdly, during the suppurative stage, in which he may die from the profuse discharge, or from pulmonary consumption induced by it. Kentish observes that very many cases prove fatal on the ninth day.

MORBID ANATOMY.—A *post mortem* examination readily accounts for the coma and laborious breathing which are such constant symptoms of fatal burns. Conjestion and serous effusion are found on the surface and in the ventricles of the brain ; and the air cells of the lungs are loaded with a thin muco-serous fluid, as in the " *suffocative catarrh of the dying*" of Laennec. The reason of the tendency to congestion in these organs has not been very well explained ; although the disorder of the lungs has been attributed to the reciprocity of function existing between them and the skin.

TREATMENT.—The treatment of burns in their early stage has been a matter of great dispute. Some authorities direct them to be treated in the same light as any other injuries which have produced an equal amount of inflammation. Thus, for a slight burn or scald, insufficient to produce any constitutional depression, they recommend the immediate application of cold in any convenient form, and its continuance until pain and inflammation have subsided.

But it had long been a popular practice to pursue a directly contrary method. It was constantly observed, that although the application of cold was most pleasurable, and continued to be so as long as it was employed unremittingly, still that if it were discontinued for a moment, the pain returned with infinitely greater force. On the other hand, it was found that if heat or other stimulants were applied to the burn, the pain although aggravated for the moment, shortly subsided, and that permanent ease was obtained much sooner than by the cooling treatment.

MR. KENTISH'S THEORIES.—These beneficial effects of stimulants (which in the ruder periods of science were supposed, as they still are by the vulgar, to depend on a dissipation or extraction of the heat) were, about forty years ago, attempted to be explained by Mr. Kentish of Newcastle, in the following manner. He assumed that the injurious effects of cold arise from its diminishing action;—and that those of heat depend on its causing an increase of action. He then shows that the treatment of frost-bites, and of burns, ought to be analogous, although reverse. And that, as is the treatment of frost-bite, we first cautiously avoid heat; but apply snow, then cold water, and so on in an ascending series until the part is able to bear an ordinary degree of heat;—that so, in treating burns, we ought at first to avoid cold; but apply a moderate degree of heat, or of some other stimulant, and proceed in a descending series, gradually diminishing the stimulant power of the applications, until the part is restored to its ordinary powers and actions.

On the merits of this as a theory, the author will not attempt to decide. Some grave writers have pronounced it to be visionary and unintelligible—and it very possibly is so. It would perhaps be a saving of trouble, if the good effects of stimulants in burns were considered as illustrations of the ultimate fact, that inflammation caused by one irritant may sometimes be dispelled by another. But as regards Mr. Kentish's *practice*, every one who has tried it fairly is decided in its favour. And its general adoption would be expedient for the following two reasons;—1st, Because it is universally admitted that slight cases get well quite as quickly under the use of stimulants as of refrigerants, and 2ndly, because of the frightful mischief that would result, if cold were applied to a severe and extensive burn by some ignoramus who had seen it used without detriment in trivial cases.

*Local Treatment of the First Class.*—In slight cases without vesica-
20

tion, the best treatment will be to apply heat, if it can be done conveniently, either by holding the part near a fire, or by dipping it in water of
112°, and continuing this until the burning pain begins to subside ; or it
may be bathed with tepid oil of turpentine, or alcohol, or æther, (which
may be warmed by putting them into a teacup, immersed in boiling water,)
and then should be warmly wrapped up in lint or cotton.   But if the surgeon prefer the cooling plan, he may apply any evaporating or refrigerant
lotion—cold water is as good as any others ; pounded ice mixed with
lard was recommended by Earle : a poultice of potato or grated turnip, is
not to be despised; but whatever is used, it must be renewed often enough
to keep up the sensation of cold.

*Of the Second and Third Class.*—The right method of treating burns
of these classes, is, to cover them entirely with some substance, gently
stimulating in its nature, and capable of entirely excluding the air and
cold; under the protection of which, in favourable cases, they will heal
without suppuration.   And Kentish's plan of first bathing the burnt parts
with tepid turpentine, then with all possible expedition applying a liniment, composed of *ung. resinæ* 3j.; *ol. terebinth* 3ss, thickly spread on lint,
and lastly, wrapping them up warmly in flannel, seems to be the most
judicious.   These dressings should be allowed to remain as long as possible, and should not be removed unless there is a profuse discharge or
bad smell from the wound.   If the vesications are unbroken, and very
tense, they should be first pricked with a needle.

If the surgeon chooses to pursue the opposite plan of treatment, he may
make use of cold applications, provided the vesicles are unbroken, and
the burn not severe and extensive enough to cause constitutional depression.   But if the vesicles are broken, a soft unguent of lard and oil should
be laid on to protect the cutis.

*Constitutional Treatment.*—If there is an urgent degree of collapse,
the measures directed in Part I. ch. i. are to be diligently adopted. . Care
should, however, be taken not to push the use of stimulants too far, lest
conjestion in the head or chest be induced or aggravated;—and, on the
other hand, not to abandon them too soon, lest the collapse return, as it
is very apt to do.   Arrowroot, and other forms of mild nutriment, must
be judiciously administered, according to circumstances.

*Use of Opium.*—If there be much pain, a good dose of opium should
be given without delay.   For children, nothing can be better than the
compound tincture of camphor, of which 3j—3ij may be given according to the age. (Each fluid drachm contains ¼ of a grain of opium.)
Yet it must be added that certain great authorities altogether condemn
its employment.   "Opium," says Larrey, "is injurious, whether used
externally or internally.   Externally it stupifies the parts, instead of exciting them to a salutary inflammation; internally, if used in considerable
quantity, it enfeebles all the organs, after producing a momentary stimula-

tion."* Travers objects to it because of its tendency to produce or increase congestion in the head. He says that " in small doses it is inefficacious, and in large ones injurious." Notwithstanding these objections, however, it may be given in moderation when demanded by urgent pain. If there be a tendency to coma, it is of course inadmissible; but then the patient will most probably perish, whether it be given him or not.

During the symptomatic fever, the bowels must be kept open by some mild laxative, such as castor oil or rhubarb; and the diet must be unirritating, but not too low. In the event of any inflammatory or congestive attack of the head or chest, purgatives, and leeches or bleeding, must be cautiously employed according to the strength.

*Treatment of the remaining Ulcers.*—The ulcers resulting from burns are very slow in healing. Their granulations are pale and flabby, and the cicatrix extremely liable to contract and become dense, hard, and cartilaginous. Thus the most serious deformities are sometimes occasioned; the chin may be fixed to the breast; the eyelids rendered incapable of closing; or a limb rigidly and immoveably bent. The cause of this disinclination to heal is not well understood; but one cause there is which may be easily detected and remedied; namely, too full a diet, which is often needlessly used on the plea of supporting the strength under the profuse discharge. "There can be no doubt," says Kentish, "that full diet and stimulants, during the suppurative stage, keep up irritation in the system, and cause the immense continued discharge by the exposed surfaces of the wounds."† And it is equally certain that many cases will rapidly get well when the diet is lowered and purgatives are administered.

There should be no hurry in removing the first dressings, but when they are removed, the succeeding applications must be suited to the state of the ulcer.

If it is irritable and painful, or hot and swelled, or seems inclined to spread by ulceration, or if small abscesses threaten to form under the skin, poultices, or the water dressing, Dover's powder at bedtime, and aperients, should be resorted to. If sloughs are tardy in separating, the case must be treated as directed at p. 109.

When the irritable state is removed, a succession of mild stimulants will be advisable; especially the zinc lotion; *ceratum calaminæ; unguentum cretæ;* simple lint; and pressure with sheet lead or strips of plaster. When the discharge is very profuse, the sore should be constantly kept thinly covered with very finely powdered chalk.

Care must be taken to counteract the tendency to contraction by frequent motion of the parts, and by fixing the skin. If the fingers are

---

* Mem. de Chir. Mil., t. i. p. 96.
† Second Essay on Burns. Newcastle, 1800, p. 64.

severely burned, it is very difficult to prevent them from adhering together, although it should be attempted by interposing lint between them,
and keeping them asunder.    It may be of some use to lubricate the cicatrized parts with pure oil.    But if, notwithstanding, contraction does take
place and form an obstacle to any necessary motion, the only remedy is
the extirpation of the cicatrix, if it can be done with safety.

SUNDRY REMEDIES.—It remains to notice divers remedies which have
acquired popularity in the cure of burns; and they all, as Mr. James
observes, either possess certain stimulating qualities, or else exclude the
influence of air and temperature.

*The liniment composed of equal parts of linseed oil and lime-water*, or
*Carron oil*, (so called because in general use at the iron-works of that
name,) is a good defensative, but has a most sordid, nauseous odour.    It
is sometimes applied after cicatrization, to prevent contraction.    *Lime-
water and milk* is an analogous preparation.    *Soap-liniment* is a good
stimulant; but is more expensive than turpentine, and not better.    *Common thick white paint* has, according to Sir C. Bell,[*] been used at the
Middlesex Hospital; but from its containing white lead, its protracted application might be hazardous.    *Copaiba* has been employed at the Exe-
ter. Hospital by Mr. Luscombe, and *Treacle* by Mr. Greenhow,[†] but
neither of the last named applications is to be compared with Kentish's
liniment.    *Flour* is a remedy very much in vogue with some people.
It should be applied thickly with a common dredger, so as to cover every
part denuded of cuticle.    *Cotton*, very soft, and finely carded, is another
popular application.    Like the flour, it is directed to be laid on the raw
surface, and to be perpetually strewed on in thick layers, so as to soak
up the discharge; but without removing any which is already applied.
The good effect of these two substances depend on the same principle.
They exclude the air, and form a soft covering, and if there is nothing
else at hand, either of them may be applied.    But they are apt to become
dry, hard, and irritating, and not unfrequently are converted into a
noisome mass of putridity and maggots.

*Vinegar.*—Mr. David Cleghorn, an Edinburgh brewer, very strongly
recommends the application of warm vinegar for the first twelve hours,
then poultices till suppuration is established, and chalk afterwards.
Although not a surgeon, he has the rare merit of writing on a surgical
subject with common sense and modesty.    He agrees with Kentish, in
recommending that stimulant applications should be applied only during
the first few hours, whilst the injury is recent.[‡]

[*] Institutes of Surgery.  London, 1838.

[†] Greenhow, Med. Gaz. Oct. 13, and Leach, Med. Gaz. Nov. 3, 1838.

[‡] Med. Facts and Obs., vol. ii.

# CHAPTER VI.

## OF THE EFFECTS OF COLD.

EFFECTS OF SEVERE COLD.—When a person is exposed to very severe cold, especially if it be accompanied with wind,—or if it be during the night,—or if he have been exhausted by hunger, watching, and fatigue, he feels an almost irresistible impulse to sleep, which, if yielded to, is soon succeeded by coma and death. During the state of coma, the body of the sufferer is found to be very pale and cold; the respiration and pulse almost imperceptible, and the pupils dilated; but the limbs are flexible as long as life remains, unless the degree of cold be very great indeed. On a *post mortem* examination, the chief morbid appearances observed are great venous congestion and serous effusion in the head.

FROST-BITE.—But if the trunk of the body be well protected, the cold may only affect some exposed part, such as the nose, ears, or extremities. The first visible effect is, that the part becomes of a dull red colour;— an effect of cold which is notoriously frequent, and which depends on a diminution of the quantity of blood conveyed by the arteries, and a stagnation of it in the veins. If the cold continue, the venous blood will be gradually expelled by a contraction of the tissues, and the part will become of a livid, tallowy paleness, perfectly insensible and motionless, and much reduced in bulk. When in this condition, a part is said to be *frost-bitten*. The patient may be quite unconscious of the accident that has befallen him until he is told it by some other person; especially if it be his nose or ear that is affected, or some other part that he does not move.

A frost-bitten part may mortify in two manners;—1st, by *direct spha-chelus*, if no reaction whatever is induced; 2ndly, by *gangrenous inflammation;* if reaction, when induced, be rendered too violent.

The degree of cold required to produce frost-bite under any ordinary circumstances of exposure must be considerably below the freezing point. Mr. Guthrie states it at ten degeees below the zero of Fahrenheit.* The natives of warm climates may be severely injured by cold that would be innocuous to the inhabitants of colder regions. Thus during the siege of Ciudad Rodrigo, when the troops were obliged to sleep on the ground without cover, three of the Portuguese actually died of the cold in one night, whilst the British escaped without being frost-bitten. But very much depends on the temperament; for according to Larrey, the phlegmatic Dutch, Hanoverians, and Prussians, suffered much more

* Guthrie, op. cit., p 111.

during Napoleon's winter campaigns than the darker and more sanguine soldiers of France and Italy.*   Those who indulge in spirituous liquors, exhausted as they are by perpetual stimulation, are much more liable to suffer than the temperate.

It is well known that a *small* part of the body may be frozen so as to be quite white, and hard, and brittle, and yet recover with proper care. This fact 'was frequently exemplified in Hunter's experiments on the ears of rabbits, and combs of cocks.   And some of the lower orders of animals may be entirely frozen and yet survive.   But it is not credible that a whole limb of a human being, much less that the whole body, could be frozen without death ensuing; although stories of such occur˙ rences have long been current amongst authors.

*Treatment.*—The indications of treatment whenever a part or the whole of the body has been exposed to severe cold, are, 1st, To produce *mode˙ rate reaction*, and restore the circulation and sensibility; 2ndly, To *avoid excessive reaction*, which would surely lead to violent and dangerous in˙ flammation.

*Of Frost-bite.*—The best remedy for a frost-bite is to rub the part well with snow.   For whilst the friction restores the circulation and sensibility, the snow prevents any excessive reaction.   After a time cold water may be substituted for the snow, and the friction may be rendered brisker.   These applications must be made in a room without a fire; and a high, or even a moderate temperature must be avoided for some time. By these means no other inconvenience will ensue, save slight swelling and tingling, with vesication and desquamation of the cuticle; although the part will remain weak and sensible to cold for some time.   X

For the *coma induced by cold* the treatment must be similar.   At first the body should be rubbed with snow;—afterwards, when its warmth and sensibility are a little restored, it should be wiped quite dry, and be rubbed with fur or flannel.   Then the patient should be put into a cold bed in a room without a fire, a stimulant enema should be administered, and a little warm wine and water, very weak, be given as soon as he can swallow.   The enema may be composed of water and salt, with a little oil of turpentine; but tobacco, which was formerly recommended by the profession in such cases, and is still popularly considered to be of great service, must not be thought of;—it would surely be prejudicial—perhaps deadly.   The after-treatment must be entirely regulated by the state of the patient;—the strength must be supported by mild cordials and nutri- ˙ ment; care being taken not to excite feverishness or headach.

The *contact of any intensely cold body* (such as frozen mercury) causes severe burning pain, followed by vesication.   It thus appears that the effects of sudden abstraction may be similar to those of too great

* Larrey, Mem. De Chir. Mill. Tom. iv. p. 111.

communication of heat. The best application is snow, gradually permitted to thaw.

VIOLENT GANGRENOUS INFLAMMATION may be caused, if heat is injudiciously applied to frozen or frost-bitten parts. It may also ensue if a part has been exposed for a long period to a *low temperature* which is *suddenly raised;*—although the cold may not have been sufficient to cause actual frost-bite, and may have been tolerated without inconvenience. A good example of this accident is narrated by Baron Larrey,* as it affected the French troops during their campaign in Poland in 1807. During the few days preceding and following the battle of Eylau, the cold was most intense, ranging from ten to fifteen degrees below the zero of Reaumur.† But although the troops were day and night exposed to this inclement weather, and the soldiers of the Imperial Guard, in particular, were nearly motionless for more than twenty-four hours, there were no complaints of its effects. On the night of the 9th of February, however, *a sudden thaw commenced*, and immediately a great number of soldiers presented themselves at the " *ambulances*," complaining of severe numbness, weight, and pricking pain in the feet. On examination, some were found to have slight swelling and redness at the base of the toes and dorsum of the foot; whilst the toes of others had already become black and dry. And in this manner, the toes, and sometimes the whole foot, perished; the mortification being so rapid that it was difficult to say whether it was preceded by inflammation or not—although it probably was so for a very brief period. The best *treatment* for such cases is the application of snow or very cold water, followed by evaporating lotions. These, if employed early enough, may prevent gangrene; or even if that have actually occurred, they should be used as long as it appears to be spreading. Subsequently, stimulating poultices and ointments should be employed to hasten the separation of the sloughs, and to promote granulation.

CHILBLAINS consist in an atonic inflammation of the skin, induced by sudden alternations of temperature; such as warming the feet and hands by the fire when cold and damp. They may present themselves in three degrees. In the *first*, the skin is red in patches, and slightly swelled; with more or less itching or tingling, or perhaps pain and lameness. In the *second*, there are vesications—the skin around being bluish or purple. In the *third* degree there is ulceration or sloughing.

*Causes.*—Chilblains are most frequent in women, children, and weakly persons generally. Some constitutions (especially those of a rheumatic diathesis) appear to be greatly predisposed to them; others are, from some unknown reason, totally exempt.

* Mem. de Chir. Mil., tom. iii. p. 61.
† From 20° to 25° below the freezing point of Fahrenheit.

*Treatment of the First Degree.*—The best treatment consists in a combination of local stimulants and depletion. When there is much heat and itching, it is an excellent plan to apply a leech;—or to make punc- tures with a needle or lancet, (or with holly-leaves, if preferred.) It would be impossible to name any stimulant that has not been recom-' mended by the public or the profession. Perhaps the best is that pro- posed by Mr. Wardrop, and consisting of *six parts of soap-liniment, and one of tincture of cantharides.* But liniments of mustard, turpentine, camphorated spirit, and ammonia;—friction with snow;—strong brine, or, in fact, any ordinary stimulant, will answer the same purpose. Whichever is chosen, it should be used cold, with considerable fric- tion, and should be strong enough to excite some increase of heat and smarting.

If there are *vesications*, care must be taken not to break them; and the liniment must be applied lightly with a feather.

If there are *ulcers or sloughs*, and they are attended with much heat, pain, and irritation, poultices are required. But as a general rule, they are too relaxing, and stimulating ointments or lotions (such as *ung. resinæ, caluminæ, zinci,* &c.) should be preferred.

---

# CHAPTER VII.

## OF THE EFFECTS OF MINERAL AND VEGETABLE IRRI- TANTS.

GENERAL OBSERVATIONS.—These substances, considered with regard to their local effects, may be divided into two classes. *First,* those which produce inflammation of the animal tissues through their tendency to *decompose* them *chemically. Secondly,* those which operate by pro- ducing *violent irritation,* but which have no power of causing chemical decomposition.

The *first class* comprehends the strong mineral acids;—the pure alka- lis, or their carbonates; sundry metallic salts, such as corrosive sublimate, nitrate of silver, and butter of antimony;—and the concentrated vegetable acids, especially the acetic and oxalic.

The *second class* includes arsenic amongst minerals, and the whole list of acrid plants, garlic, ranunculus, euphorbium, and the like,.—amongst vegetables.

ACIDS.—The decomposing agency of the concentrated acids appears to depend mainly on their affinity for water. The *sulphuric acid* blackens or *chars* the tissues in destroying them; that is, separates the water and other constituent elements, and sets free the carbon. The *nitric* turns them permanently yellow. The *hydrochloric* leaves a dead white stain. The *hydrofluoric* "is, of all known substances," says Turner, "the most destructive. When a drop of the concentrated acid of the size of a pin's-head comes in contact with the skin, instantaneous disorganization ensues, and deep ulceration of a malignant character is produced."* *Phosphorus* seems to act both by the heat disengaged in its combustion, and by the acid which is the result of it.

*Treatment.*—After injury from any of these acids, the first thing to be done is to wash it away, and neutralize it by repeated ablution with warm soap and water; then to apply poultices or any simple dressings to the ulcers that remain. The pain of these injuries is greatly increased by cold.

ALKALIS AND CAUSTIC EARTHS.—These, like the acids, appear to destroy animal matter by combining with its water. They also form a soap with the fat. Caustic potass, in the form of *liquor potassæ*, and quick lime, are the substances of this class which most frequently give rise to accidents. The *liquor ammoniæ* produces almost instant vesication and great pain when it touches the skin; it is, therefore, much to be prized as a speedy and efficient counter-irritant.

*Treatment.*—Ablution with weak warm vinegar and water, followed by poultices and simple dressings.

METALLIC COMPOUNDS.—The *bichloride of mercury* acts by its tendency to combine with albumen; and the *chloride of zinc*, and *chloride* (or *butter*) *of antimony*, probably produce their cauterant effects in a similar manner. The *nitrate of silver* is remarkable for the superficiality of its effects. It may vesicate the skin, or destroy a film on the surface of a sore, but its action does not spread. Hence, Mr. James deduces its utility in exciting adhesion, and checking spreading inflammations; erysipelas, and the like. It suffers decomposition at the moment of its contact with the animal tissue; its acid appearing to be separated, whilst the metallic oxide combines and forms a white crust with the animal matter: and this soon becomes black, because the silver loses its oxygen, and is reduced to the metallic state.

*Treatment.*—The bichloride of mercury is rendered inert by white of egg mixed with water;—the chloride of antimony is decomposed by water;—the nitrate of silver by common salt; and the chloride of zinc by a solution of an alkaline carbonate. These, therefore, would respectively be the proper applications for external injuries caused by these

* Elements of Chemistry, 5th ed. p. 377.

metallic compounds; although such cases very rarely come under the surgeon's cognizance.

*Arsenic*, if locally applied, produces inflammation, or sphacelus, not by any chemical action, but by its influence on the vital properties of the part;—it may also be absorbed into the circulation, and produce its ordinary constitutional effects as well. The *surgical treatment* of any local injury from this mineral must consist in removing it as far as possible by ablution or otherwise, and then applying poultices, or whatever other dressings may be most appropriate. Lime-water might be useful, if applied at first. Some cases, almost too horrible to think of, are recorded of the destruction of women by the local application of this poison.

ACRID VEGETABLES.—The inflammation excited by these substances requires merely soothing fomentations and emollient dressings. The smart from the sting of nettles may, it is said, be allayed by a weak infusion of tobacco, if severe enough to require any remedy at all.

If an irritating fluid have been injected into the cellular tissue, free incisions must be made, both to allow its escape, and to afford exit to pus. By this means sloughing of the skin may often be avoided, although very likely to occur when the subjacent tissue is extensively disorganized.

# CHAPTER VIII.

## OF THE EFFECTS OF THE POISON OF HEALTHY ANI. MALS, AND OF THE TREATMENT OF POISONED WOUNDS GENERALLY.

INSECTS.—The bite or sting of any insects that are met with in England are not of sufficient importance to need surgical assistance, unless inflicted in extraordinary numbers, or in peculiar situations. Mr. Lawrence[*] mentions the case of a French gentleman who was so severely stung by bees about the upper part of the chest, that he died in fifteen minutes, with all the symptoms of mortal collapse usually produced by the bite of venomous serpents. Children, if much stung by bees or wasps, may suffer severely from headach and fever. But the most common instance of danger from these insects is the alarming suffocation pro-

---

[*] Lectures, Med. Gaz., vol. v. p. 582.

duced when their sting is inflicted in the pharynx or back part of the mouth;—which sometimes happens when they are concealed in fruit, and are incautiously taken into the mouth.

*Treatment.*—If a person have been stung sufficiently to cause faintness or constitutional depression, cordials and opiates must be administered without delay. Respecting the *local treatment*, the first thing to be done is to examine the parts with a lens, and extract the stings with a fine forceps, if they have been left in the wound, as they very frequently are. Then the best remedies are those which are also most useful in burns, viz. turpentine, hot vinegar, hartshorn, spirit of wine, eau de cologne, or other stimulants. Cold applications give great relief, if used continuously. Finely-scraped chalk, flour, starch, or oil, are favourite remedies with some people. Mr. James recommends a combination of ung. hydr. fort. and liq. ammoniæ. A weak infusion of tobacco or belladonna might be worth trying. The soap liniment, or compound camphor liniment, may be used to remove the œdematous swelling that remains.

In the case of a *wasp or bee sting in the fauces*, with urgent danger of suffocation, leeches should be plentifully applied both externally and internally;—and hot stimulating gargles (especially hot salt and water) should be frequently used, in the hope of reducing the tumefaction, by causing a copious flow of blood and of saliva: but if these measures fail of affording relief, an opening must be made into the larynx or trachea.

For the bites of bugs, fleas, gnats, mosquitoes, &c., the best remedy is eau de cologne, or some other stimulant, so as to convert the itching into slight smarting. Any strong perfume will often act as a protective against these nocturnal visitants. Sweet oil rubbed over the body is said to have the same effect; a little colocynth pulp, powdered, and sprinkled about, is also said to be a sure remedy.

SPIDERS.—The most celebrated of this class is the tarantula, the miraculous effects imputed to the bite of which are too well known to need repetition here; and we can feel but little hesitation in subscribing to the opinion of Ray, " that the dancing of the *Tarantati* to certain tunes and instruments, and that these fits continue to recur yearly as long as the tarantula that bit them lives and then cease, are no other than acting fictions, and tricks to get money." We learn, however, from the least romancing of the old writers, that it produces swelling, lividity, and cramps, which were cured by scarifications and wine; and these are just the symptoms it might be expected to cause, and the most rational cure. The effects of the scorpion are similar. There is one very singular case on record, of a gentleman bitten on the penis by a spider, in America, suffering from violent vomiting, deep-seated abdominal pain, and suffocative spasms in consequence. He was relieved in thirty-six hours, by bleeding, opium, and ammonia.*

SERPENTS.—The venom of these animals operates as Fontana observed on the *vital* properties of the frame, by " destroying the irritability of the nerves, and disposing the humours to speedy corruption;" and not by any mechanical or chemical endowments. The symptoms produced vary in their nature and degree, according to the species of serpent, its degree of vigour, the frequency with which it may have bitten, and the strength of the sufferer. Some serpents can only kill small animals; the poison of some is very virulent, but soon exhausted by frequent biting; that of others is mild, but not easily exhausted; some, again, act so ener-getically on the nerves, as to cause death speedily by convulsions; others produce inflammation of the lungs; and others, whose venom is insufficient to annihilate the nervous functions at once, kill more slowly by the unhealthy or diffuse inflammation which they excite at the bitten part.

VIPER.—This is the only poisonous snake in the British Isles, but it is not often that it kills human beings. The properties of its venom have been most painfully investigated, in every possible point of view, by the Abbé Fontana;† who ascertained that it is a yellow viscous liquid, not inflammable, and neither acid nor alkaline;—that it contains no salts; and that it has no taste, except, perhaps, a slight astringent sensation if it is kept in the mouth for some time. It is not hurtful to another viper, nor does it appear to affect certain cold-blooded animals, as leeches and frogs. Moreover, it is perfectly harmless if applied to any natural mucous or cutaneous surface;—so that large quantities of it have been swallowed with impunity.

COBRA DI CAPELLO.—Dr. Russell found that this was capable of kill-ing a serpent called *Nooni Paragoodo*, but not another cobra; and that its poison was insipid when taken into the mouth, and productive of no ill consequences when applied to the eyes of chickens. The symptoms produced on animals are fainting and convulsions, but no swelling; the lungs were stuffed with blood.‡

NAIA TRIPUDIANS, hooded snake of Ceylon. Dr. Davy found that its poison tastes acrid, paralyzes the iris and levater palpebræ of fowls, when applied to their eyes, and is soon exhausted by biting. It acts chiefly on the lungs, which are found gorged with blood and serum; the

* Ray, Phil. Trans., 1698, vol. xxi. p. 57; Boccone, Musco di Fisica; Hulse, Am. Journ. Med. Sc., May 1839.

† Felix Fontana, Treatise on the Venom of the Viper; translated by Joseph Skinner. 2nd edit. Lond. 1795.

‡ Patrick Russell, M.D., F.R.S. An Account of Indian Serpents. 2 vols. folio. Lond. 1796.

symptoms being, reduction of the animal temperature and prostration of strength. According to the same authority, the *Trigonocephalus hypnale*, or *Carawilla*, has a poison that is mild, but not soon exhausted, that it produces local inflammation chiefly, and can kill frogs, but not large animals.—The *Vipera Elegans*, or tic polonga, soon causes death by convulsions; the blood is much coagulated.*

RATTLESNAKE.—This snake, unlike most others, is capable of poisoning itself. Capt. Hall made one bite itself, and it died in eight minutes. Its effects, according to Sir E. Home, may be divided into two stages, either of which may prove fatal. During the *first* which may last for sixty-two hours, the symptoms are those of great prostration of the nervous system, and contamination of the blood;—vomiting, deadly coldness, faltering pulse, the skin livid or jaundiced, bleeding from the nose, fainting fits, convulsions, and delirium. Meanwhile the bitten part swells immensely from effusion of acrid serum, and becomes mottled with blood, extravasated under the skin; and this swelling extends to the trunk. Sometimes it is attended with excruciating pain, sometimes with mere numbness or coldness. During the *second stage*, large diffused abscesses form in the swelled parts, containing bloody unhealthy pus, and sloughs of cellular tissue, and attended with low fever. After death, the body putrefies very rapidly.†

### TREATMENT OF POISONED WOUNDS.

In the first place, measures must be taken to remove the poison from the wound, or at all events to prevent its passage into the blood.

If no other means are at hand, a ligature should be tightly applied round the limb, as near as possible to the wound, and between it and the heart—so as to prevent the return of venous blood from it. Then it should be thoroughly sucked, taking care that the person who does so, has no sore nor recent abrasion in his mouth.

A better plan, however, is to cut out the bitten part as freely as may be necessary, and then to suck the wound, and bathe it thoroughly with warm water to encourage bleeding—a ligature being also applied, as in the last case.

But the best plan of all is that recommended by Sir David Barry.‡

* Davy, Physiological Researches. Lond. 1839.

† Sir Everard Home. Phil. Trans. vol. c. Case of T. Soper, who was bitten by a rattlesnake.—Hall on the poison of Rattlesnakes, Phil. Trans. vol. xxx. p. 309. Case of Mr. J. Breintal, who was bitten by a rattlesnake, reported by himself, Phil. Trans. vol. xliv. p. 147. Case of a man bitten by a rattlesnake to cure lepra, Clarke, Lancet, Dec. 15, 1838.

‡ David Barry, M. D. Experimental Researches on the influence exercised by Atmospheric Pressure, &c. Lond. 1826.

He directs, first, that an exhausted cupping-glass shall be applied over the wound for a few minutes;—next, the glass is to be taken off, and the wound freely excised;—and, lastly, the glass is to be applied again in order to promote the flow of blood, and cause the re-exudation of any of the poison that may have found its way into the neighbouring blood-ves-sels.—The cupping-glass, used in the manner we have just detailed, possesses all the efficacy, and none of the disadvantages, of ligatures;— for without interrupting the general circulation of the limb, it produces a complete afflux of all the fluids in the vicinity towards the wounded part, and entirely prevents them from conveying their contaminated con-tents towards the centre of the circulation. If the glass is applied in this manner it is far from being advantageous (as is generally supposed) to make incisions or scarifications near the wound, whether before or after its excision. For the object is to concentrate the course of the blood towards the original wound itself,—so that it may carry the venom with it as it escapes;—and this object would be counteracted by any ex-traneous incisions.

The *treatment of snake bites* during the first stage, consists first in the administration of powerful diffusive stimulants, such as hot brandy and water, ammonia, or the *eau de luce*,* to support the nervous system;— and, secondly, in the use of remedies which may be supposed to elimi-nate the poison from the blood. Thus, if there is no vomiting, it should be excited by a mustard emetic, to get rid of the vast quantity of bile that is often formed in the blood and secreted by the liver under these circum-stances; if, however, vomiting is spontaneous and too violent, it should be checked by a large dose of solid opium, and a mustard poultice to the epigastrium. But the principal remedy seems to be *arsenic*, which has long been popular for these accidents in the East Indies. It is usually administered there in the form of a nostrum, called the Tanjore pills, each of which contains a grain of it, combined with certain unknown acrid plants. The efficacy of this mineral was also fully established in the West Indies by Mr. Ireland, surgeon to the 16th regiment, who em-ployed it with perfect success in five cases of the bite of a serpent, which had previously killed several officers and men, some within six hours, and all within twelve.† He combined f℥ij. of the *liquor arsenicalis* with gtt. x. of tinct. opii., (to prevent vomiting,) f℥iß. of peppermint-water, and f℥ss. of lime-juice. This draught, which contains a grain of the arsenious acid, was given every half hour for six or eight doses, till it produced copious purging, (which was encouraged by clysters,) or

* Tinct ammoniæ comp. P. L. It contains oil of amber. Dose ♏. xxx. every half hour.

† A Letter to T. Chevalier, Esq., on the effects of arsenic in counteracting the poison of serpents. Med. Chir. Trans. 1813, vol. ii. p. 396.

till the symptoms were ameliorated. The swelled parts were well rubbed with a liniment of olive oil, turpentine, and liquor ammoniæ; and the patients, although for a time greatly debilitated, were soon able to return to their duty.

*Oil* has been very warmly recommended, both as an internal and external remedy in these cases; on what grounds it is difficult to conceive. The *fat of the viper*, a strong nauseous substance, is said to be a specific for its bite; but its efficacy is very questionable.*

If the local symptoms are very slight, stimulating embrocations, and hot fomentations, with leeches, may be sufficient. But if the swelling is rapid and extensive, or the constitution is much affected by the poison, free and extensive incisions into the swelled parts are indispensable.

The *constitutional treatment* of the second stage must be regulated by the symptoms actually present; it will most require a combination of cordials, opiates, and tonics. *Senega* and *serpentaria* have been in great repute in these cases; and of tonic stimulants they are perhaps the most useful.

---

# CHAPTER IX.

## OF THE POISONS CONTAINED IN DEAD HUMAN BODIES, AND OF DISSECTION WOUNDS.

SECTION I.—OF THE POISONS CONTAINED IN DEAD BODIES, AND OF THE INFLUENCE OF DISSECTION ON THE HEALTH.†

It appears that two distinct classes of poisons may be contained in the human body after death. The *first class* consists of certain poisons found in fresh bodies; and either produced immediately after death, or perhaps originating in some morbid condition of the soft solids and fluids that existed during life. The *second class* comprises the poisons resulting from putrefaction.

1. The *first class* of poisons appears to contain many varieties. One of the most common of them is a *gaseous emanation* of a *faint, sickly*, and indescribably *nauseous* odour. It is, perhaps, most commonly ob-

---

* Breschet says that the effects of a serpent's bite on birds can be prevented by passing a current of galvanism through the bitten part.

† The author is much indebted to a paper on this subject, read before the Medical Society of King's College, by W. Bowman, Esq., Assistant Surgeon to King's College Hospital.

served to proceed from the bodies of those who have died of fever; but this is not quite certain. This emanation is so abominably nauseous, and so sedative in its effects, that it often causes sickness and faintness in those who would be unaffected by the most advanced putrefaction. A *second variety* is that which, when inoculated into a recent puncture, and sometimes even if applied to the unbroken skin, is capable of producing the most fearful irritative and typhoid fever, with diffuse inflammation of the cellular tissue. This poison is most common in the bodies of those who have died of inflammation of the serous membranes, especially of the peritoneal inflammation attending puerperal fever. It is altogether distinct from the last, and cannot be detected by any peculiar effluvium; it is very possible, however, that they may co-exist in certain cases. Both these poisons appear to be decomposed or dissipated as putrefaction advances.

2. The *second class* of poisons, those, namely, arising from putrefaction, consist of the compounds of hydrogen, hydrosulphuric acid, carburetted and phosphoretted hydrogen, carbonic acid and ammonia, on whose chemical and sensible qualities the author need not enlarge. In the last few years an attempt has been made to persuade people that the effluvia of putrefaction are rather salubrious than otherwise, or at all events that they are not prejudicial to the health, because the workmen employed in the well-known *knackeries* of Montfauçon near Paris, as well as men who grind bones, or who are engaged in the manufacture of catgut, or candles, or leather, are in no manner inconvenienced by their offensive occupation. This dogma is sufficiently newfangled, paradoxical, and absurd, to be greedily seized upon and advocated by those who patronise the march of intellect. But although it is perfectly true that healthy persons, who use considerable exercise, and are much in the open air, and who live well but not intemperately, may be enabled to resist those noxious influences; still daily experience shows that those whose natural strength and habits of life are not so favourable to the development of their vital energies, cannot be exposed to them with impunity. Or why banish churchyards from crowded cities?

If the student of anatomy be naturally vigorous, and if he carefully avoid all other sources of indisposition, he will not find the practice of dissection to be incompatible with even a high state of health. But if it be too ardently followed, to the neglect of regular meals and sleep, it will lead to a slow and insidious disorder, consisting of a general enfeeblement of the vital powers, with marked disturbance of the digestive organs.

SYMPTOMS.—The first symptoms noticed are headach, drowsiness, and lassitude, in the evening; disturbed and unrefreshing sleep; coldness of the feet and hands, and flatulence of a fetid nature. The bowels are occasionally costive, but much more frequently the reverse; insomuch that diarrhœa is not unfrequently regarded as a test of the pupil's assiduity. The evacuations are remarkably fetid; and if, as sometimes happens, the diarrhœa is unusually severe and complicated with dysentery, they may be tinged with blood. Sometimes the upper portion of the alimentary canal is the principal seat of disorder; and instead of diarrhœa there are nausea, foul taste in the mouth, fetid eructations, want of appetite, and oppression after eating. It is not very uncommon for jaundice to occur, with or without pain in the back, fulness in the hypochondria, and other signs of hepatic conjestion. Lastly, the same causes applied more continuously and intensely, or aided by other unfavourable circumstances, may produce continued fever of various grades of malignaity.

TREATMENT.—These symptoms may, if taken early enough, be easily removed by the fresh air of the country; by aperients and alteratives, with tonics and good living. And they are to be prevented by regular daily exercise, generous diet, warm clothing, the strictest cleanliness,— and by other means for the preservation of health, with which every one is acquainted.

The *efficient cause* of this indisposition is doubtless an enfeeblement of the vital powers, principally induced by the *absorption of poisonous miasmata*. And the proofs of this absorption are so clear;—its effects on the system so marked;—and the manner in which the absorbed substances are eliminated, is so plain, that some light may doubtless be thrown on the *modus operandi* of other miasmata, which do not present themselves so palpably to the senses.

It not unfrequently happens that deleterious gases are absorbed in great quantity; either because they are present in unusual abundance, or because (as we may suppose) the vital powers of resistance are lowered. The following are instances of their effects, and of the manner in which they are got rid of by the system. A gentleman, after a hard day's dissecting, goes home:—finds himself heavy, listless, and indisposed, and with the peculiar smell of the dissecting-room clinging to him. He changes every particle of his apparel, and gives himself a thorough ablution. But in a very short time the same odour emanates from every part of him;—and it is not till after copious perspirations in the night that he is freed from the annoyance. Three gentlemen, friends of the author, dissected a fresh subject, from which proceeded the *peculiar sickly effluvium* that has been alluded to. On their return home, the weakest of them vomited;—the other two suffered from nausea and depression;—and they all had for several hours a continual sickly taste in their mouths, similar to the smell which they had been imbibing. And it is notorious that dissectors frequently recognise the smell of their subjects in the secretions of their mouths, and in the copious flatus extricated in their stomach and bowels.

From these facts it may be concluded that putrid and other deleterious

22

gases may be absorbed into the blood;—that the skin and bronchial mem‐
brane are the points of ingress;—that they may be eliminated by the skin
and mucous membranes without any alteration of their sensible qualities;
and that their elimination by the gastro-intestinal mucous membrane is
the chief cause of the diarrhœa which is such a frequent consequence of
anatomical zeal.

SECTION II.—OF DISSECTION WOUNDS.

The two most important consequences of those wounds are—1. In‐
flammation of the lymphatics; and 2. Adynamic or typhoid fever, with
diffuse inflammation of the cellular tissue.

The *causes* of these effects may be, either—1. The irritation of a tri‐
vial wound, operating on an unhealthy constitution; or, 2. Inocculation
with a morbid poison.

And the morbid poison so inoculated may be twofold; viz. 1. The spe‐
cific virus generated in recently dead subjects; or, 3. The common pro‐
ducts of putrefaction.

Of inflammation of the lymphatics, arising from these as well as from
other causes, we shall speak elsewhere. In this place we shall describe
the symptoms and treatment of the adynamic fever and diffuse cellular
inflammation.

SYMPTOMS.—The poison having gained admission into the system
through a wound, (which is in most cases so slight as to pass unheeded,)
at a period varying from six to eighteen hours subsequently, the patient
feels generally unwell; he is depressed, faint, and chilly, and complains
of lowness of spirits and nausea. These symptoms are soon succeeded
by rigors, severe headach, and vomiting;—the pulse is frequent and sharp,
but weak;—the tongue is coated, and there is the greatest restlessness
and despondency. Then the *first local symptom* appears in the form of
a most excruciating pain and tenderness of the shoulder, corresponding
to the hand that was wounded. And in most cases there soon afterwards
arises a *pustule*, on or near the wound, which sometimes resembles the
small-pox pustule, and in other cases is a flattened vesicle, containing a
milk-white serum. But this pustule may be unattended with any pain, and
the patient may be ignorant of its existence, or may not even be aware
that he has received a wound, till his attention is directed to the spot by
his attendants. As the case proceeds, the pain in the shoulder becomes
more excruciating, and is attended with fulness of the axilla and neck;—
and a doughy swelling appears on the side of the trunk, often extending
from the axilla to the ilium. At first it is pale; but it soon assumes an
eryispelatous redness, or rather a pinkish tint, like that of peach-blossoms.
The breathing now becomes difficult; the pulse quicker and weaker; the

tongue dry, brown, and tremulous; the mental distress is truly appalling, although there is seldom delirium; the countenance is haggard, and the skin is yellow; and the patient often expires before the local disease has made farther progress.

VARIETIES AND COMPLICATIONS.—These symptoms often present considerable varieties in their progress and degree of severity, and may be complicated with other maladies arising from the same, or from some coexisting cause.

1. In one small class of cases, the influence of the morbid poison is so virulent, that the patient actually *dies of the precursory fever*, before sufficient time has elapsed for any local disease to appear;—either in the axilla, or in the wound, or elsewhere. The most speedily fatal case on record, that of Mr. Elcock, was of this variety. He died in forty hours from the receipt of the dissection-wound; and the nervous commotion and mental despondency which he suffered were even parallel to those of hydrophobia. Dr. Bell, of Plymouth, died in the same manner.

2. In another (and by far the most numerous) class, the general order of symptoms is the same that we described in the text; that is, there are, at *first*, general depression and fever;—*subsequently*, diffused cellular inflammation begins in the shoulder and axilla, and spreads down the side of the trunk.

3. In a third class, diffuse cellular abscesses occur in several remote parts—the knee or elbow, for instance, as well as in the axilla, as in the case of Mr. Shekelton.*

4. In other cases the wounded finger inflames violently, and suppurates or sloughs;—or the diffuse inflammation begins at the wrist, and extends up the arm.

5. In a fifth class, inflammation of the lymphatic vessels may be confined with the peculiar depressing effects of the absorption of poison; as in the case of Mr. James, narrated in his work on inflammation.

TERMINATION AND CONSEQUENCES.—If the case do not terminate fatally at an early period, extensive and foul collections of matter form in the parts that have swelled;—and abscesses continue to gather under the skin, or between the muscles of the trunk and limbs; and from these the patient may slowly sink;—or, if he survive, his existence may be a mere burden: one or more of the fingers may perish by gangrene, the arm may remain stiff and useless, or the seeds of consumption or dropsy may be left in the system. Mr. Adam has remarked, that in most cases of recovery, every portion of the limb, between the original wound and the part first stricken with pain, was affected with swelling.†

* The case of Dr. Bell may be found in Butter on Irritative fever. Those of Mr. Elcock and Mr. Shekelton are quoted at length (with many others) in Travers on Constitutional Irritation.

† Glasgow Medical Journal, August, 1830.

In some cases, severe and protracted pains of a rheumatic character
have followed the ordinary train of symptoms.  Both Sir A. Cooper and
Mr. Abernethy suffered in this manner, and the same symptoms have
been observed by Mr. Stafford.*

MORBID ANATOMY.—The morbid appearances are those of the various
grades of the diffuse cellular inflammation.  The following may be
quoted as a fair description of an advanced stage.†  The *cuticle* covering the affected side of the trunk, vesicated and wrinkled;—the *cutis*
mottled and gangrenous in patches;—the *subcutaneous cellular tissue*, in
some parts distended with serum, in others softened and turgid with pus;
the *tissue between the muscles* of the  trunk, as well as that which separates the different muscular fasciculi, also softened and purulent;—the
*muscular fibres*, of a dirty-yellow colour, and softened;—the *axillary
glands* enlarged, but not suppurating;—the axillary *artery* and *nerves*
healthy;—but the *veins* (especially the smaller branches) dirty red, and
softened;— the brachial and median-cephalic veins of the wounded arm,
slightly red;—but the fore-arm healthy, and *no connexion whatever to
be discovered between the abrasion on the finger and the morbid parts
in the axilla*;—the *pleura* of the affected side greatly inflamed;—the
lung covered with lymph, and much serum effused into the cavity of the
chest.

DIAGNOSIS.—1. *From acute rheumatism* this disease may be distinguished by the suddenness of its invasion; by the precedence of the
constitutional symptoms; by their low typhoid type; by the depression
of the pulse; by the pain being confined at first to the axilla; by the
characters of the ensuing tumefaction; and by a knowledge of the exciting causes.

2. *From inflammation of the Lymphatics*, the diagnosis is more nice,
because that disease may coexist with this, and because it might even be
the sole effect of the same poison, (provided that it acted locally.)  In
inflammation of the lymphatics, however, the disease *begins at the
wounded part*,—which swells and becomes throbbing and painful;—the
inflammation extends in red lines up the arm to the lymphatics above
the elbow, and in the axilla; and the constitutional symptoms are at first
those of *inflammatory* fever, although they may become *irritative* and
*typhoid*, if the patient be exhausted by pain, or if matter be confined.  The
broad features of distinction may be thus stated.  The constitutional
symptoms *precede* the local, in the *diffuse cellular inflammation;* but
*follow* them in *inflammation of the lymphatics*.  In the *former* disease,
the *local affection depends upon the constitutional*; in the *latter* it is the
reverse.  Again, the two diseases are most remarkably at variance as

* Med. Chir. Trans. vol. xx. 1836.
† Abridged from the case of Mr. Young, in Duncan's paper in the Edinburgh
Med. Chir. Trans. vol. i.  Quoted also in Travers, op. cit.

regards their tolerance of blood-letting; which remedy is as eminently serviceable in cases of pure inflammation of the lymphatics, as it is positively injurious in those which arise from imbibition of poison.

PROGNOSIS.—Of the cases on record, nearly two-thirds have proved fatal. The danger will be proportionate to the violence of the constitutional symptoms;—the quickness of pulse, anxiety of mind, and prostration of strength. The cases in which inflammation begins at the injured part are much less dangerous than those in which it appears remote from it, or in several places simultaneously.

PATHOLOGY.—Some persons deny that this disease originates in the absorption of poison, and attribute it to mere local irritation acting on an unhealthy constitution.* Now it is, on the one hand, perfectly true, that severe or fatal diffuse cellular inflammation, or inflammation of the lymphatics, may be produced by the slightest conceivable injury to a vitiated habit. Witness the Plymouth Dockyard disease; and Mr. Abernethy's case of a young lady who nearly died from a prick in the finger with a clean sewing-needle. And it is equally certain that most medical students and practitioners are in a bad state of health, and consequently predisposed to suffer from such accidents. And farther, medical students are, as Mr. Colles† and every one else affirm, most liable to suffer during their third academical session, when their health has been thoroughly undermined by two previous winters of hard study, late hours, and, in some few cases, by vulgar debauchery. But there are reasons which, duly considered, place the existence and agency of a distinct morbid poison beyond all doubt.

1. It is a well-established fact, that *many individuals* are frequently inoculated from *one subject*. This happened in the well known cases of Professor Dease and Mr. Egan; and numerous instances of it are on record.‡

2. The disease most frequently arises from *fresh subjects*. Mr. Adam, in the excellent paper which we have before quoted from, has collected forty cases;—and in only two or three out of the whole number did the disease arise from a putrid subject. The most dangerous poison seems to be destroyed by putrefaction; and the disease caused by inoculation with putrid matters is in general mild, and consists of mere inflammation of the lymphatics,—although there are exceptions.

3. The *disease of which a subject died* has a manifest influence on the frequency of ill effects from dissecting it. In two-thirds of Mr. Adam's cases the disease affected a serous membrane;—and the most deadly

* Abernethy's Lectures, Renshaw's edition, p. 132. Lizars's Practical Surgery Edinburgh, ed. 1838, p. 71. See the section on *diffused abscesses* in part ii.

† Colles, Dublin Hospital Reports, vols. iii. and iv.

‡ Vide Copland's Dict., p. 304.

virus of all is contained in the bodies of women who die of puerperal fever.

4. The disease we have been describing *begins* with symptoms of constitutional disorder; and, in fact, *it may be unattended with any local disease whatever.* Consequently it cannot be said to arise from local disease, when there is none.

Lastly, it may be induced by immersion of the fingers in the fluids of a dead body, although the fingers may be quite free from wound or abrasion. A remarkable instance of this is related in the third volume of Tyrrel's edition of Sir. A. Cooper's Lectures.*

The occurrence of accidents from punctures made during dissection was frequent enough to excite considerable attention, long before the existence of a peculiar poison was proved. In one of the old histories of the conquest of South America by the Spaniards, it is said that a soldier, who had amused himself by hacking the dead body of an enemy with a sword, inflicted a very slight wound on himself with the same weapon, and died very soon thereafter; which was much marvelled at.

It merely remains to add, with regard to the pathology of this distressing malady, that the poison appears to operate both by depressing the nervous system, and by contaminating the blood;—but which of these effects it produces first, it avails little to inquire; in fact, it is not easy to conceive how one of them can occur without inducing the other.

TREATMENT.—The indications clearly are, to support the nervous system in its state of depression;—to endeavour to eliminate the poison by attention to the secretions;—and to relieve pain and tension, and promote the discharge of pus or sloughs.

As soon, therefore, as the first symptoms of indisposition make their appearance after a wound received during dissection, it will be advisable that the patient should take a mild emetic, have his feet immersed in hot water, and betake himself to a warm bed. Ten grains of ipecacuanha, with an equal quantity of the sesquicarbonate of ammonia, dissolved in a warm infusion of chamomiles, form the best emetic. After the vomiting has ceased, he should take a full dose of calomel, which may be advantageously combined with two or three grains of camphor. In an hour or two it should be followed by a purgative draught of oil of turpentine combined with castor-oil or senna, to quicken its operation, and prevent any

---

* Travers gives two analogous cases. A Mrs. Clifton died of diffused cellular inflammation following a prick. Two of her attendants became ill from the contact and effluvium of the discharge, although neither had any wound through which a poison might be inoculated. One of them suffered from acute fascial inflammation of the arm; the other from low fever, and abscess in the axilla. The latter was engaged in unfolding some sheets from which a most noisome smell proceeded, when she was all at once seized with sickness and faintness, and excruciating pain in the axilla.—*Constitutional Irritation*, p. 373, third edition.

irritation of the kidneys, (F. 18.) These remedies should be repeated,— and be aided with turpentine enemata until the bowels are fully unloaded.

The medicines subsequently given should be of a tonic and narcotic quality. If the pulse is moderately firm, and there is much thirst and headach, effervescing saline draughts; or liq. am. acet., with the strong camphor mixture, (F. 81,) may be tried. But in those cases which present a more decidedly adynamic character from the beginning;—and in all cases towards their termination, it will be necessary to administer wine, ammonia, æther, and quinine; together with whatever articles of nutriment the patient can take. It will be most urgently necessary to render the patient unconscious of his severe pain by narcotics; and the *muriate of morphia* has proved so beneficial in Mr. Stafford's hands, that it is to be preferred in similar cases. It should be given in a full dose (gr. $\frac{1}{2}$—j) at bedtime, and in smaller ones during the day;—and if the bowels have first been properly opened, it will most probably allay the pain, calm the restlessness and anxiety, and reduce the frequency, whilst it improves the tone of the pulse.

*Local Treatment.*—As soon as pain is first experienced in the axilla, numerous *leeches* should be applied, and their bleeding be encouraged by warm poppy fomentations, or poultices sprinkled with laudanum. But as soon as any distinct swelling can be detected, an *incision* should be made into it,—in order to relieve pain and tension, and to prevent the diffusion of serum or pus that may have been formed in the meshes of the cellular tissue. Incisions are the *sine qua non* of the treatment; the point on which success mainly depends; and it is most truly observed by Mr. Stafford, that in most of the cases that have hitherto occurred, if swelling or abscess formed and were not opened, the result was fatal.

If the patient survive, he should as soon as possible be removed into the country, and be put on a course of tonics and liberal diet. All the collections of matter which sometimes continue to form for months should be opened as soon as they are detected; and the ulcers that remain be dressed with stimulating lotions and bandages.

*Venæsection.*—With regard to the propriety of venæsection in this disease, there is but one opinion among the best authorities; namely that it is uncalled-for and injurious. They who recommended it do so on mistaken principles. They imagine that they have merely a local *inflammation* to treat, which, it need scarcely be repeated, is altogether an error. But experience, no less than reason, testifies to the impropriety of bleeding. It never relieves the pain, and always aggravates the nervous depression. Besides, the blood is never buffed or cupped, and the coagulum is always small in proportion to the serum. We may therefore conclude with Mr. Stafford that it is injurious, " because, in the *first* place, the nervous system has already been depressed by the introduction of the poison;—in the *second*, the fever cannot be considered simply of an inflammatory nature, but rather of an irritative or typhoid kind; and, in the *third* place, although present symptoms may be violent, yet perhaps, from the formation of abscesses, and the general reduction of the patient, he will afterwards require as much of the restorative power as possible to recover his strength."

*Calomel* is very strongly recommended by Mr. Adam and Dr. Colles, the former of whom concludes that it seems to annihilate the disease. They recommend it to be given alone in doses of gr. iij, every three or four hours, so as to salivate in thirty-six or forty-eight hours, and they say that it will do so more readily if the first few doses act on the bowels; —an effect which may be aided by purgative draughts.

PRECAUTIONARY MEASURES.—We need scarcely comment on the expediency of using some precautions in performing *post mortem* examinations, especially if the operator be out of health. The wearing of gloves, or smearing the hands with oil or lard, would be of some service, and are often recommended, but seldom practised. Sores or scratches on the fingers should be covered with adhesive plaster, or touched with the nitrate of silver to form an eschar. If the operator should puncture himself, or should suffer a scratch or abrasion to come in contact with the fluids of the subject, he should immediately wash his hands, and thoroughly suck the wound. Then a stimulant should be applied to it, in order to decompose the poison and excite a slight inflammation, which will impede absorption. Some recommend the nitrate of silver for this purpose, others oil of turpentine; Macartney speaks highly of a strong solution of alum, and Copland of a solution of camphor in concentrated nitric acid. It will also be expedient to apply the lunar caustic to the wound when the constitutional symptoms begin to show themselves, provided that it is not much inflamed.

---

# CHAPTER X.

## OF THE EFFECTS OF POISONS GENERATED BY DISEASED ANIMALS.

### SECT. I.—OF HYDROPHOBIA.

SYN.—*Lyssa, Rabies Contagiosa.*

DEFINITION.—Hydrophobia is a disease brought on by inoculation with the saliva of a rabid animal, and characterized by intermitting spasms of the muscles of respiration, together with a peculiar irritability of the body and disturbance of the mind.

SYMPTOMS IN THE DOG.—The first symptoms of rabies in the dog are an unusual shyness and melancholy. The animal avoids society, refuses his food, and seems to have lost all his vivacity; his ears and tail droop, he looks haggard and suspicious, his eyes are red and watery, and he is constantly snapping at and swallowing straws, litter, and rubbish, and licking cold surfaces, such as stones or iron. In the next stage the respiration becomes difficult, and there is a copious flow of viscid saliva, with inflammation of the fauces, and fever. The animal is by no means so *invariably* furious as is generally supposed; and it has, in the course of experiments, not always been easy to induce it to bite. Yet it may be said that there is always a greater disposition than usual to bite *if irritated;*—and in some instances there is a state of extreme rage, the animal attacking and biting indiscriminately every person and thing that comes within its reach. It has been presumed that the former milder form occurs in the domesticated and educated dog;—and that the state of uncontrollable and indiscriminate fury is met with chiefly in ill-tempered or wild dogs, and in wolves, foxes, and the other unsubjugated varieties of the canine race. Be this, however, as it may, the breathing becomes more difficult and laborious as the disease advances;—tremors and vomiting occur, and the animal is carried off in convulsions. It rarely survives the fifth day. The difficulty of swallowing water, which gives the name of the disease as it occurs in man, is very rare in animals.

CAUSES.—The cause of this malady in dogs is most frequently infection from another animal already diseased; yet it must occasionally arise spontaneously. The most probable sources of its origin are close confinement, rank unwholesome food, want of the *couch grass*, the natural medicine of the dog, and deprivation of sexual intercourse.

Besides the dog, it is probable that hydrophobia arises spontaneously in the wolf, jackall, badger, and perhaps the cat. But it may be communicated to many other mammiferous animals, and there is no doubt but that every animal capable of taking the disease, can also propagate it. This is equally true with regard to human beings as to animals. MM. Magendie and Breschet inoculated two healthy dogs on the 9th of June, 1813, with the saliva of a man who was labouring under the disease, and who died of it the same day at the Hôtel-Dieu. One of the dogs ran away; but the other was affected with decided rabies on the 27th of July following, and died of it;—and some other dogs, which it was made to bite, died also. Well-authenticated cases are recorded, in which the disease was communicated to man by pigs and horses;—and there is no doubt but that it would be so much more frequently, if it were the instinct of herbivorous animals to show their rage by biting. Breschet in the course of numerous experiments on the subject, repeatedly

23

infected dogs with the saliva of rabid horses and asses. One curious fact demonstrated by these experiments is, that when rabbits or other rodentia, and birds, are inoculated with the saliva of rabid animals, they very soon die, but without exhibiting any of the ordinary symptoms of hydrophobia.*

In the *horse* the disease commences with great distress and terror, and profuse sweating; he soon becomes frantic and outrageous, stamping, snorting, and kicking.† In the *sheep*, the symptoms are similar. An instance is recorded in which eight sheep were bitten, and became rabid;—they were exceedingly furious, running and butting at every person and thing, but did not bite. They drank freely.‡

There are several points connected with the propagation of hydrophobia, which are still involved in great uncertainty. It needs scarcely be said that the ordinary mode of propagation is inoculation of the saliva into a bite or some other recent wound. But it is not known whether the saliva itself is the poisonous agent, or whether some poisonous matter may be secreted by the mouth, fauces, or lungs, and mixed with it. This, however, is not a point of much consequence; but again, it is uncertain whether the whole solid and fluids of the animal are not poisonous also. In fact, there is some reason for believing that the disease may be communicated by the mother's milk.§ Moreover, it is probable, although not certain, that it may be communicated by contact of the saliva with the mucous membrane of the mouth, without any wound or abrasion.‖ Lastly, a point of more importance and uncertainty than any is, whether the bite of an animal in health, or of one merely enraged, may not cause the disease;—or, at all events, supposing it to be really infected with rabies, whether its bite may not be dangerous during the period of incubation, and long before the outbreak of any apparent symptoms.

SYMPTOMS IN MAN.—These may be divided into three stages. *First*, the stage of *incubation* or *delitescence*, being that which intervenes between the infliction of the bite and the first appearance of the disease. *Secondly*, the stage of *recrudescence*, or of premonitory symptoms. *Thirdly*, the progress of the disease when fully established.

*First Stage.*—The *duration of the stage of incubation* is exceedingly various. It is seldom less than forty days;—generally from five weeks

---

* Breschet sur quelques recherches expérimentales sur la rage. L'Expérience, Oct. 8th, 1840.

† Blaine's Outlines of the Veterinary Art. 2nd edit. Lond. 1816.

‡ Lancet, 1829—30, vol. ii. p. 511.

§ Two ewes were bitten by a mad dog, and died hydrophobic. One had two lambs, the other one; all three of which were seized with the disease a week afterwards, although they had not been bitten by the dog, nor, as was supposed by the mother.—Steele, Med. Gaz. Oct. 25th, 1830.

‖ Hutchinson, Lancet, Dec. 8th, 1838.

to three months. But authors are by no means agreed as to its limits. Dr. Bardsley positively denies that the malady ever comes on after more than two years from the bite; and attributes the cases said to have occurred after that time to " anomalous causes," or to inoculation from some un-suspected source. Other authors, on the contrary, seem to think that it may occur at any indefinite period—even twelve years after inoculation. Dr. Burne* relates the case of a prisoner in the Milbank Penitentiary, who died of it seven years after he was bitten. The unfortunate man had indeed kept two cats in his cell, and it is *possible* that he might have received the infection from one of them. They were, however, alive and well at the time of his decease. It must be concluded, there-fore, either that hydrophobia may come on seven years after a bite;—or that it may be communicated by animals who are to all intents and pur-poses healthy. But if a surgeon is questioned on the subject by a patient who has been bitten, it will be his duty to allay his apprehensions as far as possible. He may very safely assure him, that after six months have elapsed, the chance of the disease is very slight indeed;—and that scarcely more than a twentieth of those bitten by dogs really mad are ever affected.

*Second Stage, or Premonitory Symptoms.*—The first thing that attracts attention is a peculiar pain of the wounded part, together with slight heat, redness, and swelling. The pain is observed to shoot in the course of the nervous trunks, and has in general a rheumatic character. Sometimes, instead of it, there is a stiffness or numbness, or partial palsy. In some cases it is unattended with redness or swelling;—in others, on the contrary, the wound has thoroughly inflamed, and has broken out into suppuration afresh, although healed long before. In some instances these premonitory symptoms have not appeared at all;— or have been so slight as to pass unheeded;—in a few instances they have not appeared till after the accession of the genuine hydrophobic symptoms;—but in general they are observed from two to five days pre-vious to them.

*Third Stage.*—The first of the actual symptoms of hydrophobia is a vague feeling of uneasiness and anxiety. The patient finds himself gene-rally unwell; his mind is irritable, and his countenance gloomy;—he expe-riences a succession of chills and flushes, with transient headach; the appetite fails; there is frequently vomiting, and sometimes a well-marked accession of fever. Next, the sufferer complains of stiffness of the neck and soreness of the throat, with severe spasmodic pain at the epigastrium,— the respiration also is embarrassed, and frequently interrupted by sighing. But these symptoms are in most cases attributed to cold, and their real nature is not suspected for a day or two, till, all on a sudden, on attempt-

* Med. Gaz., April 14th, 1838.

ing to drink, the patient is seized with a fit of suffocating spasm, and manifests extreme horror at the sight of fluids.

The most prominent symptoms that henceforth present themselves, are three, viz. difficulty of breathing and swallowing;—extreme irritability of the body;—and peculiar disorder of the mind.

(*a.*) The *difficulty of breathing and swallowing* depends on spasm of the muscles of the pharynx and larynx. Sometimes the patient can swallow neither solids nor liquids; but more frequently the disability extends to liquids only; because they require a greater exertion of those muscles, and are consequently more liable to excite spasm. It is this circumstance that causes the aversion to fluids, and the alarm at the sight of them, which so generally characterize the disease. At first the spasms are excited only by attempts to swallow fluids;—then they are brought on by the sight or thought of them; or by the motions of spontaneous deglutition; but as the malady advances, they recur in frequent paroxysms,—sometimes spontaneously, sometimes excited by the slightest noise or touch. When the paroxysms have become fully developed, they cause the most frightful struggles for breath. All the muscles are convulsed;—the face is black and turgid, and the eye-balls protrude from their sockets. They may come on either during inspiration or expiration, but more frequently the latter;—the patient struggling most violently to expel the air that is confined in his chest through the closure of the larynx. In this disease, as in tetanus, the fatal termination may ensue from suffocation in the middle of a paroxysm, although it more frequently happens during an interval, from exhaustion.

(*b.*) Next to the spasm, the astonishing *irritability of the surface of the body* is the most prominent symptom of hydrophobia. The slightest impressions on the senses affect the sufferer most intensely. A look, or a sound;—the opening and shutting of the door of his apartment;—the motions of his attendants;—the reflection of light from a mirror;—the least impression on the skin; the touch of a feather, or impulse of the gentlest current of air,—are sufficient to bring on the convulsive fits, and are most earnestly deprecated by the patient.

(*c.*) The *state of mind* is in most cases extremely characteristic. There appears to be a most profound despair;—an utter incapacity for all comfort and consolation;—corresponding with the patient's haggard physiognomy and restless movements, and his hurried desponding tone of voice. He is also in general unusually talkative and verbose, as though he attempted to relieve or hide his sufferings by ceaseless conversation. But in some cases he is possessed with wild maniacal fury, and is obliged to be confined in order to prevent injury to himself or others;—whilst, as a contrary exception, it occasionally happens, that if he be originally of a strong, resolute mind, he may preserve his composure throughout; and to be the last endued with sufficient courage to attempt drinking, in spite of the impending horrors of suffocation.

PROGRESS AND TERMINATION.—When the disease is fully established, its torments are aggravated by extreme thirst; and still more by a peeuliar viscid secretion from the fauces, the irritation of which brings on the convulsive fits, and causes a perpetual *hawking* and spitting—which are very constant symptoms. Not unfrequently there is vomiting of greenish matter mixed with blood. As the disease advances, the convulsions increase in frequency and violence; there is constant restlessness and tremor;—the lips and cheeks become livid, and perpetually quiver; till at length one fit lasts long enough to exhaust the remaining strength, and release the patient from his misery. An entire and remarkable remission (perhaps from the use of medicine) sometimes occurs; and the patient enjoys perfect ease, or perhaps sleeps for some hours;—but yet the symptoms return, after a time, with aggravated violence. Again, in some cases there is a perfect calm before dissolution; " the patient becomes tranquil, and most of his sufferings subside or vanish;—he can eat, nay, drink or converse with facility; and former objects associated with the excruciating torture of attempting to swallow liquid no longer disturb his feelings. From this calm he sinks into repose, and suddenly waking from his sleep, expires."*

MORBID ANATOMY.—The morbid appearances most frequently found are, great congestion of the membranes and substance of the brain and spinal cord, with effusion of serum. Sometimes blood is extravasated around the cervical portion of the cord. The lining membrane of the fauces, œsophagus, trachea, and bronchi, are mostly highly vascular; and the lungs congested. The stomach often contains a darkish fluid, and patches of vascularity of a dark purple colour are found in it and in the intestines. But although some one or more of these morbid appearances are detected in most cases, still there is not one of them that is present invariably. The brain, spinal cord, and fauces have been found pale, and the stomach without spots. Hydrocyanic acid has been detected in the blood after death, but this is not peculiar to hydrophobia.†

PATHOLOGY.—It is quite clear, therefore, that no change of structure that has yet been discovered, can be considered essential to the existence of hydrophobia. It is true that the difficulty of breathing and swallowing may be partially accounted for by the inflammation about the fauces; and that great irritability of the surface is symptomatic of irritation of the spinal cord. But still no mere local changes can explain the mass of symptoms which must depend on a peculiar change in the blood, or nervous system, or both.

DIAGNOSIS.—The disease which we read of under the title of *sponta-*

---

* Bardsley, Cycl. Pract. Med., Art. Hydrophobia.
† Med. Gaz., 5th September, 1840.

*taneous hydrophobia,* or hydrophobia not caused by a dog's bite, consists sometimes of hysterical symptoms, sometimes of a state like delirium tremens, and sometimes of genuine phrenitis, attended with suffocative dyspnœa and great irritability of the skin. It usually occurs to hysterical women or to drunkards. Now, as we know that hysteria may stimulate any disease that can be named, nothing can be more likely than that if an hysterical or nervous person have been bitten by any dog or cat, healthy or otherwise, the fears of the consequences, and knowledge of the symptoms of hydrophobia, will suffice to bring on a stimulated attack. Or again, if a person be affected with any form of delirium after an accidental bite, what can be more likely than that hydrophobia will be the leading subject of his ravings?

But a correct diagnosis may generally be formed by attentive observation;—by endeavouring to detect the inconsistencies, as it were, that are so frequent in hysteria;—the intervals of perfect complacency and cheerfulness, if the patient can be engaged in conversation, and led to forget his malady;—and by the sudden accession and instant urgency of the false hydrophobia, compared with the more gradual accession of the real. Yet it must be confessed that the diagnosis is by no means always easy. There was a remarkable case at the Middlesex Hospital in the autumn of 1837, which at first so exactly resembled hysteria, and afterwards the delirium of cerebral irritation, or commencing inflammation, that few of the medical attendants could at first persuade themselves that it was real hydrophobia, and even some of those who believed so at first, altered their opinions afterwards. But although there was not much dysphagia, still the *irritability of the skin,—the shrinking and convulsions induced by the slightest breath of air,* and the *salivation,* enabled Dr. Hawkins to form a correct diagnosis.*

TREATMENT.—PROPHYLACTIC.—As soon as possible after the bite of a suspected animal, the whole wound should be freely and fairly cut out; and its extent should be carefully ascertained, so that the complete removal of the virus may be ensured. After this, bleeding should be encouraged by the application of a cupping glass; or the wound should be long and diligently washed in warm water; and as a last measure of precaution, especially if the bite have been irregular, (so that it is uncertain whether the excision has been complete,) the part should be cauterized by potassa fusa, or rather by nitric acid.

When we consider that substances introduced fairly into the blood may find their way all over the body in an inconceivably short space of time, (probably in nine seconds,†) it will be readily seen that excision, although performed as soon as possible after the bite may be of no avail. Yet it should never be omitted, let the interval be what it may. And one case

---

* Lond. Med. Gaz., Nov. 4, 1837. Several instructive cases may be found in the Lancet, especially one by Mr. Hodson, Lancet, 1838-39, p. 582.

† Blake, Ed. Med. and Surg. Journ., Jan. 1840.

is recorded in which it is said, that the patient was saved, although the parts were not cut out till the thirty-first day, and not till the symptoms had actually made their appearance. This, however, is doubtful.*

By some authors caustic is recommended to the exclusion of excision; especially the nitrate of silver, by Mr. Youatt. This gentleman has certainly a good right to speak in its favour, having oeen bitten four times, and having used no other preventive. But other cases are narrated in which the immediate and free application of this substance was totally useless. Whether the wound, after excision or caustic, should be allowed to heal,—or be kept open, and made to suppurate by irritating ointments,—is a disputed point. The weight of authority certainly favours the latter practice, and beyond the inconvenience it can do no harm.

As for any other preventive treatment, all that can be done is to keep the patient in as good a state of health, and in as good spirits, as possible. But there is not one of the innumerable so-called specifies that is worth a moment's trial. The Tonquin, Ormskirk, and Burling nostrums;— guaco, box, belladonna, and broom tops; all kinds of acids, alkalis, earths, and vegetables; half drowning the patient in the sea; and stewing him in hot air and vapour baths,—all of these remedies and plans have in turn been reputed infallible, and found to be good for nothing. At one time it was confidently pretended that certain vesicles appear under the tongue during the premonitory symptoms, and that if these were cauterized, the patient would be safe. But unluckily they can never be found. Mr. Youatt thinks that rue acts occasionally as a preventive with dogs, but it is very far from infallible.

CURATIVE TREATMENT.—Here we are met at the outset with the doubt whether hydrophobia can be cured at all; whether, like the plague and small-pox, it will not run its course, without the possibility of checking it. Mr. Youatt says that he believes he has occasionally prevented it in the dog, and that he has occasionally seen a case of spontaneous recovery; but that he has never cured it. And with regard to man, although it cannot be denied that a few rare cases have recovered;—still as the same remedies that were supposed to be successful in these cases, have been used again and again in others without benefit, the recoveries must fairly be considered accidental and spontaneous.

*Bleeding* has been repeatedly tried to a most enormous extent; and one case in the East Indies is said to have been cured by it: but it rarely affords even a temporary alleviation, and rather tends, by exhausting the strength, to accelerate the fatal issue. It may, however, be tried as a *palliative* if the patient be plethoric, and the face becomes very turgid during the spasms.

* Thompson, Med. Chir. Trans. vol. xiii., and Lancet, Sept. 23, 1837.

*Warm-water.*—Magendie and others have proposed, after bleeding, to inject large quantities of warm water into the veins; and it certainly is beneficial, although but for a time.

*Opium* in different forms has been given most profusely, and certainly with some success;—for whether administered by the mouth, or rubbed into the skin, or injected into the veins, it seldom fails to mitigate the patient's sufferings, although it never averts his death. This was most strikingly exemplified in the case of the Milbank prisoner, who died seven years after he was bitten. A blister was applied along the spine, and ten grains of the acetate of morphia were sprinkled on the denuded cutis. "Scarcely had one minute elapsed," says Dr. Burne, "when we observed the stare of the eyes and the dreadful alarm and anxiety of the countenance to diminish, then the violence of the spasm to abate, and the catchings in the respiration and the retching to subside; and to our astonishment this general amelioration progressed, till in four minutes the countenance had become placid, and the respiration free; the retching had ceased, and the spasms vanished." This improvement, however, did not last very long;—the symptoms returned;—a repetition of the remedy was powerless;—and the patient died. And that is the general history of the effects of opium.

The whole tribe of sedatives; *belladonna, digitalis, tobacco, &c.*, have been repeatedly tried, but with similar results. The *hot air bath* and *cold affusion*,—acids and alkalis, especially *ammonia;*—every diuretic, purgative, and sudorific that can be thought of, have succeeded no better. In one instance the *liquor plumbi diacetatis* is said to have affected a cure.

Mr. Hewitt, surgeon in the Bombay Medical Establishment, has related a single case in which the patient was saved by violent salivation. Several native soldiers and other persons were bitten one night by a wild jackall, which when killed was found to be very feeble and apparently starved, and its liver rotten and full of abscesses. A month afterwards two of the persons that had been bitten were found dead in the fields, and from the description which was given of their symptoms, Mr. Hewitt judged that they had perished of hydrophobia. Shortly afterwards, three others were seized with the disease, and came under his treatment. He induced salivation in one of them (a woman) by the most profuse administration of mercury, and she recovered; but with the other two, who were men, the same remedy was of no avail. Strangely enough, the natives of these parts were entirely ignorant that such a disease as hydrophobia existed;—a sufficient refutation of the perverse error of those who maintain that it is entirely an imaginary affection brought on by fright.[*]

---

[*] Account of the effects of the bite of a wild jackall in a rabid state, as the same occurred at Kattywar, in the East Indies, in 1822. Med. Chir. Trans. vol. xiii. 1825.

In the present state of our knowledge, the principal object in the treatment of this disease is to allay the patient's sufferings. This should be done by the external and internal administration of opium in every form, combined with other sedatives. The strength should be kept up with whatever nutriment can be taken. And if the surgeon imagines that he can give any other remedy with a chance of benefit, and without adding to his patient's sufferings, he should do so. But common humanity requires that the tortures of the disease should not be aggravated by subjecting the patient to hopeless experiments, or to the intrusion of a host of visiters.

There remains, however, one grand experiment to be made; that is to say, the production of asphyxia by the *woorali*, (as was described in the chapter on Tetanus,) and the gradual restoration of the patient to consciousness by means of artificial respiration. And there really seems to be some reason for hoping, that by thus suspending the functions of the nervous system, the effects of the poison may gradually cease without exhausting it. At all events, to use the words of Celsus, " Si nullum appareat aliud auxilium, periturusque sit qui laborat, nisi temeraria quaque via fuerit adjutus;—satius est anceps remedium experiri quam nullum."

## SECTION II.—OF THE GLANDERS.

Syn.—*Equinia.* (*Elliotson.*)

DEFINITION.—The glanders is a disease of the horse tribe, communicable to man and other animals. It is chiefly manifested by unhealthy suppuration of the mucous membrane of the nasal cavities, and pustular eruptions and unhealthy abscesses on the face and other parts.

SYMPTOMS IN THE HORSE.—It may occur in two forms, which, however, are merely manifestations of the same disease in different parts. When seated in the *lymphatic system*, it is called *farcy*—when in the *nasal cavities, glanders*. But these two forms are essentially identical; the pus of either of them will reproduce the other; and farcy always terminates in glanders, if the animal live long enough, and its progress is not arrested.

*Farcy* begins with hard, cord-like swellings of the lymphatic vessels and glands, called *farcy-buds*. These slowly suppurate, and form unhealthy fistulous sores, which discharge a copious thin sanious matter. If suffered to proceed unchecked, farcy leads to glanders, although more frequently the latter arises first.

*Glanders.*—Its symptoms are, a *continued* flow of discharge from the nostrils, which discharge is at first thick and glairy, like white of an egg; but after a time becomes opaque, purulent, bloody, and horribly

offensive, retaining, however, its viscidity.  Soon after it commences,
vesicles form on the Schneiderian membrane, which degenerate into
foul and extensive ulcers, and lead to caries of the bones.  The external
parts of the face may become gangrenous. and the animal may die in a
few days with putrid fever;—or he may perish more slowly;—the disease spreading to the lungs, and death being induced by cough, emaciation, hectic, and the formation of unhealthy abscesses all over the body.*

SYMPTOMS IN MAN.—This disease may appear either as glanders or
farcy; either of which may be acute or chronic.

(1) The *acute glanders* begins with all the symptoms that indicate
the absorption of a putrid poison.  There are general feelings of indisposition, lowness of spirits, and wandering pains; followed by fever,
furred tongue, great thirst, profuse perspirations at night, great pain in
the head, back, and limbs, and tightness of the chest.  After some days
these symptoms increase; there are severe rigours and delirium, often of
a phrenitic character; the perspirations become more profuse, and sour
and offensive, and are attended with diarrhœa of a similar character.
Then *diffuse abscesses* appear in the form of red swellings about the
joints, especially the knees and elbows—the patient complains of heat
and soreness in the throat; the tongue becomes dry and brown, the
respiration more oppressed, and the fever assumes a decidedly low
malignant character.  Next (perhaps a fortnight from the commencement of the illness, sooner or later in different cases,) a dusky, shining
swelling appears on the face, (especially on one side,) extends over the
scalp, and closes the eyes.  Then the characteristic features of the disease appear;—an offensive, viscid, yellowish discharge, streaked with
blood, issues from the nostrils; and a crop of large and remarkably hard
pustules (compared by some to those of the small-pox, and said by others
to be about the size of a pea) appears on the face.  In the mean while
the swelling and inflammation increase;—a portion of the nose or eyelids mortifies;—the discharge becomes more and more profuse and
offensive;—the pustules spread, and extend over the neck and body;
fresh abscesses form and suppurate; the thirst is most excruciating; and
low muttering delirium and tremours usher in death, much to be wished
for.

(2) The *chronic glanders* is characterized by a viscid and peculiarly
fœtid discharge from one nostril, with pain and swelling of the nose and
eyes;—and emaciation, profuse perspirations, and abscesses near the
joints, from which the patient slowly sinks.

(3) In the *acute farcy*, the patient receives the poison through a
wound or abrasion, which inflames violently, together with the lymphatics leading from it.  These symptoms are attended with considerable

* Blaine, op. cit.

fever, and are generally soon followed by the diffused abscesses, pustular eruption, and nasal discharge, that characterize acute glanders.

(4) In the *chronic farcy,* a wound poisoned by glanderous matter degenerates into a foul ulcer; the lymphatic vessels and glands swell and suppurate; abscesses form in different parts of the body; and if the disease is not cured, or does not destroy the patient first, it terminates in acute glanders.*

CAUSES.—In the horse this disease may, without doubt, arise spontaneously, when the animal is subjected to the usual influences that generate putrid poisons;—namely, close confinement and ill ventilation, especially on board ship. In man it is generally produced through inoculation of the matter into a wound. Whether the disease can be contracted by absorption of the miasmata arisiug from it, or without a breach of the cuticle, is not yet quite decided. The matter from the abscesses or nasal cavities of human beings labouring under the disease is capable of infecting both men and animals. In one of the cases published it appeared four days, in another a month, after inoculation.

PROGNOSIS.—This, in the acute disease, is highly unfavourable; the chronic, however, is sometimes, although rarely, recovered from.

MORBID ANATOMY.—The morbid appearances are the same both in man and in the horse. Clusters of white granules, or tubercles, are found in whatever tissues the disease has invaded; in the Schneiderian membrane, in the antrum and frontal sinuses, and in the vicinity of the different abscesses. The nasal cavities mostly contain a thick gelatinous secretion, and are studded with foul gangrenous ulcers, from which project fungous clusters of tubercular matter.

PATHOLOGY.—The *proximate cause* of the acute glanders appears to be a contamination of the blood with the poisonous matter. This is evident from the early depression of strength and spirits, from the profuse and fetid perspirations and purgings, from the consecutive or simultaneous appearance of the local suppurations, with their peculiarly offensive and characteristic discharge, as well as from the black and thin condition of the blood, which has lost the faculty of coagulation.—In the chronic forms the disease appears to be at first local.

TREATMENT.—The chief points to be attended to in the treatment of glanders, are, to open all abscesses as soon as they form; to syringe the nasal cavities with solutions of creosote; and to support the strength and abate the thirst with wine and soda water. Injections of creosote have cured both the acute and chronic glanders; but almost any other treatment that can be named has been found of no service. Depletion is in-

* Case of Mr. Turner, Travers, Constitutional Irritation, p. 399; case of farcy ending in acute glanders in seven months, L'Experience, Jan. 1829.

admissible. The effluvia must be counteracted by fumigations of chlorine and aromatics. In the treatment of farcy likewise, the chief points are to open all abscesses early, and support the strength. Any swollen glands should be extirpated.*

---

# CHAPTER XI.

## OF THE VENEREAL DISEASE.

### SECT. I.—OF ITS GENERAL HISTORY AND PATHOLOGY.

DEFINITION.—The venereal disease, using the term in its widest acceptation, consists in the effects of certain morbid poisons, generated and usually communicated by promiscuous sexual intercourse.

It includes two distinct diseases, *gonorrhœa* and *syphilis* which differ very widely in their nature and effects.

Both diseases present two classes of symptoms; the *primary* and the *secondary*;—the primary being the effects of the morbid poison on the parts to which it is actually applied; the secondary being the subsequent results of some general disorder of the constitution.

GONORRHŒA is an inflammation of the mucous membrane of the genitals, which is occasionally, although not very often, succeeded by various rheumatic affections, as secondary symptoms.

SYPHILIS consists, first, of ulceration of the parts to which the morbid poison is applied, and inflammation of the neighbouring lymphatics which are the primary symptoms; and, secondly, of sundry eruptions on the skin, ulcerations of the throat, inflammations of the eye, and inflammation and caries of the bones and joints, which are the secondary symptoms.

The primary symptoms of syphilis are undoubtedly contagious, and communicable by inoculation with the matter from the ulcers. The secondary symptoms, which depend on a general contamination of the constitution, are not equally communicable by inoculation, although they doubtless are so to a certain extent; but they may be communicated from

---

* Vide Elliotson's papers in the Med. Chir. Trans. vols. xiii., xviii., (*with a coloured plate*,) and xix.; the Med. Gaz., vol. xix. p. 939; the Lancet for 1831-32, vol. i. p. 698 ; Rayer, de la morve et du farcin chez l'homme; Mem. de l'Acad, de Mcd. 1837; also Med. Gaz., April 18th and 25th, 1840; and Lancet, April 30th, 1839.

the husband to his wife; from the parent to the unborn child; from a nurse to a suckling infant, and from an infant to its nurse.

There is, moreover, a third class of symptoms, which may be called *tertiary;* consisting of various eruptions, rheumatic pains, falling off of the hair, deafness, and all kinds of anomolous cachectic complaints, which are the sequelæ of syphilis when it operates on an originally bad constitution, or is aggravated by ill treatment. This vitiated state of constitution is doubtless a frequent source of stunted, sickly, and scrofulous children.

We must next lay before the reader as brief an account as possible of the various disputed opinions with regard to the history and origin of this disease.

The following are the principal questions in dispute:—namely, *First,* Was the venereal disease known to the ancients? *Secondly,* Was it imported from America? *Thirdly,* Are there more syphilitic poisons than one? *Fourthly,* Are the poisons which produce *gonorrhœa* and *syphilis* identical? *Fifthly,* Does syphilis ever arise without infection? And, *lastly,* what are the specific virtues of mercury?—These questions we will discuss *seriatim.*

I. WAS THE VENEREAL DISEASE KNOWN TO THE ANCIENTS?—(*a*) *Arguments in favour of its antiquity.*—Those who believe that it was known to the ancients argue thus. They affirm that writers on medicine from the earliest ages make mention of sundry ulcerous diseases of the genitals and of the fauces, some of which were most probably venereal. That, in particular, some of the ulcers of the genitals mentioned by Celsus correspond exactly with certain ordinary venereal sores of the present time.* That Rhazes, an Arabian writer, mentions an ulcer of the penis produced by the " *accensionem mulieris supra virum.*" That sundry foreign authors who flourished between 1270 and 1470, mention ulcers and pustules of the penis as contracted *by lying with foul women;* or with women who have ulcers,—or who have lately had connexion with one whose penis was ulcerated. But the strongest arguments of all are contained in two papers presented by Mr. Beckett to the Royal Society in 1717 and 1718, in which he contends for the antiquity of the disease in England. He proves that gonorrhœa was well known in 1162 under the terms *brenning* or *burning;*—and that certain enactments were extant, which provided that any *stew-holder* keeping a women with the *perilous infirmity of burning* should forfeit the sum of one hundred shillings. Farther, he says that John Arden, surgeon to Richard II., (1380,) defines the *brenning* to be an *inward heat and excoriation of the urethra;* and that, besides, he mentions certain " *contumacious ulcers,* which we now term *chancres.*" And, moreover, that a MS. in

* De Medicinâ, lib. vi. cap. 18.

Lincoln College, Oxford, written by Thomas Gascoigne, Chancellor of that University, and dated **1430**, states that some men (and amongst them John of Gaunt) had died of diseases caught by frequenting women. Another potent line of reasoning is founded on the circumstance, that many ancient authors state the *leprosy* of their times as being *contagious;*—and that *ulcers of the penis* and *heat of urine* were contracted by men who lay with leprous women. But it is reasonable to infer, that what they called *leprosy* was in reality *venereal disease.* Because, in the *first* place, (as Bateman says,) "there is little doubt that every species of cachectic disease accompanied with ulceration, gangrene, or any superficial derangement, was formerly termed leprous;"*—and because, in the *second* place, there is no ground for believing that *elephantiasis* (the real leprosy) is contagious at all;—and because that disease is never communicated by contact in modern times, whether in carnal conversation or otherwise;—a fact which has been ascertained by ample experience, especially at Madeira.† Mr. Beckett farther mentions the occurrence of *nodes on the bones* at those early periods; and shows that some of the so-called leprous diseases were cured by mercury, whilst real leprosy is not. Therefore those who believe in the antiquity of the venereal disease contend, that discharges from the urethra and ulcers on the genitals were known in the earlier ages;—and that they were known to proceed from fornication; although the secondary symptoms which followed them were, for the most part, not known to be venereal, but confounded with the leprosy.

(*b*) *Arguments against its antiquity.*—On the other hand, the opponents of its antiquity contend, that although ulcers or pustules on the genital organs and sundry discharges were not unknown;—still that neither in Celsus, nor in any other ancient writer, do we find mention that such maladies were *solely, or even frequently, the produce of sexual commerce;*—or that they were peculiarly *difficult to heal;*—or that they were frequently, or indeed ever, *followed by constitutional diseases.* But the most potent argument of all is this;—namely, that all at once, towards the close of the fifteenth century, whilst the French army was besieging Naples, a new and terrible disease sprang up; rebellious to every known method of treatment;—attacking high and low, rich and poor;—sparing neither *age* nor sex;—consisting of ulcers on the parts of generation in both sexes; which were speedily followed by affections of the throat and nose:—by corroding ulcers over the whole body; by excruciating nocturnal pains, and frequently by death. Whereas, "not

---

* Bateman on Cutaneous Diseases, 5th ed., pp. 304 *et seq.*

† Mr. Bacot and others who oppose the antiquity of the venereal disease, assert that leprosy is "*undoubtedly contagious.*"

one word that can be construed into any similar affection, is to be met with distinctly stated in any writer before that period."

Those, therefore, who are in favour of its antiquity, must hold one of these three opinions concerning that virulent disease of the fifteenth century;—viz. 1st, That it was a *new kind* of venereal disease;—or, 2ndly, That it was merely an *aggravated variety* of the old disease;—or, 3rdly, That it was *not the venereal disease* at all; but some malady (such as *sivvens, yaws, radesyge,* &c.) resembling it. But the consideration of the history of this new malady brings us to our second question.

II. Was it imported from America?—The greatest weight of evidence is certainly opposed to this supposition. Because no such disease is mentioned by the *very earliest* historians of the discovery of that continent;—neither is it mentioned by the earliest writers on America; and Peter Martyr, who was physician to Ferdinand and Isabella, and who was actually at Barcelona when Columbus returned from his first voyage in 1493, does not say a word as to its American origin. But besides;—of the earliest authors on the venereal disease, some attribute it to the *divine vengeance,* some to an *earthquake,* some to a *malignity of the air* caused by an overflow of the Tiber; not a few to a *celestial influx,* or *malignant conjunction of Saturn and Mars in the sign Scorpio,* or some other such astrological nonsense;—almost all refer its outbreak to the siege of Naples—but not one for the first thirty or forty years derives it from the West Indies.

Those who conceive that the new disease was *not syphilis,* found their opinion on the fact that the descriptions given by many of the oldest writers correspond pretty closely with the *yaws,* or *frambæsia* or *sivvens,* (a disease frequent enough in America,) and that like yaws it often was communicated to the *very young or old,* and to persons who did not catch it by carnal conversation.

III. Are there more syphilitic poisons than one?—(a)—*Arguments for plurality.* Carmichael and others assert, that there are various kinds of syphilitic poisons, each kind causing a peculiar primary ulcer, and a peculiar train of secondary symptoms. They say in proof of their opinions that every other morbid poison is *uniform and regular* in its effects; and that it would be "an unreasonable and unwarranted exception to a universal law of nature," if the venereal were not so also. But venereal diseases are *multiform* and *irregular;* consequently they must be caused by more poisons than one. For what other single poison can produce papular, pustular, scaly, and other kinds of eruptions?

(b) *Arguments against plurality.*—But the non-pluralists answer truly, that different eruptions may arise from one sore;—that there is no general relation between primary and secondary symptoms;—that the differences of the primary sore depend on differences of situation, treatment, &c.;—and that if arguments in favour of multiplicity of poisons be drawn from the mere appearance of ulcers or eruptions, there may be forty or fifty instead of four or five venereal poisons.*

IV. ARE THE POISONS OF GONORRHŒA, AND SYPHILIS IDENTICAL?—Hunter believed that they were identical, for he produced a chancre by inoculation with gonorrhœal matter, which was followed in three months by sore throat and eruptions. But the recent researches of Ricord show, that although the pus of a syphilitic ulcer, like any other morbid secretion, may irritate a mucous membrane and produce gonorrhœa, still that gonorrhœal matter will not produce syphilitic ulcers, and that gonorrhœa will not be followed by secondary syphilitic symptoms, unless there is also a chancre or syphilitic sore in the urethra; which was probably the case with the patient from whom Hunter took the gonorrhœal matter.

V. WHAT IS THE ORIGIN OF SYPHILIS?—There are two opinions on this subject. One is, that it is always caused by infection. Another opinion is, that it may occasionally be engendered afresh, without prior infection. Now as there must have been some causes to produce syphilis (as well as scarlatina, hydrophobia, and other animal poisons,) at first, there is no reason why the same causes may not occasionally concur to produce it again. The most probable theory is, that syphilis is occasionally produced *de novo*, if a mixture of various foul and diseased male and female secretions act upon a breach of surface in an unhealthy constitution. At least, the following facts furnish a kind of approximation to a proof of this.—Seventeen galley-slaves were inoculated with gonorrhœal matter. Slight ulcers were produced, which in five of the cases healed readily enough. But the remaining twelve patients were either scrofulous or scorbutic, or in an ill state of health, and seven of these suffered from eruptions and wandering pains.† Of the causes of gonorrhœa we shall speak in the next section.

Lastly, IS MERCURY A SPECIFIC?—Hunter not only considered that no really syphilitic disease could get well without it, but gravely upbraids human nature for doubting it. "Nothing," says he, "can show more the ungrateful and unsettled mind of man than his treatment of this medicine. If there is such a thing as a specific, mercury is one for the venereal disease." The following results, however, of experiments made by the army surgeons, and especially by Rose, Guthrie, and Hennen, will enable the reader to form a juster estimate of its capabilities. It is concluded, (1) That all kinds of primary and secondary symptoms *may* get well without mercury. (2) That out of 1,940 cases treated without it, ninety-six had secondary symptoms; and out of 2,827 treated with it, fifty-one had secondary symptoms. The average results of different experimenters, however show that there are at least *seven times*

* Carmichael enumerates *five* ; Judd *nine* ; which, however, he does not believe to be all that exist.

† P. H. Hernandez, quoted by Ricord.

as many cases of secondary symptoms, when no mercury has been given, as when it has. (3) That the secondary symptoms of cases treated without it are in general less severe, and that affections of the bones in particular are much less frequent. (4) That the average period of cure is much the same in both cases; but that relapses are more frequent when no mercury has been given.*

CONCLUSIONS.—From the foregoing details, and from various other facts on record, it may be concluded, 1st, That the venereal poison is most probably produced by the mixture of various foul and diseased secretions of the genitals,† 2ndly, That it occasionally is engendered *de novo* (*i e. without infection*) in prostitutes and others.   3rdly, That although there are no distinct *species* of syphilitic poisons, yet that there are several *varieties*;—and that different varieties prevail at different times and places, the chancre of one generation being lost in the next.   4thly, That venereal diseases existed from the earliest ages;—and that the *syphilis* of the fifteenth century was a new and virulent variety generated among the military at the siege of Naples.

SECTION II.—OF GONORRHŒA.

SYN.—Gonorrhœa virulenta; blenorrhœa; urethritis.

DEFINITION.—A gonorrhœa signifies an inflammation of the mucous membrane of the male urethra or female vagina, from the application of a morbid poison; generally during sexual connexion.

SYMPTOMS *in Man.*—The patient first experiences a little itching or tingling at the orifice of the urethra, together with a sense of heat and soreness along the under side of the penis, and slight pain and scalding in making water.   A little discharge soon exudes from the urethra: at first it is thin and whitish, but it soon becomes thick and puriform; and, when the disease is at its height, is yellow, or greenish, or tinged with blood.   The penis swells, the glans is of a peculiar cherry colour, is intensely tender, and often excoriated.   In consequence of the tumefied state of the urethra, the stream of urine is small and forked, and

---

* Vide *Aphrodisiacus*, by Daniel Turner, M. D., London, 1736; (a collection of the opinions of the early authors.) *Hunter* on the Venereal; *Hennen's* Military Surgery; *Carmichael* on Syphilis; *Bacot's* Treatise on Syphilis; *Tilley* on Diseases of the Genitals of the male; *Wallace* on the Venereal, (*Plates*); *Judd's* Treatise on Urethritis and Syphilis, (*Plates;*) *H. J. Johnson* in Med. Chir. Review; *Colles* on the Venereal; *Ricord*, Traité des Maladies Vénériennes, Paris, 1839; *Mayo* on Syphilis, Lond. 1840.

† Mr. Kingdon, at the *Lond. Med. Soc.* related a case of venereal affection generated by a healthy man and his wife. *Lancet*, May 3rd, 1838. See also Travers on the Venereal.

25

passed with much straining and with severe pain.   Other symptoms that
appear in different cases are—

1.  Long continued and painful erections.

2.  *Chordee*, a highly painful and crooked state of the penis during
erection.   Hunter says that there are two kinds of it—the inflammatory
and spasmodic.   The *inflammatory* arises from a deposite of lymph in the
*corpus spongiosum urethræ*, which glues together the cells, and prevents
their distention; so that when the penis is turgid with blood, it is bent at
one part, and horribly painful.   " 'The *spasmodic chordee*," says Hunter,
" comes and goes, but at no stated times; at one time there will be an
erection entirely free from it, at another it will be severely felt; and this
will often happen at short intervals."

3.  *Tenderness or soreness* of all the *parts in the vicinity of the genitals;*
of the groins, inside of the thighs, perinæum, and testicles.

4.  There may be severe *irritation*, or actual *inflammation of the urinary organs;*—producing great pain in the perinæum, and spasm of the
accelerators and other muscles during micturition, so as to interrupt the
stream of urine, and cause the most exquisite agony;—or irritation of the
bladder, with very frequent desire to make water, and great pain in doing
so, which lasts for some time afterwards, as though from spasm of its
muscular coat;—or there may be pain in the loins, scanty urine, tenderness of the abdomen, vomiting, and other signs of severe irritation of the
kidneys.

5.  *Hæmorrhage* from the urethra;—which may be either an *exhala-
lation* of blood from the distended capillaries, or an actual *laceration of
the vessels* when stretched by violent erection.   The loss of blood generally gives relief.

6.  *Inflammation* and obstruction of the *mucous follicles* of the urethra,
which may suppurate and burst either into the urethra, or externally; or
both.

7.  *Inflammation* of the *lymphatic glands* of the groin; constituting
*sympathetic bubo*.

8.  *Gonorrhœa spuria, vel externa*, or *balanitis*—inflammation and
suppuration of the sebaceous follicles around the *corona glandis*; with or
without excoriations.

9.  *Phymosis*, or *paraphymosis* may easily arise, owing to the swelled
condition of the *glans* and prepuce.   When the latter is œdematous, it
presents a curious semi-transparent appearance called *crystalline*.

10.  *Inflammation of either testicle.*

VARIETIES.—Gonorrhœa varies extremely in its severity.   It is always most severe in first cases, and in patients who are very young, or
who possess irritable or scrofulous constitutions.   In such cases it may
be attended with extreme fever and constitutional disturbance, and may

even prove dangerous to life by leading to extensive abscesses in the neighbourhood of the bladder.*

But, after repeated attacks the urethra becomes as it were inured to the disease, and each subsequent infection is more trivial. In these cases the discharge is the first symptom, and precedes the pain and scalding. In some rare instances the constitutional affection is extremely anomalous, and characterized by severe and continuous rigors.

MORBID APPEARANCES.—On dissecting a urethra affected with recent gonorrhœa, the mucous membrane is found red and swollen, and the follicles or *lacunæ* enlarged and filled with pus. The inflammation appears always to be most vivid near the orifice, and, except during the most acute stage, does not extend more than two or three inches from it.

CONSEQUENCES.—1. When gonorrhœa is left to itself, it gradually declines in severity, and is succeeded by a *gleet*, or thin mucous discharge, which is often very obstinate. 2. Repeated gonorrhœa may lead to *stricture* of the urethra; 3, to irritability of the bladder; 4, to a hard, dense, semi-cartilaginous state of the corpus spongiosum urethræ; 5thly, it may be followed by an attack of *gonorrhœal rheumatism;* pain, tenderness, and swelling of the joints, especially the knees and ankles, and fever. This generally attacks young people of a delicate strumous habit.

CAUSES.—We have defined gonorrhœa to be an inflammation and purulent discharge from the urethra, produced by infection from a similar disease. But inflammation and purulent discharge from the urethra may be produced by many other causes, some of which have no connexion with sexual matters. Thus—

(*a*) In the first place, discharges resembling gonorrhœa may be caused by *local violence.* The author some time ago treated a most obstinate case of this description, brought on by galloping several miles on a horse without a saddle. The patient was a married gentleman, with a constitutional tendency to irritation of the mucous membranes; during the treatment he suffered from a severe attack of rheumatism. The introduction of bougies; blows on the perinæum;—violent bending of the penis during erection; and long travel in a jolting vehicle over bad roads, are well authenticated causes of similar cases.† (*b.*) Urethritis with discharge may be produced by various *disorders of the constitution.* It has been a symptom of *rheumatism;* and not unfrequently it precedes a paroxysm of *gout.* It may be caused by *sympathy with irritation of other parts.* Thus it may be occasioned by *piles;*—and it has been known to accompany the cutting of a tooth several times in the same patient. (*c.*) A discharge is liable to occur in patients affected with *stricture;*—and to recur in those who have been long habituated to it, upon

---

* For cases, *vide* Judd, op. cit. p. 70.

† *Vide* Judd, op. cit p. 32.

any neglect of their health, exposure to severe cold, or *inordinate fatigue,* or *excess in food, wine,* or *venery.* (*d.*) Lastly, discharges are sometimes (although rarely) occasioned by the *use of particular medicines.* *Guaiacum* and cayenne pepper have been named as some.

Again, a man may contract a pretty severe discharge from a woman who is perfectly chaste, and has not been previously infected by a third party. Thus—(*a.*) The *menstrual fluid* is capable of causing urethritis with violent scalding and chordee, and followed by swelled testicle—and a considerable degree of irritation may be produced by the vaginal secretions, just previous to menstruation.* (*b.*) Similar consequences sometimes ensue if the female be affected with *leucorrhœa,* or with any other discharge of any sort whatever.

DIAGNOSIS.—The question next follows, whether there is any means of distinguishing the *simple gonorrhœa;* that is a discharge which does not arise from sexual connexion, or which a man contracts from some accidental malady in a clean chaste woman, from the *venereal gonorrhœa* or *clap,* caught from an infected prostitute. The answer is, decidedly not. The disease of the urethra, however produced, is the same in its nature, the same in its symptoms, and requires the same treatment.

The grand diagnostic sign laid down by writers,† whereby to distinguish *simple gonorrhœa* from *venereal gonorrhœa,* is the comparative mildness of the former, and the absence of acute inflammation. But this, although frequently, is by no means invariably the case. And the author can testify that in some of the non-venereal cases the pain, scalding, and other inflammatory symptoms may be of great severity, and of long continuance, and that they may be followed by rheumatism, which is so frequent a consequence of genuine venereal gonorrhœa. But if the patient strongly deny that his malady can arise from impure connexion, and if his character place his statement above suspicion;—if the existence of some one of the foregoing causes can be ascertained, and especially if it be known that he have suffered from it before in like manner, it will be right to pronounce the case *not venereal;* and more especially if the patient be married, or be in circumstances which would render any imputation on his continence either disgraceful or ruinous. Again, if, as Mr. Bacot observes, " a discharge come on only a few hours after connexion; and if it have continued several days without inflammatory symptoms; if the patient has been liable to some discharge after any excess of venery or of wine;—in all such cases the probability is, that the patient labours under some other diseased condition of the urethra, and that although the intercourse of the sexes may have been the exciting cause, still there may be no imputation on the cleanliness of the female."‡

But it is most important to observe, that although discharges may arise

---

* Judd, p. 24.          † Titley, op. cit. p. 186.          ‡ Bacot, op. cit. p. 101.

from many causes besides connexion, and although some discharges may arise from connexion with chaste women, yet that every one of them is capable of exciting a similar discharge in a healthy person.

These observations will go far towards solving another question that is frequently asked, viz. What is the danger of conveying infection when the discharge is very small in quantity, or when it is merely gleety and mucous?

The surgeon should inform the patient that the more virulent the disease, the greater is the danger of communicating it; but that, however slight the discharge, there still will be some risk. If, however, the patient be determined to run that risk he should cleanse the urethra first by making water and syringing it thoroughly with a mild astringent lotion. It is a well-established fact, that the contact of matter is indispensable to the propagation of the disease; consequently, by removing the matter, the hazard will be diminished. A person may have received the infection, but cannot communicate it previous to the appearance of discharge.

The time at which the disease appears after infection from a morbid poison is the fourth or fifth day. The later it appears, the less severe it generally is; but in some very trivial cases the discharge often comes on immediately after connexion.

GONORRHŒA IN THE FEMALE.—This, unless the patient is very young and delicate, is a much more simple disease than it is in the male; since the parts affected are less complex in formation, and less important in function.

The *symptoms* are much the same. Heat and pain in making water; tenderness and soreness, especially in walking, uneasiness in sitting, and muco-purulent discharge. On examination, the parts are found swelled and red, and if the case is severe, there may be excoriations or minute aphthous ulcerations. Sympathetic enlargement of the inguinal glands, and abscesses in the mucous follicles, are occasional complications.

*Acute inflammation of the vaginal mucous membrane*, from whatever cause induced, has precisely the same symptoms as acute gonorrhœa from infection. It may occur in the youngest children from local violence of any sort; or from sympathetic irritation;—teething, costiveness, worms, or any other disorders of the alimentary canal.—*Leucorrhœa*, or *fluor albus*, may in general be distinguished from gonorrhœa by the absence of heat or pain in micturition; and by the pain in the back, pallid countenance, irregular menstruation, and signs of exhaustion and debility which generally accompany it. Yet a profuse gonorrhœal discharge will cause the same appearances.

As we have recently insisted, all discharges, however produced, are contagious. If, however, a woman has a discharge, or has communicated one, the surgeon must observe some caution before he casts any reflection

on her chastity.  And after all, both in the male and female, whatever the
cause, the treatment is the same.

PROPHYLACTIC TREATMENT.—Immediately after a suspicious connexion, it will be prudent to make water so as to cleanse the urethra, and
then perform a thorough ablution with soap and water.  If the patient is
subject to gonorrhœa, it will also be worth while to wash out the front
part of the urethra with a syringeful of some astringent lotion.

CURATIVE TREATMENT.—The remedies for gonorrhœa are threefold;
first, antiphlogistic measures, to get rid of inflammation; secondly, certain
diuretics which have a peculiar sanatory influence on inflamed mucous
membranes; and thirdly, injections to wash away the discharge, and alter
the action of the inflamed capillaries.  These different remedies are to be
combined in various degrees in different cases.

Supposing it to be a first attack in a young irritable subject, with considerable pain and frequency of micturition, the patient should be confined
to the house for two or three days, if his avocations permit of it.  Ten or
a dozen leeches should be applied to the perinæum; but not at bedtime,
unless the surgeon wishes to be called up in the night to stop the bleeding.
The penis and scrotum should be supported by a suspensory bandage, and
be kept constantly wet with a cold or tepid lotion.  The glans penis
should be protected from irritation by a piece of lint spread with sperma-
ceti ointment.  The diet should be moderate, to the entire exclusion of
fermented liquors, and the patient should drink barley-water, linseed tea,
gum water, and other mucilaginous fluids.  But it is far from advantageous to increase the quantity of urine too much, or cause the patient
to make water often; because the act of micturition is accompanied with
very great suffering.  The scalding will be relieved by combinations of
alkalis and sedatives (F. 19, 83;) and by fomentation with *tepid* water,
or a *tepid* bath; but the bath should not be *hot*, nor even warm, otherwise
it will excite the circulation and bring on erections.  The bowels should
be opened with a dose of calomel at night, and some castor oil in the
morning; and it is advisable to give half a grain or a grain of calomel, with
gr. one-eighth of tartar emetic, and gr. x. of Dover's powder; or F. 7,
every night whilst there is much pain and chordee.  The mercury is not
necessary as a specific, but it is highly useful to check the inflammatory
symptoms.  At the same time copaiba or cubebs should be given as soon
as possible, but not before the patient is free from fever.

If the patient is very plethoric, and suffers greatly from pain and fever,
and has a hard pulse and white tongue, and if there be tenderness of the
abdomen, pain in the back, or other signs of irritation of the urinary organs, it may be right to take blood from the arm; and to administer calomel, opium, and antimony pretty freely.

Urgent inflammatory symptoms having been got rid of, and the ordinary
nightly pain being provided against by the foregoing measures, the re-

maining treatment consists principally in the administration of copaiba or cubebs, and the use of injections, the patient being enjoined to live regularly, and to abstain from violent exercise, fermented liquors, and other excitants.

Copaiba is best administered in the form of emulsion, F. 20, or in the *gelatinous capsules;* the cubebs may also be conveniently combined with alkalis, as in F. 84, 85. Both these remedies are capable of producing very unpleasant effects. They may purge and gripe excessively;—in which case a laxative of rhubarb and magnesia, followed by chalk and opium, should be given;—and the copaiba, or cubebs, when resorted to, should be administered in small doses, combined with opium or hyoscyamus. Sometimes they cause great fever, with furred tongue, sickness, headach, and a rash;—which may be removed by low diet and laxatives, with care to avoid cold. Many attempts have been made to diminish the nauseous taste of these medicines, and especially of copaiba, by making alkaline solutions or extracts;—but this object is never attained without a sacrifice of their efficacy. The solution of chloride of lime has been used as a substitute, in doses of ♏ x.—xxx; but it has not proved of much efficacy.

It may be added, that copaiba and cubebs seldom agree well with young delicate subjects, with light complexions.

Injections are certainly the remedies most to be depended on in gonorrhœa; but their use requires some precautions, as they may very easily cause swelled testicle or retention of urine, if used injudiciously.

If the patient applies at the very commencement of the disease, when he begins to suffer from the premonitory irritation, and the discharge is just appearing, it is a good plan to inject the urethra once a day with a strong injection, (such as a scruple of alum, and the same quantity of sulphate of zinc, to four ounces of water—or eight grains of nitrate of silver to the same quantity of water,) and also to use an injection, one-fourth of that strength, several times a day. This local treatment, together with low diet, aperient medicine, and abstinence from exercise and stimulants, will cut short many cases in three or four days.

During the acute stage, the prudence of using injections will depend in some measure on the constitution of the patient;—for it is decidedly not safe to use them with young, delicate, irritable subjects, and most especially whilst there is any tenderness of the glands of the groin, or any aching in the spermatie cord or testicles. And it will depend, in the next place, on the degree of medical control which the patient can submit to. For injections may be used much more early and freely with a hospital patient who keeps his bed, or with a person who is able to stay at home and apply leeches, than with a young gentleman who lives with his family, is obliged to conceal his malady, and to partake of his ordinary avocations, and appear at the dinner-table. So that as a general rule it is best to refrain from them till the inflammatory symptoms are mitigated by the antiphlogistic remedies before mentioned.

But as soon as the chordee is a little abated, the patient should use an injection of nitrate of silver (gr. ii. ad $\mathfrak{Z}j$.) every night at bed-time, and a weak injection of alum four or five times a day. By these means the discharge will probably soon become thin and bloody, and then cease altogether. If this does not succeed, other injections, F. 21, 22, 23, 36, 37, may be tried in succession; but both the injections and the copaiba or cubebs should be continued for a few days after the discharge has ceased.

TREATMENT OF COMPLICATIONS.—Painful erections and chordee may be relieved by bathing the parts with tepid or cold water, and the diaphoretic powder at bed-time; and if the chordee lasts long, a little mercurial ointment and extract of belladonna should be smeared on the part at bedtime. According to Hunter, the spasmodic chordee is benefited by bark. Hæmorrhage may be checked by cold, and pressure on the urethra. Inflammation of the mucous glands of the urethra is to be treated by leeches and poultices. An opening must be made if the swelling obstructs the flow of urine, but not otherwise. Swelling of the glands in the groin may generally be removed by rest, and a few leeches.

TREATMENT OF CONSEQUENCES.—*Gleet* is often a very tedious complaint, and requires a judicious and long-continued treatment. If it is the sequel of repeated gonorrhœa, and is accompanied with no appreciable derangement of the health and strength, it may be got rid of by a course of remedies that act on the urinary organs, together with most temperate habits of living. Copaiba, either alone or combined with astringents;—F. 86, 87; oil of turpentine; F. 90; cantharides, especially in combination with zinc, (F. 88,) or steel, F. 89, are the most useful remedies. The bowels should be kept properly open, but saline purgatives should be avoided. If the patient wants to make water oftener than natural, and there is an uneasy sensation in the urethra afterwards, and the urine deposites a mucous cloud, buchu and uva ursi (F. 91) will be advisable. The occasional passing a smooth metallic bougie, large enough to fill the urethra without stretching it, will also be of material service. It is also highly useful in these cases to inject the urethra with cold water from an elastic bottle, twice a day. If the health is materially enfeebled by debauchery or mal-practices, affusion of cold water on the genitals, cold sea-bathing, bark and steel, good living, and perfect chastity of body and mind, are the necessary remedies.

A *scirrhous or semi-cartilaginous condition* of the corpus spongiosum urethræ is always extremely difficult to get rid of. The frequent introduction of bougies, and friction with ointments of mercury or iodine,—warm bathing, and the internal use of Plummer's pill and iodine, afford the best chance of relief. Cases are recorded in which portions of osseous matter have been removed from the septum penis by incision.*

*Gonorrhœal rheumatism* must be treated on the same principles as common rheumatism;—if severe, by bleeding; otherwise the bowels should be well cleared by calomel and black draught, and the colchicum should be given in doses of ♏ xx. of the wine with magnesia, every four or five hours, and a dose of Dover's powder at bed-time. In the chronic stage, F. 7. at bed-time;—sarsaparilla, bark, volatile tinct. of guaiacum, sea air, tonics, and warm bathing, are the remedies.

THE TREATMENT OF GONORRHŒA IN THE FEMALE must be conducted upon precisely the same principles. During the acute stage, rest in the recumbent posture, leeches, anodyne fomentations, frequent ablution, lubrication with lard or cold cream—and very frequent sponging with a weak solution of alum, a piece of lint dipped in which should be inserted between the labia; with laxatives and diaphoretics, are the measures to be adopted, until heat, pain, and tenderness subside; afterwards injections may be used with much greater freedom and benefit than in the other sex. Those of acetate of zinc and nitrate of silver appear to be the best; and they should be continued for some time after all discharge has ceased. But much greater liberties may be taken with the vagina than with the male urethra; and the disease may often be stopped at once, without risk, by the application of the solid nitrate of silver, as recommended by Jewel and others. It should be applied, however, either *before* the inflammatory symptoms have attained any height, or after they have subsided. *Terebinthinate medicines* (copabia, &c.) may be given, although they do not much good. Abscesses or other complications are rare; but if they occur, they must be treated on general principles.

SECTION IV.—OF PRIMARY SYPHILITIC ULCERS.

GENERAL DESCRIPTION.—Primary syphilitic ulcers or chancres may be caused by the application of the syphilitic virus to any surface, mucous or cutaneous, entire, wounded, or ulcerated. Their most frequent *seat* is the genitals;—and in men they are more frequently than otherwise found on the inner surface of the prepuce, or the furrow between the prepuce and corona glandis, or the angle by the frænum;— obviously because those spots are most convenient for the lodgment of filth. It is notorious that persons with a long prepuce, whose glans is habitually protected by it, and covered with a delicate semi-mucous membrane, are more liable to suffer than those whose glans is uncovered and clothed with a denser cuticle. The *time* at which venereal sores appear is usually said to be from the third to the tenth day after in-

* Titley, p. 175.

26

fection ; but it is more probable, as Ricord observes, that the syphilitic virus operates progressively from the first moment of its application, and that the ulcer is fully formed by the fifth day; although it may not be perceived by a careless person till later. The average duration of a syphilitic ulcer produced by inoculation is, according to Wallace, twenty-five days.

Primary syphilitic ulcers present very many varieties. These varieties depend,—1st. On the peculiar sore from which infection was received; because every kind of sore, and especially the phagedænic and fungous varieties, have a tendency to reproduce their like. 2ndly. On the state of constitution of the patient, and degree of inflammation which is present. 3rdly. On the situation; and, lastly, on the local treatment.

It is impossible in this work to collate and describe the innumerable varieties of syphilitic ulcers that are spoken of by authors. For practical purposes it will suffice to consider them under three heads. 1st, the Hunterian, or indurated chancre; 2ndly, the common or non-indurated chancre; and 3rdly, chancres complicated with sloughing or phagedæna.

1. THE HUNTERIAN CHANCRE, or indurated ulcer, is generally found on the common integument or on the glans penis. It may begin either as a pimple, or as a patch of excoriation which heals up, leaving the centre ulcerous. It is nearly circular;—deep and excavated; the base and edges are hard as cartilage, but the hardness is circumscribed;—there is little pain or inflammation;—its colour is livid or tawny;—it is never so hard nor excavated when on the body of the penis as on the glans.

It is this form of ulcer which is ordinarily produced when the pus of a chancre is inoculated into the sound skin for purposes of diagnosis. Supposing the inoculation to have been performed with the point of a lancet. During the first twenty-four hours, the puncture reddens. In the second and third days it swells slightly, and becomes a pimple surrounded by a red areola. From the third to the fourth day, the cuticle is raised by a turbid fluid into a vesicle, which displays a black spot on its summit, consisting of the dried blood of the puncture. From the fourth to the fifth day, the morbid secretion increases and becomes purulent, and the vesicle becomes a pustule with a depressed summit. At this period the areola, which had increased, begins to fade, but the subjacent tissues become infiltrated and hardened with lymph. After the sixth day, if the cuticle and the dried pus which adheres to it be removed, there is found an ulcer, resting on a hardened base; its depth equal to the whole thickness of the true skin, its edges seeming as if clean cut out with a punch—its surface covered with a grayish pultaceous matter, and its margin hard, elevated, and of a reddish brown or violet colour.*

* Ricord, op. cit., p. 89.

2. The Common, or non-indurated chancre, is most frequently found in the inner surface of the prepuce. It may be said to have four stages. In the 1st, it is a small itching *pimple* or *pustule*, which bursting, displays,—2ndly, a foul *yellowish or tawny sore*, attended with slight redness and swelling, and spreading circularly. It may or may not be covered at first with a dirty brown scab. In the third stage it throws out indolent fungous granulations;—except it be situated on the *glans*; (for the *substance* of the glans penis has no power of throwing out graunlations, although its surface may;) and is usually stationary for a little time after it has ceased to ulcerate, and before it begins to heal. In the 4th stage, it *slowly heals*; cicatrization being preceded by a narrow vascular line. The cicatrix is often red and indurated;—swelled, if on the prepuce; but depressed, if on the glans, from want of granulations. It is exceedingly liable to ulcerate afresh. If the ulcer be seated near the frænum, it is almost sure to perforate it.

One *sub-variety* has been termed by Mr. H. J. Johnson the *multifarious sore*;—because the discharge is so infectious that it excites fresh ulcers on the sound skin. Another sub-variety is described under the term *excoriation sore, aphthous sore, or superficial sore*; a circular, shallowish sore, much resembling an excoriation, not ulcerating deeply. Finally, an *excoriation* or a *fissure* of the prepuce may be infected, and may be followed by secondary symptoms. But if ulceration does not spread, it will be very difficult to say whether it is a venereal ulcer, or merely a common fissure or excoriation obstinate in healing; for, in both cases, it may appear yellowish and indolent. Inoculation is the test.

3. Chancre complicated with Phagedæna or Sloughing.

(*a*) *Phagedænic chancres* are extremely rapid in their progress, and highly painful; their surface yellow, and dotted with red streaks, their shape irregular; their edges rugged or undermined; the surrounding margin of skin swelled, and sometimes red or livid; and the discharge profuse, thin, and sanious. Sometimes these ulcers eat deeply into the substance of the penis; sometimes they undermine the skin extensively; and sometimes they extend in one direction whilst they heal in another.

(*b*) *Sloughing phagedæna* affecting chancres requires no observations on its symptoms distinct from those made at page 97.

Simple or sloughing phagedæna may affect chancres or open buboes for two reasons. 1st, If the constitution be irritable and broken down by debauchery, night watching, exposure to cold and damp, or by the profuse administration of mercury, or by confinement in the foul pestiferous air of a hospital. Hence it is liable to occur to soldiers, sailors, prostitutes, and bakers;—the last-named class of individuals being obliged to work in the night. 2ndly, They may probably be produced by some peculiar acrimony of the venereal virus. There is reason for believing that intercourse between foreigners gives rise to a very destructive kind of poison. The venereal secretions of the Portuguese women appear to have been horribly deleterious to the British soldiers during the Peninsular war, who gave the expressive name of *The Black Lion* to the sloughing sores that resulted from connexion with them.

(*c*) Chancres may be affected with *simple acute inflammation* leading to gangrene, from violent local irritation, such as horse exercise.

CHANCRE IN THE URETHRA.—Ricord has proved satisfactorily, that this is the cause of the secondary syphilitic symptoms which were formerly attributed to gonorrhœa. The existence of chancre in the urethra may be suspected, if in a case of gonorrhœa the discharge is very capricious, sometimes thin, scanty, and bloody, sometimes thick and profuse; and if the pain is confined chiefly to one spot. But it can only be proved, either by the ulcer being visible at the orifice, or by inoculation with the matter.

SYPHILITIC ULCERS IN THE FEMALE require no distinct observations. They do not usually cause so much distress as in the male, but they are very slow in healing, especially if interfered with by the urine. When situated high in the vagina they may cause no symptoms at all, except perhaps a mucous discharge, and can only be detected by the speculum.

DIAGNOSIS.—The ordinary means of distinguishing a syphilitic ulcer are, that it is seated on the genitals; that it has followed a suspicious connexion; that it is probably circular, with hardened base and elevated edges; and above all, that if treated with simple applications merely, it is extremely difficult to heal. But none of these characteristics are infallible. The surest test is that of *inoculation*, which has been brought into great repute by Ricord. If some of the pus of a real chancre, taken whilst it is extending and before it begins to heal, be inoculated into the skin of the thigh, it will produce a regular chancre there, after the manner we have already described (p. 202.) It may be right to adopt this practice in some few cases where the propriety of giving mercury is doubtful; but the sore produced by inoculation must be destroyed by lunar caustic as soon as its character is decided.

AFFECTIONS THAT MAY BE MISTAKEN FOR CHANCRE.—This is the most convenient place for describing the nature and treatment of various affections that may be mistaken for chancre.

1. *Gonorrhœa externa*, or *balanitis*, is an inflammation of the surface of the glans and inside of the prepuce, with profuse purulent discharge, and excoriation of the cuticle. It generally affects dirty people with long prepuce, and is caused either by the acrid secretions of the part, or by contact with unhealthy secretions in the female. Sometimes, however, it occurs to cleanly people whose health is disordered. The thick profuse discharge, the peculiar smell, the superficiality of the excoriations, and their appearance immediately after connexion, distinguish this complaint from chancre; and a little opening medicine, common soap and

water, and any mild astringent lotion, will suffice to cure it. Lime-water is the best lotion if there is much inflammation, and a grain of corrosive sublimate to an ounce and a half of lime-water if there is not. If the cure is not effected in two or three days, the excoriations should be touched with nitrate of silver. Sometimes balanitis is attended with very great inflammation and fever, and with *phymosis*, from the great swelling of the prepuce; and the pain may be so severe and gnawing, as to make the surgeon uncertain whether there is not a plagedænic ulcer concealed by the foreskin. The thick discharge, and the pain being general and not confined to one spot, form the chief means of diagnosis; and repeated injection of warm-water and astringent lotions under the foreskin are the remedies.

2. *Minute aphthous-looking points*, sometimes in clusters, sometimes surrounding the glans; some of them healing, whilst others break out. They are totally devoid of pain; and, although they may last a long time, do not lead to ulcers. They are best treated by washes of *arg. nit.* or *cupr. sulph.* and alteratives.

3. *Herpes præputialis**  begins with extreme itching and sense of heat. The patient examining the part, finds one or two red patches, about the size of a split pea. On each patch are clustered *five or six minute vesicles*, which, being extremely transparent, appear of the same red colour as the patch on which they are situated. In twenty-four or thirty hours the vesicles become larger, milky, and opaque; and on the third day they are confluent and almost pustular. If the eruption is seated on the inner surface of the prepuce, the vessels commonly break on the fourth or fifth day, and form a slight ulcer with a white base and rather elevated edges. If this ulcer be irritated by caustic or otherwise, its base may become as hard as that of a chancre. If left to itself, it mostly heals in a fortnight;—sooner if situated on the external skin. The *cause* of this complaint is either some derangement of the digestive organs, or irritation within the urethra, which should be ascertained by the bougie. It is very liable to recur in the same individual, which of course, if known, will greatly aid the diagnosis. *Treatment.*—A little dry lint, or gold-beater's skin, at first, and subsequently a very weak lotion.

4. *Psoriasis præputii*, painful, irritable and bleeding cracks or fissures around the edge of the prepuce,—best treated by ung. hydr. nitr. dil.

SECTION IV.—OF THE TREATMENT OF PRIMARY SYPHILIS.

PROPHYLACTIC TREATMENT.—It need scarcely be said, that after a suspicious connexion, a thorough ablution should be performed with soap and water; and if there are any fissures or excoriations about the genitals, they should be washed with a strong solution of alum.

---

* Bateman on Cutaneous Diseases, 5th ed., p. 238.

*Local Treatment.*—It seems to be pretty well established, that if a chancre last for a few days only there will be no fear of secondary symp" toms. If, therefore, a patient applies as soon as he perceives the chancre, it will be advisable to touch it thoroughly with a stick of nitrate of silver, and destroy it; then give an aperient, enjoin rest and low diet, and wrap the penis in rag dipped in warm water, to prevent inflammation. But if the sore has lasted more than a week, the nitrate of silver will not act deeply enough to destroy it effectually; and the potassa fusa, or strong nitric acid, must be employed instead. If a small chancre is situated at the edge of the prepuce, it may occasionally be cut out.

. But neither of the foregoing plans can be adopted with safety, if the chancre is inflamed, the patient feverish, or if there is any local swelling or tenderness in the groin. When this is the case the treatment cannot be too soothing. Weak black wash on lint will then suffice. After" wards, during the indolent and granulating stages, the sore may be treated with astringent lotions, and be touched occasionally with nitrate of silver or sulphate of copper.

*Constitutional Treatment.*—If there are none of the contra indications that will be mentioned presently, the patient should take mercury. Not that it is absolutely necessary in all cases, or that the venereal disease cannot get well without it, but that it affords a more decided security against secondary symptoms. But before doing so, it will be right to open the bowels by blue pill and black draught;—and to prescribe low living, rest, and saline medicines, *till local pain and inflammation and any general disorder of the system have been removed.* A *warm bath* or two may also be useful. If the patient be young, plethoric, and a countryman, it may be right to *bleed* him; but great care must be taken not to induce weakness;—and neither this nor any other measure should be needlessly adopted from motives of mere routine.

Then the object is to induce a *gentle* mercurial action, and maintain it *long enough.* Five grains of blue pill should be given every night and morning; and if no effect on the mouth is produced by the fourth day, the dose at night should be doubled. This will rarely fail, in another day or two, to produce the desired effect;—viz. *slight soreness and sponginess of the gums,* with a *slight* increase of the saliva. It must be observed, that the only *use of salivation* is to show that the system is affected. It should be steadily maintained for four or five weeks, and until the sore has healed and all hardness of the cicatrix has vanished. If the mouth become *too sore,* the dose should be lessened;—if the soreness *subside too soon,* it may be increased; or two or three doses of calomel may be added. Mean while the patient should live regularly, but not too low:—he should avoid all excess of food or wine, and acescent vegetables, and every thing likely to disorder the bowels;—his clothing should be rather warm, so as to keep the skin perspirable;—and, above all, he should most sedulously avoid fatigue, cold, wet, and night air.

The *strong mercurial ointment* is not so likely to disorder the bowels as the blue pill, but it is more troublesome, and might fatigue a feeble patient injuriously. The dose is from ʒß—ʒj;—to be rubbed in daily upon the inside of the thighs or arms till it disappears. The morning is the best time for doing it, as the skin is then softer; it should be rubbed on different limbs successively; the patient wearing the same drawers both by night and day. If the skin becomes irritated, it should be well washed and bathed. If the patient is too weak to rub in himself, it must be performed by a servant, whose hands should be protected by a pig's bladder, well softened in oil and tied round his wrist. If *calomel* is preferred, two or three grains may be given every night, combined with a little opium: but it is more apt to purge, and should only be used in cases where that effect would not be objectionable.

THE ILL EFFECTS OF MERCURY that require to be guarded against are as follow: 1. *Griping and purging;*—which are to be obviated by combining a small quantity of opium or hyoscyamus with the blue pill, and giving occasionally a draught with P. rhæi ƷŽj, tinct. ejusd. fʒj, tinct. opii ♏xx. ap. menth. fʒx. It is far from uncommon for a slight attack of *dysentery* to occur, especially about the time that salivation commences; there being sickness and severe griping, with frequent straining and ineffectual attempts to go to stool. This should be treated by the draught just mentioned, followed by opiate enemata and the warm bath;—the mercury being omitted for the time.

2. *Sore throat;* redness of the whole fauces, and sloughing or ulceration of the tonsils with fever. In this case the mercury must be discontinued, till leeches, gargles, and aperients have set the throat to rights;—and then it may be resumed in smaller doses.

3. *Violent salivation.* This may be caused by a too liberal use of the remedy; or by a sudden check to the cutaneous secretion by cold and damp. It is, however, very common to meet with persons who are salivated by the smallest quantities conceivable; and every practitioner should make a point of ascertaining this, before he prescribes mercury for any new patient. The *symptoms* of severe salivation are, swelling and inflammation of the salivary glands, cheeks, tongue, and fauces, with a flow of peculiarly fetid saliva, and ulceration or even sloughing of the gums. The best *local applications* for this state are, a few leeches to the Stenonian ducts on each side;—and gargles of brandy and water, to which a little of the solution of chloride of lime may be added, (F. 39, 40, 92.) The bowels should be cleared by mild aperients; and as soon as fever has abated, the patient should have a good diet and tonics. Change of air, and especially removal from the venereal wards of a hospital, are

indispensable. If the salivation is very obstinate, repeated blisters should be applied behind the ears, and to the throat.*

4. *Eczema mercuriale* (*Eczema rubrum, Erythema mercuriale, hydrargyria*) consists of patches of redness and inflammation, which appear first in the groins, axillæ, and flexures of the limbs, and then spread over the trunk. These patches are covered with minute vesicles, which soon burst, discharging a thin acrimonious fluid, and leaving the surface excoriated, and exceedingly painful and tender. The discharge often becomes profuse and fetid, and the affected parts much swollen and fissured. It generally lasts for ten days, but may remain for many weeks.† *Treatment.* Warm bathing, mild and unctuous applications, aperients, diaphoretics, salines, and opiates, during the early stages;—subsequently, bark or sarsaparilla, and the mineral acids. Dr. Colles has described another and less severe form of eruption, which resembled the itch, except that the intervals between the fingers are free from it; the treatment is the same. When a *patient who is disposed to these affections reverts* to the use of mercury, the doses should be small, combined with hyoscyamus, and he should carefully avoid heat, violent exercise, and every thing else that excites the cutaneous circulation.

5. *Erethismus mercurialis* consists in a tendency to palsy of the heart. The symptoms are great depression of strength; anxiety about the præcordia, dyspnœa, frequent sighing, weak and tumultuous action of the heart;—frequent sense of suffocation, disturbed sleep, and faintness upon any exertion; which faintness may prove fatal. *Treatment.* Removal to a fresh atmosphere; stimulants; especially the mistura moschitonics; and good living.‡

If during the mercurial course any *febrile or inflammatory attack* arises, it is a general rule to discontinue it until such a state has been removed. And if the *patient become thin and feeble;* losing his appetite and strength, complaining of disturbed sleep, night sweats, cough, or any other symptoms indicative of debility, his diet must be generous, and sarsaparilla or cinchona and other tonics must be liberally administered; and if these symptoms persist, notwithstanding the mercury is given in diminished doses, it must be relinquished altogether.

If the *patient is very easily salivated,* the doses must be very small at distant intervals, and the strength must be well supported by tonics and

---

* Dr. Macleod, relates two cases of coma following the sudden cessation of salivation; one fatal; the other cured by reproducing it. Lond. Med. and Phys. Journ. vol. lvi. p. 231.

† One variety, *hydrargyria maligna*, now almost unknown, is attended with typhoid fever. Eight out of fourteen cases died. Alley on Hpdrargyria. Lond. 1810.

‡ Vide Dr. Bateman's case. Med. Chir. Trans. vol. ix.

good living. If, on the other hand, as sometimes happens, the *mercury seems to make no impression* on the system, the patient may be bled and purged;—should use the warm bath, and live low. But the doses must not be very much increased, lest they suddenly induce violent salivation, or *erethis mu*

There are some *patients whom it is scarcely advisable to subject to a mercurial course*, viz. those naturally labouring under, or strongly disposed to, *consumption* or *scrofula;* or who are extremely debilitated, or who are liable to the erethismus.

For these and other cases in which mercury is unadvisable, the *iodide of potassium* has been proposed as a substitute; in doses of gr. iii.—v. ter die. It produces a great flow of urine. In over doses, it causes sickness, salivation and emaciation; with symptoms of violent cold in the head and swelling of the eyes.

*Sarsaparilla and guaiacum*, as combined in the *compound decoction of sarsaparilla*, appear to maintain the secretions, especially those of the skin and kidneys, to increase nutrition, and allay morbid irritability of the nervous and circulating systems. Hence they are admirable remedies for debility during or after a mercurial course; and for the multifarious variety of symptoms that arise when the health is broken down as well by the disease as by its remedy.

The *gangrenous chancre (when occurring in healthy subjects, with firm pulse,)* requires to be treated by the early and free abstraction of blood; and then the bowels having been opened, and the pulse being reduced, opium should be given pretty freely in combination with salines and antimonials. The poppy fomentation is the best application at first, and the balsam of Peru, or nitric acid lotion subsequently, to assist in throwing off the sloughs. The ulcer which remains is usually healthy, and is very seldom followed by secondary symptoms; therefore *there is no need of mecury unless the sore begin to ulcerate*, (there being nothing in the general health to account for it,) or unless *secondary symptoms* appear.

The *phagedænic and phagedæno-gangrenous chancres* must be treated according to the state of the system. If there be fever and thirst, with a full habit and harsh pulse, blood should be drawn at first; if, however, the constitution is broken down, and the pulse quick and feeble, opium should be given freely; —and if the application of a strong solution of opium do not stop the phagedæna, the diseased surface must be destroyed by strong nitric acid, as directed at p. 100. Mecury is inadmissible when chancres are affected with inflammation, sloughing or phagedæna.

If *phymosis* is present, and there is a discharge from under the prepuce, and it cannot be turned back, the existence of an ulcer will be detected by local hardness and tenderness. Whilst there is any inflammation, leeches and poultices must be applied, and milk and water, or a mild

27

saturnine lotion, should be injected frequently between the prepuce and glans. The prepuce should be slit up, if the tumefaction is so great that it threatens to slough; but not otherwise. If phymosis be caused by *small ulcers at the edge of the prepuce,* (which sometimes occur during the healing of venereal sores,) they should be touched with *arg. nit.,* or *cupri sulph.,* or *ung. hydr. nitrat.*

As soon as the *frænum has been perforated* by an ulcer, it should be completely divided.

*Chancre in the urethra* must be treated as gonorrhœa; but if its nature is decided, a course of mercury should be given.

### SECTION VI.— OF BUBO.

DEFINITION.—Bubo signifies an inflamed lymphatic vessel or gland leading from a venereal ulcer.

CAUSES.—Any local irritation will, in certain habits, cause inflammation of the lymphatics; in gonorrhœa, for instance, the glands in the groin are apt to swell. But the genuine syphilitic bubo arises from absorption of the poisonous secretions of a chancre; and the ordinary time of its appearance is, just as the ulcerative stage of the chancre is ceasing.

VARIETIES.—(1.)—*Bubo of the penis* consists of an inflamed lymphatic vessel on the penis.

(2.) *Acute bubo* at the groin generally affects only one gland, and pursues the course of an ordinary acute abscess. The cellular tissue between the gland and skin is the seat of suppuration.

(3.) *Indolent or chronic bubo* very commonly affects more than one gland. It occurs in weak, scrofulous habits, and especially in persons worn out by the improper administration of mercury. The glands slowly enlarge; suppuration is slow and imperfect, and commences at several points. The skin is long before it inflames, but when it does so, a large tract of it becomes of a dusky bluish tint, the matter spreads widely:— and at last large portions of skin perish by ulceration or sloughing, leaving an extensive sore that may be months in healing.

DIAGNOSIS.—If a bubo at the groin affect one gland only, and that above Poupart's ligament, it is most probably caused by chancre on the penis, provided there be one. But if many glands are swelled, and they are below the level of Poupart's ligament, the swelling is probably caused by mere irritation. But the only sure diagnosis of a syphilitic bubo is, that if the matter taken from it be inoculated, it will produce a chancre; or that the sore produced by opening the bubo, presents the elevated edges and copper-coloured margin of a chancre. As, however, every bubo is attended with some common inflammation of the cellular tissue, the surgeon should recollect that some of the matter taken when it is first opened, may not cause chancre by inoculation.

A gland in the groin (or elswhere) may inflame and form an acute abscess, without there being any chancre to account for it. Such cases were once explained on the supposition that syphilitic poison might be absorbed from the skin without causing ulceration. But whether this may happen or not, the surgeon should not give mercury for such cases unless decided secondary syphilitic symptoms appear.

TREATMENT.—1. The *acute* bubo must be treated as an acute abscess. The first indication is to procure resolution ;—by rest ;—purging with calomel and black draught ;—salines, low diet, leeches, and warm or cold applications, according to the patient's choice. The applications to the chancre should be soothing, and mercury, if being administered, should be at once given up. Sometimes, it is true, a rapid exhibition of it causes a rapid disappearance of the bubo ;—But more generally it hastens suppuration, and it certainly predisposes to subsequent spreading ulceration. It may easily be resumed afterwards. Even if matter does form, the surgeon should be in no haste to evacuate it;—but should endeavour to procure its absorption by repeated leechings, and cold discutient lotions, with aperients, attention to the health, and change of air. When the case becomes chronic, frictions, bandages, &c., may be used to remove any swelling that remains.

But if the matter increases, and the skin is inflamed and shining, a puncture should be made, and the case be treated as an acute abscess under the same circumstances.

2. In treating the *indolent bubo*, the general health must be amended by every possible means; tonics, the acids, sarsaparilla; change of air, and especially a sea voyage ;—with occasional leechings and cold lotions, when demanded by an aggravation of heat and pain. If these measures fail, and matter forms, and the skin is becoming bluish and thin, a blister may be applied;—or the diseased skin may be rubbed with *arg. nit.*; which measures will either promote absorption, or at least stimulate the parts to a healthier action. But if the matter continue to increase, the swellings should be opened either by rubbing it with *potassa fusa;*—or by applying the nitrate first and then opening it with a lancet;—either plan having the advantage of causing diminution of the swelled glands, and preventing the spread of ulceration. Mercury should not be given ;—except, perhaps, in alterative doses towards the close of the case.

In treating the sore formed by opening a bubo, the first thing is to get rid of the loose red skin. This may be done (as soon as the part is becoming indolent and swelling is abated) by cutting it away with scissors, or by the potassa fusa. A solution of nitrate of silver is the best dressing afterwards.

*Sinuses*, if they are not soon healed by stimulating injections, must be slit up.

If the ulcer become *inflamed*, or *irritable*, spreading by ulceration, or if it be attacked by *sloughing*, or *phagedæna*, (which may destroy the patient by exhaustion, or by laying open the femoral artery,) the same treatment must be adopted that has already been directed for similar ulcers.

## SECTION. VI.—OF SECONDARY SYPHILIS.

The symptoms of secondary, or constitutional syphilis, generally occur about six weeks after the primary symptoms;—sometimes a fortnight, sometimes not for months. For some time before their appearance, the patient is generally thin and wan;—looks dispirited;—his eyes are heavy;—and he complains of want of appetite and sleep, and of rheumatic pains.

The effects of constitutional syphilis are usually first manifested upon the skin and mucous membrane of the throat, and then upon the bones. We shall first describe these several local affections, and then the treatment of secondary syphilis generally; but syphilitic affections of the eye and testis, which generally accompany those of the throat, will be treated of in the chapters that are particularly devoted to those organs.

SYPHILITIC ERUPTIONS vary in degree from the slighest discolouration to the most inveterate ulcers. 1. In the mildest form, the skin is mottled and stained in irregular patches of brownish red colour; which are caused by a slight swelling and vascular injection. A greater degree of the same derangement will produce *syphilitic psoriasis*, in which the skin is raised in copper-coloured blotches, covered with scabs of hypertrophied cuticle. Or there may be an eruption of *papulæ* or pimples, varying in size from a pin's head to a pea. These eruptions are succeeded merely by scabs or exfoliations of the cuticle.

2. *Scaly Eruption (Lepra syphilitica)* is an aggravated variety of the preceding. It begins with an eruption of copper-coloured blotches, which become covered with scales of enlarged cuticle;—these are succeeded by scabs, and when they fall off, by shallow ulcers with copper-coloured edges.

3. *Vesicular Eruption, (Rupia.)* Large flattened bullæ, filled with serum, which gradually become purulent, and finally dry into scabs, under which the skin is ulcerated. The ulcers spread under the scabs, and the latter become remarkably thick from successive additions.

4. *Pustular Eruption. (Ecthyma.)* Large prominent pustules, with a copper-coloured base, leading to ulcers.

5. *Tubercular Eruption.* Board, red, inflammatory tubercles, forming most frequently at the alæ of the nose, or on the cheeks. They gradually pustulate, and are succeeded by deep irregular ulcers, terminating in puckered cicatrices.

*Condylomata* are soft red fungous elevations of the surface of the skin, generally situated about the anus, or between the scrotum and thigh, or at other parts where two cutaneous surfaces are in contact. They are covered with a thin cuticle, and often exude a copious thin discharge, which is doubtless occasionally contagious. They generally occur together with psoriasis or lepra.

SYPHILITIC SORE THROAT.—1. The mildest variety is a superficial excoriation of the mucous membrane of the tonsils or some other part of the month or fauces, corresponding to psoriasis on the skin. The parts affected are swollen and sore; sometimes red and raw, and sometimes covered with a whitish secretion. This state may be succeeded by a superficial ulceration.

2. The *excavated* ulcer looks as if a piece had been scooped out of the tonsil. Its surface is foul and yellow, its edges raised, and ragged, and swelled. There is remarkably little inconvenience from it, and very little constitutional affection, unless it be attended with eruption likewise.

3. The *sloughing* ulcer begins as a small *aphthous* spot, which rapidly ulcerates, and is attended with great pain and fever. The surface of the ulcer is covered with an ashy slough, and the surrounding mucous membrane is dark, livid and swollen. The lingual artery may be opened by the spread of the ulceration, and the patient may die of haemorrhage, unless the common carotid is tied.

SYPHILITIC ULCERATIONS of the nose and palate commence with ulcerations of the mucous membrane, similar to those of the throat, which may denude the periosteum, and then produce exfoliation of the bones, with profuse fœtid discharge and odious deformity. Ulceration of the nose generally begins with a sense of heat, and dryness, and snuffling.

*Syphilitic ulceration of the larynx* is mostly caused by an extension of ulceration from the palate. It is characterized by tenderness, great huskiness of voice (which frequently degenerates into a mere whisper,) suffocative cough, and expectoration of bloody purulent matter;—there is great loss of flesh and strength, and life is often terminated by suffocation.

SYPHILITIC DISEASE OF BONE most frequently attacks the tibia, ulna, os frontis, and other superficial bones. It commences with tenderness of the affected bone, and severe pain, which begins in the evening, and lasts almost all night, but ceases in the daytime. The pain is shortly accompanied with oblong swellings, called *nodes*, arising from infiltration of the periosteum with lymph and serum. Next, a quantity of serum is effused between the periosteum and bone, producing a fluctuating tumour. If the disease advance, the bone (which from the first is swelled) becomes carious, matter forms between it and the periosteum; extensive exfoliations ensue; the patient suffers severely from the pain and discharge; and if the disease be seated on the head, (in which situation it is called *corona veneris,*) death may ensue from irritation of the dura mater, or protrusion of the brain through apertures in the skull. Such aggravated cases are fortunately, however, now very rare; although common enough when mercury was supposed to be the only means of stopping the ravages of the disease.

DIAGNOSIS.—There is often some difficulty thrown into the surgeon's way, by the denial of patients that they have ever had any primary symptoms. If, however, the patient has a copper-coloured eruption, a sore throat, falling off of the hair, and a general faded unhealthy look, and these disorders are of recent date, and cannot be attributed to any causes connected with diet or residence, the probability is that they are syphilitic.

TREATMENT.—In the first place, if a venereal eruption and sore throat is ushered in with pain in the chest and other febrile or inflammatory symptoms; it will be necessary to give aperients, and saline medicines with antimony, and to restrict the diet, and confine the patient to the house. The warm-bath will also be highly useful.

When the febrile state has vanished, if the patient has never taken a course of mercury;—or if he has been subjected to an imperfect course of it for the primary symptoms;—and his constitution is sound, he may take mercury after the manner directed in the last section. If, under its use, the strength and general appearance are improved, so much the better;—but if the patient gets thinner, weaker, and haggard, and suffers from chills or feverishness, or if his ulcers become irritable and phage-dænic, it must be given up. The corrosive sublimate in very small doses, and not carried to the extent of affecting the mouth, will often be of great service when a full course of the mineral is inapplicable. F. 30.

The iodide of potassium is the remedy next in efficacy to mercury, and should be administered when the former is deemed inexpedient. Sometimes it is useful to combine it with iodine, F. 74.

Sarsaparilla, F. 56, 57, is a remedy that may almost always be used with advantage. It may be combined with corrosive sublimate or the iodide of potassium; or may be administered after a course of those remedies, to restore the flesh and strength. The mineral acids, especially the nitric; F. 29;—sedatives, especially hyoscyamus and conium; F. 93;—and tonics, F. 1, 2, 3, 26, 31, will be all of service in protracted cases. In these the surgeon will find it necessary to change and vary his remedies repeatedly. The main object should be to improve the general look and condition of the patient, and never to push a remedy, if it does not manifest harm, under the vague idea that it is a specific.

*Local Treatment.*—For syphilitic eruptions, the warm, vapour, and sulphur baths will be often expedient. Obstinate patches of lepra or pimples may sometimes have their removal hastened by ung. hydr. nitratis diluted, or the ung. hydr. precipitati albi. Itching eruptions may often be relieved by a weak lotion of corrosive sublimate. Ulcers must be treated according to their condition—whether inflamed, irritable, or indolent. In general, weak mercurial applications, black wash, or weak red precipitate ointment, answer best.

Condylomata are treated like warts.—Vide Part iv. chap. 2.

For the common excoriated sore throat, any soothing detergent gargle will do—F. 39, 40. When there are ulcers, it is advisable to use gargles of corrosive sublimate;—(gr. i. ad. ℥iv.;) and when the ulcers are indolent they may be touched with the *linimentum æruginis*. *Mercurial fumigation* is also occasionally of benefit. It is effected by putting a scruple of red sulphuret of mercury on a heated iron in a proper apparatus, and inhaling the vapour—a heated penny-piece in a teacup will answer the purpose.

Ulceration of the larynx is occasionally benefited by similar fumigation; but of course mercury so as to affect the mouth is almost always injurious;—as it is in other cases of rapid ulceration. Sarsaparilla, and sedatives; blisters to the throat and occasional leechings; and the operation of tracheotomy, if the breathing becomes much embarrassed, are the necessary measures.

The pain of nodes is often relieved by blisters, and so are rheumatic pains of venereal origin. In disease of bone, the use of mercury requires the greatest caution, and is only admissible if the patient has a sound constitution, and has never taken a course of it. It is peculiarly noxious when there is caries of the bones of the nose. When nodes are very tense and full of fluid, it may be necessary to puncture them, but it should be avoided if possible. If during secondary syphilis, the nose becomes tender or painful, the greatest benefit will be derived from the application of one or two leeches twice or three times a week to the inside of the affected nostril. At the same time, the patient should take plenty of sarsaparilla, with small doses of iodide of potassium, and should have the benefit of country air, and a nutritious diet. By these means, any farther mischief will sometimes be averted. If, however, ulceration does occur, it is of the utmost consequence to remove any loose or carious portions of bone, as soon as possible.

SYPHILIS OF CHILDREN.—When a man labours under constitutional syphilis, he may communicate it to his wife and offspring. The consequence is sometimes that the infant dies about the fourth or fifth month, and the woman miscarries repeatedly. Sometimes a child is born weakly and shrivelled, with hoarse voice, discharge from the nostrils, and copper-coloured blotches or ulcers, especially about the anus and pudenda. Sometimes, again, it is born healthy, but these symptoms appear a month afterwards. Lastly, a child may be infected with primary syphilis during its birth.

The parents in these cases should take a course of mercury, and be treated in other respects for secondary syphilis. And for the children, the best plan is to rub ten grains of mercurial ointment daily into the axilla, or soles of the feet, till the symptoms disappear.

# PART IV.

## OF THE INJURIES AND SURGICAL DISEASES OF VARIOUS TISSUES, ORGANS, AND REGIONS.

---

## CHAPTER I.

### OF THE DISEASES OF THE SKIN.

#### SECTION I.—CARBUNCLE AND BOIL.

DEFINITION.—A carbuncle signifies an unhealthy inflammation and sloughing of a circumscribed portion of the cellular tissue.

SYMPTOMS.—It begins with a hard, circumscribed, livid red swelling, and with severe burning, smarting pain. Its most prominent part soon becomes soft and *quaggy*, and numerous small ulcerated apertures form on it, which give exit to a thin discharge, compared by Sir A. Cooper to flour and water. These ulcers gradually unite, and form a considerable opening, from which a slough of cellular tissue is slowly protruded; and when that is separated, the parts may granulate and heal. The most usual situations of carbuncle are the back; the nape of the neck, and the nates. The tumour may vary in size from that of a half crown to that of a small plate.

Carbuncle is always an evidence of a vitiated state of the blood and disorder of the digestive organs; and it usually afflicts elderly people of bloated frame and intemperate habits. It is sometimes attended with considerable fever, and almost always with loss of appetite, flatulence, and unhealthy secretion of the liver. And it may be attended with great danger to life, if the patient is very old, or weak;—or if the carbuncle is very large, and seated on or near the head.

TREATMENT.—The objects of the local treatment are, to afford a free exit to sloughs and discharge, and to excite the diseased tissues to healthy suppuration and granulation. In the first place, therefore, a free

incision should at once be made completely through the tumour;—and if the tumour is extensive, it should be scored across by a second incision at right angles to the first. Then warm poultices should be applied; and if there is much atony about the system, the yeast poultice, F. 46, or linseed meal poultice mixed with a little port wine, or beer-grounds, or unguentum resinæ, will be advisable. Stimulating ointments and lotions, especially the nitric acid lotion F. 17, will complete the cure.

The indications for the constitutional treatment are, first, to evacuate and correct the secretions of the alimentary canal. This is to be effected by purgatives, which should be given in repeated doses, till the motions become light yellow and bilious, instead of dark, grumous and offensive;—or, at all events, as long as the patient feels lighter and better under their use. If the patient is tolerably vigorous, calomel and the black draught will suffice; but in general it will be better to use a few doses of blue pill, and the warmer aperients, such as rhubarb, and decoction of aloes, F. 8. Very often an emetic, composed of a scruple of ipecacuanha, followed by a cupful of warm camomile tea, will be of service. If there is much fever and a pretty good pulse, the patient may take the liq. am. acet., or effervescing saline draughts;—but more frequently, bark with the mineral acids, or ammonia, or camphor, or small doses of opium, (F. 1, 2, 3, 26,) will be necessary to support the strength; together with wine, beef-tea, &c. In fact, in no case must the patient be reduced too much.

BOILS are miniature carbuncles. The best plan is to cut them through as soon as possible, poultice for a day or two, and then apply stimulating plasters; such as the empl. galbani vel ammoniaci; cobbler's wax will do as well. The general health should be attended to in all cases, and the diet be regulated. If they continue to come out in successive crops, alteratives must be tried; such as, Plummer's pill; sarsaparilla; saline or sulphureous mineral waters, and sea-bathing;—but the liq. potassæ, or sodæ carb., in moderate doses three times a day, are generally considered of most utility. " I was myself always troubled with boils," says Hunter, " until I took forty drops of this lixivium (of soda) night and morning in milk for two months, when all by boils disappeared, and I have since had no return of them."*

SECTION II.—TUMOURS.

I. THE COMMON VASCULAR SARCOMA, or *simple ɪfleshy tumour,* is a yellowish-white, firm, fleshy, or fibrous mass;—with few blood-vessels;— often surrounded with a coat of condensed cellular tissue;—and sometimes containing irregular patches of bone or cartilage.

---

* Lectures in Palmer's Ed., vol. i. p. 610.

28

Its *formation* is supposed to be owing to the organization of lymph. In *external character*, it is a firm, lobulated tumour, circumscribed, moveable, and free from tenderness, unless accidentally inflamed. It is also free from pain, unless it press on some sensitive part. It grows slowly but steadily, and when it has attained considerable bulk, the veins on its surface become enlarged and tortuous. As to its consequences, *first*, it may last the whole life of the individual, without any ulterior consequences. Or (2) it may, by its enlargement, inflame the skin, and then slough out entirely. (3) It may produce sundry inconveniences, or even death, by pressure on various parts. Or (4) it may become the seat of malignant ulceration. It is known from abscess or inflammatory tumour by its *slow*, but *steady*, and *painless* enlargement. From scirrhus it is known by the absence of lancinating pain, and of the cancerous cachexia. But as it may degenerate into cancer, the proper *treatment* is extirpation with the knife.

II. The Fatty Tumour consists of lobulated masses of fat, very slightly vascular, and contained in a cyst of cellular tissue. In *external character*, it is a softish, lobulated, painless tumour, feeling like fat. Its *growth* is slow, but progressive; and it may attain enormous bulk, even forty pounds. Its *terminations* may be the same as those of the last-mentioned tumour, and its *treatment* should be also the same.

*Operation.*—An incision—rather too long than too short—should be made along the tumour, and through its cellular cyst. If the skin adhere to it, (but not otherwise,) a portion may be removed by two elliptical incisions. Next, the tumour should be removed as rapidly as possible, partly by cutting its cellular adhesions, partly by tearing them with the finger. Then the wound should be examined to ascertain that extirpation is complete;—and after bleeding has ceased it should be closed, and healed by the first intention. Sometimes fatty tumours may be removed by passing a seton through them, so that they may waste away in suppuration. This method is more tedious and painful than excision, but it may be adopted when it is an object to avoid a long cicatrix.

III. Encysted Tumours, or *Wens*, occur most frequently under the skin of the head. They consist of a sac, smooth on its internal surface, and containing various matters;—sometimes like curd or rice, (such tumours being formerly called atheroma;)—sometimes like suet, (steatoma;)—sometimes like honey, (meliceris;)—sometimes mere water;—sometimes hair, or matter like horn. These tumours are painless, rounded, elastic, circumscribed, moveable, and they fluctuate indistinctly. They enlarge slowly and steadily.

*Treatment.*—If inconvenient, extirpation is the only remedy. *Punctures, setons, injections*, or any means for obliterating them by exciting inflammation, are very hazardous;—because these cysts (like all new textures) are liable, if irritated, to take on malignant action. Ointments of iodine, or other substances for creating absorption, are perfectly use-less, and may be mischievous. If, however, the tumour consist, as it occasionally does, of an enlarged and obstructed follicle of the skin, its aperture (a little black spot) should be looked for, a probe may be passed into it, and the contents be squeezed out as often as necessary. Other-wise, a straight, double-edged, pointed bistoury should be thrust com-pletely through the tumour, then the cut edge of the sac should be seized with forceps, and the whole of it be dissected out.

IV. The Painful Subcutaneous Tumour is a small hard body, rarely larger than a pea or coffee-berry, seated immediately under the skin, liable to fits of excruciating pain, and supposed to be formed in the substance of a nerve. It must be extirpated. The removal of such a tumour from the breast has cured an obstinate hysteria.*

SECTION I.—TUMOURS.

I. General Hypertrophy.—The skin may grow into pendulous flaps or ridges, which, if inconvenient, are to be removed by incision.

II. Tumours of Cicatrices.—Under the term *keloides*, Dr. Warren describes a tumour consisting of a thick patch of skin, white and insensi-ble, and resembling the cicatrix of a burn. It is most frequently, but not always, found to grow on the site of some old cicatrix, and it is said that the coloured races of mankind are peculiarly liable to this kind of hyper-trophy of cicatrices. Extirpation with the knife is the only remedy.†

There is another affection, which Mr. Cæsar Hawkins has designated the *warty tumor of cicatrices*, which occasionally appears on old scars. " There appears, in the first place, a little wart, or warty tumour in the cicatrix, which is dry and covered with a thin cuticle, but which soon becomes moist, and partially ulcerated, like the warts of mucous mem-branes, from which a thin and semi-purulent fluid is secreted. In this stage it gives no pain nor inconvenience." After a time the warts are converted into a more solid tumour like fungus hæmatodes, very vascular, and easily bleeding when touched. And this finally (according to the principle laid down in the Chapter on Ulceration, p. 76) ulcerates or sloughs, forming a foul excavated ulcer, with fresh growths of warts around it, which may destroy the patient by its constant irritation and discharge. This affection belongs to a class termed semi-malignant, (see the next section.) The remedy is extirpation with the knife; or amputa-tion of the affected limb, if the diseased growth is very extensive; and the patient may be confidently assured, that if thoroughly extirpated it will not return.‡

---

\* Wood in Edinburgh Med. Chir. Trans., vol. iii. Lond. Med. Gazette, vol. vi. p. 59.

† Warren on Tumors, p. 40.

‡ Cæsar Hawkins, Med. Chir. Trans., vol. xix.

III. WARTS consist of elongated papillæ of the cutis, clothed with cuticle. When the cuticle is thin, which frequently happens when the warts are situated where two surfaces of skin are contiguous, the warts are *soft*, and may exude a serous discharge. They may be produced by local irritation, but very frequently they arise and disappear without any assignable cause. Warts are frequently relics of venereal sores, but although they may be produced by infection, they require no mercury. The best remedies for destroying them are stimulants;—argenti nitras— liq. hydrarg. oxymur.—tinct. ferri sesquichloridi, liq. plumbi diacetatis— pulv. sabinæ—ltq. arsenical.—liq. aluminis comp.—or the juice of the spurge, or of the sumach. If their shape permit, they may be snipped off or tied;—or if in very inconvenient situations, (as about the finger nails,) may be cut out;—but the surface from which they grew requires some astringent to be frequently applied, in order to prevent their reproduction.

IV. CORNS are growths of thick and hardened cuticle, and are produced when the skin, situated over some projecting point of bone, is irritated by frequent pressure or friction. It need scarcely be said that their usual seat is on the joints of the toes, and that tight boots or shoes are their usual cause. They are divided into two kinds, the hard and the soft. Hard corns are situated on the surface of the foot, where the cuticle can become dry and hard; whilst, if corns are situated between the toes, the cuticle is soft and spongy. Moreover, according to Sir B. Brodie, when a corn is completely formed, a minute bursa is developed between it and the cutis vera.[*]

*Treatment.*—The best plan is to extirpate the corn as soon as possible, and this may often be conveniently effected in the following manner. The foot should be bathed in hot water every night and morning, and the corn should be continually covered with a plaster, consisting of equal parts of soap plaster and oil, spread on kid leather. When the corn has become soft and sodden by these means, an oblique incision should be made with a lancet completely round it, and converging to its centre;—but without cutting deeply enough to wound the skin. When enough of it has been detached in this manner, it should be twisted round with a pair of forceps, till the root is pulled out. If this cannot be done, some palliative means must he tried. The feet should be bathed every day, and the corns should always be kept covered with the above-mentioned plaster, or with common emollient ointment; because it is a great object to have them soft and pliant, not hard and dry. The application of several plasters of thick soft leather, each having a hole punched in it to receive the corn and relieve it from pressure, is a very useful device. But if the corn is on the sole of the foot, it must be covered with a piece of adhesive plaster spread

---

[*] Brodie, Lecture on Corns, Med. Gaz. vol. xvii. p. 775; Key on Bunion, Guy's Hosp. Rep. vol. i. p. 416.

on linen, before the circular plasters are applied, otherwise the weight of the body will cause the flesh to bulge into the holes, and cause much pain in walking. Sometimes it is useful to put a sole of felt into the shoe, with a hole in it to receive the corn. At the same time, the corn should be frequently shaved down with a blunt knife or a rasp; and its exfoliation may be hastened by rubbing it with nitrate of silver, or liniment of ammonia, or by touching it with a hair pencil dipped in strong nitric acid, or the chloride of antimony. The soft corns between the toes are generally more painful than the others; the nitrate of silver is the best application. When a corn inflames, and the bursa between it and the skin suppurates, the pain is often most excruciating, and only to be relieved by paring it down, and letting out the fluid. It need scarcely be added, that the proper way to prevent corns is to wear boots or shoes properly adapted to the shape and size of the foot. Women in particular should not wear their shoes too low, so as to throw all the pressure of them on the toes. But if people chose to sacrifice comfort to what they fancy elegance, they must suffer for their folly.*

V. Horny Tumours are formed by an inspissation of the matter of the sebaceous follicles, and are easily removed by two small incisions.

SECTION II.—MALIGNANT AND SEMI-MALIGNANT AFFECTIONS.

These may be of two orders. *First*, the *really malignant* formations, depending on constitutional vice, implicating the glands, and appearing in several remote organs. To this class belongs scirrhus, which when it affects the skin is generally propagated to it fiom some neighbouring scirrhous gland. But it occasionally commences in the skin originally, as a small hard indolent lump, which gradually degenerates into cancerous ulceration.

*Secondly*, the *semi-malignant* ffec tions ; which although incurable if left to themselves, destroying the tissues in which they are situated, spreading progressively and destroying the parts in their vicinity, and finally fatal to life from their constant irritation, still are not really malignant;—because they do not attack the lymphatics, do not appear in several remote organs simultaneously, and do not return, if effectually removed. (Vide p. 120.) To this class belong the following:—

I. The Cancerous Ulcer (*Lepoides*) occurs on the face or neck of old people, especially below the under eyelid. It begins with a flat, brown, irregular crust, like a wart;—which falling off displays an ulcer with slightly elevated edges, but no hardened base. Its progress is slow; it is unaccompanied by hæmorrhage, and it occasionally cicatrizes for a

---

* Bunions will be treated of, under the head of Bursæ, in the next chapter.

time. *Treatment.* The knife. In some few cases, arsenic, or the chloride of zinc, may be used instead.*

II. LUPUS is a destructive ulceration of the face, commencing on one
side of the nose. There are two forms; 1st, the genuine lupus, *herpes
exedens,* or *noli me tangere;* and 2ndly, the *herpes,* or *lupus non exedens.*

1. *Lupus exedens.*—A portion of the skin of the face (mostly on or
near the *alæ nasi*) inflames, swells, and becomes of a bright red tint.
The swelling frequently occurs in the form of one or more *tubercles.*
The inflamed surface sooner or later becomes excoriated, and secretes an
ichorous matter which dries into a scab. After a time, a painful, foul,
excavated ulcer forms;—variable in its progress, sometimes stationary, or
partially cicatrizing;—but, in the end, destroying the flesh of the nose and
cheek; and causing caries and exfoliation of the bones;—till the patient,
a horrid spectacle, dies worn out with pain;—his eye dropping from its
socket into the chasm made by the destruction of the cheek. This affection mostly occurs to adults;—especially if of weakly scrofulous habits,
vitiated by intemperance and gross feeding.

2. The *lupus non exedens* is a milder form, and attacks scrofulous
children. It begins with shining tubercles, which ulcerate; but the ulceration has a tendency to spread *widely,* rather than *deeply;*—causing prodigious deformity by the successive ulceration and puckered cicatrization
of the face.

*Treatment.*—The indications are, 1st. To correct the general health;—
and abate inflammation;—by opening the bowels;—by keeping up the
secretions;—by allaying the irritation, and promoting appetite and digestion;—by regulating the diet; and by the application of poultices, or narcotic soothing fomentations, whilst pain and inflammation are acute. A
course of Plummer's pill, alkalis, and sarsaparilla, will generally be of
great service. The liq. arsenicalis in small doses may also be tried.
2ndly. To alter the diseased action by various stimulants. If ulceration
has not commenced, the part should be rubbed frequently with nitrate of
silver, so as to keep it constantly covered with a black crust. If ulceration has commenced, the nitrate may be applied in the same manner;—
or in the form of a lotion. But the best applications for ulcerated lupus
are the arsenical. Now, arsenical applications should be either *very
weak* or *very strong*; they should either produce *mild stimulation* or
*sphacelus.* They should either be so weak as not to do any harm if
absorbed into the blood; or so strong as immediately to kill the part they
are applied to, and so render it incapable of absorbing them. The weak
may be tried first;—in the form of a lotion composed of ʒi—ʒiv liq.
arsenical. ad. ʒij aquæ, in order to act as a mild stimulant and alterative.

* Cæsar Hawkins in Med. Chir. Trans. vol. xxi.; Warren on Tumours, Boston,
1837.

3rdly. But if these measures do not speedily succeed, the diseased surface must be destroyed by escharotics, of which arsenic and the chloride
of zinc are the best. The *arsenic* may be applied in the form of ointment or solution (Ʒi. ad. Ʒi) on lint, suffered to remain four or five hours.
The *chloride of zinc* is a highly deliquescent salt, and is therefore ingeniously recommended by Mr. Ure, who introduced its use into this country, to be combined with two parts of fresh burned plaster of Paris.
This may be made into a paste with a little water, and be spread on
the diseased surface for four or five hours. It causes severe pain for
eight or nine hours, which, however, may be relieved by opium.
When a suspicious tubercle is increasing rapidly, but not ulcerating, it
should also be destroyed with the chloride; but in this case, the cuticle
should first be removed with the liquor ammoniæ. Caustic pastes may
also be made with two parts of powdered *potassa fusa*, and one of soft
soap;—or of three parts of quick-lime, and two of dry soap, moistened
at the time of using with spirits of wine;—or of three parts of caustic potass
and two of fresh burned lime incorporated in a hot iron mortar. The
last is called the Vienna paste; the lime is useful in correcting the deliquescent and diffusive power of the potass. When either of these
caustics is used, the neighbouring sound parts should be protected by
layers of sticking plaster. After the sloughs have separated, which
generally happens in from six to twelve days, according to their depth,
the surface must be treated with a weak solution of nitrate of silver; but
if there appears any return of the ulcerative process, the caustic must be
applied again.[*]

---

# CHAPTER III.

## OF DISEASES AND INJURIES OF MUSCLES, TENDONS, AND BURSÆ.

I. ATROPHY OF MUSCLES.—Two forms of atrophy of muscles may
come under the surgeon's observation. The first, which may be called
*rigid atrophy*, is a state in which the muscle becomes short, rigid, and
inextensible; and it generally, by its shortening, causes various displace-
ments and deformities of the parts to which it is attached;—thus clubfoot
is a consequence of this condition of the muscles of the calf.

---

[*] Ure on Lupus and the Chloride of Zinc, Med. Gaz. vol. xvii. and xviii.; and Cyclop. Pract. Surg., Art. Cauterants; Earle, Med. Chir. Trans., vol. xii.; Travers, ib·
vol. xv.

*Causes.*—This state of rigid atrophy may be a sequel of various circumstances.   1st. It may be induced by *long inactivity* of a muscle;—
thus, after long-continued disease of the knee, the flexor muscles of the
ham may become shortened and inextensible, keeping the joint permanently bent, and often dragging the tibia off from the condyles of the
femur.   2ndly. It may be a sequel of a species of *subacute inflammation*,
which occasionally affects muscles or their investing fasciæ, and which is
attended with pain, tenderness, and spasm.   3rdly. It may be a sequel of
*habitual spasm*, by whatever cause produced.   4th. It may arise from
*defective innervation;* that is, from a want of nervous energy.   It sometimes happens, that after a fever, one arm, or one leg, or both legs, are
suddenly or gradually deprived of the power of motion.   The affected
member is always chilly; its skin is numb: it is imperfectly nourished,
and decreases in bulk; if the patient is young, it ceases to grow in proportion with the other parts of the body; and its flexor muscles become
affected with this form of rigidity, so that the joints are immoveably bent
and contracted.

TREATMENT.—In the earlier stages this affection may be relieved in
various ways.   By cupping, fomentations, or the steam bath, and subsequently blisters over the affected muscles, if there is any evidence of
local inflammation.   By purgatives and other constitutional measures,
if spasm appears to arise from disordered bowels or any other sympathetic source.   By stimulating frictions, affusion with cold water, passive
exercise, shampooing, extension upon splints by bandages, and electricity or galvanism, if it arise from want of nervous energy, or if, arising
from any other cause, it has become chronic.   But, in cases of long
standing, the only remedy that can be relied on is *division* of the affected
muscle or its tendon; by which means the divided parts will retract,
they will unite by lymph, and will consequently be lengthened, and then
extension and the other measures may be pursued with greater vigour
and efficacy.   (For farther illustrations, refer to Clubfoot and Wry
Neck.)

ACUTE ATROPHY.—In this affection, one or more muscles rapidly
waste away, and their wasting is attended with severe pain, especially
in the course of their nerves.   This complaint is rare, and apparently
incurable.*

II. RUPTURE OF MUSCLES AND TENDONS.—This is an accident which
is frequently caused by violent muscular contractions; especially if, after
illness or long inactivity, the muscles are subjected to sudden and severe
exertion.   The muscles which are most frequently ruptured, are the
gastro-cnemius and biceps flexor cubiti; but more frequently the tendons

---

* Two cases of it are given in Mayo's Pathology, p. 117.   The author witnessed
one some years ago.

give way, especially the tendo achillis, and flexor tendons of the wrist. "It occasionally happens," says Mr. Liston, "to gentlemen of mature years, who, forgetting these, join in the sports of youth as they were wont to do; suddenly they suppose that some one has inflicted a blow on the leg from behind—their dancing is arrested, the foot cannot be extended, and the nature of the case is forthwith evident to the most careless observer."[*]

The *symptoms* of this accident are, sudden pain, or sometimes an audible snap, loss of the motion peculiar to the muscle, and a depression at the ruptured part, which may be felt with the fingers. The reparation is effected by the effusion and organization of lymph, like the callus of broken bone.

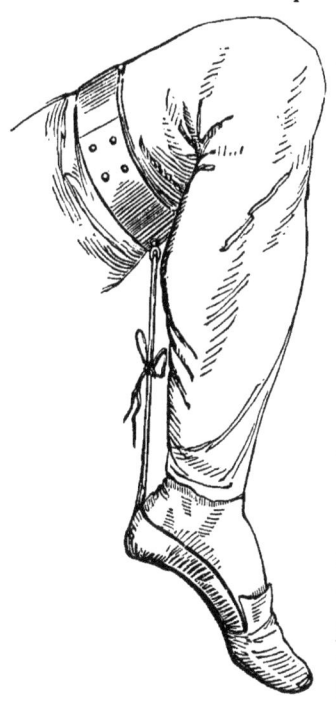

*Treatment.*—The main point is to keep the injured muscle in a state of constant rest and relaxation, so that the severed ends may be in close approximation, and to prevent any violent extension till the union is firmly consolidated. Pain and inflammation must be counteracted by leeches, and cold or warm lotions. For the ruptured tendo achillis nothing can be better than the apparatus depicted in the adjoining cut, which is taken from Mr. Liston's Practical Surgery. For rupture of the extensors of the thigh, the limb must be placed in the same position as in fracture of the patella. If the biceps is ruptured, the elbow must be kept bent to its utmost;—if the tendons about the wrist or fingers, the fore-arm must be confined by a splint. After three or four weeks of this rest, the surgeon may use *passive motion;* that is, may bend and extend the joints of the injured limb with his hands several times successively. But the patient must be cautious in using the muscle for a long time; and (if it be the tendo achillis) must walk with a high-heeled shoe for two or three months; so that the recent callus may not be stretched and lengthened, which would cause permanent weakness.

III. STRAINS.—A strain signifies a violent stretching of tendinous or ligamentous parts, with or without rupture of some of their fibres. It produces instant severe pain, often attended with faintness; and great

---

[*] Liston, Practical Surgery, 3rd. ed. The following woodcut is taken from Mr. Liston's work.

tumefaction and ecchymosis; with subsequent weakness and stiffness. If the part is not kept at rest, or if the knee or some other large joint is affected, there will be great pain, inflammation, and fever, that may lead to serious or even fatal results.

*Treatment.*—The most essential measure is perfect rest; and to ensure this, if the case is at all serious, the part must be confined by a paste-board splint. Warm fomentations generally give more relief than cold lotions. If inflammation run high, or a large joint is affected, leeches, or bleeding, and general antiphlogistic measures, must be adopted. Subsequently the indications are to procure absorption of thickening and extravasation by friction with stimulating liniments, moderate exercise, and bandages, especially the caoutchouc or flannel bandage. If the case is severe, it may be expedient to apply a succession of blisters, or the other remedies directed for chronic inflammation of joints.

V. Acute Inflammation of Fasciæ, and Whitlow.—Acute inflammation of fascia is generally caused by punctured wounds:—especially by puncture of the fascia of the biceps during venesection;—and by punctures of the fingers, inflammation of the tendinous sheaths of which is called *the-cal abscess; paronychia gravis,* or *tendinous whitlow.* It is attended with severe, tensive, throbbing pain; exquisite tenderness; slight, but tense and resisting swelling; and very great constitutional disturbance. It may lead to suppuration;—the matter extending itself along muscles and tendons—from the fingers to the fore-arm—causing sloughing of the tendons—severe irritative fever—life often obliged to be saved by amputation—or the limb if preserved stiff and useless.

*Treatment.*—If the pain and tension increase, notwithstanding the employment of leeches, fomentations, and purgatives, *free incisions* must be made through the inflamed parts; in order to give vent to matter, if it have formed—or by creating a free discharge of blood, to prevent its formation. If the finger be the part affected, it should be freely laid open with a scalpel. If matter have extended into the palm, the incision should be continued along the metacarpal bone till it freely gushes out. It is better not to cut into the spaces *between* the metacarpal bones, (unless matter points there very decidedly indeed) for fear of wounding the digital artery. If it be necessary to slit up the palmar fascia, a cut should be made over the head of a metacarpal bone, in order that a director may be passed under it.

Whitlow.—There are three varieties of whitlow or paronychia. 1st, the fascial which we have just described. 2ndly, the *cutaneous; i. e.* inflammation of the skin of the last phalanx; with burning pain, and effusion of a serous or bloody fluid under the cuticle. 3rdly, the *subcutaneous;* with greater pain and throbbing, and suppuration *under* the skin.

*Treatment.*—Search should be made for thorns or other foreign particles sticking in the skin; and leeches, purgatives, fomentation in very hot water;—pressure, so as to stop the arterial pulsation in the inflamed part, or the application of arg. nitras, may be tried in order to cause resolution. But in general the complaint may be cut short much more easily by an incision;—which should be rather long, otherwise it may be closed by fungous granulations; and the matter may burrow and do fresh mischief. Tonics and alteratives (as recommended for boils) are mostly of service.*

VI. Subacute Inflammation of Fascia.—Subacute inflammation sometimes affects the fasciæ of the fore-arm, hand, and neck; producing pain and tenderness, with spasm of the subjacent muscles. *Treatment.*— Leeches, fomentations, blisters, mercurial camphorated liniments, F. 25; vapour bath; very small doses of colchicum and Dover's powder at bed-time, with a purge in the morning; or blue pill administered so as to cause incipient ptyalism.

VII. Tumours on Tendon and Ligament.—Small tumours about the size of a pea are apt to form on the tendons or fascia. Sometimes they follow a strain; and they have been knewn to occur on the palmar fascia after a good day's work at the oar; but they often arise without any assignable cause. If indolent, as they often are, they may be left to themselves, and they will probably disappear. If painful, leeches, blisters, and frictions with mercurial ointment or liniment, are the proper remedies.

VIII. Chalkstone Tumours are composed of the lithate (or urate) of soda; a white insoluble substance, which in gouty subjects is frequently deposited in the texture of the bones, joints, and cellular tissue;—but most frequently into the cellular tissue that environs the tendons of the feet or hands. The tumours which this substance forms are not always inorganie, but may be permeated by exquisitely sensible threads of cellular membrane. After remaining indolent for a variable time, they inflame the superjacent skin, and cause the formation of ulcers that are extremely obstinate, and discharge vast quantities of the concretion. They must be treated with simple dressings. It is rarely expedient to meddle with these tumours with the knife; but if any one be very inconveniently situated, and be perfectly indolent, it may be extirpated. The wound must be expected to heal very slowly.

IX. Ganglion and Tumours of Bursæ.—The simplest affection of bursæ and of the synovial sheaths of tendons, is excessive secretion of synovia, and consequent tumefaction, to which the name of ganglion is given. A recently-formed ganglion is an indolent fluctuating tumour, transparent enough to permit the light of a candle to be seen through it. It contains a clear synovia; but tumours of those bursæ which may be formed by friction such as the bursa that forms the swelling of bunion, do not con-

* Vide James, op. cit., and a paper in the Edin. Med. and Sur. Journ. 1828.

tain synovia, but a viscid, semi-fluid substance, like the crystalline lens. The ordinary situation of ganglion is, of course, that of the various bursæ;—on the patella, or olecranon; or on the inner side of the head of the tibia; or the angle of the scapula; but most frequently about the wrist and fingers. When the general sheath of the flexor tendons at the wrist is affected in this way, it forms a remarkable tumour, which projects in the palm of the hand, and also above the wrist, but is bound down in the middle by the anterior annular ligament of the carpus. When ganglion has lasted sometime, or has been subjected to inflammation, the synovial membrane becomes thickened, the contained fluid turbid and mixed with flakes of lymph, and the tumour loses its softness and transparency. The ordinary cause of ganglion is a twist or strain of some kind, or irritation from pressure or friction.

*Treatment.*—The best plan of treating recent non-inflamed ganglion seems to be, to puncture it with a cataract-needle, or fine-grooved needle, so as to empty the sac, and form an aperture by which its contents may henceforth pass into the cellular tissue and be absorbed. As soon as the sac is emptied, constant pressure should be applied by means of compress and bandage, which may be wetted with cold lotion if agreeable. The punctures must be repeated when necessary. 2. If this plan fails, recourse may be had to friction with mercurial and other stimulating liniments; or Scott's ointment, F. 25, or blisters, with the view of exciting absorption. 3. In obstinate cases it is a good plan to dissect out the cyst of the ganglion—provided that it is formed of a mere bursa, (as over the patella or olecranon,) and has no connexion with the sheaths of tendons. 4. But if the bursa is large or deeply seated, as over the angle of the scapula, it should be punctured with a lancet, when it may probably inflame and suppurate, and heal up like an abscess. 5. In obstinate cases, especially if the cyst is much thickened, Mr. Key recommends a puncture to be made, and a few threads of silk to be passed through the sac as a seton. This will create great suppuration and constitutional disturbance for a time, but it will destroy the secreting power of the sac, and effect a radical cure. The less, however, that the sheaths of the *flexors* of the wrist are meddled with, whether by puncture or seton, the better. Mr. Wickham strongly recommends the vapour bath, or local steam bath, (vide p. 59,) as a means of getting rid of thickness and stiffness after these operations. Lastly, any rheumatic or gouty tendency should be corrected by proper medicines.

X. Acute Inflammation of the Bursæ is most frequently exemplified in the affection called the *housemaid's knee,*—which is an acute inflammation of the bursa, that intervenes between the patella and skin,—common enough in that class of females, from kneeling on hard damp stones. It causes very great pain, swelling, and fever; it may be distinguished from acute inflammation of the synovial membrane of the knee-joint, by observing that the swelling is very superficial, and in front of the patella, which is obscured by it; whereas, in inflammation of the synovial membrane of the knee, the patella is thrown forwards, and the swelling is most prominent at the sides. *Treatment.*—Rest, leeches, fomentations, and purgatives; by which if the pain and swelling are not relieved, it must be punctured, and treated as an acute abscess.

XI. Loose Cartilages are sometimes formed in the synovial sheaths of the foot and hand. Their origin, symptoms, and treatment are the same as when they are found in joints.

XII. Bunion. A bunion signifies a painful swelling of the inner side of the ball of the great toe. It consists of a bursa developed between the skin and the projecting bone, and of a thickened state of the ligaments of the metatarsal joint of the great toe, which is always distorted, and thrown outwards, instead of being in a line with its metatarsal bone, as it ought to be. It seems to be produced, partly by the use of tight boots, which cramp the toes together, and force the great toe outwards, in order to make the foot fashionably pointed;—and it is partly a consequence, as Mr. Key has shown, of a weak, flattened state of the foot, which throws the extremity of that metatarsal bone forward, and the toe outwards. The ligaments of the joint are thus stretched and thickened, the joint is rendered unnaturally prominent, and subjected to pressure and friction, a bursa forms over it, and there is a constant state of tenderness and pain, subject to fits of inflammation. *Treatment.*—The patient must wear proper shoes, so arranged as not to press on the tender part. Mr. Key recommends the great toe to be kept in its proper place by means of a partition in the stocking like the finger of a glove, and a partition of strong cow's leather fixed in the sole of the shoe. A mercurial plaster on soft leather often gives great comfort. If the bursa inflame, it must be treated by rest, leeches, and poultices, in order to avoid suppuration and the necessity of a puncture, which is sure to lead to an inveterate fistula; for which Mr. Key says that a weak solution of creosote is the best application.

* Vide Key on Bunion, Guy's Hosp. Rep. vol. i.; Wickham, Cyclopædia Pract. Surgery, *Art.* Bursæ.

# CHAPTER IV.

## OF THE DISEASES AND INJURIES OF THE LYMPHATICS.

ACUTE INFLAMMATION of lymphatic *glands* has already been exempli-fied when speaking of bubo. The inflamed gland enlarges rapidly, and forms a hard, tense swelling, with great pain and fever. If it suppurate, the matter is formed in the cellular tissue around it, or between it and the skin, and the case proceeds as an acute abscess. This affection may be caused, (1.) By constitutional disorder, like acute abscesses. (2.) By local violence, such as blows or kicks. (3.) By the irritation or absorp-tion of acrid matter from ulcers, venereal or otherwise. (4.) By simple injuries, a clean prick, for instance, in persons whose health is deranged. (5.) By punctures inoculated with some irritant fluid, perhaps from a putrid body.

When the disease arises from ulcers or punctures, the inflammation generally begins in the absorbent vessels leading to the glands, which appear as red lines under the skin, and feel hard, cordy, and tender.

Inflammation of the lymphatics, when a consequence of dissection wounds, may be distinguished from the typhoid malady arising from the same cause, (Part iii. Chap. ix.) by the simple inflammatory character of the constitutional symptoms. It begins with swelling and festering of the original wound, from which red lines extend up the arm. In trivial cases, these may stop at, or may not even reach the elbow; and there may be very little or no febrile disturbance. But, in severe cases, the glands in the axilla swell and become exquisitely painful;—there is great fever; the pulse is rapid, full, and hard;—matter is formed; and if it be confined by fasciæ, and not evacuated by art, the nervous system may sink under the excruciating pain, and the patient may die. If the matter is discharged, he recovers his health without much diffi-culty. A comparison of these symptoms with those of the other affec-tion will readily show their intrinsic difference,—although, as was before said, it is very possible that both may be combined.

*Treatment.*—Acute inflammation of the lymphatics arising from local injury, from constitutional causes, or from the irritation of ordinary ulcers, must be treated by leeches, fomentations, purgatives, and the other local and general antiphlogistic measures, that require no comment. If it be produced by slight injuries, whether in dissection or otherwise, the original wound should be dilated, and then be assiduously fomented;

lunar caustic should be applied to the skin over the inflamed lymphatic vessels, and the bowels should be cleared. If the axillary glands are affected, and the pulse is full and hard, venesection should be performed, and even repeated according to its influence on the pain and on the pulse;—calomel should be frequently administered, and the swelled parts should be covered with leeches and fomentations. Incisions should be made early wherever matter is suspected to exist, or is likely to be formed—and when fever abates, the patient's health should be recruited by tonics and change of air, and care must be taken to prevent the formation of sinuses.

CHRONIC GLANDULAR TUMOURS may arise from simple chronic inflammation—from sarcomatous transformation—from deposite of scrofulous tubercle, and from scirrhus or other malignant disease:

(1.) *Chronic inflammation* causes a tender swelling, with aching pain, and slight redness of the skin. It may be caused by any slight irritation in the course of the lymphatics, but is more frequently constitutional. *Treatment.*—Repeated leechings, cold lotions, and aperients, followed by alteratives and tonics.

(2.) *Glandular sarcoma* consists in the transformation of one or more glands (especially in the neck) into sarcomatous tumours, whose characters and treatment have been before described, (page 217.) These are to be distinguished from scrofulous tumours by the circumstance, that one or two glands only are enlarged, and that they grow slowly but steadily;—whereas in scrofula a whole cluster is enlarged, and they are subject to fits of swelling and subsidence, from constitutional changes or atmospheric vicissitudes. From scirrhus and fungus medullaris they may be distinguished by attention to the diagnostic signs of those maladies.

# CHAPTER V.

## OF THE DISEASES AND INJURIES OF BONE.

### SECTION I.—OF THE DISEASES.

I. SIMPLE EXOSTOSIS signifies a tumour formed by the hypertrophy or irregular growth of bone. These tumours are hard, indolent, and irregular, and mostly situated on the upper part of the humerus, or on the lower part of the femur, near the insertion of the adductor magnus. Their *shape* is sometimes broad and flat; sometimes rounded and prominent, with a narrow neck. Their *structure* is that of ordinary bone, either dense like the cortical substance, or porous like the cancelli. They cause no pain, unless they happen to press on nerves or arteries; but when growing from the internal surface of the cranium or orbit, they of course give rise to the most serious evils. Their *cause* is generally un-known; sometimes, however, they can be traced to pressure or a blow. They sometimes appear during growth, and spontaneously disappear.

*Treatment.*—In the first place, an attempt may be made to procure absorption of the tumour by means of blisters, friction with ointment of mercury or iodine, and mercurial plasters. F. 25. Sometimes (espe-cially if the complaint follow a blow) a moderate course of mercury, so as barely to affect the mouth, will be effectual. If these measures do not succeed, the tumour must be removed by operation. If it is globular, with a narrow neck, it may be cut down upon, and be sawn or chiselled off. But supposing that its base is broad, so that this cannot be done, its periosteum may be shaved off; after which it will probably perish by necrosis, or else waste away. Inflammation must be guarded against after these operations; for it may possibly affect the whole bone, and the joints at either extremity, and lead to very disagreeable consequences.

II. Rickets is a disease of scrofulous children, consisting in a general feebleness of the body, with atrophy of the bones.* Their cortex is thin, and their internal structure very spongy: the cells large, and filled with gelatinous fluid;—sometimes the bones are as soft as cartilage. Of course they are unable to support the weight of the body, without bend-ing and producing deformity. In moderate cases, the ankles only may be a little sunk, or the shins bent, or the spine curved; but in aggravated cases the physiognomy and general appearance are very peculiar. The stature is short; the head large, with a very protuberant forehead; the face peculiarly triangular, with a very sharp-peaked chin, and projecting teeth; the chest narrow and prominent in front, whence the vulgar term *pigeon-breasted;*—the spine variously curved; the pelvis distorted in such a manner that the three points of support, viz. the promontory of the sacrum, and the two acetabula, are pressed together, rendering the cavity perilously small for childbearing, and the limbs are crooked, their natural curves being increased. But after puberty it is astonishing how firm the bones become, and, in particular, how they are strengthened by strong ridges developed on their concave sides.

*Treatment.*—The health must be invigorated by the measures pre-

---

* Atrophy of bone may be *concentric* or *excentric.* In the former it is shrunk in size; in the latter, it is feeble in tissue, and lighter in weight, but may preserve its original size. Atrophy, again, may be general, as in rickets and mollities ossium; or partial, when it depends on some local cause, as from want of exercise, deficient nervous influence, or insufficient supply of arterial blood, or sometimes after inflam-mation.—Vide T. B. Curling on Atrophy of Bone, Med. Chir. Trans., vol. xx.

scribed for scrofula.  The child should not be permitted to stand or walk, if its legs are weak, but should be made to crawl on the carpet, and be carried about in the air; or at all events, when not using exercise, it should recline on a sofa.  Mechanical supports, stays, irons, &c., are of use when the debility is partial, care being taken that they do not press injuriously on one part whilst supporting another.

III. MOLLITIES OSSIUM (*Malacosteon*) is a disease of adult age.  In some cases the bones are reduced to a mere shell, thin as a wafer, and filled with fat, in others they are soft, reddish, and spongy.  This malady is incurable.  It is mostly connected with some palpable disorder; such as fetid sweats, enormous deposites in the urine, or cancer, of which it is a very frequent attendant.*

IV. ACUTE INFLAMMATION of bone most frequently attacks the femur or tibia in children, and is usually attributed to cold.  It frequently affects more than one bone, but does not often involve the articular extremities.

*Symptoms.*—The patient is seized with violent shivering and fever, and with deep-seated severe pain, and great swelling of the affected limb, the skin of which displays a kind of erysipelatous redness.  Matter soon forms, burrows amongst the muscles, and at last points in several places.  Sometimes the patient is destroyed by the violence of the constitutional derangement, or sinks under the profuse suppuration that follows; but more frequently life is preserved, and the bone left in a state of *necrosis*.  On examination of cases that have proved fatal, or that have been subjected to amputation, the shaft of the bone is generally found separated from the epiphyses, and partially or entirely separated from its periosteum; and patches of newly-formed bone are deposited upon its surface, and between the layers of the periosteum.

*Treatment.*—Aperient and febrifuge medicines, with leeches and cold lotions, should be assiduously employed at first.  As soon as flunctuation can be detected anywhere, an opening should be made; and it is better to do so too soon than too late.  When a free exit is provided for the matter, a bandage should be applied to prevent its accumulation.  If the patient seem likely to sink, in spite of tonics and nutriment, from the extreme discharge, the affected limb must be amputated.

V. CHRONIC INFLAMMATION of bone is most frequently the result of some constitutional disorder, and generally attacks several bones simultaneously.  It is denoted by slow enlargement, tenderness, weight, and pain.  If caused by injury, it may lead to necrosis; but in general it produces no organic change, save irregular enlargement.

*Treatment.*—The general health should be improved by change of air, alteratives, and tonics, especially Plummer's pill, or hyd. c. crcta, in

---

* Such bones contain very little earthy matter, and their animal matter is so perverted that it yields no gelatine, which it need scarcely be said is the chief animal constituent of healthy bone.

small doses every night, and the iodide of potassium, with sarsaparilla. F. 56, 57. The local measures are repeated leechings and fomentations as long as there is tenderness or much pain; with Scott's ointment F. 25, or blisters subsequently.

VI. INFLAMMATION OF THE PERIOSTEUM generally occurs on the subcutaneous aspect of thinly-covered bones; especially the tibia, ulna, clavicles and os frontis. It produces oval swellings, called *nodes*, through an infiltration of lymph and serum into the periosteum, or between it and the bone. If acute or mismanaged, it may lead to suppuration, and caries or exfoliation of the bone; but more frequently it causes merely a superficial deposite of rough bone. It may sometimes be caused by mechanical injury, or exposure to cold; but far more frequently it is a consequence of disorder of the health, especially of a venereal taint, or the too free use of mercury.

*Treatment.*—For the acute, leeches, fomentations, purgatives, diaphoretics, and colchicum in doses of ♏ xx. of the wine every six hours; or gr. ii. of the iodide of potassium at the same interval. Calomel may be given in doses of gr. ii., with half a grain of opium every night, if the constitution has not been injured by any previous profuse administration of it. For the chronic, the same treatment as for chronic inflammation of bone. The severe nightly pain is, after the application of leeches, best relieved by renewed blisters. An incision is sometimes necessary if matter form between the periosteum and bone, and no measures succeed in producing its absorption and allaying the pain; but it very often happens, especially in venereal cases, that mercury, (if not previously administered to excess,) or the iodide of potassium, sarsaparilla, and blisters, will accomplish those objects.

VII. ABSCESS is a rare consequence of inflammation of bone. A cavity lined with a vascular membrane, and filled with pus, is formed in the substance of the bone, generally the tibia, which may or may not be unusually dense around it. Abscess may be suspected when, in addition to permanent inflammatory enlargement and tenderness, (which may have lasted for years,) there is a fixed pain at one particular spot, aggravated at night, and unrelieved by any remedy.

*Treatment.*—When there is good reason to suspect the existence of abscess, the bone must be laid bare by a crucial incision, and an opening be made with a trephine at the precise seat of pain; it may, if necessary, be deepened with a chisel. After the pus is evacuated, the wound must be left to granulate and cicatrize.

VIII. NECROSIS.—This term, although signifying the death or mortification of bone generically, is yet usually restricted to one form,—in which part of the shaft of a cylindrical bone dies; and is enclosed in a case of new bone. The term *exfoliation* signifies necrosis of a thin superficial layer, which is not encased in any shell of new bone.

1. Necrosis is a frequent consequence of inflammation of the shafts of long bones in children, especially of the femur and tibia.

*Pathology.*—The bone dies;—its periosteum and the surrounding cellular tissue become infiltrated with lymph, which speedily ossifies, forming a new shell around the dead portion, and adhering to the living bone above and below it. The dead portion, (technically called the *sequestrum,*) generally consists of the circumference of the shaft only, and not of the entire thickness; for the interior of the shaft seems to be atrophied and absorbed after the death of the exterior. The inside of the sequestrum is usually rough, as if worm-eaten. In the majority of cases the *epiphyses,* or articular extremities, are fortunately unaffected. After a time, if the *sequestrum* is removed by art or accident, the newly-formed shell contracts, its cavity is abolished, and it gradually assumes the shape and function of the former bone.

*Symptoms.*—After acute inflammation, the bone remains permanently swelled; and the apertures, which were made for the discharge of matter, remain as sinuses, from which many sensitive, irritable granulations shoot. These sinuous apertures in the skin correspond to holes in the shell of new bone, (technically called *cloacæ;*)—and if a probe be passed into them, the *sequestrum* may be felt loose in the interior; or at least the probe will strike against dead bone.

*Treatment.*—The indication is to remove the *sequestrum.* Any hope of its being absorbed or extruded by any natural process, is quite nugatory; and to permit it to remain, is but to condemn the patient to a perpetuance of disease and deformity. As soon, therefore, as the shell of new bone is sufficiently strong, a free incision should be made so as to expose its surface, and it should be made at a part where *cloacæ* exist, or where the bone is nearest the surface. Then the new shell must be perforated with the trephine, or with Hey's saw, or with a pair of strong bone forceps;*—and the sequestrum must be drawn out. If it cannot be extracted entire, it should be divided with strong forceps. If the sequestrum be small, or the cloacæ large, the former may perhaps be extracted without any operation; and one way of enlarging the cloacæ is to dilate the sinuses in the skin, and keep them open with tents of lint. Necrosis of the articular extremities, or of the tarsus or carpus, involves the joints, and requires amputation.

2. Exfoliation signifies the mortification and separation of a superficial layer of bone, without the formation of a shell of new bone, as in necrosis. It is generally caused by some mechanical or chemical injury, or by stripping off the periosteum. Not, however, that stripping off the periosteum is invariably followed by exfoliation; for the bone may remain red and m$_{oist}$, and throw out granulations; whereas, if it be about to exfoliate, it becomes white and dry.

* The chloride of zinc has also been used to make a hole in the new shell.—Vide p. 222.

*Treatment.*—A lotion of weak nitric acid may be useful; and the exfoliating portion should be removed as soon as it can be detached.

IX. CARIES is an unhealthy inflammation of bone, essentially producing *softening*, and probably leading to ulceration and suppuration.

*Pathology.*—The bone is soft and red; its cells are filled with a red serous or thick glairy fluid;—and in scrofulous cases there is also a deposite of more or less tubercular matter. The bone, when macerated and dried, looks soft and spongy; eaten into hollows, and thrown into irregular elevations, at the site of granulations.

*Symptoms.*—"The external character of the limb," says Mr. Mayo, " is the same in necrosis and caries. The bone appears enlarged, and one or more sinuses open from it at points that are soft, and red, and sunken." If a probe is passed into these, it will readily break down the softened texture of the carious bone which yields a gritty feel.

*Causes.*—Caries most frequently attacks bones of a soft, spongy texture; such as the vertebræ, the round and flat bones, and the articular extremities of long bones. Its genuine cause is some constitutional disorder; scrofula, syphilis, or mercury.

*Treatment.*—The indications are two-fold;—to rectify constitutional disorder, and to remove the local disease. The former object must be accomplished by change of air, tonics and alteratives, and the measures that have been directed for scrofula and syphilis, supposing the caries to be connected with those maladies.

If it can be done, the best local remedy consists in freely exposing and removing the whole of the diseased portion of the bone by the chisel or trephine. If this cannot be done, lotions of the dilute nitric or phosphoric acids may be tried. Caries of the articular extremities or bones will be considered together with diseases of the joints.

### TUMOURS OF BONE.

Of the various tumours of bone, some depend on an hypertrophy of its normal structure, or on the enlargements incident upon inflammation and its consequences. These have been sufficiently described in the preceding paragraphs. Others, which depend upon the development of advantitious tissues in or upon bone, remain yet to be noticed; and they are of two orders: the non-malignant and the malignant; the former of which we shall treat of first.

1. *Tumours from extravasated blood.*—Mr. Travers* describes a case in which, after a blow, the clavicle enlarged into a firm oval elastic tumour; which, when punctured by a grooved needle, yielded a few drops of dark grumous blood. The whole bone was extirpated. On axamination, it was proved that the tumour had evidently originated in a rup-

* Med. Chir. Trans., vol. xxi.

ture of the vessels of the bone, and an extravasation of blood into the cancelli. By the pressure of this blood, and a continuance of the extravasation, the bony tissue was expanded and absorbed; and the cancelli were converted into chambers filled with dark solid coagula. The tumour was invested by the periosteum.

2. *Osteo-aneurism.* This consists in that disease of the capillaries of the bone, which is' called *aneurism by anastomosis,* as will be described in the chapter on the arteries. The bone affected is generally the tibia just below the knee. The patient complains of a sudden pain in the part. This is followed by a painful swelling, and all the veins of the leg are observed to be very tense and full. After a time, the whole limb becomes dark red, and painful; and the tumour becomes distinctly pulsatory. On examination, it is found to be composed of a tissue filled with clots of blood in concentric layers, and each clot communicating with a dilated artery; the bone of course expanded, thinned and absorbed, as in the last case. This disease is rare. Ligature of the main arterial trunk of the limb, or amputation, are the remedies.

3. *Cartilaginous exostosis, enchondroma,* (Müller.) This growth is described by Müller as a firm spheroidal tumour consisting of masses of true cartilage embedded in a fibro-membranous cellular structure. When boiled, it yields a variety of gelatine, termed *chrondrine.* It may be developed in the centre of a bone, or on its surface. In the former case, it causes the bone to expand and be absorbed before it, till at last it is covered by a mere shell. This tumour ordinarily affects only one bone; and is occasionally found in the glands, especially the parotid. It is not malignant; for although incurable, and although by its continued growth it may distend the skin, and cause ulceration, and wear out the constitution by the irritation and discharge, still it does not return it thoroughly extirpated.

4. *A hard fibrous or fibro-cartilaginous* tumour, containing bony spiculæ, may be developed in the substance, or on the surface of bone, especially of the superior or inferior maxillary.

5. *Hydatids* are occasionally developed in bone.

MALIGNANT TUMOURS.

6. *Osteo-sarcoma* is described as a form of cartilaginous growth, containing numerous cysts filled with a reddish fluid, and having a kind of skeleton composed of thin papery plates and spiculæ of bone, dispersed arborescently like coral through it. This is malignant, because, after amputation of the tibia for this disease, it has appeared on the stump of the femur.

7. *Medullary sarcoma* is perhaps the most frequent malignant disease

of bone. Its characters have been already described. " It generally,"
says Mr. Mayo, " arises in the cancellous structure; it is therefore usually
attended with considerable pain, for the growth of the tumour is rapid,
and the shell of the bone has to be partly absorbed, partly mechanically
forced open from within."

8. *Scirrhus* in bone is generally a concomitant of the disease in the
breast, or in some other part. The femur is the bone most frequently
affected, and is often fractured in consequence of the scirrhous deposite and
atrophy of its proper texture. (Vide p. 124.)

The chief points which distinguish the malignant from the non-malignant tumours, are, their greater rapidity of growth; the greater pain with
which they are accompanied, their greater softness at some points than
at others; their tendency to involve and become blended with the skin and
other adjacent tissues, (a sure characteristic of malignant growth,) and the
existence of the malignant cachexia.—(Vide p. 123.)—But as it is often
impossible to distinguish these two classes of tumours from each other, or
from inflammatory enlargements, it is satisfactory to know that the early
treatment of them all is the same. The same measures that will cure the
curable affections, will check the incurable. They are, repeated leeching,
mild mercurial alteratives, sarsaparilla with small doses of the iodide of
potassium, and change of air and other general tonics. If these measures
fail, the only recourse is amputation or extirpation; which may be performed with confidence of a cure as regards the non-malignant growths.
But the extirpation of truly malignant growths, to be effectual, should be
very early, and very complete, a partial removal being to use Mr. Liston's
words, an " unmeaning and utterly useless cruelty."*

### SECTION II.—OF FRACTURE GENERALLY.

The term *fracture*, with its varieties simple and compound, transverse,
oblique, and comminuted, requires no definition.

EXCITING CAUSES.—The exciting causes of fracture are two: mechanical violence, and muscular action. Mechanical violence may be *direct*
or *indirect*. It is said to be *direct*, when it produces a fracture at the part
to which it is actually applied; as in the instance of fracture of the skull
from a violent blow. It is said to be *indirect* when a force is applied to
two parts of a bone, which gives way between. This is exemplified in
the case of fracture of the clavicle from a fall on the shoulder. The
sternal end of the bone is impelled by the weight of the body, and the

* Vide Sir A. Cooper on Exostosis, in Cooper and Traver's Surgical Essays;
Brodie on Abscess in Bone, Med. Chir. Trans., vol. xvii.; Müller on Tumours, by
West; Breschet sur des Tumeurs Sanguines; and Liston on Tumours of Mouth and
Jaws, Med. Chir. Trans., vol. xx.

acromial end by the object it falls against; and the bone, acted upon by these two forces, gives way in the middle.

The bones most commonly fractured by muscular action, are the patella and olecranon; but the humerus, femur, or any other bone, may give way from this cause, if preternaturally weak.

PREDISPOSING CAUSES. There are certain circumstances which render the bones more liable than usual to be broken. These are (1.) *old age*, which renders the bones soft and brittle; the earthy matter being deficient in quantity, and the animal matter having lost its elasticity. (2.) *Disuse*, as in bed-ridden people. (3.) Certain diseases, as *mollities ossium* (p. 233) and *cancer* (p. 124.) (4.) *Original conformation*; the bones of some people being exceedingly brittle, without any assignable cause.

REPARATION.—The reparation of fractures is produced by the effusion and organization of lymph. But this process varies considerably as it occurs in different bones.

1. After fracture of ordinary bones, a quantity of lymph is effused into the cellular tissue around the broken part. This, in two or three weeks, becomes converted into a cartilaginous capsule, called a *provisional callus*, which completely surrounds the fracture, and adheres firmly to the bone above and below it. In two or three weeks more, the provisional callus ossifies;—and then the use of the bone is restored. But at this time the ends of the fractured bones are not *directly* united; and if the provisional callus were removed, they would still be separable;—in the course of five or six months, however, ossific matter is gradually deposited between them, and the provisional callus is absorbed.

2. But after fracture of the *cranium, olecranon, patella, cervix femoris*, or any bone invested with synovial membrane, no provisional callus is formed. If the broken parts are kept in the very strictest apposition, bony union will certainly occur in two or three months. But if a portion of the skull be removed;—or if after fracture of it, or of the other bones in the same category, the divided parts be not kept in the closest apposition, the lymph effused will be converted into ligament, which very slowly ossifies.

There has been much dispute as to the source of the lymph which ossifies and forms the *callus*, or new bone by which fractures are united. Some persons have asserted that it is effused by the bone or its medullary membrane, others by the periosteum, and others by the cellular or other tissues around. The fact is, that all three of them are capable of secreting a lymph which will ossify. But when it proceeds from the bone alone, as after fracture of the skull, reparation is very slow. Whereas, when a provisional callus is formed. all the tissues indiscriminately around the fracture seem to participate in the effusion of the lymph, and the union is rapid. Morever, if any ordinary bone, a rib, or the clavicle for instance, (which if fractured would unite by a provisional callus) be extirpated, the lymph which is effused by the surrounding tissues will most probably form a new bone.*

SYMPTOMS.—The essential symptoms of fracture are three. (1) *Deformity*, such as bending or shortening, or twisting of the injured limb. (2) *Preternatural mobility*,—one end of the bone moving independently of the other, or one part of it yielding when pressed upon. (3) *Crepitus*,—a grating heard and felt when the broken ends are rubbed against each other. But it must be recollected that if the broken parts are displaced, they must be drawn into their natural position, otherwise no crepitus will be detected. In addition to these symptoms, there will be more or less pain, swelling and helplessness of the injured part.

It is important in every case to know the causes which produce displacement and deformity after fracture, because it is necessary to counteract them carefully during the treatment. They are three. (1) *Muscular action;* which produces various degrees of bending, shortening, or twisting in different cases. (2) The weight of the parts below, which, for instance, causes the shoulder to sink downwards, when the clavicle is broken. (3) The original violence which caused the fracture, as when the ossa nasi are driven in.

TREATMENT. The general indications for the treatment of fracture, are *first*, to procure union, which is accomplished by keeping the parts at rest, and in apposition; and, secondly, to prevent deformity. For the latter purpose, certain appliances must be used, which will counteract the various causes of displacement that were enumerated in the preceding paragraph. Displacement from muscular contraction must be obviated by keeping the part (if possible) in such a position that any offending muscle may be relaxed; and by using mechanical means of extension and support.

The *general* method of treating fractures may be thus described. In the *first* place, the limb must, if possible, be put in a position that will relax the principal muscles that cause displacement. In fracture of the upper end of the radius, for instance, the elbow should be bent to relax the biceps; and in fracture of the olecranon it should be straight, so as to relax the triceps.

*Secondly*, the fracture must be *reduced* or *set*: that is to say, the broken parts must be adjusted in their natural positions. For this purpose, the upper end of the limb must be held steadily, whilst the lower is *extended*, or drawn in such a direction as to restore the limb to its proper length and shape. The extension should be made firmly, but gradually and gently, otherwise it will aggravate the muscular spasm which it is intended to overcome.

---

* Vide a paper by the author, containing an account of some experiments on the restoration of bone, by Dr. Heine, Med. Gaz., July 29, 1837; Troja de novorum ossium regeneratione, Paris, 1775; Bransby Cooper, Guy's Hospital Rep. 1837.

*Thirdly*, it is usual to bandage the whole of the fractured limb from its extremity. This is done for the double purpose of preventing œdema, and of confining the muscles, that they may not contract and disturb the fracture. The many-tailed bandage is highly useful for fractures of the leg or thigh.

*Fourthly*, it is necessary to use some mechanical contrivances to keep the limb of its natural length and shape, and prevent any motion at the fractured part. It is usual to employ *splints* of wood, carved to the shape of the limb. The surgeon should measure the sound limb which corresponds to the injured one, and select splints that are long enough to rest against the condyles or other projecting points at its extremities. These must be *padded*, and pads are easily made of loose tow wrapped up in pieces of old linen. The splints, when ready, should be firmly bound to the limb with pieces of old bandage; leather straps and buckles are very inconvenient.

Several substitutes for wooden splints have been brought into use of late years. One of the most popular and convenient of these is the *gummel*, or *starched* bandage, or *appareil immobile*; on which a French-man has written a large book. It consists merely of layers of bandage, lint, or linen imbued with a mucilage of starch or gum or arrowroot; which, when dry, form a remarkably light, firm and unyielding support. Another contrivance of the same nature, invented by Mr. Alfred Smee, and called the *moulding tablet*, will often be found a very simple but efficacious auxiliary. It is composed of two layers of coarse old sheeting, stuck together with a mixture of gum arabic and whiting. It is easily prepared by rubbing very finely powdered whiting with mucilage of gum arabic till it acquires the consistence of thick paste, and then spreading this on the surface of the sheeting, which is to be doubled on itself; it dries without shrinking, and becomes remarkably hard and tough; and may readily be softened by spunging it with hot water, so that it may be adapted with the greatest accuracy.*

Some practitioners, instead of applying splints immediately, place the limb on a pillow, and merely apply leeches or cold lotion for the first few days, or perhaps for a week, and resort to splints after the inflammatory stage has passed over. But it appears to be far better, in every case, at once to use measures, by splints or otherwise, for keeping the fracture immoveable. "If" says Mr. Liston, "the limb is laid loosely on a pillow, in an easy position, as it is by some thought or said to be, and no efficient means are employed to prevent the spasmodic action of the muscles, the startings of the limb, the jerkings of the broken ends, the displacement of the fragments; then assuredly, in spite of all local and general measures, there will arise frightful swelling, pain, tension, and

* Lond. Med. Gaz. Feb. 1839.

heat; the intermuscular tissue will be gorged with blood, and the ciren-
lation of the limb roused to a dangerous and alarming degree."*

The remaining treatment of simple fracture must be conducted on
general principles. Cordials to restore the patient from the shock of the
injury; the catheter, if he cannot make water, which is common after
fractures of the leg; opiates to allay pain and muscular twitching;
aperients, if they can be given without disturbing the fracture; cold
lotion, if agreeable; and leeches or bleeding very rarely indeed, to allay
excessive inflammation, must be employed at the discretion of the prae-
titioner.

If, through any mismanagement a fracture has united crookedly, an attempt may be made to bend the callus, and restore the right shape. Such
a proceeding may easily be effected before the fourth week, and it has
been successful at the sixth month.†

SECTION III.—OF NON-UNION AND FALSE JOINT.

The cases in which bony union is not produced within the usual time,
may be divided into two orders. (1) Those in which the reparative
process is *very slowly or not at all set up.* (2) Those in which it is *set
up, but ·frustrated.*

1. The *causes* of non-union, or slow union, in the first order, are mostly constitutional. Old age, debility, gout, and cancer;—the supervention
of an acute disease, and pregnancy: which last seem to act by producing
a determination of blood to other parts.

2. *Secondly,* the restorative process will be frustrated if the fracture is
subjected to *motion* and *disturbance.* And the lymph which should have
constituted a callus is either converted into ligament, which unites the
broken extremities, or else a *false joint* is formed; the ends of the bone
being tipped with cartilage and synovial membrane, and surrounded with
a ligamentous capsule. (Vide p. 64.)

TREATMENT.—In recent cases, the first thing to be tried is the application of some apparatus which will ensure perfect rest, perfect apposition, and pressure of the broken ends against each other. Should this
not succeed after a fair trial of two months, means must be adopted to
excite the adhesive inflammation around the fracture. This may be done
by rubbing one end of the bone against the other;—or by making the
patient walk on the limb, which must be first well supported with splints;
and then the apparatus should be again firmly applied for six or eight
weeks.‡ If this also fail, the *ultima ratio* consists in converting the

* Practical Surgery, p. 65.
† Syme, Ed. Med. and Surg. Journ., Oct. 1838.
‡ Amesbury, Syllabus of Lectures on Fractures, &c., with plates of apparatus.

simple into a compound fracture; viz. by passing a seton between the broken ends—or by cutting down on them, and shaving or sawing them off, or applying caustic to them. All these measures require caution, as they will produce great constitutional disturbance and profuse suppuration;—the seton is that which is most convenient, and most commonly employed. An incision should be made on each side down to the bone, taking care to avoid the nerves and vessels; a seton of coarse thread should then be passed between the fractured ends, and should be allowed to remain eight or ten days, after which the part must be put up immoveably in splints. It sometimes happens that union will be expedited by permitting the broken ends to overlap each other a little. If the want of union can be attributed to any peculiarity of constitution, alteratives should be administered; thus a case is reported in which mercury given to ptyalism effected a cure after the seton had failed.*

A few instances are known in which the callus, after union was completed, inflamed and became absorbed, so that the fracture was disunited again. Leeches and blisters to the part proved effectual remedies.† A recent callus is also sometimes absorbed during fever; and it used to be common enough in the sea scurvy.

SECTION IV.—OF COMPOUND FRACTURE.

DEFINITION.—A simple fracture may be attended with a wound; but unless the wound communicates with the fracture, the latter is not compound.

CAUSES.—Fracture may be rendered compound. (1) By the same injury which broke the bone. (2) By the bone being thrust through the skin. (3) By subsequent ulceration or sloughing of the integuments.

DANGERS.—These are threefold. (1) The shock and collapse of the injury, which may prove fatal in a few hours, especially if much blood has been lost. (2) Inflammation, fever, and tetanus. (3) Hectic or typhoid fever, from excessive suppuration.

QUESTION OF AMPUTATION.—In order to decide upon the necessity of this operation, the extent of the injury and the restorative powers of the patient must be most carefully examined. If the bone is very much shattered and comminuted;—if the fracture extend into a joint, especially the knee;—if the soft parts are extensively torn or bruised;—if, in particular, the skin has been torn away, so that the wound cannot be closed; or if it be so injured that a large tract of it must slough;—if the patient is very old;—or much enfeebled, either by previous disease, or present loss of

---

* Guy's Hosp. Rep. No. 5.        † James, Address in Prov. Med. Trans. 1840.

blood;—if the collapse of the injury is excessive and permanent;—amputation is probably requisite.  Of course more may be hazarded with a
young patient; or with an old person of a spare, firm habit, who has always been healthy and temperate, than with one who is bloated and plethoric, and in the constant habit of enfeebling his vital powers by over-
stimulation and animal indulgence.

*Laceration of arteries* is a dangerous complication both of simple and
compound fracture.  It is detected by the great flow of blood, if there be
a wound; and if not, by a rapid, diffused, and dark-coloured tumefaction
of the limb, with coldness and want of arterial pulsation in the parts below.  If it be the *femoral*, amputation will most probably be required,
because the vein may have been injured also;—if any other, (the anterior or posterior tibial, for instance,) it may be secured;—provided that
there is no other valid cause for amputation, and that the required incision
will not too much aggravate the injury to the soft parts.  But, *cæteris pa-
ribus*, this accident is always an additional reason for amputation, if there
be other circumstances rendering it probably expedient. ·

If amputation be decided on, it must be performed before the accession of fever and inflammation, as was observed in the chapter on gunshot wounds, (page 147.)

TREATMENT.—If it be determined to save the limb, it must first be
placed in a proper position, and then the fracture must be reduced.  If
a sharp end of bone protrude, and it cannot easily be returned or kept in
its place, it should be sawn off.   Any loose fragments or splinters of
bone should be at once removed; and if necessary, the wound may be
dilated for this purpose.  If suffered to remain, they greatly aggravate
the inflammation and danger of tetanus, and may produce long-continued disease of the bone.  After reduction, the great object is to produce adhesion of the external wound, so as to convert the compound
fracture into a simple one, and the best application is a piece of lint dipped
in blood, or in warm water, and covered with oil silk;—then bandages
and splints are to be used; but, if possible, the splints should have apertures corresponding to the wound, so that it may be dressed without
disturbance to the whole limb.  When inflammation and swelling come
on, the bandages must be loosened, and cold be applied if agreeable.
Opium, with antimony and saline draughts;—laxatives or enemata, if
they can be given without disturbance;—and sometimes, though very
rarely, bleeding, are the general remedies.   The catheter should be
used if required.  The great object in the subsequent treatment is to
prevent the lodgment of matter by sponging and pressing it out carefully at
each dressing, and applying compresses to prevent its accumulation, and,
if required, by making openings for its discharge.   But if, notwithstanding the employment of tonics, wine, and good diet, the patient

seem likely to sink under the discharge and irritation, amputation is the last resource.

SECTION V.—OF PARTICULAR FRACTURES.

I. FRACTURES OF THE OSSA NASI, AND OF THE MALAR AND SUPERIOR MAXILLARY BONES, may be produced by violent blows or falls on the face, or by gunshot injuries.

*Treatment.*—Any displacement of the fractured portions should be rectified as soon as possible, by passing a strong probe or female catheter up the nostril, and by manipulation with the fingers. A depressed fragment may often be conveniently raised by passing one blade of a dressing forceps up the nostril, and applying the other externally, so as to grasp the fragment between them. Some practitioners are in the habit of introducing tubes or plugs of oiled lint, in order to keep the fragments in their places; but this appears to be unnecessary, and is very irritating. A plug of lint may, however, be requisite to check profuse hæmorrhage. If the fracture is compound, any loose splinters should be carefully removed. The great swelling, ecchymosis, bleeding from the nose, and headach, with which this injury is followed, will require to be combated by bleeding or leeches, purgatives, and cold lotions, and spoon diet; and if collections of matter form, they should be opened without delay. If there are symptoms of pressure on the brain, and the vomer seems depressed, it should be carefully drawn forwards.

II. FRACTURE OF THE LOWER JAW may be caused by violent blows. Its most usual situation is at the middle of the horizontal ramus. Sometimes in children (though rarely) it occurs at the symphysis, and still more rarely at the angle, or in the ascending ramus.

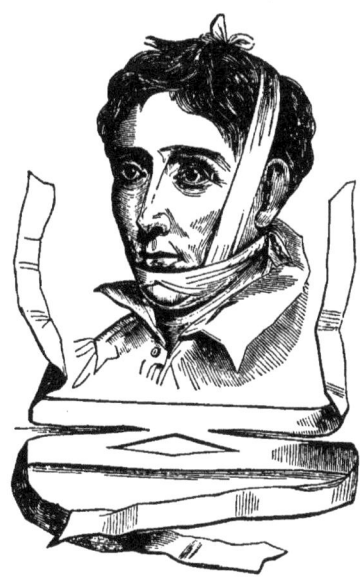

*Symptoms.*—It is known by pain, swelling, inability to move the jaw, and irregularity of the teeth, because the anterior fragment is generally drawn downwards. On removing the chin, whilst the hand is placed on the posterior fragment, crepitus will be felt; and the gums are lacerated and bleeding. The diagnosis of fracture of the *ascending ramus* will often be obscured by the great swelling. Great pain and difficulty of motion are the chief signs.

*Treatment,* 1st, *by the four-tailed bandage.*—A piece of pasteboard, softened in boiling water, should be accurately fitted to the jaw, and then a four-tailed bandage should be applied. This is made by taking a yard and a half of wide roller, and tearing each end longitudinally, so as to leave about eight inches in the middle, which should have a short slit in it. The chin is to be put into this slit, and then two of the tails are to be tied over the crown of the head, so as to fix the lower jaw against the upper, and the other two are to be fastened behind the head. The teeth on either side of the fracture may be fastened together with dentists' silk. It is occasionally useful to place a piece of cork, grooved above and below, between the molar teeth on each side, especially if any of the teeth at the fractured part are deficient. Sometimes a tooth falls down between the broken parts; a circumstance which should be looked to, if there is much difficulty in fitting them together.

2ndly, *By apparatus.*—If the above simple means do not suffice to keep the fractured parts in contact, Mr. Lonsdale's apparatus should be used;—and perhaps it would be well to adopt it in all cases, after the primary swelling and tenderness have subsided. It affords perfect support, and yet allows of free motion.* The patient for the first fortnight must be fed entirely with gruel, broth, arrowroot, &c. The cure generally occupies five or six weeks.

III. FRACTURE OF THE CLAVICLE is most frequently *situated* at the middle of the bone, and it is *caused* by falls on the arm or shoulder, more frequently than by direct violence.

*Symptoms.*—The patient complains of inability to lift the affected arm, and supports it at the elbow;—the shoulder sinks *downwards, forwards,* and *inwards;*—the distance from the acromion to the sternum is less than it is on the sound side;—and the end of the *sternal* fragment of the bone projects as though it were displaced, although it is not so in reality, but merely appears to be so, in consequence of the sinking of the shoulder and of the outer fragment.

*Treatment.*—The shoulder must be raised, and must be supported in a direction *upwards, backwards,* and *outwards.* The broken parts may

---

* Lonsdale on Fractures. Lond. 1838. It consists of a grooved plate of ivory to fit the teeth; and a wooden plate adapted to the base of the bone. These two plates are fastened together by screws.

be *reduced*, either by putting the knee between the scapulæ, and drawing the shoulders backwards; or by placing the elbow close to the trunk and a little forwards, and then pushing it upwards. To support the parts during the cure, the most common apparatus is,

(1.) The *stellate*, or *figure of* 8 *bandage*, depicted in the adjoining cut. In the first place a thick wedge-shaped pad must be put into the axilla, with the large end uppermost. Then a long roller must be passed over each shoulder alternately, and be made to cross on the back. In the next place, the arm must be confined to the side by two or three turns of the roller; and lastly the elbow (which should be brought more

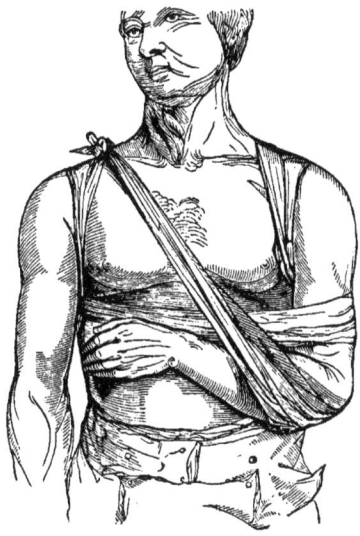

forward than is represented in the cut) should be well raised by a sling, which is also to support the fore-arm. It will be noticed, that the shoulder is kept *up* by the sling, *out* by the pad, and *back* by the bandage. In ordinary cases the patient may be allowed to walk about in a week or ten days, and the cure will be completed in a month or five weeks.

If, however, there is any difficulty in maintaining a proper position, the patient must be confined to bed; and some additional apparatus be employed. The simplest is a straight splint across the shoulders, to which the shoulders are to be bound by the figure of 8 bandage; or a splint shaped like a T, of which the horizontal part is bound to the shoulders; and the vertical part passes down the back, and is confined by a belt round the abdomen.

Besides these there is the *clavicle bandage*, which consists of two loops for the shoulders, attached to two pads resting on the scapulæ, which are drawn together by straps and buckles (it is little, if at all, better than the figure of 8 bandage)—and *Amesbury's apparatus*, which, although very complex, seems constructed in a manner that prevents all possibility of displacement. If nothing else will do, it should be procured at an instrument-maker's.

IV. FRACTURES OF THE SCAPULA.—The *body* of this bone may be broken across by great *direct* violence. The symptoms are, great pain in moving the shoulder, and *crepitus;* which may be detected by placing one hand on the acromion or spinous process, and moving the shoulder or the inferior angle with the other. *Treatment.*—A roller must be passed round the trunk, and a few turns be made round the humerus, so as to fix the arm to the side, and prevent all motion. Bleeding, or at all events purging and low diet, will be required to avert inflammation of the chest.

FRACTURE OF THE NECK OF THE SCAPULA may be caused by blows or falls on the shoulder, but it is a rare accident. The line of fracture is generally oblique, so that the articular surface and coracoid process are detached from the body of the bone.

*Symptoms.*—The shoulder appears sunk, and the arm lengthened; the acromion is unusually prominent, and the deltoid dragged down and flattened; the head of the humerus can be felt in the axilla; and on placing one hand or one ear on the acromion, and moving the shoulder, crepitus may be detected. Crepitus may also be felt on pressing the coracoid process,—which is situated deep below the clavicle, between the margins of the pectoral and deltoid muscles. The accidents with which this fracture is most likely to be confounded are fracture of the neck of the humerus, and dislocation of the shoulder joint; the symptoms of which should be carefully studied and compared. The existence of crepitus, and the fact that the surgeon can move the shoulder freely, (although with great pain,) are the chief points of diagnosis between this accident and dislocation.

*Treatment.*—The shoulder must be supported by the same sling, bandage, and pad, that are used for fracture of the clavicle; but a short sling from the axilla of the injured side, to the opposite shoulder, should be used in addition to the long sling from the elbow to the shoulder. Union may occur in seven weeks. Bleeding, leeches, purgatives, rest in bed, and warm fomentations, will be necessary for the contusion with which this fracture is accompanied.

FRACTURE OF THE ACROMION is known by a flattening of the shoulder, because the fractured portion is drawn down by the deltoid; and by an evident inequality felt in tracing the spine of the scapula. It may be distinguished from any dislocation, by noting that the humerus may be freely moved in any direction, and that, on slightly raising the shoulder, the fragment is restored to its place.

*Treatment.*—The same bandages, &c. are to be applied as for fracture of the clavicle; but great care must be taken to raise the elbow thoroughly, so that the head of the humerus may be lifted up against the acromion, and keep it in its place. Moreover, no pad must be placed in the axilla; otherwise the broken part will be pushed outwards too much. Union is generally ligamentous, owing to the difficulty of keeping the parts in strict apposition.

*Fracture of the Coracoid Process* is a rare accident, *caused* by sharp blows on the front of the shoulder.

*Symptoms.*—The patient is unable to execute the motions performed by the biceps and coracobrachialis, that is to bring, the arm upwards and forwards;—and motion or crepitus of the detached process may be felt by pressing with the finger between the pectoralis major and deltoid, whilst the patient coughs or moves his shoulder.

*Treatment.*—The humerus must be brought forwards and inwards, so as to relax the biceps and coracobrachialis, and must be confined to the trunk.

V. FRACTURE OF THE HUMERUS.—*Fracture of the shaft* will be known at a glance by the limb being bent, shortened, and helpless, and by the crepitus felt when it is handled.

*Treatment.*—The fracture may be reduced by drawing the elbow downwards, whilst the shoulder is steadied. Then the whole limb, from the hand upwards, is to be evenly bandaged. Next, a long padded splint should be placed on the inner side of the humerus, one end of it pressing against the axilla, the other against the inner condyle; three other splints are to be placed on the other sides of the limb, and are to be fastened by tapes;—lastly, the limb may be confined to the side for the sake of greater security, and the hand be supported by a sling; but the *elbow* must not be *raised up;* otherwise the fracture will be liable to be displaced.

*Fracture of the neck of the humerus* is caused by great direct violence, and is attended with much swelling. It may occur either at the *anatomical* neck;—and is, *above* the tubercles;—or, at the *surgical* neck, or just *below* them. The former form occurs sometimes to children, but the latter is by far more frequent.

*Symptoms.*—Pain and incapability of moving the arm. The shoulder seems flattened, but there is no hollow below the acromion, as there is in dislocation. The head of the bone may be felt in its socket, and the broken end of the shaft in the axilla. On grasping the former, the elbow may be moved independently of it, and crepitus may be felt.

*Treatment.*—The same splints, bandages, &c., are to be used as in the last case; and a pad to be placed in the axilla. The fore-arm should be *lightly* supported with a sling, but neither in this nor in the last case should the elbow be forcibly raised. The great secret in managing both is to get a good purchase against the axilla and the inner condyle with the innermost splint.

32

It is a good plan in fractures of the upper part of the humerus, as soon as pain and inflammation are abated and the patient is able to leave his bed, to apply a large piece of pasteboard, or of Mr. Smee's gummed sheeting, or of the soft leather sold for splints, all over the shoulder, and down the outer side of the arm to the elbow, instead of the outer splint; but the inner splint must in no case be dispensed with.

Fracture of the lower extremity of the humerus may present many varieties. (1) There may be an *oblique fracture above the condyles;*—which usually happens to children. The radius and ulna, with the lower fragment, are drawn upwards and backwards as in dislocation:—but the natural appearance of the parts is restored by extension. (2) Either *condyle* may be broken off; and the fracture may or may not extend into the joint. (3) There may be one fracture *between the two condyles,* and another separating them both *from the shaft.* All these injuries may be distinguished from dislocation of the elbow by noticing that the motions of the joint are free, and are attended with crepitus above the elbow;—and that the length of the forearm, measured between the condyles of the humerus and the lower extremities of the radius and ulna, is the same as on the sound side.

*Treatment.*—The patient must be confined to his bed for some days; with the arm on a pillow, and leeches and lotions be employed to reduce the inflammation and swelling. After this, the arm should be bandaged, and a piece of pasteboard, gummed sheeting or leather be softened in water and applied to the elbow, which should be bent. Besides this, an *angular splint* should be employed. It is composed of two pieces joined at a right angle;—one of which is placed behind the upper arm, and the other below the forearm. *Passive motion* of the joint should be commenced in a fortnight or three weeks;—but the patient should be warned that it is very difficult to avoid all deformity and loss of motion.

VI. FRACTURES OF THE FOREARM. *Fracture of the olecranon* may be *caused* by direct force, or by violent action of the triceps muscle.

*Symptoms.*—The patient easily bends his limb, but has great pain and inability in straightening it. A hollow is felt at the back of the joint, because the broken part is drawn from half an inch to two inches up the arm; but sometimes, when the ligaments are not torn through, this displacement may be very trifling, or altogether absent.

*Treatment.*—The limb should be placed in a straight position, and leeches, &c., be used till swelling and tenderness subside. Then the forearm having been bandaged, the olecranon should be drawn down as much as possible, and the roller, continued from the forearm, should be passed around above it, and then back again about the elbow in a figure of 8 form. Then the whole upper arm should be rolled in order to prevent contraction of the triceps; and a splint must be placed in front, so as to keep the arm straight. Passive motion should be commenced in three weeks. Union will be ligamentous.

Compound fracture of the olecranon is far from an uncommon consequence of violent blows or falls on the elbow; and it is often followed by
protracted disease of the joint. The part must be bathed and fomented;
the wound be closed as it best may; the water-dressing be applied, and
the elbow be kept straight and motionless with a splint;—leeches, &c.
must be used to reduce inflammation, and when the wound is healed, and
the joint free from active disease, *passive motion* must be employed to
restore it to its proper uses.

Fracture of the *coronoid process* is very rare. It is caused by the action
of the brachialis muscle. Mr. Liston gives a case of it which occurred
to a boy of eight years old, and was caused by his hanging with one hand
from the top of a high wall.

*Symptoms.*—Difficulty of bending the elbow, and dislocation of the
ulna,—the olecranon projecting backwards.

*Treatment.*—The arm must be bandaged, and kept at rest in the bent
position. Union will be ligamentous.

Fractures of the *shafts of the radius and ulna*, together or singly, are
known by the ordinary signs of fracture, especially by the crepitus felt
on fixing the upper end, and rotating or moving the other. The objects
in the treatment are to prevent the fractured ends of either bone from
being pressed inwards towards the interosseous space, and to prevent the
upper fragment of the radius from being more *supinated* or *everted* than
the lower.

*Treatment.*—The fracture is easily reduced by extension from the
wrist and elbow. Then the elbow being bent, and the forearm placed
in a position intermediate between pronation and supination—(that is to
say, with the thumb uppermost) one splint should be applied to the flexor
side, from the inner condyle of the humerus to the palm of the hand; and
another from the outer condyle of the humerus to the back of the wrist.
Both splints should be well padded along their middle, so that they may
press the muscles into the interosseous space, and prevent the bones from
coming together. If the radius alone is broken, especially near its lower
extremity, the hand should be permitted to drop downwards; but if the
ulna alone, or if both bones be fractured, the splints should extend to the
ends of the fingers, and the hand be kept in a *line with the forearm;* and,
besides, a third slight splint may be applied to the ulna. Some practitioners, instead of placing the thumb uppermost, place the forearm *quite
supine*, with the palm uppermost;—then having reduced the fracture,
apply one splint below from the olecranon to the fingers' ends:—and
another above from the bend of the elbow to the wrist. But this plan has
no particular advantage, and does not allow the flexor and pronator muscles to be relaxed.

After the first week, the splints may be removed and the starched
bandage be substituted. A dry roller is to be first applied from the hand

to a little above the elbow. This is to be covered with several layers of roller imbubed with starch; but the part should still be supported by a splint till the starched rollers become dry. The cure is generally complete in a month or five weeks. It must be recollected that the bandage must not be applied too tightly, so as to press the fractured extremities towards the interosseous space.

Fracture of the *lower extremity of the radius* is often a very awkward accident, because the lower fragment is dragged amongst the flexor tendons by the pronator quadratus. This fracture is generally situated half an inch or an inch above the wrist-joint, and is caused by falls upon the hand. The accompanying figure shows the appearance after the accident; the hand, with the lower fragment being drawn upwards and backwards by the extensor tendons. It somewhat resembles dislocation of the wrist;

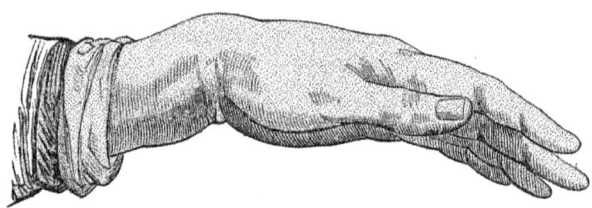

but it may be distinguished by attending to the relative positions of the styloid process of the radius, and the root of the thumb. It sometimes happens that the posterior rim of the articular surface of the radius is obliquely broken off, and the hand partially dislocated backwards.* These fractures must be treated as the other fractures of the forearm, but care must be taken to apply pads against the projecting points of the fractured bone, so as to keep them in their places. Passive motion must be commenced early.

VII. FRACTURES OF THE HAND.—The *carpus* is rarely fractured without so much other injury as to render amputation necessary. Fracture of the *metacarpal bones*, or of the *phalanges*, will be readily recognised. No part of the hand should be amputated unless positively necessary, and even one finger should be saved if it can be done.

*Treatment.*—For fractures of the carpus, metacarpus, or first phalanges, it is a good plan to make the patient grasp a ball of tow or some other soft substance, and bind his hand over it; or the hand may be supported on a flat wooden splint, cut into the shape of the thumb and fingers. If one finger only be fractured, it may be confined by a thin lath or pasteboard splint. It must be recollected that the palmar surfaces of the metacarpal and digital bones are concave. They must therefore be slightly padded before they are bound to any flat surface, or they will unite crookedly.

* Barton, Philadelphia Med. Examiner, Nov. 7, 1838.

VIII. FRACTURE OF THE RIBS is generally situated in their anterior half, and is generally caused by *direct* violence; such as blows; the bone giving way at the point struck. Sometimes, however, it is caused by *indirect* violence; as for instance, when the chest is violently compressed between two points. In 1837, several people were crushed to death in a crowd in the Champ de Mars in Paris, and many of them were found to have several ribs broken in this manner. Sometimes, in old subjects, one or more ribs are broken by violent coughing.*

*Symptoms.*—Fixed lancinating pain, aggravated by inspiration, coughing, or any other motion. By tracing the outline of the bone, or by placing the hand or the stethoscope upon it, crepitus may be felt during the act of coughing or inspiration, and the patient is sensible of it likewise. If the fracture be situated near the spine, or if the patient be very corpulent, it may be difficult to detect fracture with certainty, but this is of little consequence; for in every case when a patient complains of pain on inspiration after a blow on the chest, the treatment is the same.

*Treatment.*—The indications are, (1) To *prevent all motion* of the ribs, by passing a broad flannel roller;—or a towel fastened with tape round the chest so tightly, that respiration may be performed solely by the diaphragm;—(2) to *obviate inflammation* of the chest, and diminish the arterializing duties of the lungs by bleeding, purging, rest in bed, and low diet. *Opiates* should be given for pain and cough.

If several ribs are broken on each side, it may happen that no bandage can be borne, and the case becomes highly serious. Quietude and depletion are the only remedies.

*Emphysema*, a swelling caused by the presence of air in the cellular tissue, is an occasional complication of this fracture. It is produced in the following way. The extremities of the fractured rib perforate both *pleuræ*; and wound the lung. In the act of inspiration, air escapes from the lung into the cavity of the pleura, and from thence through the wound in the *pleura costalis* into the cellular tissue of the trunk. *Emphysema* forms a soft tumour, that crepitates and disperses on pressure.

*Treatment.*—Provided the air escapes freely from the cavity of the chest, little inconvenience results, and if the skin merely be very much distended, it may be punctured. But if the air accumulate in the pleura and compress the lung, which will be known by great dyspnœa and a hollow sound on percussion, and if the breathing is not relieved by free depletion, an aperture must be made into the chest to let the air escape. —See the chapter on the Injuries of the Chest.

IX. FRACTURE OF THE STERNUM. *Symptoms.*—Crepitus may be felt during inspiration or other movements of the trunk, and displacement (if any) can be detected by examination.

---

* See an interesting paper on Fracture of the Ribs, by M. Malgaigne, in the Arch. Gen. de Med. 1838, quoted in Forbes, Rev., vol. vii. p. 554.

*Treatment.*—The same as for fractured ribs.

_ X. FRACTURE OF THE PELVIS can only be caused by most tremendous violence, and are generally attended with some fatal complication;—such as laceration of the bladder or rectum, or of the great arteries or veins. The only thing to be done is, to place the patient at perfect rest, and in as easy a position as possible;—to keep a catheter in the bladder; to make incisions if urine is extravasated into the perineum, and to treat any symptoms that may arise. There are some cases of fracture of the os innominatum passing through the acetabulum, and caused by falls on the hip, which might be mistaken for fracture of the cervix femoris. In some cases stated by Mr. Earle,* the foot was everted, but not shortened; and there was loss of prominence of the trochanter; but the limb could be turned freely outwards, which motion is highly painful after fracture of the neck of the femur. The diagnosis will be guided chiefly by the crepitus felt on applying the stethoscope to the ilium, and by examination per anum. The patient must be kept on a fracture-bed. One of Mr. Earle's cases was cured in eight weeks. Fracture of the *os coccygis,* or of the lower extremity of the sacrum, may be caused by violent kicks or falls;—the former may occur during parturition to women who have children after the coccyx is united to the sacrum. The loose portions must be replaced by introducing the finger within the rectum, and the bowels must be kept relaxed, so that no disturbance may be occasioned by hard stools.

XI. FRACTURE OF THE FEMUR present many varieties, which must be carefully studied; because, as Pott observes, " they so often lame the patient, and disgrace the surgeon." We must, therefore, treat separately of fractures of the neck of the femur; of the shaft just below the trochanters; of the centre of the shaft, and of the condyles.

Fracture of the *neck of the femur* may occur either within the capsular ligament, or external to it. The fracture *internal to the capsule* is the more common, and is generally caused by *indirect violence;* that is, by a slight force acting on the lower extremity of the limb, as happens in slipping off the curbstone; sometimes, however, it is produced by falls or blows on the hip. It is very rare in persons under fifty; but very common in old people, especially in old women; because, in addition to the changes which all the bones experience in advanced life,—the thinness of the cortex, sponginess of the cancelli, deficiency of the bone earth, and loss of elasticity of the animal matter,—the neck of the femur is always peculiarly atrophied; it is *shortened,* and *sunk* from the oblique to the *horizontal* position;—changes that cannot fail to render it more easily fractured.

* Earle, Fractures of the Pelvis, Med. Chir. Trans., vol. xix.

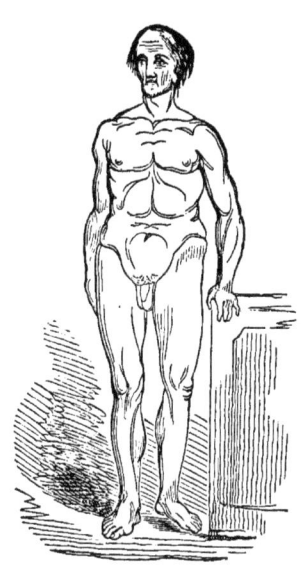

*Symptoms.*—After a blow or fall, the patient finds himself unable to stand, and complains of great pain, increased by motion, and principally seated at the upper and inner part of the thigh. The leg is from half an inch to two inches shorter than the other;—the foot is turned outwards;—the heel rests in the interval between the ankle and tendo achillis of the other leg; *crepitus* may be detected if the hand or the stethoscope be placed on the trochanter, whilst the limb is *drawn to its proper length* and rotated; the trochanter generally projects less than on the other side, and the limb may generally be freely moved, although with great pain, especially if it is abducted. It may be mentioned, that the shortening very often does not occur till some days after the accident; and sometimes it is very trivial, or even wanting, if the fractured parts are locked together. Moreover, in some cases, the limb is turned inwards instead of outwards. But in any case, when an old person has tumbled down, and complains of pain in the hip, and is unable to stand, this fracture should be suspected, and be carefully looked for, although there may be no apparent shortcuing.

Fracture of the neck of the femur, internal to the capsular ligament, very rarely unites by bone; for the following reasons: *First.* Because of the inadequate nutrition of the upper fragment, which is only supplied by the small vessels of the *ligamentum teres. Secondly.* Because the fracture, being separated from the cellular tissue by the capsular ligament, cannot be assisted by a provisional callus, which (as has been described at p. 239) is secreted by the tissues surrounding the fracture. Yet is remarkable that bone is often deposited on the outside of the capsular ligament, both after this fracture and after disease of the joint; which bone is equivalent to the callus formed after an ordinary fracture; but is in this instance prevented by the capsular ligament from aiding in the work of reparation.[*] *Thirdly.* Because the fractured, surfaces cannot be easily kept in appositiou, or pressed against each other. *Fourthly.* Because the patients, being old, have neither time nor constitutional vigour sufficient to effect the cure. So that in general this fracture either unites by ligament, or,

---

[*] Instances of this may be seen in a preparation given by Mr. Earle to the Hunterian Museum, and marked 137.249 F.; and also in one in the King's College Museum, referred to in Mayo's Pathology.

more commonly, does not unite at all; but the stump of the cervix becomes rounded and covered with a smooth porcellaneous deposite, and
plays in a socket formed by the hollowing and absorption of the head.
Yet it may unite by bone, if the patient is young, and if the fractured
surfaces can be kept in tolerable apposition.   Mr. Stanley gives a case
happening to a boy of eighteen, in which this fracture united firmly by
bone in two months, as was proved by dissection, although the case had

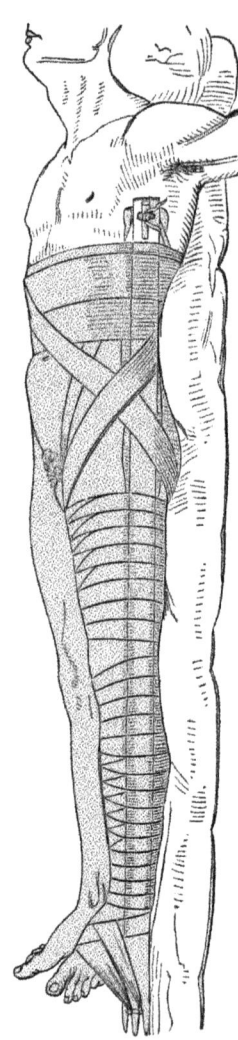

been mistaken for a dislocation, and the limb
had been forcibly extended, and otherwise
treated unfavourably for the union.*

Fracture *external to the capsular ligament*
resembles the last in many general features,
but differs in the following points; 1. It is
always caused by *direct* violence.   2. It
may occur to persons of any age.   3. It is *not
attended with so much shortening and eversion*.   4. *Crepitus* is much more easily felt.
5. It may very easily unite by bone, if the
patient's age or other circumstances do not
prevent it.   6. It is caused by direct violence,
and therefore is attended with great fever,
pain, and swelling—sometimes enough to
prove fatal;—whereas in fracture internal to
the capsule, caused by falls on the feet, there
is very little local or constitutional disturbance after the first week.

*Treatment.*—If the patient is old and feeble, no attempt should be made to procure
osseous union; both because it would be unavailing, and because the patient's little rem-
nant of health and strength would be sacri-
ficed by the long confinement that would be
necessary.   But he should be kept in bed
for a fortnight, till pain and tenderness abate;
(the most comfortable posture is generally
on the back, with the knees supported by
pillows;) then he may get up and crawl about
with crutches; and in time he will regain a
tolerable use of the limb, especially if not

---

* Stanley, Med. Chir. Trans., vol. xviii.—See also nine cases of this fracture by
Mr. Howship, ib. vol. xix.: and the whole subject fully discussed in Sir A. Cooper
on Fractures and Dislocation of the Joints, seventh ed., 1831.

very corpulent. The sole of the shoe must be made thick enough to counteract the shortness of the limb.

But if the patient is young and vigorous, an attempt must be made to procure either a union by bone, or at least by a short firm ligament; and there are two modes of treatment, viz. Amesbury's fracture-bed, and the long straight splint.

The *fracture bed* consists of four parts, something like a W. The body is placed on the first;—the second is appropriated to the thighs, and must be made of a proper length for them;—the legs are to hang over the third, which must also be made of a proper length;—and the fourth is a footboard. There is a hole to admit of evacuations; and the patient can be so confined as to prevent any motion of trunk or body, together or singly. Both thighs must be bandaged;—the trochanter must be supported with a pad,—a long splint should be placed on the outside of the thigh—and the two limbs should be fastened together. By these means union may probably occur in two or three month; or even if ligament form, it will be short.

The object of the long straight splint is to overcome the resistance of all the muscles by extension, instead of averting it by relaxing them by position. The common straight splint of Dessault extends from the pelvis to the foot, and has a footboard with straps, &c. at the bottom. But the simple splint employed by Mr. Liston, and depicted in the adjoining cut, which is taken from his Practical Surgery, appears to be better. It is a simple deal board, of a hand's breadth for an adult, but narrower and slighter for a young person. It should reach from opposite the nipple to four or five inches below the foot. At its upper end it has two holes, and at its lower end two deep notches; with a hollow for the outer ankle. " A pad of corresponding length and breadth is attached by a few pieces of tape; a roller is split at the end, and having been tied through the openings in the top part of the splint, is unrolled so far, and fixed for the time to the lower end of the pad. The apparatus thus prepared for application is here represented." The limb must now be gently extended from foot and pelvis to its proper length, and must be bandaged from the foot to the hip. The splint is next applied to the outside of the limb; the roller before spoken of must be repeatedly passed round the instep and ankle, and through the notches, so as to secure the foot, and must then be carried up the leg. A perinial band, composed of a large soft handker-

33

chief, padded with tow and covered with oiled silk, must be put round the groin, and be fastened firmly to the holes at the top of the splint; and, lastly, a few turns of broad bandage are to be passed round the trunk.* The disadvantage of this plan, compared with the former, is supposed to be, that the perineal band tends to draw the fractured parts asunder. But more depends on the surgeon in every case than on the splint; and a man who watches his patient properly, and keeps him in a comfortable posture, and corrects any deviation as soon as it occurs, will be success-ful with either.

Fracture of the femur *just below the trochanters* is liable to be fol-lowed by great deformity and non-union, because the upper fragment is tilted forwards by the psoas and iliacus muscles.

*Treatment.*—The best plan is to place the patient on a fracture-bed, with the trunk and thighs bent at a very acute angle, so as to relax the offending muscles.

Fracture of the *shaft* of the femur requires no observations as to its *causes* or *symptoms.*

*Treatment.*—(1.) The first apparatus that we shall notice is the *double inclined plane.* It consists of two pieces like the letter A;—one for the thigh, the other for the leg, with a board to fasten the foot to. The whole limb must be bandaged;—the *thigh-piece* must be made accurately to correspond to the distance between the tuber ischii and the bend of the knee;—and then one splint is to be placed from the *great trochanter* to the *outer condyle*;—a second, from the ramus of the pubes to the inner condyle; and a third on the anterior surface of the limb. Perhaps it is a good plan to apply a fourth splint, from the *tuber ischii* to the *bend of the knee*, before placing the patient on the plane. Both legs should be bandaged. The disadvantage of this plan is, that the patient's *bottom* sinks in the bed, and thus the upper fragment is tilted forwards.

(2.) A second plan is that of Pott.† It consists in laying the patient on the affected side, the thigh at right angles to the trunk, and the knee bent—with a many-tailed bandage and four splints, applied between the different points of bone that have just been mentioned. The disadvan-tages of this plan are, first, that the patient soon turns round on his back, dragging the upper fragment away from its right place; and, secondly, that the pressure on the great trochanter may cause sloughing, &c. The first evil may be prevented simply by watching the patient, and telling him to turn round on his belly rather than on his back, if he wishes to shift his position. The second may be remedied by placing him on his back, at the end of a fortnight, with his knees bent up and supported by pillows.

(3.) A third plan is that of the long straight splint before described. Which of these three plans is the best, every surgeon must decide for

* Liston, op. cit. p. 88.          † Pott, Chirurgical works, vol. i. p. 365.

himself. The author prefers the second; but believes that a careful surgeon will succeed with either of them.

If *both thighs* are broken, a fracture-bed should be employed;—or, if the surgeon has not one, the patient should be placed on his back, with four splints to each thigh, and his knees drawn up, and supported by pillows.

When the lower end of the femur is fractured obliquely downwards and forwards, the sharp end of the upper fragment is apt to pierce the extensor muscles, and the lower fragment to be dragged down into the ham by the gastrocnemius.

*Treatment.*—Firm extension must be kept up with the double inclined plane and splints;—and the knee must be well bent, to relax the gastrocnemius.

*Fracture of the condyle into the knee-joint* mostly happens to old persons, and not unfrequently proves fatal. If much *comminuted*, or if *compound, amputation* will be necessary. Otherwise, the limb should be placed *straight*, so that the head of the tibia may keep the fractured parts in their places;—lotions and leeches should be used to prevent inflammation;—and afterwards a pasteboard splint. *Passive motion* should be commenced in five weeks.

XI. FRACTURE OF THE PATELLA is generally transverse, and is *caused* by sudden contraction of the extensor muscles attached to it;—as, for instance, when a person who has his knee much bent under him, and is in danger of falling, tries to save himself by throwing the body forwards.

*Symptoms.*—Inability to straighten the knee, and separation of the fractured parts, which can be readily felt.

*Treatment.* The limb must be laid straight, with the foot much raised on a single inclined plane. The joint should be steadied with a slight pasteboard splint, and leeches and fomentations be used till inflammation subsides;—and then, as soon as it can be borne, some apparatus may be employed to keep the broken surfaces as nearly in contact as possible. The most common consists of one pad, or strap, or bandage placed above the patella, and a similar one below it;—the two are then approximated by longitudinal straps, or bandages, passing between them. But the best apparatus conceivable is that invented by Mr. Lonsdale; for it causes no circular constriction of the limb whatever. If the parts can be kept in *complete apposition*, the union may be bony;—if not, it will be ligamentous; it is however, a great object to have the ligament as short as possible. *Passive motion* may be begun in six weeks.

*Longitudinal or comminuted* fracture of this bone, being caused by direct violence, will be attended with great inflammation;—which being subdued, the parts must be kept in their places by bandages and pasteboard splints. *Compound* fracture will generally require amputation;—unless the *wound is very small;*—the skin not injured enough to slough or ulcerate;—and the constitution very good.

XII. FRACTURES OF THE LEG.—The ordinary fractures of the leg may be readily distinguished by careful examination. There are several methods of treatment.

(1) *By the tailed bandage and splints.*—The injured leg being laid on its outer side, the fracture is reduced by extension from the knee and ankle. Then a many-tailed bandage is applied, after the manner represented in the cut. This bandage is easily made thus.—Take a piece of roller, long enough to reach from the knee to the foot, and to overlap

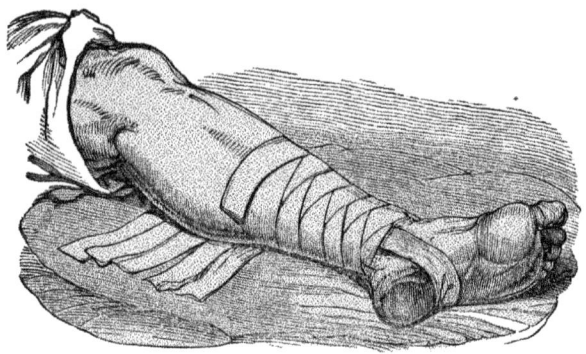

about one-third of the leg besides. Cut another roller into pieces of the proper length, and lay them across the first at right angles, in such a manner that each shall overlap one-third of the preceding one; these transverse pieces are to be stitched to the longitudinal one, and then the bandage is ready for use. One splint, well padded, should be applied to the outer side of the limb; another to the inner side; and if there is any projection of either fragment, it should be kept in place by a third slight splint to the shin. The outer splint should have a foot-piece, which should be carefully padded in such a manner as to prevent the foot from turning either inwards or outwards, especially the latter. There is a very useful rule, which should be attended to in all cases of injury below the knee: it is, *to keep the great toe in a line with the inner edge of the patella.*

(2) By *the double inclined plane*, represented in the adjacent cut, from

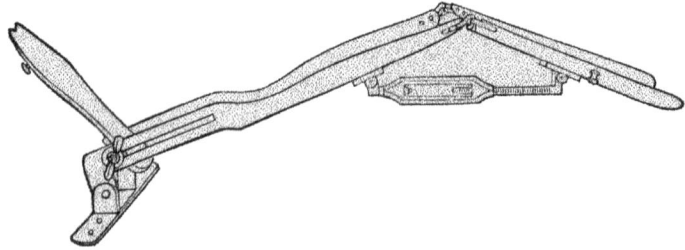

Mr. Liston's "Practical Surgery," or by some of the numberless varieties of it in existence. Before its application, it must be made to correspond to the length of the sound limb, and must be well padded.

(3) By the *junks.* This very simple but efficient contrivance consists of a piece of old sheeting, with a bundle of reeds rolled together from either end. But it is more easy to comprehend it from seeing it once than from a page of description.

(4) *By the starched bandage.*—In most cases of fracture of the leg, unattended with any particular complication, it is expedient to permit the patient to leave his bed at the end of a week, with the fracture supported by the starched apparatus. First of all, a dry bandage should be applied from the foot half way up the thigh; then a piece of stout pasteboard, softened in boiling water, should be accurately adapted to the limb on each side; and the outer piece should be made to overlap the heel. In the next place, the hollows about the ankle and tendo achillis should be well padded with tow; and then four or five layers of roller must be put on, thoroughly imbued with mucilage of gum or starch; and lastly a dry roller. When this has become dry, (which will be in a day or two,) the patient may get up, and move to his chair or sofa, but the foot must be suspended from his neck by a sling; and he must be particularly cautioned not to attempt to move it by its own efforts.

For fracture of the head of the tibia into the knee-joint, the treatment is the same as for fracture of the condyles of the femur. The limb should be placed straight, so that the end of the femur may act as a splint, and keep the broken parts in their places. The whole limb should be raised, so as to relax the extensor muscles of the knee; and this should be done in *all cases of fracture of the upper end of the tibia* (for which, consequently, the treatment by splints, with the knee bent, is inapplicable.) Pasteboard splints and starched bandages should be applied, to keep the joint motionless; but they should not cover the front of the knee so as to interfere with the leeches, fomentations, &c., that will be necessary to reduce the inflammation. *Passive motion* should be commenced in five weeks.

*Fracture of the lower end of the fibula,* about three inches above the ankle-joint, is not an uncommon accident, and is caused by twists of the

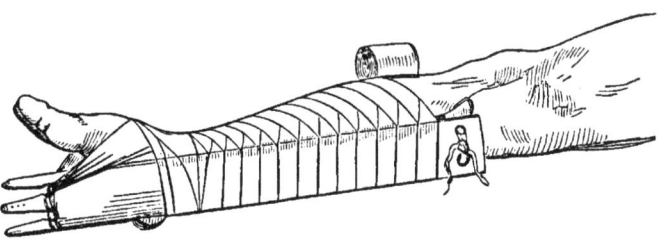

foot, or by jumping on uneven ground. Fracture of the internal malleolus may occur in the same way; and one or the other of these fractures commonly accompany dislocation of the ankle. They may either be treated as the other fractures of the leg, or with the straight splint here shown, which is a diminutive of the straight thigh splint before described. It is to be applied to the side opposite the fracture.

*Compound fractures* of the leg are to be treated on the principles already laid down for the treatment of compound fracture in general.

XIII. FRACTURES OF THE FOOT will often be attended with so much other mischief as renders amputation expedient. But an attempt should be made to save part of it;—especially the ball of the great toe. Pasteboard splints and other contrivances must be used to preserve the proper position;—and if matter forms, there should be no delay in freely dividing the dense fasciæ of the foot, to let it escape.

---

# CHAPTER VI.

## OF THE DISEASES AND INJURIES OF THE JOINTS.

### SECTION I.—OF THE DISEASES OF THE SYNOVIAL MEMBRANE.

I. ACUTE INFLAMMATION of the synovial membrane (or *synovitis*) may be produced by *local* or by *constitutional* causes. The former are blows, strains, mechanical injuries, and especially penetrating wounds, and cold. The latter are, the rheumatic and gouty diatheses, and the morbid state of the constitution produced by syphilis or the abuse of mercury;—sometimes, also, this disease is a sequel of gonorrhœa. It very seldom attacks young children. The joint most frequently affected is the knee.

*Symptoms.*—In the most acute form, the symptoms are severe aching pain in the joint, aggravated by the slightest motion; great swelling *occurring immediately after the pain;* redness and tenderness of the skin, and fever, which is often violent and alarming.

The swelling is peculiar, and it is distinctive of the disease. It is occasioned by a rapid effusion of fluid into the synovial cavity; and, consequently, if the joint is superficial, it fluctuates freely. It is always most prominent where the joint is least covered by ligament, and, consequently, the shape of the joint is always altered. When the knee is affected, the patella is protruded forwards, and there is a great fulness at each side of it, and at the lower and front part of the thigh. In the elbow, the swelling is most distinct above the olecranon, and in the hip and shoulder there is a general fulness of the surrounding muscles.

*Prognosis.*—This disease is much more serious when it affects one joint solely; and more particular when it arises from local injury, (especially a penetrating wound,) than when it affects many joints, and arises from constitutional disorder. The danger to life, in any case, will be proportionate to the severity of the febrile symptoms, and the rapidity and sharpness of the pulse; delirium, or typhoid symptoms show great peril.

In severe cases, moreover, the membrane may suppurate, and the cartilage ulcerate, and the patient may often esteem himself lucky in recovering with the joint permanently anchylozed and immoveable; whilst milder cases will be merely followed by a stiffness that may be gradually removed by treatment.

*Morbid anatomy.*—In recent cases, of great severity, the synovial membrane is found red, the joint filled with turbid synovia, mixed with flakes of lymph, or with pus, and portions of the membrane, and perhaps of the cartilage, ulcerated.

*Treatment.*—In all cases arising from injury, the joint, or rather the whole limb, should be confined by a splint, so as to keep it perfectly motionless. This is indispensable; for the joint cannot be kept motionless without it. The other measures are, *bleeding* from the arm, if the patient is robust, and the joint important; if not, leeches in abundance *to* the joint, or cupping *near* it; ice, evaporating lotions, or warm poppy fomentations, according to the patient's choice; purgatives in moderation, and not given so as to disturb the part by frequent motions; salines; calomel, with opium and antimony, in moderate doses every four hours, till the mouth begins to suffer, and opiates at night to relieve pain. A warm poultice of camomile flowers, boiled till they are quite soft, will generally be found more soothing than cold applications. Blisters, it need scarcely be said, are inapplicable during the acute stage.

When the disease is manifestly connected with rheumatism—when it is attended with red sediment in the urine and acid perspirations, and affects several joints, and extends to the synovial sheaths of tendons, colchicum should be administered, F. 95. But when only two or three joints are affected, or when there has been a manifest translation of the disease from some internal part, or from one joint to another, Sir B. Brodie prefers the use of calomel and opium, in moderate doses, till the mouth is affected. When there is a tendency to gout, and the patient complains of grinding, excruciating pain, as if the joint were torn asunder, the colchicum is also the main remedy. In syphilitic cases (which will be known by the patient's general history, by his wan, peculiar appearance, and most likely by the existence of papular or other eruptions, vide, p. 212,) mercury may be tried, if it has never before been given to excess; but if it has, or the constitution is broken down, recourse may be had to the iodide of potassium in doses of gr. iii. ter die, with a small dose of colchicum and opium at night; and sarsaparilla should be given in abundance. **F. 56. 57.**

II. CHRONIC INFLAMMATION of the synovial membrane is characterized by *swelling* of the joint, of the same nature that attends the acute form, and by a dull aching *pain*, accompanied with a sense of weakness and relaxation, and not unusually aggravated by pressing the articular surfaces against each other. The swelling always comes on in a few days after the pain; and sometimes, in cases of an indolent character, it is the only symptom present; these cases are called *hydrops articuli* or *hydrarthus*. If the disease proceed, the synovial membrane and surrounding tissue become thickened and gristly, and the swelling loses its softness and fluctuation; and, in neglected cases, the inflammation will lead to ulceration of the cartilages and destruction of the joint. The *causes* are the same as those of the acute form, of which it may be a sequel.

*Treatment.*—The indications are, first to correct constitutional disorder; secondly, to reduce inflammation; and thirdly, to produce absorption of the effusion and thickening, and restore the part to its proper uses.

In the first place, therefore, if the complaint is constitutional, and depends on gout, it must be treated by colchicum and warm aperients, especially the decoction of aloes and alkalis, F. 8, 9, 95, 99. If the habit is rheumatic, colchicum, or the iodide of potassium, must be resorted to; and in most cases, especially those following syphilis or gonorrhœa, warm bathing, change of air, sarsaparilla, and a most carefully, regulated diet, avoiding all heavy, innutritious, acescent, or indigestible substances, will be indispensable.

Secondly, in cases arising from local injury; whilst there is any activity about the inflammation, (especially an increase of aching pain at night,) the part should be confined by a splint or starched bandage, and should be bathed with cold lotions, and blood should be repeatedly taken by leeches or cupping.

The third indication is to be fulfilled by *counter-irritation*, beginning with blisters, which are as serviceable in the chronic as they are detrimental in the acute disease. They should be applied in succession, and be quickly healed up; and should not be put too near the joint, if it is superficial, as the knee. The strong acetum cantharides will often be found a very convenient substitute. After the blistering, when the activity of the disease has subsided, the tartar-emetic ointment, F. 38; the linimentum hydragyri, or liniments of cantharides, ammonia, and turpentine, F. 14; the *douche*, or affusion with hot water; the vapour bath, and passive motion, will complete the cure. But all stimulating applications and passive motion must be at once abandoned, if they cause an aggravation of heat and pain. The ointment of Scott, F. 25, the *ceratum hy-*

*drargyri comp.* of the pharmacopœia, is one of the most useful applications for the convalescent stage of this and other chronic diseases of
joints. If it is applied thus: the surface of the joint, having been first
washed with camphorated spirit, should be covered with the ointment
thickly spread on lint; next, adhesive plaster should be evenly applied in
strips, so as to form a complete casing for the joint; and lastly a bandage.
The starched bandage may be substituted for adhesive plaster. When
the knee is bandaged in this way, the adhesive straps should be arranged
so as not to press too tightly on the patella.

III. ABSCESS IN JOINTS.—If, after acute or chronic inflammation, a
joint becomes very much distended, and there is constant pain, unmiti-
gated by remedies, and considerable constitutional excitement, suppuration of the synovial membrane may be fairly suspected. The first
thing to be done under these circumstances is to make a puncture with a
grooved needle, and examine the fluid that exudes. If it is serum, two
or three more punctures may be made, and an exhausted cupping-glass
be applied over them; and by these means the part may be very safely and
expeditiously relieved of a considerable quantity of fluid. If it is pus, a
free opening should be made with a lancet, in a depending position, so
that the matter may run out easily; the joint should be placed on a splint
in the most easy and convenient posture: the general health should be
amended by tonics, alteratives, and proper diet; and then, in favourable
cases, a cure will be effected by *anchylosis*. But if the suppuration and
constitutional disturbance increase, the limb must be amputated.

It has been mentioned in several previous chapters, that a rapid effusion of pus into the joints and other parts is a frequent occurrence in
glanders, phlebitis, puerperal fever, diffuse cellular inflammation, dissection wounds, and other cases in which the blood is contaminated by a
morbid poison. The part becomes red and painful, and very soon afterwards is found to be filled with pus. The only local treatment consists
of a free incision in a depending position, and a splint, with a bandage
to prevent accumulation of matter.

IV. PULPY FUNGUS consists in the conversion of the synovial membrane (generally of the knee) into a thick pulpy substance of a light
brown or reddish brown colour, intersected by white membranous lines.
It produces, after a time, ulceration of the cartilages, caries of the bones,
wasting of the ligaments, and abscesses in various places.

*Symptoms.*—Gradually increasing stiffness and swelling of the
joint, *without pain*;—the swelling less regular than that of chronic inflammation;—and not fluctuating, although so soft and elastic that it
seems to do so.

*Treatment.*—The progress of the disease may be retarded by rest and
antiphlogistic measures; but, after a longer or shorter duration of the in-

34

dolent stage, ulceration of the cartilage and hectic come on, and the patient can only be saved by amputation.*

V. Loose Cartilages commence as little pendulous growths upon the synovial membrane, which becomes accidentally detached.

*Symptoms.*—They can be felt, when they present themselves at the surface of the joint;—and when they get between the ends of the bones, which they are very apt to do during exercise, they cause sudden excruciating pain and faintness, followed by inflammation.

*Treatment.*—If possible, the cartilage should be fixed by bandages, so as to prevent it from getting between the bones;—otherwise it must be removed. The patient should be confined to his bed for two or three days before, and for several days after the operation. The cartilage should be well fixed;—its coverings slowly divided;—then it must be taken out with a tenaculum;—the wound be closed;—and the greatest care be taken to prevent inflammation.

VI. Pendulous Fleshy or Gristly Tumours may produce many of the symptoms of loose cartilages. They may, perhaps, be distinguished by being less hard. They have been extirpated from the knee, but of course with very great hazard to life.

### SECTION II.—INFLAMMATION OF THE CELLULAR TISSUE.

Inflammation of the cellular tissue around a joint is a peculiar affection, particularly described by Mr. Wickham, an author of great experience on the joints. It commences with a tolerably firm swelling, various in extent;—attended with slight obtuse pain, and caused by a deposition of lymph, which renders the tissue hard and brawny. As it increases, the skin becomes distended, white, and shining, and the pain and constitutional distress extreme. After this *adhesive stage* has lasted an uncertain number of months, suppuration occurs at one or more points; and the abscesses burst through the synovial membrane, and cause irreparable disorganization of the joint.

*Treatment.*—Leeches or cupping, and cold lotions, followed after a time by Scott's ointment (F. 25.) Mr. Wickham deems counter-irritants and friction injurious.†

### SECTION III.—THE LIGAMENTS.

Weakness and elongation of ligaments must be remedied by mechanical support. Authors have described a form of inflammation of the liga-

---

* Brodie on Diseases of the joints, 4th, edit. p. 72.

† Wickham on the Joints, p. 84, Winchester, 1833. See also Nicolai, quoted in Coulson on the Hip Joint, p. 85.

ments of joints characterized by great pain from motions that shake or twist them.* It must be treated like the subacute facial inflammation, p. 227.

SECTION IV.—THE CARTILAGE.

The affections of cartilage in which the surgeon is interested, are its absorption or atrophy, and ulceration: of which there are several varieties.

I. The cartilage of the joints of elderly persons is sometimes partially absorbed, so as even to denude the bone;—but both the cartilage itself and the exposed surface of bone are quite healthy. This state may exist without producing any symptoms, except, perhaps, a slight grating.

II. Articular cartilage is occasionally converted into a soft fibrous or villous structure. This change seems sometimes to be mere atrophy, sometimes the forerunner of ulceration.

III. ACUTE ULCERATION of cartilage is a frequent accompaniment of that acute inflammation and suppuration of the synovial membrane which follows penetrating wounds. The cartilage rapidly disappears, but the exposed surface is healthy, and if the patient escape with life, it readily granulates and heals. Sir. B. Brodie and Mr. Mayo relate several cases of acute idiopathic ulceration of cartilage " attended not with effusion into the joint, but with suppuration or œdema external to it," and rapidly followed by anchylosis; but such cases are rare.

IV. CHRONIC ULCERATION of cartilage is one of the most important affections of joints, and ought to be carefully studied. It generally affects persons of bad, scrofulous constitutions, between the age of puberty and thirty-five;—and is usually ascribed to cold, or to neglected injury. It is generally an *idiopathic* or *primary* affection,† but it may also be a consequence of previous caries of the bone; as will be described in the next section;—and it may also follow the chronic inflammation of the synovial membrane, if neglected.

*Symptoms.*—For the first few weeks (or perhaps months) of this disease, the patient only complains of slight occasional rheumatic pains, and trifling lameness of the joint. After a time, the pain increases in severity, especially at night, and it is generally referred to one small spot, deep in the joint, and is compared by the patient to the gnawing of an animal. Moreover, it is usually accompanied by an aching of some other part of the limb;—thus, when the hip or elbow is affected, there is an aching of the knee or wrist;—but it is important to notice, that both the pain in the affected joint, and the sympathetic remote pain, are always aggra-

* Mayo's Pathology, p. 79.

† Whether it always commences with an inflammation of the synovial membrane, is another question. If it does, it must be with a very different form from that which produces the ordinary effusion of synovia.

vated by motion of the joint, and by pressure of the articular surfaces against each other.   As the disease proceeds, the suffering becomes most excruciating, and is attended with painful spasms and starting of the limb during sleep; so that the patient's rest is broken, his spirits exhausted, and his appetite and general health rapidly impaired.   At first the pain is unaccompanied with any swelling; in fact, this symptom never appears in less than four or five weeks, and often not for as many months; and when it does appear, it is slight; and as it depends on an infiltration of the tissues *around* the joint, and not on effusion *into* it, the shape of the joint is unaltered.

*Terminations.*—In fortunate cases, that are subjected to judicious treatment at an early stage, the ulceration may be arrested, and the diseased surfaces will throw out lymph and heal; or very probably the lymph effused by two opposite ulcerated surfaces will unite, and *anchylosis* will be produced.*   But, in unfavourable cases, the ulceration proceeds and lays bare the bone, which becomes carious, and can be heard to grate on the least motion;—suppuration occurs into the joint, and numerous tortuous abscesses form around it, so that the surrounding soft parts are disorganized;—the joint, which has long been immoveably bent by the flexors, becomes dislocated by their continued action, owing to the destruction of the ligaments—and the patient, unless amputation is performed, dies exhausted with hectic.

The *prognosis*, in the first stage, that is, before swelling has occurred, may be favourable; but after swelling has existed for some time, the patient will be fortunate in recovering with anchylosis; and after suppuration, he will (especially if an adult) be almost certainly compelled to suffer amputation.

*Treatment.*—The first and most indispensable measure is *perfect rest;* which must be ensured by confining the joint with a starched bandage, or splint of undressed leather.   The splint or bandage should have apertures in it to allow the application of counter-irritants.   (2.) Occasional *leeching* or small cuppings, in the early stages, when the pain is severe.   (3.) *Counter-irritation* either by a seton, or caustic issue, or the actual cautery.   If the knee is affected, an issue may be established on each side of the head of the tibia.   Sir B. Brodie recommends, in these cases, that the issue should be kept open by rubbing the sore occasionally with

---

* The ulcerated portion of cartilage is sometimes supplied by a dense membrane. "I cannot," says Brodie, "assert that this membrane is never ultimately converted into the true cartilaginous structure.   In other cases a compact layer of bone is generated on the carious surface."   In others there is found "a thin layer of hard semi-transparent substance of a gray colour, and presenting an irregularly granulated surface."   Sometimes, lastly, the head of the bone is covered "with a crust of bony matter, of compact texture, of a white colour, smooth, and like polished marble."   Brodie on the Joints, 4th ed. p. 168.

caustic potass, or the sulphate of copper, rather than by peas. The actual cautery is exceedingly efficacious, and not half so painful in reality as might be imagined. The manner of applying it is described elsewhere.* For children, blisters answer very well; and it is better to keep one blister open than to apply a succession of them. Sir B. Brodie has shown, that tissues, when long established, sometimes irritate the constitution, bringing on a return of the pain which they relieved at first, and which will again depart if they are healed up. It is a practical rule, therefore, to give up issues for a time, before condemning a joint to amputation. (4.) The strength, if enfeebled, must be repaired by bark and the mineral acids, and especially by sarsaparilla, and pain must be relieved by opiates. Occasionally, a cautious course of Plummer's pill is of service. (5.) When abscess forms, there need be no haste in opening it; but if the skin becomes very much distended, it may be punctured, and the part be wrapped in a fomentation cloth, so that the matter may gently exude. No rough squeezing is admissible. If the puncture heals, another may be made when necessary—if it remains open, it should be made large enough to let the matter flow out freely as soon as it is secreted. The case must then be treated as described at p. 265.

## SECTION V.—ARTICULAR CARIES.

CARIES OF THE HEAD OF A BONE is not an uncommon cause of ulceration of the adjacent cartilage and disorganization of the joint. The affected bone is found to be soft, red, and vascular, and deficient in earthy matter, so that it is easily cut or crushed; its cancelli are filled with a reddish fluid, and in scrofulous cases a cheesy matter is deposited in them. Owing to this softened state of the bone, the cartilage peels off it readily. This disease most frequently affects the knee, elbow, and small bones of the carpus and tarsus;—it is very common in scrofulous children, but rare after thirty. An advanced stage gives rise to what was formerly called *spina ventosa;*—that is, the extremity of the bone becomes greatly enlarged, but is hollowed out into a mere shell by suppuration in its interior. The *symptoms* are nearly the same as those of ulceration of cartilage;—that is, fixed pain, extending to different parts of the limb;—aggravated by motion, and unaccompanied at first by swelling. In scrofulous cases there is a remarkable absence of pain, except during the formation and bursting of abscesses.

*Treatment.*—This is also nearly the same that is required for ulceration of cartilage. The chief dependence is to be placed on *perfect rest;* and on the various measures that have been directed for the treatment of scrofula. (p. 114.) *Issues* are not advisable in genuine scrofulous cases, as a general

* Refer to the Index.

rule; but they are of great service when the pain is severe and continuous.
Small *leechings* may be also occasionally expedient to relieve pain. *Abscesses* should in general be left to burst of themselves. *Amputation*
need not be so hastily performed in general in this disease as in the last—
both because the patient has a greater chance of recovery with anchylosis;—and because it seems probable that disease of the lungs or mesentery is sometimes suspended or averted by the continuance of a (not very
severe) disease in the extremity. The author believes that it will agree
with the experience of most surgeons, that those members of a scrofulous family are least likely to be consumptive at puberty, who have suffered from scrofulous affections of the skin or glands in early youth. If,
however, the pain is so serious that it exhausts the strength and spirits,
the part must be amputated; because the continuance of so severe an outward disease might induce the very same disease in the lungs or mesentery, which a more moderate degree might avert.

DIAGNOSIS.—It may be useful to present a concise view of the differences of the three principal chronic diseases of joints, as regards their two
principal symptoms—viz. pain and swelling. The *pain* in chronic synovitis is not very severe; it usually increases for ten or fourteen days,
and then declines;—and it is not *immediately* aggravated by motion, or
by pressure of the articular surfaces against each other. In *ulceration of
the cartilage*, the pain is very severe; continuous and exhausting, and increases as the disease advances, becoming greater after the occurrence
of swelling; moreover, it is attended with sympathetic pain of some other
part of the limb, and is always aggravated by motion. In *articular caries*
in scrofulous cases, says Brodie, "there is not that severe pain which
exhausts the powers and spirits of the patient," as in ulceration of cartilage;—but it must be confessed, that in cases occurring to adults there is
very little difference in this respect.

The *swelling* in *chronic synovitis* comes on in the course of a few
days; it fluctuates freely, and alters the form of the joint. In the other
two affections it does not come on till after some weeks or months, and
it does not alter the shape of the joint. Mr. Wickham believes that in
most affections of bone there is a great tendency to erysipelas of the superjacent skin, and believes that this may sometimes be a criterion of
caries. On this account, issues (as they are less irritating to the skin)
are to be preferred to setons, in treating the last-named disease.


SECTION VI.—ANCHYLOSIS.


ANCHYLOSIS or immobility is a frequent consequence of serious injuries and diseases of joints; therefore, whenever it is likely to happen, the
affected joint should be placed in the position which will be the least inconvenient for it to preserve. The elbow should be placed at a right an-

gle; the wrist straight; the hip and knee a little bent; and the ankle at a right angle to the leg. There are three varieties of anchylosis.

(1.) The *spurious* or *false* anchylosis, which depends on thickening and deposites into the synovial membrane and ligaments, and rigidity of the muscles. The extensor muscles are apt, in almost all cases where the joint is diseased, to become paralyzed and wasted; and the flexor muscles to fall into the state of *rigid atrophy* (p. 223;) becoming short, inextensible, and very probably dislocating the joint, by their continued traction. This form of alchylosis is very common after synovities. *Treatment.*—Daily vigorous friction with stimulating liniments over the extensor muscles;—vapour baths or the local steam bath—shampooing— and passive motion—that is to say, the joint to be every day bent and extended with a gentle degree of force, not sufficient to cause much pain. If one or more rigid muscles seem to be the main obstacles, their tendons should be divided.

(2.) *Ligamentous* anchylosis signifies the union of two articular surfaces by ligament, and is an occasional consequence of compound dislocation, and of ulceration of cartilage. It only admits of very gentle treatment by passive motion, especially if it follow disease.

(3.) *Bony anchylosis* is produced when the lymph that is effused after destruction of cartilage ossifies. It is incurable, except by sawing through the bone, and then establishing a false joint, as after fracture. This has been successfully accomplished by an American surgeon, in case of anchylozed hip-joint; but, of course, it is so serious an operation that it must not be undertaken inconsiderately.

## SECTION VII.—OF DISEASE OF THE HIP-JOINT.

This joint is exceedingly liable to chronic disease, and there are certain peculiarities in the symptoms which render it expedient to devote a section to it in particular. The usual forms of disease are the chronic ulceration of cartilage in the adult, and scrofulous caries of the head of the femur in children. The symptoms and consequences of both are nearly the same.

*Symptoms.*—The disease begins with slight occasional pain, and more or less lameness in the gait. As it advances, the pain becomes very excruciating in the cases of ulceration of cartilage, whilst in those of scrofulous caries it is comparatively trifling; but in both forms it is felt chiefly in the knee; and in the scrofulous caries, this pain in the knee may be the only symptom complained of; nay, there may even be some swelling there. The criterion, however, is, that if the surgeon moves the hip-joint, or if he jerks the femur upwards against the acetabulum, great pain will be felt in the hip, and the pain in the knee will be greatly aggravated. There is also tenderness in the groin, and behind the great tro-chanter, and sometimes swelling of the inguinal glands; and the nates of the affected side soon becomes wasted and flabby.

But the chief characteristics of hip disease are certain alterations that occur in the length of the limb. In the first stage the limb acquires an apparent increase of length, which is accounted for in different ways by different authors. (1.) One opinion is, that it is produced by effusion into the cavity of the joint, and consequent protrusion of the limb out-wards and downwards. (2.) Mr. Wickham explains it by supposing that in the first stage of the disease there is a spasmodic action of the glu-tæi and rotator muscles, by which the limb is drawn a little away from its fellow. The surgeon in comparing their lengths, naturally approxi-mates the sound limb to the diseased one, instead of disturbing the latter, and thus, as the sound limb is carried over the median line, it seems to become a little shorter, and the diseased one seems, by comparison, *ap-parently lengthened.* (3.) Sir B. Brodie explains it by showing that when the patient stands upright he rests his whole weight on the sound limb, and stretches out the other in advance merely to steady himself; and that, in consequence of this repeated attitude, the pelvis on the dis-eased side becomes habitually depressed. But whatever explanation be adopted, it must be remembered that the lengthening is apparent, and not real; because the distance from the spine of the ilium to the patella is the same on both sides.

In a subsequent stage of the complaint, the limb becomes apparently shortened. This shortening is attributed by Mr. Wickham to a prepon-derating action of the psoas and iliacus which draw the limb up across the other. And this explanation is rendered probable by the fact that spasmodic action of those muscles is capable of simulating dislocation of the hip.* But it is sometimes caused by the patient's attitude, as is ex-plained in the quotation from Brodie in the next page. This shortening is functional, and is easily removed, if the disease is checked. But if the disease proceed, it is succeeded by another kind of shortening, caused either by the destruction of the neck of the femur, by caries, or (as is more commonly the case) by the destruction of the acetabulum and capsular ligament, and dislocation of the bone upwards by the muscles. The deformed appearance caused by this dislocation is well exhibited in the adjoining sketch, taken from a patient under the care of Mr. Ferguson in the King's College Hospital; it also shows the apparently broad and large, but really wasted and flattened form of the nates.† The effect of

* Kluyskiens, "l'Experience," Oct. 29, 1840. Case of spasmodic affection simu-lating dislocation of the hip.

† It also excellently illustrates the following passage from Brodie, relating to the cause of the *apparent shortening* which succeeds the *lengthening* in the early stage:— In " a few cases, where the patient is in the erect position, it may be observed that

the altered length of the limb in distorting the spine is also seen. Some-

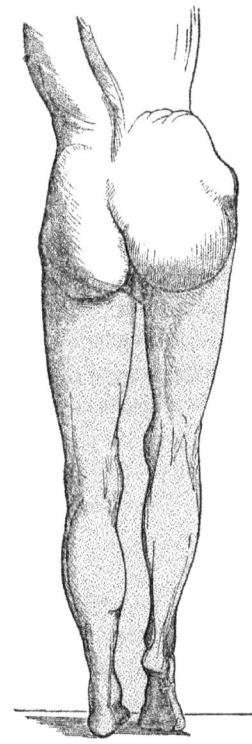

times the limb is turned inwards, as in dislocation on the dorsum ilii; or outwards, as in fracture of the neck of the femur; this is accidental. This organic shortening is usually soon followed by abscess, which may burst on the thigh or the groin, or into the pelvis or rectum; and from this stage it is exceedingly rare for an adult to recover, although, in the case of children, the prognosis is not unfavourable, if the strength is pretty good.

*Diagnosis.*—The ulceration of cartilage may be known from caries of bone by various distinctions, which have been before pointed out. The great pain caused by pressing the femur against the acetabulum will distinguish either disease from sciatica; and they may be distinguished from inflammation of the synovial membrane of the hip by the fact, that the pain in the latter complaint is referred to the upper and inner part of the thigh, and that it is not aggravated by standing on the limb.

*Treatment.*—This must of course be the same in principle as the treatment of other diseased joints. *Perfect rest* must be enforced by a starched bandage, or leather splint, or by confining the patient to a fracture-bed; at all events he should not be permitted constantly to lie on the sound side, otherwise the distortion of the spine, and danger of dislocation, will be enhanced. When the stage of shortening has commenced, great comfort and advantage may often be derived from keeping up constant extension of the limb by means of a weight attached to the thigh above the knee, by a cord which passes over a pulley at the end of the bed. *Cupping* will be of great service in the early stages. But the principal dependence is to be placed on *counter-irritation* by means of an issue behind the great trochanter, or at the anterior edge of the tensor, vaginæ femoris, or by a seton in the groin; and these measures should not be neglected, even though suppuration has commenced. Abscess must be treated in the manner directed for large chronic abscess, at p. 80.

the foot which belongs to the affected limb is not inclined more forward than the other, but that the toes only are in contact with the ground, and the heel raised, at the same time that the hip and knee are a little bent." Op. cit. p. 134.

35

## SECTION VIII.—WOUNDS OF JOINTS.

*Symptoms.*—A wound may often, but not invariably, be known to have penetrated a joint, by the escape of synovia, in the form of small oily globules.

*Treatment.*—The object is to avert acute inflammation of the synovial membrane, which might prove fatal. If, therefore, the part wounded be the knee, and if the skin be torn or injured so that the wound cannot be closed, or so that it is certain not to unite by adhesion, and if the patient's constitution be bad, amputation should be performed at once. Otherwise, the wound should be carefully closed with a piece of lint dipped in blood;—the joint should be kept quite motionless on a splint;—and every local and constitutional measure be adopted, to avert or subdue inflammation.

## SECTION IX.—OF DISLOCATION GENERALLY.

*Symptoms.*—The symptoms of dislocation are two;—(1.) *Deformity;* there being an alteration in the form of the joint;—an unnatural prominence at one part and a depression at another, together with lengthening or shortening of the limb. (2.) Alteration of the mobility of the joint, which is most frequently rendered stiff and motionless.

*Causes.*—Dislocation may be caused by mechanical violence;—or by muscular action. And the circumstances that enable muscular action to produce it are,—a peculiar position, (as when the jaw is very much depressed;)—paralysis of an antagonist set of muscles;—elongation of ligaments;—or fracture or ulceration of some process of bone. Thus ulceration of the acetabulum permits the head of the femur to be dislocated upwards; and fracture of the coronoid process permits the ulna to be dislocated backwards.

*Morbid Anatomy.*—Dislocation is generally attended with rupture of ligaments, which may readily unite and heal by the adhesive inflammation. If the dislocation be left unreduced, the lymph thrown out around the head of the bone in its new situation becomes converted into a new socket and ligaments, and a very useful degree of motion is often acquired. Mean while the old socket gradually becomes filled up.

*Diagnosis.*—Dislocation may be distinguished from fracture, 1. by the *absence of crepitus.* For although a slight *crackling* is often perceptible, owing to an effusion of serum into the cellular tissue, it can hardly be mistaken for the *grating* of fracture. 2. By the circumstance that mobility is *increased in fracture, diminished in dislocation.* 3. By *measurement* of the bone supposed to be broken, which, if broken, will be most probably shortened. 4. By the *patient's age;*—for fractures near joints are most common in the young, dislocations in the adult.

*Treatment.*—The reduction of dislocations may be effected by fixing the part from which the bone has been dislodged;—whilst the dislocated limb is extended in such a manner as to draw the head of the bone into its socket, and in such a position as to relax as many of the opposing muscles as possible. After reduction, leeches, cold, and purging must be used to prevent inflammation, and the joint should be kept at rest till any laceration of its ligaments may have healed, otherwise the dislocation may be perpetually recurring. But it will be necessary, before attempting reduction, to diminish the resistance offered by the muscles, if those which surround the affected joint be large, or if the patient be robust and plethoric. Bleeding to faintness; immersion in a hot bath (100 to 106 F.) for half an hour, and the exhibition of half-grain doses of tartar emetic, are the requisite measures. But they may be often avoided, if the reduction can be effected before the patient has recovered from the faintness consequent on the injury.

COMPOUND DISLOCATION is a dangerous accident, because of the acute synovial inflammation, rapid ulceration of cartilage, and violent constitutional disturbance, with which it is liable to be followed. The necessity of amputation will depend on precisely the same contingencies as in compound fracture;—old age;—bad constitution;—shattering of the bone;—extensive bruising or laceration of the integuments, so that the wound cannot be closed;—laceration of large blood-vessels;—or if it be the knee joint. If the limb is to be saved, the dislocation must be reduced;—if the end of the bone protrude through the skin, and render reduction difficult, it must be sawed off, or the aperture must be slightly dilated;—the wound must then be closed, and covered with a piece of lint dipped in blood;—and the case be treated as a wounded joint.*

SECTION X.—OF PARTICULAR DISLOCATIONS.

I. DISLOCATION OF THE JAW may be caused by a blow on the chin, when the mouth is wide open, or by spasm of the pterygoid muscles,

---

* Dislocations, especial'y of the large joints, sometimes occur from elongation of their capsules and ligaments, the consequence either of impaired nervous power, or of a mild kind of inflammation, whether rheumatic or not, by which, without any evident change in the organization of tissues, their property of resistance becomes so much impaired that they will yield considerably to an extending force.—See remarks and cases by Mr. Stanley, in a paper "On dislocations of the Hip Joints, accompanied by elongation of the Capsules and Ligaments." F.

by which the articular condyles are drawn over the transverse root of the zygomatic process.

*Symptoms.*—The mouth fixedly open;—the chin protruding forwards;—and a prominence felt under the zygomatic process. If one side only is dislocated, the chin will be turned towards the opposite.

*Treatment.*—The surgeon should wrap a napkin around his thumbs, and place them at the roots of the coronoid processes behind the molar teeth;—then he should press them downwards and backwards, elevating the chin at the same time with his fingers. Or he may place the handle of a fork on the last molar teeth, and depress them with it, using the upper teeth as a fulcrum. Or a piece of cork may be put between the molar teeth in order to act as a fulcrum, whilst the chin is elevated. After reduction, the chin must be confined for a week or two by a *four-tailed bandage.*

II. DISLOCATIONS OF THE CLAVIOLE.—The *sternal extremity* of this bone may be dislocated *forwards* by blows on the shoulder. It can readily be felt on the anterior surface of the sternum. The *treatment* is in all respects the same as for fractured clavicle. Dislocation of this end of the bone *backwards* has been caused by curvature of the spine. It has produced so much pressure on the œsophagus as to threaten starvation, and, in consequence, has been extirpated by Mr. Davie of Bungay.

The *outer extremity* of the clavicle may be dislocated *upwards* on the acromion. The shoulder is sunken and flattened; and, on tracing the

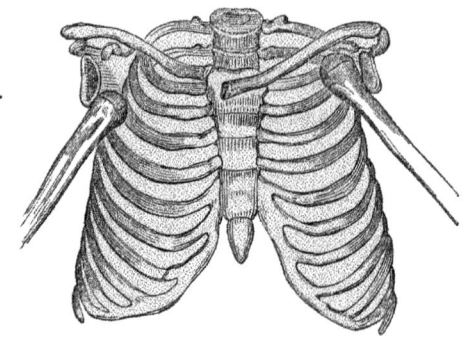

spine of the scapula, the end of the clavicle can be left upon the acromium. The outer extremity of the clavicle has also been known to be dislocated *under* the acromion by a kick from a horse on the shoulder.*

*Treatment.*—Same as for fractured clavicle. The preceding cut is intended to show dislocation of the outer end of the clavicle upwards,

---

* Forbes's Rev. vol. vi.

and of the humerus downwards, on the right side; and dislocation of the sternal end of the clavicle forwards, and of the humerus forwards, on the left side.

III. DISLOCATION OF THE SHOULDER JOINT may occur in four directions. The head of the humerus may be thrown downwards, forwards, and backwards, or may be partially dislocated against the coracoid process.

(1.) In the dislocation *downwards* or *into the axilla*, which is the most common, the head of the bone rests on the axillary plexus of nerves, between the subscapularis muscles and the ribs.

*Symptoms.*—The arm is lengthened;—a hollow may be felt under the acromion, where the head of the bone ought to be;—the shoulder seems flattened;—the elbow sticks out from the side;—and the head of the bone can be felt in the axilla, if the limb be raised; although such an attempt causes great pain and numbness.

*Diagnosis.*—There are three fractures liable to be mistaken for this dislocation: viz. fracture of the *acromion*;—of the *neck of the scapula;*—and of the *neck of the humerus.* The first two may be known by the facility with which the form of the joint is restored by raising the limb, and by the crepitus felt on doing so. In fracture of the *cervix humeri*, the limb is *shortened*, instead of being lengthened as it is in dislocation;—there is not so much vacuity under the acromion;—and the rough angular end of the shaft may be felt in the axilla, instead of the smooth head of the bone.

(2.) In the dislocation *forwards*, the head of the humerus may be felt under the clavicle. The arm is shortened;—the elbow projects backwards;—the acromion seems pointed, and the head of the bone cannot be felt under it.

(3.) In the dislocation *backwards*, the head of the bone may be felt on the dorsum scapulæ; and the elbow projects forwards.

(4.) The head of the bone may be *partially dislocated*, being thrown partly off the glenoid cavity against the coracoid process. The symptoms are, projection of the acromion and a hollow under it, although not so much as after entire dislocation; cramps of the hand, and difficulty of moving the shoulder.

TREATMENT.—There are five methods of reducing the first or downwards form of dislocation.

(1.) By *simple extension.* A jack-towel is to be passed round the chest, both above and below the shoulder, so as to fix the scapula well; this should be held firmly. Another should be fastened round the arm, above the elbow. Extension should then be made by the latter;—the patient sitting on the floor, his elbow being bent, and the humerus being raised and carried forwards, so as to relax the deltoid, supra-spinatus, and biceps muscles. When extension has been made for some minutes, the surgeon should lift the head of the bone, and it will frequently return with a snap.

(2.) The extension may be performed in the same direction with the aid of the *pulleys;*—recollecting always that they are not to be used in order to exert *greater force,* but to exert it *more equably.* A damp bandage should be applied round the elbow to protect the skin before the strap of the pulleys is attached.

(3.) By *the heel in the axilla.* The patient lies down on a bed, and the surgeon sits on the edge. He puts his heel (without his boot) into the axilla, to press the head of the bone upwards and outwards, and at the same time pulls the limb downwards by means of a towel fastened round the elbow.

(4.) According to *Malgaigne's method,* the patient lies down, and the surgeon sits above and behind him;—that is to say, facing the position which is requisite for reduction by the heel in the axilla. The scapula is well fixed, by placing one hand or foot upon the shoulder, or by passing a jack-towel over the shoulder, and fixing it to the opposite corner of the bed;—then the elbow is raised from the side, and drawn straight up by the head, till the bone is thus elevated into its socket.

(5.) By the *knee in the axilla.* The patient being seated in a chair, the surgeon places one of his knees in the axilla, resting the foot on the chair. He then puts one hand on the shoulder to fix the scapula, and. with the other depresses the elbow over his knee.

The dislocation *forwards* may be reduced by the *heel in the axilla,* or by *extension* with the jack-towel or pulley. But the extension must be made in a direction downwards and backwards. For the dislocation backwards, extension should be made forwards. The partial dislocation forwards may be reduced by simple extension.

After reduction a pad should be placed in the axilla, and the arm and shoulder be confined for some days with a figure of 8 bandage, a few turns of which should confine the arm to the trunk. Warm fomentations —perhaps leeches—and subsequently frictions, will relieve the pain and swelling. The more weak and flabby the patient, or the oftener the dislocation has occurred, the longer will confinement be necessary, in order to allow of a complete consolidation of the ruptured ligament. In fact, when the dislocation has occurred more than twice, an apparatus consisting of a clavicle bandage, with a broad band round the head of the humerus, should be worn for some months, so as to restrain the motions of the joint.

It has been before directed that this and all other dislocations should be reduced as soon as possible after the injury. If the reduction has been delayed till the muscles have fixed the part, and the patient is robust, it will be necessary to bleed or administer tartar emetic, and to make a long, slow, and gentle, but unremitting extension by the pulleys.

When the extension has been continued some time, the surgeon may gently rotate the limb by the fore-arm, or lift the head of the bone; and during the whole operation the patient's attention should be diverted as much as possible to other objects. If the dislocation has lasted some time, there will be still greater necessity for a preparatory bleeding, purging, and the warm bath, and for a tedious operation. Sir A. Cooper's opinion is, that a reduction ought not to be attempted after three months.

IV. DISLOCATION OF THE ELBOW presents six varieties. Both radius and ulna may be dislocated, (1) Simply backwards; or (2) backwards and inwards; or (3) backwards and outwards. (4) The ulna by itself may be dislocated backwards;—and the radius by itself either (5) backwards, or (6) forwards.

(1.) When both radius and ulna are dislocated *backwards*, the elbow is bent at a right angle, and is immoveable. The olecranon projects much behind;—a hollow can be felt at each side of it, corresponding to the greater sigmoid cavity;—and the trochlea of the humerus forms a hard protuberance in front. The conoroid process rests in that fossa of the humerus which naturally contains the olecranon.

(2.) In dislocation of *both bones backwards and outwards*, the coronoid process is thrown behind the external condyle; and in addition to the preceding symptoms, the head of the radius can be very plainly felt on the outer side of the joint.

(3.) The dislocation *backwards and inwards* is known by a great projection of the outer condyle, in addition to the symptoms of the first variety.

(4.) In *dislocation backwards* of the *ulna solely*, the olecranon is much projected backwards;—the elbow is immoveably bent at right angles, and the fore-arm is much twisted and pronated.

The *treatment* of these four varieties is the same. Reduction may be effected, *first*, by fixing the lower end of the humerus whilst the fore-arm is drawn forwards; or *secondly*, the surgeon may bend the elbow forcibly over his knee; or *thirdly*, (if the case be quite recent,) he may forcibly straighten the arm, so as to make the tendon of the biceps pull the *trochlea* of the humerus back into its place.

(5.) The head of the *radius alone* may be *dislocated forwards*, being thrown against the external condyle. The hand is prone, the elbow slightly bent, and, in bending it more, the head of the radius can be felt to strike against the front of the humerus. *Treatment.*—Simple extension from the hand, the elbow being straight.

6. Dislocation of the *radius backwards* is very rare. The head of the bone can be felt behind the outer condyle. *Reduced* by simply bending the arm, which should be kept bent for three weeks.

*Diognosis.*—These dislocations of the elbow may be readily distinguished from fractures, (1) by the impaired mobility of the joint, and by the absence of crepitus; (2) by measuring the length of the humerus from its condyles to the shoulder;—which, in dislocation, will be equal to that of the sound limb, but will be diminished in fracture of the lower extremity of the humerus.

·V. DISLOCATIONS OF THE WRIST may readily be distinguished by the altered position of the hand, which is thrown either backwards or forwards if both bones be dislocated, or twisted if one only be displaced,— and by the alteration of the natural relative position of the styloid processes of the radius and ulna with the bones of the carpus. They are seldom unaccompanied by fracture of the lower extremity of the radius. They are reduced by simple extension.

VI. DISLOCATIONS OF THE HAND.—The *os magnum* and *os cuneiforme* are sometimes partially dislocated through relaxation of their ligaments, and form projections at the back of the hand, which must not be mistaken for ganglia. *Treatment.*—Cold affusion, friction and mechanical support.

Dislocations of the *thumb, fingers,* and *toes,* are difficult of reduction in consequence of the strength and tightness of their lateral ligaments,

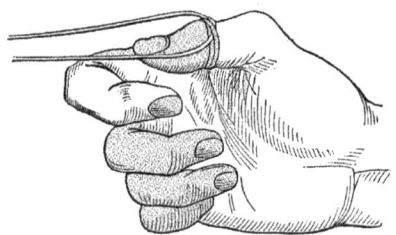

and the small size of the part from which extension can be made. A firm hold may be obtained by means of a piece of tape fastened with the knot called the *clove hitch,* represented in this figure. Extension should be made towards the palm, so as to relax the flexor muscles. · But " before the reduction has been effected," says Mr. Liston, " it has been in some cases even found necessary to divide one of the ligaments; the external is most easily reached; it is cut across by introducing a narrowbladed and lancet-pointed knife through the skin at some distance, and directing its edge against the resisting part."

VII.—DISLOCATIONS OF THE RIBS.—The costal cartilages may be torn from the extremity of the ribs, or from the sternum;—and the posterior extremity of the ribs may be dislocated from the spine by falls on the back; but these accidents are very rare. Any displacement must be rectified if possible, and the same local and constitutional treatment be adopted that was prescribed for fracture.

VIII.—DISLOCATIONS OF THE HIP JOINT may occur in four directions;—besides two others that are exceedingly rare.

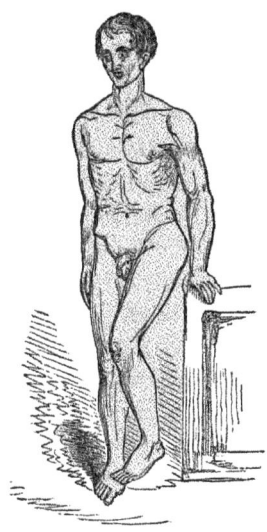

1. Dislocation *upwards on the dorsum ilii* is most frequent. *Symptoms.*—The limb is from an inch and a half to two inches and a half shorter than the other;—the toes rest on the opposite instep;—the knee is turned inwards, and is a little advanced upon the other; —the limb can be slightly bent across the other, but cannot be moved outwards; the trochanter is less prominent than the other, and nearer the spine of the ilium;—and if the patient is thin, and there is no swelling, the head of the bone can be felt in its new situation.

*Diagnosis.*—Fracture of the *cervix femoris* may be distinguished from this dislocation by the greater *mobility*, and by the limb being *turned outwards*, and by *extension*, which restores it to its proper length.

*Treatment.*—In the first place, it will be requisite to diminish the force of the muscles by means that have been already mentioned. Then the patient being placed on his back, his pelvis should be fixed by a strong girth or towel passed between the pudendum and thigh, and fixed to a wall or post. A linen roller should next be applied to the lower part of the thigh, and over it the strap belonging to the pulleys;— which last are to be fixed to the wall or some other firm object. Then

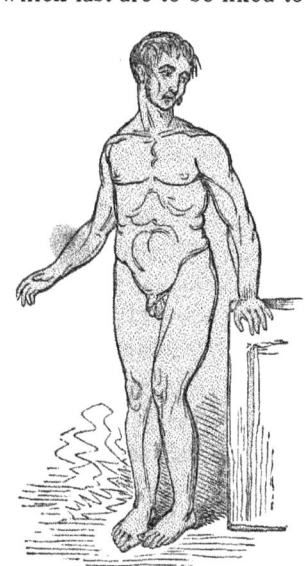

extension is to be made in such a direction as *to draw the thigh across the opposite, a little above the knee.* After a little time, the surgeon should gently rotate the limb, or lift the upper part of it, and the head of the bone will probably return to the acetabulum. The patient should then be carefully moved to bed with his thighs tied together.

2. The dislocation *backwards* (in which the head of the femur is thrown *into the sciatic notch,* or on the *pyriformis*) is known by the following symptoms. The limb is shortened from half an inch to an inch:—the toes rest on the ball of the great toe of the other foot;—the knee is advanced and turned inwards, but not so much as in the last case; the trochanter is rather behind its natural position, and the head of the bone can scarcely be felt. *Treatment.*—Pulleys are required, as in the last case; but the patient should be placed on his side, and the

36

limb be drawn across the middle of the opposite thigh. After a little while the upper part of the limb should be lifted by means of a napkin, so as to raise the head of the bone over the edge of the acetabulum.

3. In the dislocation *downwards*, the head of the bone is thrown into the *thyroid foramen*, or on the *obturator externus*. The *symptoms* are as follow:—the limb is lengthened one or two inches;—it is drawn away from the other;—the toes point downwards and directly forwards;—and the body is bent forwards, because the psoas muscle is on the stretch. *Treatment.*—The object is to draw the head of the bone outwards, and rather upwards. There are two methods of effecting this. In the first place, the patient may be laid on his back on a bed, with one of the bed-posts

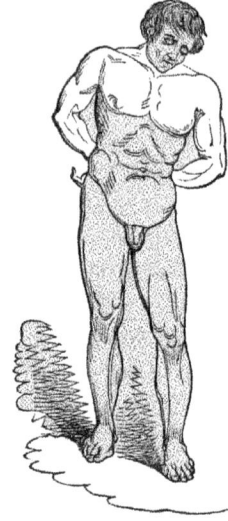

between his thighs, and close up to the peri-næum. Then the foot may be carried inwards, across the median line;—so that the bed-post, acting as a fulcrum, may throw the head of the femur outwards. But the foot must not be *raised*, otherwise the head of the femur may slip round under the acetabulum into the sciatic notch. (2.) Or the pelvis may be fixed by straps, and the pulleys be applied to the upper part of the thigh, to draw it outwards: whilst the knee is at the same time pulled downwards and inwards.

4. In dislocation *upwards and forwards*, (on the pubes,) the limb is shortened about an inch;—it is drawn away from the other, and the foot points directly outwards; the head of the bone may be plainly felt below Poupart's ligament;—and by this circumstance this dislocation may be distinguished from fracture of the cervix femoris. *Treatment.*—The patient is to be laid on the sound side;—extension should be made with the pulleys in a direction backwards and outwards;—and after it has been continued a little time, the head of the bone should be lifted over the edge of the acetabulum by means of a napkin.

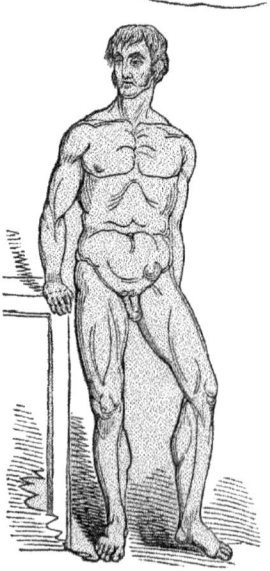

Besides these, a dislocation directly upwards, and one directly downwards, have been known to occur, although very rarely. In a case of dislocation directly downwards, recorded by Mr. Keate, the limb was lengthened three inches and a half, and was fixed and everted; the trochanter was sunk; and the head of the bone, close to and on a level with the tuberosity of the ischium, where it was capable of being moved under the finger. In a case of dislocation directly upwards, that was examined by Mr. Travers jun. some time after the accident, the limb was completely everted and slightly moveable; and the neck of the bone lay between the two anterior spinous process of the ilium; so that when the patient was erect, the limb seemed to be slung or suspended from this point. The diagnosis must in such cases be guided by an attentive examination of the deformity that is present, and by the absence of any symptoms of fracture.*

Sir Astley Cooper has decided that eight weeks is the latest period after which it is justifiable to attempt the reduction of a dislocated hip, except in persons of extremely relaxed fibre or of advanced age; and numerous instances are on record of death from abscesses or phlebitis, occasioned by violent extension at a later period.

IX. DISLOCATION OF THE KNEE.—Dislocation of the *tibia from the femur* is not very common; and when it does occur, is rarely complete. In most cases the tibia is thrown backwards towards the ham. The deformity and impediment to motion will enable the practitioner to distinguish the accident;—and if there be no complication requiring amputation, the displacement must be rectified by simple extension, and the knee be kept at rest till inflammatory symptoms have subsided.

*Dislocation of the patella* may occur either inwards or outwards; more frequently the latter. The symptoms are, that the knee cannot be bent, and that the bone can be felt in its new situation. This dislocation may be caused either by mechanical violence, or by a sudden contraction of the extensors of the thigh.† There is, in general, no difficulty in reducing it by means of the finger and thumb, if the knee is straight and the leg raised. A case is recorded, however, in which the patella was turned round, so that its inner edge rested on the outside of the trochlea of the femur, and its outer edge was immediately under the skin. The surgeon was unable to reduce it by any means, even although he divided the extensor tendon; and the patient died in eleven months, in consequence of his wounding the joint. Mr. Mayo relates a similar case, in

* Vide a paper on Rare Dislocations of the Hip-joint, in the Med. Chir. Trans. vol. xx. by Mr. Travers jun.

† As some surgeons appear to be skeptical as to the existence of this accident, it may be expedient to subjoin the following case. December 6th, 1838. Miss H., aged 22, whilst playing at blind man's buff, fell to the ground. I was immediately sent for, and found her lying on the floor, faint and sick, and complaining of a most excruciating pain in the left knee. On examination I found the patella partially dislocated towards the outer side, and easily replaced it, which produced immediate relief: but the patient was confined for a fortnight with acute inflammation of the joint.

which he succeeded in overcoming the difficulty by bending the knee to the utmost, so that the patella was drawn out of the groove in which it was lodged.

The patella is dislocated upwards after rupture of the tendon by the extensor muscles. This must be treated as fracture of the patella.

X. DISLOCATION OF THE ANKLE may occur in four directions. (1.) Dislocation of the *tibia inwards* is the most common. It is attended with fracture of the lower third of the fibula, and may be known by the sole of the foot turning outwards;—the inner edge turning downwards;—and great projection of the internal malleolus. (2.) Dislocation of the *tibia and fibula outwards* is attended with fracture of the internal malleolus, and may be known by the sole of the foot turning inwards. In dislocation *forwards*, the foot appears shortened, and the heel lengthened;—in dislocation *backwards*, the reverse. The first and two last of these dislocations are generally attended with fracture of the fibula, a little above the external malleolus; but this is not invariably the case.

*Treatment.*—The patient must be laid on the affected side, and the knee must be bent, (to relax the gastrocnemius,) and be firmly held by an assistant. The surgeon must then grasp the instep with one hand, and the heel with the other, and make extension, (aided by pressure on the end of the tibia,) till he has restored the natural shape and mobility of the parts. Then the limb must be *put up* with a short splint or starched bandage, in the same manner as a fracture of the lower part of the leg, taking care to keep the great toe in its proper line with the patella. Vide p. 261.

*Compound dislocation of the ankle* must be treated according to the rules laid down for the general treatment of compound dislocation. The necessity of amputation must also be estimated by the same rules. If the end of the tibia protrude, and its reduction be difficult, or if it be fractured obliquely, it had better be sawn off. This measure, by shortening the limb, diminishes muscular spasm, and prevents the constitutional irritation arising from ulceration of the cartilage.

XI. DISLOCATIONS OF THE FOOT.—The tarsal bones may be dislocated from each other in various ways. The astragalus may be thrown either inwards or outwards;—moreover it has been known to be completely shot out from under the tibia, and under these circumstances has sloughed out, or has been dissected out by the surgeon, leaving the limb tolerably useful. The five anterior tarsal bones may be dislocated from the os calcis and astragalus. The os cuneiforme internum may be dislocated upwards by the tibialis anticus muscle—the metatarsal bones from the tarsal, and the toes from the metatarsal. In any of these cases, the proper position of the parts must be restored as much as possible by pressure and extension, and be preserved by bandages; but reduction will often be very difficult, if not impossible.

# CHAPTER VII.

## OF INJURIES AND DISEASES OF ARTERIES.

SECTION I.—OF WOUNDS OF ARTERIES.

SYMPTOMS.—An artery may be known to be wounded by the flow of blood;—which is profuse;—of a florid colour,—and ejected *per saltum;*— that is to say, in repeated jets, corresponding to each beat of the pulse.

PATHOLOGY.—It must be evident that the bleeding from wounded arteries must necessarily be profuse and dangerous, because from the nature of their coats they remain open and patulous, and do not collapse as the veins do; and because of the perpetual current of blood impelled by the heart. Hence it is important at first to study the means by which arterial hæmorrhage is arrested, and those by which the wound is permanently closed; as well as the different effects of different kinds of wounds.

There are four processes employed by nature for the temporary suppression of arterial hæmorrhage. In the first place, the divided orifice *contracts* more or less; and 2ndly, it *retracts* into its cellular sheath. The 3rd process is the *coagulation* of the blood in the arterial sheath and in the wound, thus obstructing the farther exit of blood; and 4thly, there is the faintness induced by hæmorrhage, which both checks the current of blood from the heart, and gives the blood an increased disposition to coagulate.

Now if a *very large* artery, such as the femoral or subclavian, is wounded, and if the aperture in it is large, and the flow of blood is in no manner opposed, the loss of blood will be so rapid as to occasion death almost instantaneously. But if the wound in the artery is very small it may be closed firmly by coagulated blood during syncope, and the patient may survive.*

If the artery is of the second order, as the humeral or tibial, the bleeding will most probably cease for a time through the influence of the four processes that we have just spoken of. But in the course of some hours, when the faintness has passed off, the coagula in the orifice of the vessel will most probably be dislodged by the recovered impulse of the heart's action, and the bleeding will recur again and again, so that the

* A Case is quoted in Forbes' Rev. vol. vii. p. 254, in which a patient lived a year after a wound in the ascending aorta.

patient will very likely die of it, unless it be checked by art. In some cases, however, the orifice of the vessel may become permanently closed in the way that we shall mention directly.

If the wounded artery is small, as the digital or temporal, the hæmorrhage, though pretty brisk for a time, will generally soon cease spontaneously and permanently in the following manner.

Supposing the artery to have been *completely divided;* its orifices will *contract,* and will *retract* into the sheath, which also will be plugged with coagula. Thus then the bleeding is checked for the time. But shortly the adhesive inflammation is set up;—a yellowish green, tough lymph is effused, and fills up the contracted orifice of the vessel;—that part of the artery which intervenes between the wound and the nearest branch, gradually contracts in the shape of the neck of a champagne bottle;—the blood coagulates within it, adheres to its internal surface, and becomes organized into a cellulo-fibrous tissue;—and, finally, the impervious portion of the artery degenerates into a fibrous cord, and is gradually absorbed.

It must be evident that a *puncture or partial division* of an artery, is much more dangerous than complete division; because the two principal natural means of arresting hæmorrhage,—namely, the *contraction* and *retraction,* are prevented;—and the bleeding can only be obstructed by the coagulated blood in the wound. Under these circumstances, three things may happen. In the first place the aperture, if longitudinal or very small, may in favourable cases be closed by the adhesive inflammation, the artery remaining pervious. The uniting lymph, however, is very liable to be dilated into a *false aneurism.* Or, secondly, the channel of the artery may be obliterated by lymph or coagulated blood. Or, thirdly, bleeding may recur perpetually, till the undivided part of the vessel ulcerates, or is divided by art. From these details may easily be gathered the reason why, when a small artery has been partially divided, (as the temporal in arteriotomy,) it is judicious to divide it completely.

When an artery is *torn across,* it contracts almost immediately, and becomes quite impervious, so that an arm or leg may be torn off by a shot or by machinery, without any loss of blood from the axillary or tibial arteries. For this reason, there is no hæmorrhage from the umbilical cord of young animals, which is either torn or bitten through by the mother. Lastly, it will be readily seen that division of arteries which are diseased, or which are situated in condensed and inflamed tissues, so that they cannot contract or retract, will be followed by profuse bleeding.

TREATMENT.—The first indication is to stop the flow of blood, until measures can be adopted for arresting it permanently. This may be done by placing a finger on the orifice of the bleeding vessel, or by grasping it between the finger and thumb, if the wound is large and open;—or, by making pressure on the wound itself;—or by pressing the trunk of the artery above, against a bone;—or by applying the *tourniquet;*\* or in default of that, a handkerchief may be passed round the limb, and be twisted tightly with a stick. The *permanent measures* are, ligature—torsion —pressure—cold, and styptics.

LIGATURE.—When a ligature is tied tightly upon an artery, it divides the middle and internal coats, leaving the external or cellular coat enclosed in the knot. Then the following series of phenomena occurs. The cut edges of the internal coats unite by adhesion;—the blood between the point tied and the nearest collateral branch coagulates and adheres to the lining membrane;—the ring of the cellular coat enclosed in the ligature ulcerates;—the ligature comes away in from five to twenty-one days, (sooner or later according to the size of the vessel;)—and, finally, that portion of the artery which is filled with coagulum shrinks into a fibrous cord.

Now it must be observed that the efficacy of the ligature depends on two things. (1st) On the *adhesion of the cut surfaces* of the internal coats of the artery;—and in order to promote this, the *ligature should be small and round*, (*dentists' silk* is the best material,) so as to divide them smoothly and evenly.†

(2ndly) On the *adhesion* and *organization of the blood* in the artery between the part tied and the nearest branch. Now, although the adhesion of the internal coats alone *may* be sufficiently strong to resist the current of blood, and prevent bleeding when the external coat ulcerates and the ligature comes away;—still it must be recollected that the place of this adhesion is close to the ligature;—that the ligature is necessarily removed by ulceration of the cellular coat;—that this ulceration is attended with suppuration;—that owing to this suppuration the adhesion might be broken up,‡—and that consequently it will be expedient to have a long coagulum of blood above the ligature, and to make its adhesion to the artery as firm as possible.

Hence the important rule, *never to tie an artery immediately below a branch;*—and in tying it, to *disturb it as little as possible;*—in order not to tear through the vessels which it receives from its sheath, and on which the nutrition of its coats, and their capabilities for adhesion, depend.

The manner of tying an artery is simple enough. If the wound is large and open, as after an amputation, the orifice will generally be readily seen, and very likely will project a little. It should be taken hold of with a forceps, and be gently drawn out, and then an assistant should tie the

---

\* The tourniquet is described in the chapter on Amputations.

† J. F. D. Jones, M. D, Treatise on Hæmorrhage and the Ligature. Lond. 1805.

‡ Manec says it is always so. On the Ligature of Arteries, translated by Garrick and Copperthwaite. Halifax, 1832.

ligature round it as tightly and smoothly as possible in a double or tre-
ble knot.   If the bleeding orifice cannot be drawn out with the forceps,
it may be transfixed with the *tenaculum;*—but in some cases, where it
is deeply seated or cannot be found, or is contained in a dense consolidated tissue, it is necessary to pass a curved *needle and ligature* through
a considerable thickness of the flesh, and tie it all together.  This, however,
should never be done if it can be avoided.   In all cases where it is possible, the artery alone should be included in the ligature.   After tying, one
end of the ligature should be cut off, and the other be made to hang out
of the wound.

When an artery is completely divided, it is necessary to tie both orifices;—or if it is wounded, but not divided, a ligature must be placed by
an aneurism needle both above and below the wound; after which the
intermediate part may be cut through.   But this is not of much couse-
quence.   It is necessary to observe, that in all cases when it is possible,
*a wounded artery must be tied at the wounded part;*—and not in the
trunk above.   When the wound is not large enough to expose the artery,
it should be lengthened by an incision upwards and downwards;—and it
is better, as Mr. Guthrie insists, to cut even through thick muscles, than
to tie the trunk of the artery above the wound.*   When the artery is
diseased and brittle, the ligature should be large, and not tied so tightly,—
otherwise it may cut through entirely.

2. Torsion is performed by drawing out the vessel, fixing it by a pair
of forceps a quarter of an inch from the end, and then twisting the end
round and round till it will not untwist itself.   There is no English authority for applying this method to large arteries, but it may be useful
enough when many minor vessels bleed after the extirpation of a tumour.

3. Pressure is a means of suppressing hæmorrhage that may be resorted
to when the ligature is either deemed unnecessary, or when it cannot be
applied.   Thus it is applicable to wounded arteries of small size situated
immediately over bones; as the temporal;—or to arteries that cannot be
tied because they lie very deeply; as the external carotid in the parotid
gland;—or to arteries that are so diseased that a ligature will not hold.
The pressure must be confined as much as possible to the bleeding orifice, and should be effected by a *graduated compress*; *i. e.* one composed
of several pieces gradually decreasing in size, the smallest being on the
wound.   It is also a good plan to apply pressure to the course of the
trunk, above the wound.   Moreover, when pressure is to be relied upon,
the whole limb should be securely bandaged from its extremity, in order
to diminish its entire circulation, and it should be placed in a raised
position.   When the palmar arch is wounded, one compress may be
placed on the wound, and another on the back of the hand;—a paper

* Guthrie on Diseases and Injuries of Arteries, p. 254.  Lond. 1830.

knife or strong slip of wood may then be laid on each compress transversely across the hand, and their ends be firmly tied together.

4. COLD is applicable to cases of bleeding from numerous small vessels. If there is a general oozing from a stump after amputation, a cloth dipped in cold water may be twisted over the face of it. *Exposure to cold air* will sometimes suffice to check hæmorrhages from the vagina and rectum.

5. STYPTICS are of various kinds. 1. Some of them check hæmorrhage by opposing a mechanical obstacle to the exit of blood;—as the *agaric*, and other porous substances which entangle it;—2, others act by coagulating the blood;—3, or by causing contraction of the bleeding vessels;—4, or by exciting the adhesive inflammation and formation of granulations. The tinc. ferri. mur.; a saturated solution of alum;—turpentine, and nitrate of silver, are the best.* They are applicable to the same cases as cold and pressure;—that is, when the bleeding vessels are very numerous and small. The *actual cautery*, which is the most potent styptic of all, has two operations. If the iron be *red hot*, it stops bleeding mechanically by burning up the orifices of the vessels, but the bleeding is liable to return when the eschar separates. It is better, therefore, to use the iron at a *black heat*, for then it excites the adhesive inflammation; and is very efficacious for arteries that either cannot be tied, or that are too diseased to hold the ligature. A *pinch with the forceps* will often cause small vessels to cease bleeding. There are certain other methods that have been proposed for obliterating arteries, which act by causing effusion of lymph on their inner surface, and coagulation of blood in them:—such as applying a ligature for a few hours, and then removing it;—or passing needles through them;—but these are not to be depended on.†

*Medical Treatment.* In cases of arterial hæmorrhage, which there is any difficulty in restraining by ligature or otherwise, it will be necessary to keep the patient in the recumbent posture, and on low diet; and to keep down the heart's action by lead, F. 60, henbane, or opium.

SECONDARY HÆMORRHAGE may occur under the following seven circumstances. 1. It often happens that in a few hours after a wound has been bound up, and the patient put to bed and become warm, sundry small arteries bleed. This case is easily managed. The wound must be opened; any vessels must be tied that require it;—the surface should be sponged with cold water, and then be exposed to the air for a few hours. 2. There may be a *general exudation* of blood from a wound, owing to

---

\* Kreasote is one of the best styptics we have. I have known it to be applied to a wound of the finger on a person of the hæmorrhagic diathesis—with the effect of arresting an alarming bleeding which nothing else would staunch. F.

† When the lining membrane of an artery is wounded, or is inflamed in a moderate degree, the blood always has a tendency to coagulate upon it, or to deposite adhesive lymph upon it.

some disorder of the circulation. Its *causes* are described in the chapter on the hæmorrhage, p. 66, and on Gunshot Wounds at p. 144, and the *treatment* at p. 147. 3. Hæmorrhage may occur from *sloughing* of an artery, as also mentioned at page 144. 4. From *ulceration* spreading through the arterial tunics. 5. It may occur from imperfect closure of an artery when a ligature separates. This may be owing to some disease of the vessel, which renders it prone to ulceration; —or to a coarse, thick, ill-applied ligature that has bruised the internal coats instead of cutting them evenly;—or to a disturbance of the artery in its sheath. In the last three cases the only remedy is to cut down upon and tie the bleeding orifice;—or if that cannot be done, or the vessel be too diseased to hold the ligature, and pressure and styptics fail, the trunk must be tied above. 6. Hæmorrhage is apt to come from the lower orifice of a divided artery, if only the upper one has been tied. In this case the blood *wells* out in a continuous stream, but not with the arterial *saltus*;—and it is not quite so florid as that which comes from the other end. 7. Hæmorrhage is likely to occur from either orifice, if the operation for *aneurism* is applied to a wound of an artery;—that is, if the trunk at a distance be tied instead of the wounded parts.\* For these two cases the ligature is the remedy.

THE HÆMORRHAGIC DIATHESIS is a peculiar constitutional defect, which seems to consist in deficient contractility of the arteries. The slightest wound bleeds almost uncontrollably, and life may be lost through the most ordinary surgical operation. If the existence of this diathesis be ascertained, surgeons would do well to refrain from operations with the knife on the individual possessing it. In a case of congenital phymosis, in an individual of this kind, which fell under Mr. Liston's care, he very judiciously employed the ligature instead of the knife. There is a case quoted in Forbes's Brit. and For. Med. Rev., Jan. 1840, of four children who possessed this diathesis. They were born of healthy parents; their skins were white and complexions fair;—they were very subject to fever with ecchymosis; their blood was very fluid, but coagulated in the usual manner; violent coughing easily produced hæmoptysis or epistaxis, and any slight injury caused ecchymosis of the skin. One died at twenty months from biting his tongue; another at eight years from general mucous hæmorrhage, and a third at twelve from epistaxis.

SECTION II.—OF INFLAMMATION OF ARTERIES.†

This is rather an uncommon and obscure disease. There are three

---

\* Guthrie, op. cit. p. 248.

† Guthrie, op. cit. Mayo, Pathol., p. 447. Copland, Dict., art. Arteries; and Hodgson on Diseases and Injuries of Arteries, Lond. 1815, p. 5.

forms of it. 1. *Subacute Arteritis* (*Phlegmonous Arteritis*, Guthrie) is a local form of inflammation, not extending any great distance. It produces redness and thickening of the artery, with effusion of lymph into its cavity, and coagulation of the blood within it. The *symptoms* are, tenderness of the affected artery, with violent pain, numbness, absence of arterial pulsation, and tendency to gangrene, in the parts supplied by it. *Treated* by local and general antiphlogistic measures;— taking care to support the circulation of any part that threatens to slough.

2. *Acute Arteritis* (*Erysipelatous or diffused Arteritis*) has a tendency to spread, and involve the arterial system generally, and to produce rapid suppuration, and it is almost invariably fatal. It may be idiopathic, or may be caused by a wound. It is known by very violent fever, and great throbbing of the arteries; succeeded by symptoms of irritative or typhoid fever; with livid vesications on different parts of the body. If the disease originate in a wound, there will probably be gangrene. *Treatment* must be antiphlogistic, without reducing the patient too low.

In a case of severe and rapidly fatal inflammation of the chest, the aorta was found to participate in the inflammation, and there was an effusion of adherent lymph on its inner surface, nearly blocking up the left subclavian artery. This is believed to be not an uncommon cause of embarrassed circulation towards the close of acute inflammation in the chest.

A curious case is recorded by Mr. Crisp, (Lancet, 1835–6, vol. i. p. 534,) of what seems to be rheumatic arteritis. A girl, aged 22, suffered from violent fever, fainting. profuse perspirations, great pain in the limbs, and tenderness in the course of the arteries. After some days, no pulse could be felt in the axillary from an inch below the clavicle, or in the popliteal. Both feet became gangrenous, especially the left, which was amputated below the knee eight months afterwards; at the time of the operation no pulse could be felt in any of the extremities. Very little blood came from the larger arteries, and that not *per saltum*, but the smaller vessels bled profusely. On examination of the leg, the arteries seemed smaller than natural, but not otherwise diseased.

3. *Chronic Arteritis* may be supposed to be one cause of thickening, softening, and ossification of arteries.

SECTION III.—OF ANEURISM.

DEFINITION.—An aneurism is a sac filled with blood, and communicating with an artery, by the rupture or dilatation of which it has been produced.

VARIETIES.—In the first place, a distinction must be made between *aneurism*, which consists of a dilatation of an artery, for a *part only* of its circumference; and the *general dilatation*, which consists of a bulbous expansion of all the arterial tunics for the whole of their circumference, and which differs from true aneurism in containing no *laminated coagula*.

Then there are three kinds of aneurism. *First*, the *true* aneurism, which consists of a sac formed by one or more of the arterial tunics.[*] *Secondly*, the *false* aneurism, which is formed after a puncture of an artery by a dilatation of the adhesive lymph by which the puncture was united. *Thirdly*, the *diffused* aneurism; which is formed when an artery is lacerated by a fractured bone, or ruptured by a blow, without a wound in the skin; or when an artery is punctured, and the wound in the skin heals up speedily. In either of these cases, the blood escapes into the cellular tissue, which forms the sac of the aneurism. Besides these kinds, authors speak of a *sacculated* aneurism; that is, one which is formed into pouches by an unequal dilatation of their parietes;—and of a dissecting aneurism, that is to say, one in which the blood finds its way between the arterial tunics, and may even open into the artery at another part.

PATHOLOGY.—The formation of aneurism is preceded by some disease of the artery. Its internal coat may be thickened and converted into a hard cartilaginous or a soft pulpy substance. Or there may be a deposite of ætheroma, that is, a thick, soft pultaceous matter like very thick pus, between the internal and middle coats. Or, lastly, there may be a deposite of a brittle calcareous substance (composed of phosphate of lime) in the substance or on the outer surface of the inner tunic. This earthy matter may be deposited in spots, or scales, or rings, or projecting spiculæ; and in the arteries of elderly people is very common.

The most general opinion is, that aneurism generally commences by a laceration of the internal and middle tunics of the artery, when diseased and brittle; but that it may also commence by a dilatation of all three of the tunics at some diseased spot. This is the opinion of Hodgson. Scarpa, however, asserts, "that there is only one form of this disease;—that, namely caused by a rupture of the proper coats of the artery, and an effusion of arterial blood into the cellular sheath which surrounds the ruptured artery."[†] Let the aneurism, however, commence as it may it gradually dilates under the constant pressure of the heart's impulse, and forms a sac, communicating with the trunk of the artery by a distinct rounded opening. It soon becomes lined with coagulated blood,

---

[*] It may be remarked that some authorities call all aneurisms false which do not consist of all three arterial tunics.

[†] Scarpa on Aneurism, by Wishart, Edin. 1808, p. 113.

deposited in distinct concentric laminæ, of which the outer ones are the palest and firmest;—and whether it was originally formed or not of all the three tunics, certain it is, that the two internal ones soon become absorbed and disappear. Sometimes aneurisms commence, by the blood finding its way into small cysts or abscesses that are developed between the coats of the artery.

SYMPTOMS.—If an aneurism be seated in the neck or limbs, it appears as a tumour in the course of an artery, and pulsating with it. If it be small, and not filled with coagulum, pressure on the artery above will render it flaccid, so that it may be emptied by pressure;—and the blood returns into it afterwards with a peculiar vibratory thrill or *bruissement*. The patient will very often say that it commenced after some violent strain, when something appeared to give way. In the chest, an aneurism will be principally known by an unnatural pulsation felt by the patient, and detectable by the stethoscope;—together with symptoms of disordered circulation and respiration. In the abdomen, aneurismal tumour may be felt through the parietes.

DIAGNOSIS.—Tumours situated over arteries, and receiving pulsation from them, may be distinguished from aneurism by noticing, 1st, that they do not pulsate at first, when they are small;—whereas aneurisms do so from their earliest formation. 2ndly, that a tumour may often be lifted up from the artery, and that then it will cease to pulsate. 3rdly, That aneurisms are generally soft at first, and become hard subsequently;—tumours are generally the reverse. 4thly, That tumours *cannot be emptied by pressure;*—and that no alteration is made in their consistence by compressing the artery above. 5thly, *Enlarged lobes of the thyroid gland* may be distinguished from aneurism of the carotid by their slipping up out of the fingers, along with the larynx, in the act of deglutition. 6thly, *Psoas abscess* may be known from aneurism by the precursory pain and weakness in the back; and by its disappearance when the patient lies down.

PROGRESS.—As an aneurism enlarges, its coats become thinner, but are strengthened by the adhesion of the parts around. As the enlargement proceeds, these are gradually absorbed;—bone offers no resistance, but is absorbed as well;—cartilage (especially the intervertebral) is, from its elasticity, longer in yielding; but at last the tumour reaches the skin and distends it. Inflammation succeeds;—the skin becomes red, then livid and vesicated;—and sloughs. When the slough separates, a fatal bleeding ensues;—sometimes in a gush enough to destroy life at once, although more frequently the blood oozes away slowly. But an aneurism may burst into a mucous canal;—or into a serous cavity; (although then the aperture is formed by a laceration, and not by sloughing)—or into a vein, with, of course, a fatal disturbance of the circulation if the vein be large:—or it may cause death by pressure on the trachea or œsophagus, without bursting.

SPONTANEOUS CURE.—In some fortunate cases a spontaneous cure occurs. 1st, It may occur in consequence of the coagulation of the blood contained in the sac, and the conversion of the aneurism into a firm tumour. In some cases, however, the sac does not become quite obliterated, but the coagula become thick and firm enough to resist farther distention. Nature generally endeavours to aid this process by enlarging the collateral circulation, and by setting up the adhesive inflammation so as to thicken the artery and obstruct its current. It has happened that a portion of clot has been detached from the interior of the sac by some accidental violence, and has effected a cure by blocking up the opening into the aneurism. 2ndly, The aneurism has sometimes sloughed, or has been involved in a large abscess; and the artery participating in the inflammation has become obstructed by effusion of lymph, or by coagulation of the blood in it. 3rdly, The artery has become obliterated by an accidental pressure of the aneurism upon it;—or by the pressure of blood escaping from it on its bursting into the cellular tissue, as sometimes happens.

CAUSES.—The *predisposing* cause of aneurism is some constitutional tendency to arterial disease. The *exciting cause* may be, strong emotion of the mind;—violent exertion of the body, or local injury. Men are very much more subject to it than women;—and it is said that sailors, porters, and those who use the upper extremity, are most liable to aneurism of the axillary artery;—but post-boys and others who exert the lower extremity, to poplitæal aneurism. It is most frequent between the ages of thirty and fifty.

TREATMENT.—The indications are to stop the circulation through the aneurism, and to produce coagulation of the blood within it.

*Surgical Treatment.*—If the aneurism throbs painfully, and is rapidly on the increase, and the patient is plethoric, a moderate quantity of blood may be abstracted once or twice; and then, if it can be done, the great measure is, to tie the artery between the aneurism and the heart. The operation should neither be performed too near the aneurism, so as to place the ligature on a portion of the vessel that is diseased;—nor too far from it, lest the circulation through it be kept up by means of collateral branches. After the operation, the temperature of the limb falls two or three degrees;—but in a few hours it rises rather higher than that of the opposite limb, because the blood is forced to circulate through the superficial capillaries. Subsequently it sinks again rather below the natural standard. Therefore the patient should be placed in bed, with his limb in an easy position; wrapped up, to preserve its circulation; and though it become rather swelled, (which is not unlikely,) cold must on no account be applied.

When a ligature cannot be applied between the aneurism and the heart, it has been proposed to tie the vessel on the distal side; and this operation has been performed with success in cases of carotid aneurism, by Mr. Wardrop and others. But Mr. Guthrie shows that this operation does not act as the (Hunterian, or) ligature between the aneurism and the heart does, by stopping the circulation through the aneurism; but by " giving rise to inflammation in the aneurism, and in the artery both above and below it, and that unless it does this, it fails." It is therefore a dangerous and uncertain operation, and should only be performed where the tumour increases rapidly, and cannot be checked by any other means.

After the operation the limb may become gangrenous, in the same manner as described at p. 144. If the gangrene spread beyond the fingers or toes, amputation should be performed above the level of the ligature.

Any other local measures, such as the application of *pressure* to the aneurism, or to the trunk above it,—or of *ice*, may have done good in some cases, but more frequently the reverse.

The *medical treatment* that must be resorted to when no operation can be performed, consists in measures that reduce the heart's action, without lowering the vital energies too much. *Bleeding* may be performed occasionally, if the patient is plethoric, and the tumour increase rapidly, with violent pulsation;—but it should never be carried to faintness. The *diet* should be light. *Bodily or mental exertion* and *fermented liquors* should be rigidly abstained from. Much benefit may be derived from digitalis in moderate doses. But the most useful remedy is the *acetate of lead* given in doses of gr. ½—i ter die, with half that quantity of opium, and a draft containing acetic acid, F. 60, 61. This medicine seems to have the faculty of rendering the blood coagulable, and of diminishing the caliber of the arteries. It used to be mentioned in terms of commendation by Mr. Green in his lectures at King's College, who gave some cases of its efficacy.* But it must be recollected that *frequent bleeding* and too *rigid starvation* will increase the irritability of the heart and arteries, and render the system incapable of forming healthy lymph; and that consequently they will prevent the desired changes in the aneurismal sac. Particular care should be taken not to administer drastic purgatives; because they invariably cause a great excitement and throbbing of the arteries.

DIFFUSED ANEURISM may be caused by rupture or laceration of an artery without a corresponding wound of the skin, so that the blood escapes into the cellular tissue. It is known by a rapid dark-coloured swelling of a limb soon succeeding an injury;—perhaps fluctuating, and

---

* See also a case of aneurism of aorta caused by acetate of lead in large doses, Arch. Gen. de Med., Sept. 1839.

sometimes pulsating, together with coldness, numbness, and absence of pulsation in the parts below. For this, as well for the *false aneurism*, formed by dilatation of the cicatrix of a wounded artery, the operation for ordinary aneurism is inadmissible; but the wounded part must be exposed, and a ligature be placed above and below it, as was directed in a former page.

ANEURISMAL VARIX is produced when an artery is punctured through a vein, and they adhere together, the communication remaining permanent. The vein becomes enlarged and tortuous, and presents a vibrating thrill at each pulse.

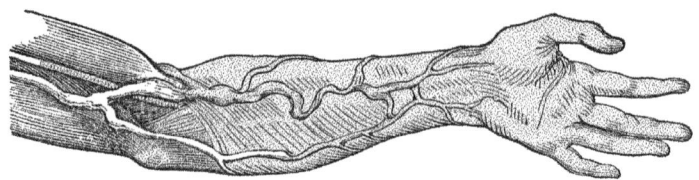

VARICOSE ANEURISM is said to exist, when an artery has been punctured through a vein, and a false aneurism has formed between them, opening into both, and formed of lymph that was effused between them. These two cases need not be interfered with, unless they enlarge rapidly, or cause inconvenience. If they do, a ligature must be placed both above and below the wound of the artery.

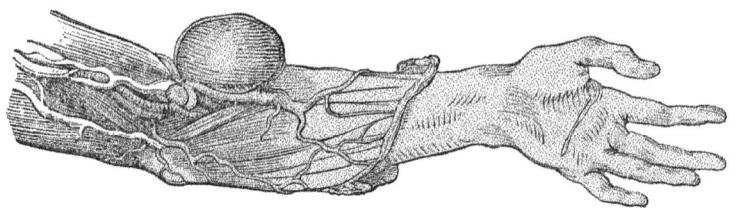

SECTION IV.—OF ANEURISM BY ANASTOMOSIS AND NÆVUS.

ANEURISM BY ANASTOMOSIS is a pulsating tumour, generally situated in the subcutaneous tissue of the head or neck, or sometimes in the orbit. It is formed of several enlarged and tortuous arteries, accompanied with many dilated veins, which feel like a bundle of worms.

NÆVUS is a similar affection, consisting apparently in an enlargement of very many small arteries, which form a kind of erectile tissue. It appears soon after birth as a small red shining spot in the skin. This in many cases remains stationary, and gives no farther trouble; but more commonly it enlarges, and forms a soft, dusky red, and pulsatory tumour, the skin covering which is so exceedingly thin, that profuse bleeding may occur from the slightest abrasion. Nævus may, however, like aneurism by anastomosis, be seated under the skin, which may not be implicated. This affection, like the preceding, may remain long stationary;—or it may ulcerate or slough, and cause the patient's death by repeated hæmorrhage.

The symptoms of large nævi, and of aneurism by anastomosis, are the same. " Some of these tumours," says Mr. Liston, " communicate a thrill to the fingers; they can be emptied to a certain extent by uniform and continued pressure, or by interrupting the circulation, and are instantly filled on permitting the blood again to flow into or towards them. The large ones pulsate synchronous with the heart's action. They are much increased in size by any thing that increases the activity of the circulation; as the cries of children, and the violent exertion of adults. On the application of the stethoscope, pulsation is heard as in common aneurismal tumours, and a sound which differs from that of the common aneurism, being loud, rough, and whizzing, and which being once heard can never be mistaken.

TREATMENT.—The treatment of these affections comprises two kinds of measures—first, such as act by obliterating the distended vessels— secondly, extirpation.

If the red spot of incipient nævus in infants is frequently well rubbed with nitrate of silver, it will very often disappear. If a nævus is small, an attempt may be made to excite the adhesive inflammation in it by performing *vaccination* on its surface,—(which generally fails,)—or by passing a *seton* through it, (taking care that the threads are large enough completely to fill the aperture made by the needle,)—or by *breaking up its substance* with a red-hot needle;—or by *injecting* a weak solution of zinc. sulph. into it by means of Anel's syringe;—or by *pressure*, if it be seated over a bone;—or by the application of the concentrated nitric or sulphuric acids. But all these measures are very uncertain. The seton seems to be the best of them, and may be resorted to when it would be dangerous to attempt extirpation. Moreover, the operation of injecting a nævus with an irritating fluid has been known to cause the instant death of a child by convulsions.

As a general rule, therefore, the entire extirpation of these tumours is the best plan; and it may be done either by the knife or by ligature. If it is done with the knife, two elliptical incisions should be made, to include the whole of the diseased growth, and a little of the sound tissues around. For, to use Mr. Guthrie's words, " it cannot be too forcibly impressed on the mind of the surgeon, that if the diseased part be cut into, the bleeding will be terrific and difficult to stop."

But it is generally considered that the ligature is the safest and best method. The most convenient form of using it is to pass two or three needles crucically through the base of the tumour, and then twist a strong

38

silk ligature firmly round beneath them.    Or instead of this, two or more
double ligatures may be passed through the base of the tumour, with a
curved needle which has its eye at its pointed extremity, and then the
tumour may be strangulated by tying the adjacent threads together.    The
tumour may be punctured before the threads are finally tightened, but in
every case the constriction should be made as tight as possible.    If the
skin is not implicated, it may be dissected back in flaps before the ligatures are passed.

Another method analogous to extirpation, is the division of all the soft
parts around the tumour.    This was once done successfully by Mr. Lawrence, in an aneurism by anastomosis on the finger.    He divided all the
soft parts, except the tendons and thecæ.    But in other cases it has been
unavailing.

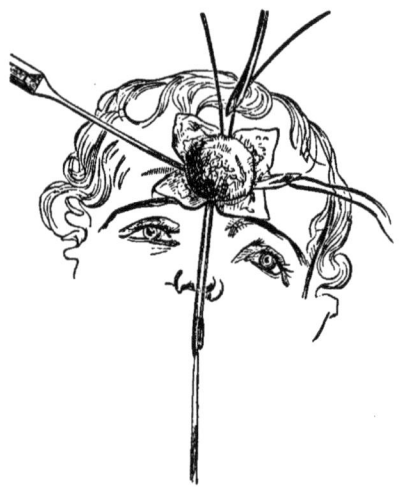

If the disease is inaccessible to any of these means, (as in the orbit,)
and increase rapidly, ligature of the common carotid (or of any other
large trunk supplying it) is the only resource, but it is dangerous and
not often successful.*

* Vide Curling's Pathological Lectures in Med. Gazette, July 1838.   Lawrence,
Med. Chir. Trans. ix. 216; and a fatal case of convulsion during the operation for
nœvus by injection, Med. Gaz. vol. xxi. p. 529.

# CHAPTER VIII.

## OF INJURIES AND DISEASES OF VEINS.

I. Wounds.—The hæmorrhage from wounded veins is not in general dangerous, unless from some large and deep-seated trunk, or from a large varicose vein on the leg. It may in ordinary cases be restrained by pressure and a raised position. But if there is any difficulty in the matter, it will be necessary either to apply a ligature, (which, however, should always be avoided if possible,) or to keep up unremitting pressure on the bleeding point with the finger. The latter practice was resorted to "in the case of his Excellency William Prince of Orange, who, in his hurt by the Spanish boy, as my Lord Bacon relates, when the internal jugular was opened, could find no way to stop the flux of blood, till the orifice of the wound was hard compressed by men's thumbs, succeeding for their ease one after the other, for the space of forty-eight hours, when it was hereby stanched."*

II. Inflammation of Veins, or Phlebitis, is a very important disease, of which there are two forms, the *subacute* and the *acute*. The Subacute Phlebitis is not a very serious disease, and generally affects the veins of the leg, especially if varicose. The *Symptoms* are tenderness and hardness of the affected vein, more or less swelling around it, œdema of the parts below, and painfulness of the limb generally. After it has subsided, the vein is usually felt hard as a cord; because, as was explained in a previous page, inflammation of a blood-vessel causes the blood within to coagulate, which, with the lymph that is effused, renders it impervious. *Treatment.*—Rest, with the limb in an elevated position;—leeches;—fomentations, or cold lotions, according to the patient's choice;—and purgatives;—subsequently, friction with camphorated oil, and bandages. If the limb is very œdematous, it may be punctured with a grooved needle.

III. Acute Phlebitis is a most dangerous, and generally a fatal disease. It is generally caused by wounds of veins,—venesection, for example—if irritated and not permitted to heal; or by tying veins;—more rarely it is caused by bruises and other injuries unattended with an open wound. It is a frequent concomitant of malignant puerperal fever, phlegmonous erysipelas, and diffused cellular inflammation; to which diseases it is remarkably analogous, both in the form of constitutional affection which attends it, and in being frequently caused by confinement in the unhealthy wards of hospitals. Vide p. 84.

* Turner, op. cit, vol. 1. p. 346.

*Symptoms.*—The symptoms are, repeated shiverings, rapidity of the pulse, anxiety of the countenance, and depression of spirits, and more or less swelling and tenderness over the course of the affected veins. In many cases, the tongue soon becomes furred, brown, and dry, or black; the pulse exceedingly rapid and weak; the prostration of strength and spirits extreme; the skin sallow;—then bilious vomiting and low delirium come on, and are followed by death, perhaps in two or three days from the commencement of the attack. In other more protracted cases, great swelling and redness occur over the inflamed veins, and abscess forms, which, if punctured, is found to contain clots of blood mixed with pus. But the most characteristic termination of this disease is the formation of *consecutive abscesses*. The patient remains low, with an anxious sallow countenance, rapid pulse, and yellow tongue; and suddenly complains of excruciating pain in the shoulder, knee, or some other joint, which is rapidly succeeded by a copious formation of pus;—and this abscess is followed by others in the other joints, or in the lungs or liver, which ultimately cause death.

*Pathology.*—At an early period of the disease, the lining membrane of the affected vein is found deeply red, and a little lymph is effused at the seat of injury. Subsequently, the vein is plugged with coagulated blood and lymph, mixed either with real pus, or with pus-like fluid formed of softened coagulum, which was mentioned at p. 69. In cases which do not terminate very early, some portion of the vein is formed into an abscess, by the effusion of lymph above and below the inflamed part; and this abscess soon communicates with the cellular tissue by ulceration. The extreme malignity of the constitutional affection which accompanies this disease, used to be accounted for by supposing that the inflammation travelled along the great veins to the heart. Mr. Arnott, however, in his very elaborate paper on this subject in the 15th volume of the Medico-Chirurgical Transactions, showed that this was a mistake; because the inflammation is generally found to stop abruptly at the juncture of some collateral branch with the inflamed vein. The more probable supposition is, that the whole of the blood is contaminated by contact with the inflamed part, and by admixture with its secretions; and that this contaminated state of the blood is the source of the great constitutional depression, as well as of the *consecutive* abscesses that are so often formed. We may refer to a former page, (72,) where we have shown that these abscesses are not universally to be accounted for by the theory of an absorption and deposition of pus; because (as Sir B. Brodie very fully proved in his Clinical Lectures at St. George's Hospital in 1839) they may occur after injuries which have not given rise to any formation of pus,—as well as in cases such as phlebitis, glanders, or snake-bite, in which pus is copiously formed, and is very probably mixed with the blood.

*Treatment.*—The principal things to be done in this almost hopeless malady are—to apply numerous re-lays of leeches—and fomentations to the part affected—to open all abscesses early—to open the bowels moderately—to allay restlessness and pain;—and to support the strength by nutriment, such as beef-tea and arrow-root. Relief is also generally afforded by a flannel bandage. As to any other measures, stimulating or lowering, they must be employed according to the exigencies of each particular case. *Bleeding* may occasionally be of service when the patient has a robust unimpaired constitution; but in many cases it would only accelerate the fatal issue; nay, excessive bleeding seems occasionally to be a main cause of the disease. *Mercury* may be resorted to generally, unless there is very great depression indeed. *Wine* and bark should be used, if the pulse is very feeble.

IV. Varix signifies an enlarged and tortuous state of the veins, which are generally thickened, rigid, and divided into irregular pouches, with their valves incapable of preventing the reflux of blood. This state may be *caused* by any thing that retards the venous circulation;—such as occupations that require a standing posture; or pressure from loaded bowels or the gravid uterus. It is most frequently *seated* in the lower extremities, scrotum, and rectum.

Varicose veins on the leg produce several troublesome consequences. (1) In the first place, they occasion great pain, weight and fatigue upon taking much exercise, or remaining long in an erect posture. (2) They frequently cause ulcers or excoriation of the skin, as described at p. 96. (3) Sometimes a vein becomes exceedingly thin, and bursts; causing profuse and dangerous hæmorrhage, inasmuch as there might be no valves between the part ruptured and the heart. (4) Occasional inflammation occurs, with clotting of the blood in the affected vein;—which may, perhaps, give rise to abscess.

*Treatment.*—This may either be *palliative* or *radical.* The palliative consists of measures adapted to prevent farther enlargement, and induce contraction of the distended veins. If one or two trunks only are affected, it may be sufficient to apply pieces of leather spread with soap plaster firmly over them;—but if many smaller veins are enlarged, the whole limb should be well supported with a calico or caoutchouc bandage, or laced stocking, which should be applied in the morning before the patient rises. Friction with lin. hydrargyri;—or with iodine ointment;—the application of tincture of iodine, repeated blisters, and electric sparks, have been supposed to accelerate the cure. Constipation should always be provided against; and when the patient is not taking exercise, the leg should be placed in a raised position.

But if these means fail, and the patient is subject to urgent inconvenience, the radical cure must be resorted to; that is to say, the diseased veins must be obliterated; and there are three methods of doing it. (1) *Bro-*

*die's plan.* A long curved, narrow-pointed knife, like a bistoury, but cutting on the convex edge, is introduced by the side of the vein, and carried horizontally with its flat surface between it and the skin. Then the convex edge is turned towards the vein, in order to cut through it, as the knife is being withdrawn. (2) By *caustic*, after the method introduced by Mr. Cartwright, and improved by Mr. Mayo. A very narrow slip of skin, across the vein, is destroyed by means of a paste of potassa fusa and quicklime. This will most probably cause *subacute inflammation* of about an inch of the vein, with coagulation of the blood and obliteration of its canal for the same extent.

(3.) By the *needle.* Three or four fine needles, such as are represented at p. 130, are to be introduced at three or four places, either altogether behind the vein—or else through both coats, so as to transfix them once or twice—the latter way is the best. Then a piece of silk is to be twisted round each needle with moderate tightness, after the manner of the twisted suture, and the points of the needles are to be cut off. The effects of this proceeding will be, that the circulation through the vein will be obstructed, and its lining membrane *subacutely* inflamed by the pressure of the ligature. Subacute inflammation of a blood-vessel has been more than once shown to be followed by coagulation of the blood within it, and adhesion of the clot to its parietes; which will of course obliterate the vein. The needles may be withdrawn as soon as the vein becomes hard and painful;—the patient should of course be confined to his bed during the process. But it sometimes happens, as M. Bonnet has particularly shown, that an obliteration caused by the mere adhesion and organization of coagulum is ineffectual, because the coagulum is reabsorbed; which may render it necessary to divide the vein, either by the knife, or by a second application of caustic after the slough formed on Mr. Mayo's plan has separated, or by applying the ligature over the needles so tightly that the vein may be divided by ulceration.*

* Arnott in Med. Chir. Trans., vol. xv. Lee, ibid. Mayo, Pathol.; Copland and others in Med. Gaz., July and August 1838. Bonnet, quoted in Brit. and For. Med. Rev., Jan. 1840.

# CHAPTER IX.

## OF INJURIES AND DISEASES OF THE NERVES.

I. COMPLETE DIVISION of a nerve is attended with palsy and loss of sensibility in the parts which it supplies. The nerve, however, will readily unite in the same manner as bone or tendon, and sensibility and motion will return. Sensibility has begun to return in three weeks, and the power of motion in four weeks after division. A nerve may also recover its functions after a small piece of it has been removed. Sometimes, however, the divided ends, instead of uniting, shrink and become bulbous, as they do in a stump after amputation.

II. PARTIAL DIVISION.—If a nerve is partly divided, leaving some fibres on the stretch, as sometimes happens in venesection, very disagreeable consequences may ensue; such as immediate severe pain, recurring in paroxysms, and shooting in the course of the nerves; violent spasms, or palsy of the limb;—fits of epilepsy;—and great disorder of the digestive organs. The same symptoms may also ensue if a nerve have been bruised, or compressed, or stretched;—or if it have been divided, and its extremity have become implicated and compressed in a cicatrix. This not unfrequently happens after amputation, and produces excruciating pain, with spasm and retraction of the muscles of the stump, causing it to become conical. *Treatment.*—If these symptoms come on *immediately* after a wound, so that it is probable that a nerve has been partly divided, an incision may be made so as to divide it completely. If, however, they appeared whilst a wound was healing, it is the best plan to remove the cicatrix entirely. But it unfortunately happens, that neuralgic pains, though produced by a local exciting cause, do not always cease on its removal. Very disagreeable consequences, in the shape of palsy, or numbness, or spasm, sometimes ensue, if a nerve is subjected to pressure—as for instance, the pressure of crutches on the axillary nerves—or to a blow, such as people often meet with on the ulnar nerve above the elbow;—or to a violent stretch. Leeches, blisters, and the application of mercurial or tartar emetic ointment, are the chief remedies.

III. INFLAMMATION OF NERVES is known by pain and tenderness, with fever if acute. *Sciatica* is an example of rheumatic inflammation of the sciatic nerve. The local and general treatment must be antiphlogistic, according to circumstances.

IV. TUMOURS in nerves may produce every local and general symptom of nervous irritation. The *painful subcutaneous tumour* is one instance. Iodine, counter-irritation, and the other means of exciting absorption, may be tried;—but if they fail, as they most likely will, the tumour must be extirpated, provided that it be not intimately embedded in the substance of a large nerve such as the sciatic, the division of which would paralyze a limb.

V. NEURALGIA, or TIC DOULOUREUX.—This affection may be *defined* to be severe pain affecting the nerves, not necessarily produced by organic lesion. It occurs in paroxysms of very severe pain, mostly of a plunging, lancinating character, shooting in the course of the nerves. It most frequently attacks persons of middle age, female sex, and comfortable circumstances.

*Causes.*—The exciting causes may be of two orders. (1.) There are some which act upon the nerve that is the seat of pain. Thus neuralgia may be produced by wounds and other injuries, as before related;—by tumors;— by spiculæ of bone pressing on the nerve, (which is a frequent cause of facial neuralgia;) or by some disease in the brain or spinal cord at its origin.

(2.) It may be caused *sympathetically* by influences that act upon distant parts, or on the system at large;—as, for instance, by loss of blood and debility;—by wet and cold;—by irritation of the skin from eruptions or wounds;—by carious teeth;—by disorders of the alimentary canal;— sometimes by diseases of the urinary or other internal organs;—lastly, by *malaria.* When arising from malaria, it is generally *intermittent,* like other diseases arising from the same source, and occurs at regular intervals. But all intermittent neuralgia is not necessarily caused by malaria; because this as well as other nervous affections, may occur only at stated periods, although caused by a local source of irritation that is permanent.

The *nature* of the complaint is apparently *functional* derangement. The suddenness of its accession and departure,—and the absence of organic change in nerves that have been affected for years, prove that it is not essentially inflammatory;—although inflammation of a nerve, when existing, may doubtless be an exciting cause.

The most common forms of neuralgia are,—the *Supraorbital Neuralgia, Brow Ague* or *hemicrania,* which is usually caused by malaria;—neuralgia of the *superior* and *inferior maxillary* nerves, which is often caused by diseased teeth, or disease of the bony canals through which those nerves pass;—and neuralgia of the ear, mamma, and testicle, which will be treated of elsewhere; it may also attack the extremities, or any internal organ.

*Treatment.*—The *indications* are three. *First,* to remove all local sources of irritation; *secondly,* to amend any disorder of the constitution that can be detected; *thirdly,* to palliate pain.

In the *first* place, therefore, the whole course of the affected nerve, should be thoroughly examined, and if there be a cicatrix, or tumour, or wound—or a carious tooth; or an abscess, or ulcer, or hernia, or aneurism, measures should be taken for their removal. In cases of neuralgia of the extremities, if there is any tenderness, or other reason for suspecting inflammation of the nerve or its sheath, leeches and blisters, followed by liniments, (especially F. 24,) or tartar emetic ointment applied in the course of the nerve, combined with proper constitutional remedies, may effect a cure. The head, and particularly the spine, should be well scrutinized; and if any pain or tenderness, or other genuine sign of congestion or disease, is detected, it should be removed by cupping, the warm bath, and blisters, or the tartar emetic ointment.

*Secondly.* The state of the constitution must be regulated in the same manner as was directed in the treatment of chronic inflammation. If there be paleness of the lips, emaciation, and debility, iron, bark, and other tonics may probably be given with advantage. Inquiry should always be made in these cases for piles, menorrhagia, or other weakening ailments. On the other hand, bleeding and low diet have cured cases attended with hard full pulse and plethora. In all cases, the appetite, the tongue, the biliary and alvine secretions, and the state of the uterine system, should be investigated. In the brow ague and other cases arising from malaria, quinine should be freely administered; and if it fails, the liq. arsenicalis, or the extract of nux vomica, in doses of gr. $\frac{1}{4}$ ter die, may be tried. In cases of a rheumatic or gouty character, colchicum, F. 96, will be of service. But all lowering remedies, and especially mercury, should be used with the utmost care and hesitation.

*Thirdly;* but if no cause whatever can be detected;—or if detected it cannot be removed;— or if, as frequently happens, even though removed, its removal fail to cure the disease, an *empirical* and *palliative* plan of treatment is the only resource. A course of *purgatives; tonics,* especially the carbonate of iron, and oxyde or sulphate of zinc; *mercurials; sarsaparilla; valerian* and other *fetid stimulants; narcotics;* any remedies, in fact, that have been known to do good, may be tried in succession; taking care, however, not to impair the constitution by giving them at random. Opium, morphia, hyoscyamus, belladonna, conium, stramonium, or prussic acid, given internally; friction with ointments, or alcoholic solutions of veratria, strychnia, or aconitina ($\mathfrak{z}$ss ad $\mathfrak{z}$i)—sprinkling gr. $\frac{1}{4}$—two-thirds of morphia or strychnia, on a newly blistered surface; or inoculating it under the cuticle—galvanism, acupuncture, issues, or the moxa, generally afford some relief, and sometimes completely cure. *Division of the nerve,* with or without *excision* of a portion, is the last resource. It produces instant ease;—which, however, lasts but a short time; and the oftener it is repeated, the more transient are its effects.

39

Sometimes, after repeated division, the pain is as severe as ever, although the part may be quite numb and insensible.

VI. ANOMALOUS NERVOUS AFFECTIONS.—The same local and constitutional causes that give rise to neuralgia, may also occasion every other symptom that can be produced by functional nervous disorder; such as rigid and permanent spasm, (as in wry-neck) or twitching and convulsion of muscles;—difficulty of swallowing and performing evacuations, owing to spasm of the œsophagus, of the sphincter ani, or of the perineal muscles;—sneezing, dumbness, stammering, thirst, and affections of the sight and hearing. The treatment must be conducted on the same principles.

VII. HYSTERICAL NEURALGIA.—Hysterical females are liable to suffer from various obstinate maladies which simulate serious organic disease. In particular they are exceedingly subject to severe and permanent pain and tenderness of the joints; (especially the knee or hip;) with weakness of the limb, and inability to use it;—or to pain and tenderness of the spine, with perhaps spasms, or weakness of the legs, tympanites of the belly, and palsy of the bladder;—symptoms, in fact, of ulcerative disease of joints or spine, that might mislead careless practitioners; more particularly as they are often attributed to some injury. These cases may be known by observing that the patients are young females, perhaps newly married, most likely (but not invariably) subject to irregular menstruation, torpid bowels, and coldness of the extremities;—or perhaps to well marked fits of hysteria. Not uncommonly some intimate friend has laboured under a similar complaint just previously. The pain is greatly aggravated by motion or pressure;—but it seems to be principally seated in the skin; and the patient shrinks from the least touch;—whilst, if her attention be engaged elsewhere, a somewhat rude examination may be made without complaint. The pain often prevents the patient from sleeping, but once asleep, she may continue so for hours. There may be some degree of swelling, but it is puffy and diffused,—and comes and goes capriciously. These complaints may last many years in defiance of all treatment, and then may vanish suddenly without assignable cause;—or perhaps from some strong impression on the nerves,—fright or fanaticism. Sometimes the patient labours under an obstinate contraction of some joint; perhaps the hip, or the finger; which very likely goes off quite suddenly, and transfers itself to another joint.

*Treatment.*—Any detectable disorder of the digestive or uterine systems should be removed. The patient should have fresh air, generous living, and plenty of occupation for body and mind; she should be encouraged to take exercise, notwithstanding pain and weakness; and to resume as far as possible the habits of a healthy person. The shower bath;—the mistura ferri, or the ammonio chloride in doses of gr. ii.; the sulphate of zinc in small doses with ext. anthemidis—or the ammonio sulphate of copper in doses of gr. ⅛ ter die, may be given with benefit if the circulation is languid; and quinine may be of use if the pain is periodic. The bowels should be kept open by nightly doses of the warmer aperients, such as aloes, or colocynth, with assafœtida, cajuput oil, or the compound galbanum pill. Acidity of the stomach must be counteracted by soda or magnesia; and inaction of the liver by occasional doses of the blue pill. Deficiency or excess in menstruation should be properly looked after. " Sometimes," observes Sir B. Brodie, " the symptoms have abated under the use of active purgatives; or of valerian combined with bark and ammonia, or of injections of assafœtida." F. 96 is one of his prescriptions for these cases. He also recommends warm fomentations; especially one composed of sp. rosmarin. ℥iss and mist. camph. ℥viss, or of lin. camph. ℥iv, with ext. belladon. ʒii. Occasional leeching may be of service, but counter-irritants should be avoided. If the limb at any time become very hot, it should be sponged with tepid lotions;—but if cold, it should be wrapped up warmly in flannel and oiled silk.* Amputation in these cases is useless and cruel.

# CHAPTER X.

## OF INJURIES OF THE HEAD.

### SECTION I.—WOUNDS OF THE SCALP.

Wounds and contusions of the scalp, be they ever so slight, are not to be neglected. For they may be followed by erysipelas;—or by inflammation and suppuration under the occipito-frontalis, or within the cranium, that might easily prove fatal. It may be observed, that sutures are generally inexpedient;—that although there be considerable arterial hæmorrhage, ligatures should be avoided, if it can be restrained by pressure;—that if a flap of the scalp is nearly or even quite detached, it should be carefully washed, and returned to its place, avoiding sutures and pressure by bandages and plasters;—that if a blow on the head causes an extensive and increasing extravasation of blood under the scalp, rendering it evident that an artery has been divided by the blow, the exact situation of the injured vessel should, if possible, be ascertained, and

* Vide Brodie on the Joints, 4th ed. p. 311. Brodie on Local Nervous Affections, Lond. 1837. Rowland on Neuralgia, Lond. 1838.

pressure be applied there;—that early and free incision must be made in the event of suppuration under the occipito-frontalis;—but that if blood be extravasated there, its absorption is to be promoted by bleed-ing, cold, and low diet; and no incision is to be made, unless positively necessary.

SECTION II.—CONCUSSION OF THE BRAIN.

DEFINITION.—Concussion (commonly called stunning) signifies an interruption of the functions of the brain, induced suddenly by mechanical injury, and not necessarily attended with organic lesion.

SYMPTOMS.—More or less diminution of consciousness, sensation, and voluntary motion, with feebleness of the pulse. There are two degrees of it. (1.) In ordinary cases, the patient lies for a time motionless, unconscious, and insensible; if roused and questioned, he answers hastily, and instantly relapses into insensibility; after a time, he moves his limbs as if in uneasy sleep, and vomits, and frequently recovers his senses instantly afterwards;—remaining, however, giddy, confused, and sleepy for some hours. (2.) In the more severe degree the patient is profoundly insensible, the surface pale and cold, the features ghastly, the pulse feeble and intermittent, or perhaps insensible, and the breathing slow, or per-formed only by a feeble sigh, drawn at intervals.

*Vomiting* is an important symptom. It is not present in very slight cases, nor in very severe ones; and its occurrence is mostly an indication of approaching recovery.

CONSEQUENCES.—(1.) Concussion is occasionally succeeded by a pe-culiar state of insensibility, which may last some days. The patient lies as if in a tranquil sleep; his pulse is regular; but on the slightest exertion it rises to 130 or 140, and the carotids beat vehemently;—when roused he answers questions, but immediately relapses into unconsciousness. Some patients in this state resemble somnambulists; they may get out of bed, bolt the door, shave, or make water, but still are insensible to what passes around. (2.) Concussion may be followed by death, from failure of the hearts action. (3.) It generally leads to more or less inflammation. (4.) It may leave a very infirm state of the health and intellect;—im-pairment of the memory, or of the senses, especially of smell and hear-ing; and a constant tendency to inflammation, and to extravagant actions after drink or any other excitement.

PATHOLOGY.—The brain is often found bruised, or ecchymosed, or la-cerated; but still concussion may be fatal, without any injury that can be detected by dissection.

PROGNOSIS.—It is not often that concussion proves fatal, unless there is also a fracture of the skull or extravasation of blood within it. But the danger will be great, if the pulse and respiration continue feeble for some hours.

DIAGNOSIS.—Concussion may be thus distinguished from the insensibility arising from compression of the brain. In concussion the insensibility comes on *immediately* after the accident;—in compression it *may* come on after an interval. In concussion the pulse is weakened; and the greater the insensibility 'the weaker it will be;—in compression the pulse *may be* full and hard, and the skin hot. Stertorous breathing is rare in concussion, frequent in compression. The pupil in the former is variable, sometimes contracted, sometimes dilated, but yet in severe cases insensible to light;—in compression it is almost always dilated and insensible. The rise of the pulse on any exertion is another distinctive symptom of concussion.

TREATMENT.—The *indications* are: (1) to recover the patient from insensibility and collapse; (2) to prevent inflammation; (3) to restore any faculties that may remain impaired.

1. If the depression be very great, and the pulse very low, warmth may be applied to the surface, and ammonia may be held to the nostrils, and be administered internally. But in general the patient should be left to recover by himself, because, in case of laceration of the brain, stimulants would increase the effusion of blood.

2. After reaction has taken place, the patient (unless too young or feeble) should be bled;* at all events, the bowels should be freely acted on, and perfect rest and low diet should be observed. If the pulse become hard and frequent, and if the patient complains of pain or tightness in the head, the bleeding and purgatives should be repeated as often as may be necessary, with saline and antimonial draughts in the intervals; and the head should be shaved and kept wet with evaporating lotions. As a general rule, after any severe blow on the head, the patient should observe a cautious antiphlogistic regimen for a month or six weeks— carefully keeping himself free from all fatigue, intemperance, and excitement.

3. In order to remove headach, deafness, giddiness, squinting, loss of memory, tinnitus aurium, and other remote consequences of concussion, a course of mild alterative mercurials;—repeated blisters, or an issue or seton;—the shower-bath, change of air, general friction of the surface, and a most regular diet, are the remedies.

* Whether the patient has recovered his consciousness or not, he should be bled; if the pulse become hard, and the skin hot. But bleeding is not a remedy for concussion itself:—it merely removes its consequences; and if employed during a depressed state of the circulation, may induce epileptic convulsion, or perhaps death. In every case of sudden insensibility, whether from disease or accident, the vulgar clamorously demand that the patient should be bled; but the surgeon must be very ignorant or very weak if he yields to their wishes.

SECTION III.—COMPRESSION FROM EXTRAVASATED BLOOD.

SYMPTOMS.—The symptoms of compression of the brain are those of apoplexy. They are insensibility; general palsy, (sometimes, but rarely, confined to one side;) dilated and insensible pupil; slow, labouring pulse; skin often hot and perspiring; retention of the urine, through palsy of the *detrusor urinæ;* involuntary discharge of fæces through palsy of the *sphincter ani;* and stertorous breathing, owing to palsy of the *velum pendulum palati.* Sometimes, however, the pupils are contracted, and sometimes one is contracted and the other dilated.

CAUSES.—Compression (surgically considered) may be produced by three causes. (1.) By extravasation of blood. (2.) By fracture of the skull. (3.) By suppuration within its cavity.

The *symptoms of compression from extravasated blood* generally show themselves in the following manner. The patient receives a blow, and becomes stunned and insensible from the concussion, with extremely feeble pulse and cold skin. After a while he recovers his senses;—but again in an hour or two he becomes sleepy, confused, and insensible; with slow stertorous breathing, slow pulse, and dilated pupils. These symptoms closely correspond with those of one form of apoplexy, called the *ingravescent ;* in which the patient suddenly feels an acute pain in the head, caused by the bursting of a blood-vessel, and becomes sick and faint —in fact, suffers from concussion. Then he recovers his senses—but shortly afterwards, as the extravasation from the ruptured vessel increases, becomes quite comatose.

On the other hand, if a large quantity of blood is extravasated rapidly, the symptoms of compression may immediately succeed the insensibility of concussion without any interval of consciousness.

The blood may be situated, (1) between the dura mater and skull; and if in large quantity, it proceeds from laceration of a branch of the middle meningeal artery; (2) between the membranes; (3) in the substance of the brain.

TREATMENT.—The head should be shaved and examined, and if there is no sign of fracture, the case must be treated as one of apoplexy; the *indications* being to avert inflammation, and procure absorption of the blood by bleeding, cold applications to the head, purgatives, and calomel in repeated doses. Frequently a puffy swelling arises after a day or two, and points out the seat of the blow. If the symptoms are not relieved by the above measures, the last resource is trephining;—which operation should be performed at the seat of the injury, if that is known,—or if that is not known, it should be done where any puffy swelling arises;— or lastly, if there is no puffy swelling, it should be done over the middle meningeal artery;—and if one side is more palsied than the other, it should be done on the other, because, as is well known, injury of one side of the brain produces palsy of the opposite side of the body.* The trephine should be rather large. That extravasation only which is between the dura mater and skull admits of relief by this operation; and blood, if found there, must be carefully removed by a sponge, but the dura mater must not be punctured to search for it, unless fluctuation is very palpable indeed. The skull is said always to be white and bloodless at the seat of effusion between it and the dura mater, because it is deprived of its supply of blood from that membrane. This, therefore, is an important diagnostic sign; and in a desperate case it might be advisable to cut through the scalp, and examine the bone at any part where mischief is suspected to exist.

SECTION IV.—FRACTURE OF THE SKULL.

Fractures of the skull are divided, (1) into those which consist of a mere crack or fissure without displacement; (2) into those in which the fragments are displaced or depressed. Fracture most frequently occurs at the part where the injury was received;—but it may in some cases be seated exactly opposite; this is called *counter-fissure.* *Fracture of the base of the skull* is the most dangerous kind. It is caused when the patient falls from a height, and pitches on his head; the basilar process being snapped through by the weight of the whole body, which tells upon it through the spinal column. In these cases there is frequently a copious venous hæmorrhage from the ears, in consequence of laceration of the sinuses at the base of the brain. This is a most unfavourable symptom; although a slight hæmorrhage from the ears, or nose, or mouth, may depend on an insignificant rupture of the membrana tympani, or of the mucous membrane of those parts. These cases mostly terminate fatally, although there is one instance of recovery on record.

1. *Simple fissure* requires no treatment apart from that of the concussion, compression, or scalp wound, with which it may be accompanied.

2. *Fracture with depression* may be *simple or compound;* the compound being that which is attended with a scalp wound exposing the fracture.

(*a.*) *Simple fracture with depression* may be ascertained by a careful examination of the shaved scalp, when, if it exist, there will be felt a depression at one part, with a corresponding edge or projecting ridge near it. Sometimes a coagulum of blood under the scalp conveys the feeling of a sharp elevated ridge of bone;—it may be known, however, by yielding to firm pressure with the finger. But although there may be a real fracture with depression, still there may be no compression of

---

* Provided the injured part be the anterior-superior portion of the cerebrum.

the brain; because the outer table may merely have been driven into the diploe, or the outer wall of the frontal sinus may have been broken in. The former accident (i. e. fracture of the outer table only) can only happen to a patient of middle age, because the diploe neither exist in infancy nor old age;—the latter will be known by the escape of air, when the nose is blown forcibly, either into the cellular tissue of the forehead, or out of the wound if there be one. *Treatment.*—In a case of *simple* depressed fracture, if there are no symptoms of compression, (and there sometimes are not,) and if the patient is conscious and rational, no incision should be made through the scalp, nor should the trephine be immediately resorted to;—but he should be bled, purged, and kept under the strictest antiphlogistic regimen; and then perhaps recovery may be completed without the slightest appearance of compression, and inflammation be averted. Even if there be *slight* symptoms of compression, the same plan is to be adopted, in the hope that they may be removed by free depletion; but if they are severe, or if they do not yield to depletion, the depressed bone must be elevated by trephining. In children, whose bones are soft and thin, great indentations and depressions may be produced without fracture. They are to be treated upon the principles already laid down; and if the bowels are kept well open, they may not cause any bad symptoms whatever, and the bone may rise in time to its proper level.

(*b.*) In the case of *compound* fracture of the skull with depression of bone, whether there are symptoms of compression of the brain or not, the bone must be elevated. If possible, it should be done with the elevator; but if one piece of the bone is wedged in under another, a *small* aperture should be made with the trephine, in order to make room for employing the elevator. If any pieces of bone are perfectly loose and detached, they must be removed; but not if they have a pretty good adhesion to the pericranium and dura mater.


SECTION V.—WOUNDS OF THE BRAIN, HERNIA CEREBRI, &c.


*Wounds of the dura mater* add very considerably to the danger of compound fractures of the skull, both from the risk that inflammation may spread over the surface of the arachnoid, and from the greater chance of hernia cerebri. Hence this membrane should never be indiscreetly wounded. If the arachnoid is wounded as well, the danger is less, because granulations then speedily shoot up, and close the communication between the wound and the cavity of the arachnoid.

*Wounds of the brain*, whether incised or lacerated, are not of necessity attended with any mental or bodily disorder, besides that which arises from the concussion, compression, or inflammation that may accidentally be present. Instances are numerous in which portions of the brain have been lost without any ill consequences at the time or afterwards. But yet Sir B. Brodie has observed in some cases a greater degree of mental confusion than usually attends concussion, and in others spasmodic twitchings of the muscles.

If *foreign bodies* are embedded in the brain, the danger will be materially augmented. But it is a rule laid down by the best authorities, that no foreign body, whether a portion of the skull or not, is to be removed, if the removal will add in the least to the irritation or injury.

The *treatment* of these wounds consists in the preventing of inflammation;—and in causing the wound to cicatrize without the formation of *hernia cerebri*.

HERNIA CEREBRI.—When a portion of the skull has been removed, the brain, impelled by its arterial circulation, may protrude through the aperture in the form of a rounded tumour, styled *hernia* or *fungus cerebri*. If the dura mater is still entire, it very probably sloughs under the constant pressure of the protruding brain. The tumour consists of brain, in which more or less clotted blood and lymph are effused, and of fungous granulations. As it increases in size, it suffers constriction from the aperture through which it passes, and sloughs; but is speedily succeeded by a similar growth, which undergoes the same processes, till the patient dies of the irritation. *Treatment.*—In order to prevent this affection, a well-regulated pressure, just sufficient to afford a natural support, should be made upon the brain by means of compresses of soft lint oiled, in all cases where the skull is perforated. If the fungus has already protruded, the best application is liq. calcis, with which the lint may be wetted. If this fail, and the degree of pressure requisite to prevent increase cause symptoms of cerebral oppression, the part should be shaved off level with the scalp, and any farther growth be prevented by the liq. calcis and lint, and pressure, as before.

## SECTION VI.—INFLAMMATION OF THE BRAIN.

GENERAL DESCRIPTION.—Inflammation of the brain rarely makes its appearance till a week after an injury, frequently not till three weeks, or even later. Its symptoms and progress are very various; sometimes sudden, violent, and soon terminating in destructive suppuration;—sometimes slow, insidious, and unsuspected, till suddenly manifested by fatal coma or palsy.

SYMPTOMS.—*First stage.* The patient complains of pain in the head, aggravated by heat, motion, and any thing that causes excitement of mind or body, together with a disagreeable sense of languor or weakness, confusion of ideas, quick pulse, disturbed sleep, nausea and want of appetite, and alternate flushing and paleness. *Second stage.* These symptoms having lasted a day or two, there comes on a violent riguor, followed by burning heat of the skin;—the pulse is hard and frequent;—the carotid and temporal arteries pulsate vehemently;—the headach becomes most intolerable and throbbing, the pupils are contracted;—light is insupportable to the eyes, and sound to the ears;—the tongue is dry, the bowels obstinately costive, and the stomach rejects every thing with frequent retching. Besides these symptoms, violent delirium or convulsions come on at intervals, or perhaps coma. If they are unrelieved, the *third stage* soon follows. The pulse loses its force, and becomes either slow and oppressed, or excessively rapid; and squinting, low delirium, convulsions, or palsy, soon usher in death. Rigors, followed by squinting, dilated pupil, stertorous breathing, coma, and palsy, are indications of suppuration.

Certain changes on the outside of the head, also accompanying the mischief that is going on within. Supposing the injury which is the cause of the inflammation to have been accompanied with a wound which up to the occurrence of the inflammation has been going on well—to use the words of Pott,—" the sore loses its florid complexion and granulated surface, and becomes pale, flabby, glassy, and painful; instead of good matter, a thin gleet is discharged from it; the lint with which it is dressed sticks to all parts of it; and the pericranium, instead of adhering firmly to the bone, separates all round from it to some distance from its edges." The bone, moreover, becomes white, dry, and bloodless; because the nutrient vessels that naturally pass from the dura mater to the skull are cut off, in consequence of the inflammation or incipient suppuration of that membrane. If there be no wound, still the scalp presents the puffy swelling that has been before spoken of. If the dura mater is exposed, it at first appears of " a dull sloughy cast, and smeared over with something glutinous;" and subsequently is covered with matter.

Pathology.—It is believed that if the membranes and surface of the brain be inflamed, there will be greater pain, and a greater disposition to delirium and convulsions;—but that in inflammation of the cerebral substance there will be an early tendency to coma and palsy.

Prognosis will be unfavourable if the malady have advanced to its second stage, and is not promptly relieved by depletion.

Treatment.—Upon the first appearance of the symptoms, bleeding should be performed, (perhaps from the temporal artery or jugular vein,) to the approach of faintness; the bowels should be most freely opened, and the head be shaved and kept cool and elevated. If they do not yield, the bleeding should be repeated as often as may be necessary; leeches should be freely employed, and from two to six grains of calomel, with a quarter of a grain of tartar emetic, (not enough to cause vomiting,) should be given every two or three hours. The remedies for the third stage are blisters to the head or its vicinity;—mustard cataplasms to the feet;—terebinthinate or stimulant enemata;—and trephining, if suppuration is indicated by symptoms of compression, or by the above-mentioned state of the wound. The trephine should be large, and if the matter be seated between the dura mater and skull, it may afford relief, although it rarely does.

*Abscess in the brain*, or that form of disorganization which is called *softening* or *ramollissement*, (which appears to be a modification of gangrene,) may be very remote consequences of injury; not occurring perhaps for years. Their *symptoms* are very obscure and insidious. Occasional headach; general loss of health and strength; impairment of the memory or other mental faculties; quick pulse, and furred tongue; disorder of the eyes or ears; sense of constriction, or of coldness in the scalp, or of creeping in the limbs, with numbness, are the most frequent. But these are succeeded by sudden convulsions, or palsy, or coma, from which the patient soon dies, although he may perhaps recover for a time. *Treatment.*—Blisters, issues, setons, or the tartar emetic ointment;—mercurial alteratives;—purgatives;—occasional depletion;—shower-baths;—the most regular diet, and avoidance of every kind of excitement of mind or body, are the remedies in case mischief is suspected. After the occurrence of palsy or decided other symptoms, blisters;—leeches, if the pulse is strong enough, and there is pain or heat in the head—purgatives, and enemata. But if the patient is low and feeble, he must be supported by mild nutriment and stimulants of the diffusive kind, especially the preparations of ammonia.

## SECTION VII.—TREPHINING AND PARACENTESIS.

I. TREPHINING.—The apparatus requisite for this operation comprises a large and small trephine, a straight and curved Hey's saw, and an elevator—besides a good scalpel, and the other instruments which every surgeon is supposed to have in his pocket.

There are four cases which may require this operation. 1. Fracture of the skull with depression of bone. 2. Extravasation of blood under the skull. 3. Suppuration of the dura mater. And lastly, occasional cases of epilepsy arising from the irritation of a diseased spot of the skull. For the first and last cases, the trephine should be quite small, so as not to sacrifice more bone than is absolutely necessary; but when the operation is intended for the relief of suppuration or extravasation, the trephine should be quite large, so as to afford a free exit to the fluid.

Supposing it to be a case of depressed fracture. In the first place, the bone, if not already laid bare by a scalp wound, must be exposed by an

incision in the shape of a V, or T. Then perhaps some loose fragment
may be picked out, or a projecting point may be sawn off with a Hey's
saw, that will enable the surgeon to raise the depressed portion with the
elevator. But if this cannot be done, a circular piece, consisting of the
edge of the depressed bone, and of the adjoining bone under which it
has been wedged, must be removed. The pericranium being shaved off
from the part which is to be perforated, the surgeon applies the trephine,
and works it with an alternate pronation and supination of the wrist, and
when it has made a circular groove deep enough to work in steadily, he
takes care to withdraw the centre pin. He saws on steadily and cautiously, pausing frequently and examining the groove with a probe, to
ascertain whether it has reached the dura mater, and when it has, he
introduces the elevator to raise the circular piece of bone. He must be
particularly careful to fix the centre pin, and the greater part of the circumference of the instrument, on firm bone,—and by no means to press
heavily, whilst sawing, on any piece that is loose or yielding. The saw
will be known to have reached the diploe by the escape of blood with
the bone-dust;—but it must be recollected that the diploe neither exists
in children nor in the aged. The trephine should not be applied in the
course of the sutures, nor over the lower part of the frontal or occipital
bones, if it can be avoided.

II. Paracentesis Capitis, or puncture of the head, is an operation
that sometimes is resorted to in hopeless cases of hydrocephalus in children, when all medicine fails of checking the effusion of water, or of
causing it to be absorbed. It has been particularly recommended by
Dr. Conquest, who has performed it in nineteen cases, out of which he
succeeded in saving ten. The operation merely consists in introducing
a very fine trocar or grooved needle perpendicularly to the surface,
through the anterior fontanel, as far as possible from the longitudinal
sinus. When two or three ounces of fluid have escaped, the puncture
should be carefully closed, and moderate support be applied to the head
by bandages. If the child becomes faint, it must be kept in the recumbent posture, and have a few drops of salvolatile. The operation may
be repeated at intervals of two or three weeks.*

* Vide Dr. Watson's Lectures in the Med. Gaz. for March 1841.

# CHAPTER XI.

## OF THE DISEASES AND INJURIES OF THE SPINE.

I. LATERAL CURVATURE.—Curvature of the spine presents many varieties, some of which arise from mere debility, whilst others are caused by the destruction of portions of the spinal column by disease. We shall first describe that distortion which arises from debility of the bones, ligaments, and muscles, and which is so exceedingly common in this country in young females of the middle and upper classes, from about the age of ten to sixteen.

*Symptoms.*—The first thing that attracts attention is a projection of one scapula, or of one side of the bosom, or an elevation of one shoulder, (most commonly the right,) which are popularly, but erroneously, supposed to be *growing out.* On examination, the spine is found to be curved like an italic *f*;—the right shoulder projecting, and the right side of the chest and the left hip being unnaturally convex;—whilst the chest on the left side and the loins on the right are correspondingly curved inwards. This affection is readily caused by occupation or postures that tax one side of the body more than the other,—if at the same time the patient be subjected to want of exercise, or other influences that deprive the muscles and ligaments of their natural elasticity and vigour.

*Treatment.*—Attention must be paid to the following circumstances; viz. position, exercise, and rest. (1) In the first place, the patient must be watched, in order to find out from what particular attitude or habit the distortion takes its rise. Standing on the right leg is the most frequent, for in this posture the left side of the loins is thrown upwards, and the patient is obliged to raise the right shoulder to keep the body perpendicular. A habit of raising the right shoulder whilst writing, or drawing, or playing the harp, or riding on horseback,—or of sleeping constantly on one side with too high a pillow,—or the abominable custom of wearing dresses made low on the chest, so that the patient hitches her frock up on one shoulder and lets it fall off the other, are also occasional causes. And all of these, and every other one-sided posture, should be vigilantly prohibited. (2) The patient should take free exercise in the open air, whether walking or riding, or indulging in any games or sports, such as the dumb-bells, the skipping-rope, drawing a light garden roller, hopping, or carrying weights in the hands. The *club exercise*, introduced by Mr. Angelo into the regular cavalry training, is extremely advantageous.* It consists in a series of exercises for the arms, whilst a club or loaded stick about two feet long, and from two to seven pounds in weight, is held in each hand. In this, as well as in using the dumb-bells, or other exercises performed in a standing posture, the heels should be closed, the feet at an angle of 60°, the knees straight, the belly thrown back, (so that it may not be strained,) the chest forwards, and the shoulders square; and whilst both sides are duly exercised, the weaker one should be principally brought into play. (3) These exercises should never be carried so far as to fatigue, and after using them the patient should lie down on her back on a flat inclined plane, although an easy posture on a bed or sofa, or on the floor, will do as well. She should never be forced to stand longer then is perfectly agreeable, and when sitting, should rest herself well against the back of the chair. Her seat should be wide enough to reach to the knees, and the feet should be well supported. These measures, combined with tonics, especially steel, F. 63, good diet, country air, bathing, friction of the back with horse-hair gloves, and attention to the health, may be sufficient to cure incipient cases, and to palliate severer ones.

*Curvature from Rickets.*—There is another form of curvature from debility, which chiefly affects young children of the lower orders, and arises from *rickets*. It is readily distinguished by the general rickety aspect of the patient, (vide p. 232,) and by the distortion of the limbs that is also present, as well as by the circumstance that the spine is not simply curved laterally as described above, but is often curved directly forwards;—the seat of this curvature being the upper part of the back;— or perhaps it may be curved backwards.

There are four other measures which must occasionally be resorted to for the cure of these and the other severer degrees of spinal distortion, viz. the recumbent position—mechanical support—mechanical extension —and division of some of the spinal muscles.

1. The *recumbent position*, continued for a length of time, is a measure which has been most disgracefully abused by certain spine-quacks; insomuch that poor wretches who have applied to them to be cured of a mere distortion of the back, have, after many months of confinement, been sent away broken in health, and incapable almost of moving a limb. In slight cases the patient need only lie down for a short time after taking exercise; in order to relieve the spine from the weight of the body whilst its muscles are fatigued. In severer cases, the patient should

* Vide proposed Regulations for the instruction &c. of the Cavalry. Part I. Published by Authority. Lond. 1832. Page 11. A judicious system of gymnastic exercises for girls is a desideratum. Walker's " Exercises for Ladies " is in many parts unfit for the perusal of young females, and contains one or two exercises that are positively injurious.

never be permitted to *sit* or *stand* upright; she should, however, walk out daily in the open air; but when *not walking* should *lie down.* She should, moreover, be provided with some exercises for the arms, which may be used whilst lying down. But a continuance in the recumbent position, without rising at all, is only necessary under one circumstance —and that is, if the curvature increases very fast, and is so abrupt at one point that it begins to compress and irritate the spinal cord, and produce spasms or palsy of the legs.

2. *Mechanical support* by means of stays, or other contrivances made to receive the weight of the trunk at the axillæ, and transmit it to the hips, are of service in many cases; but all circular constriction of the body, as with the common female stays, is an evil.

3. *Extension* of the spine longitudinally, may be effected by fixing the pelvis or feet to the bottom of an inclined plane or couch, and the armpits to the upper part of it; then there must be some contrivance by which the couch may be very gently lengthened. Or something may be done, by pulling at the arm on the convex side of the chest, whilst one foot of the operator is pressed against that side of the chest, and the other against the pelvis. These measures may do good if not abused.

4. *Division of spinal muscles.*—Lastly, there are some cases, in which the difficulty is either entirely caused, or chiefly kept up, by over-action of the muscles on one side, which, as modern experience has taught us, may be relieved by dividing those muscles. Such was a case, treated by Mr. Child, in which the deformity was contracted by using the right arm inordinately in pulling a printer's press,—and in which the right trapezius and rhomboids, which were much hypertrophied, were cut through. It will readily be seen that the muscles to be divided are the transverse ones, (the trapezius, rhomboids, and levator anguli scapulæ,) on the convex side of the curvature, and the longitudinal one s,(sacro-lumbalis and longissimus dorsi,) on the concave side. The operation is easily performed. The muscle to be divided must be put on the stretch, and a puncture be made with a sharp-pointed bistoury on one side of it. A blunt-pointed curved bistoury is then passed under the muscle, (with of course its flat side towards it,) till its point is felt under the skin at the other side; and as the bistoury is being withdrawn, the musele is to be cut through. In a case operated on by Mr. Whitehead of Manchester, in which the sacro-lumbalis was divided, there were some troublesome spasms of the muscles of the other side—but they yielded to opium.*

* Vide Guerin, Gazette Médicale, July 29, 1839 ; Child, Med. Gaz., 27 Nov. 1840; and Whitehead, Med. Gaz. 4 Dec. 1840.

The operations noticed in this paragraph and unfortunately sanctioned by Mr. Druit, deserve to be characterized as he has justly done those barbaıous ones which have lately been performed for the cure of stammering. This " may truly be styled muscle-cutting gone mad." F.

II. Angular Curvature (Pott's curvature) is produced, as the adjoining cut
shows, by caries of the bodies of the
vertebræ, or ulceration of the intervertebral substance. The symptoms in an
advanced stage are threefold, 1. Pain at a
particular part of the back, aggravated
by motion,—great tenderness on pressure; and a peculiar dead sickening
sensation like that of a carious tooth,
if a smart blow be struck on the part with
the knuckles. 2. Curvature of the trunk
forwards, and projection of the spinous

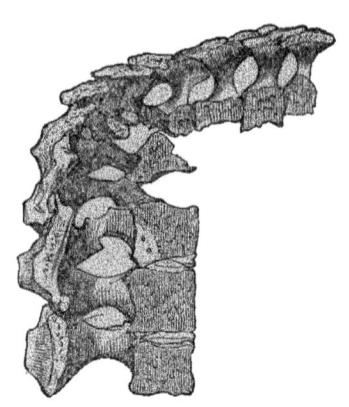

processes of the diseased vertebræ backwards, in consequence of the
destruction of their bodies.* 3. Pain, numbness, coldness, spasms, or
palsy of the extremities, (stumbling in walking is an early symptom,)—
or signs of visceral disorder, such as costiveness, flatulence, incontinence
or retention of urine, or an alkaline or albuminous state of that fluid.
This third class of symptoms, it will be readily seen, are caused by
irritation or compression of the spinal cord. If the disease be seated
in the cervical vertebræ, palsy of one or both arms generally precedes
palsy of the legs or disorder of breathing. Caries of the dorsal vertebræ
is attended with constrictions of the chest or upper part of the abdomen.

*Consequences.*—1. In favourable cases, abscesses, if they form, are
healed, or their matter is absorbed; the diseased bones collapse, and the
patient recovers with more or less deformity, which is of course incurable. 2. In some fatal cases the patient dies suddenly from two or three
of the diseased vertebræ giving way and crushing the spinal cord,—or
from dislocation of the odontoid process, owing to ulceration of its ligament,—or from the bursting of abscesses into the spinal cord, or into
some visceral cavity; but more frequently death is caused by the slow
irritation and exhaustion, caused by the formation of psoas or lumbar
abscesses.

*Diagnosis.*—This affection must not be confounded with its hysterical
counterfeit spoken of in the ninth chapter. It may readily be distinguished from distortion arising from debility by noticing that the curvature is abrupt and angular, whereas in the latter affection it is gradual
and rounded, and implicates nearly the whole spine. It may be distinguished also by the tenderness and pain; and by the symptoms of irritation of the spinal cord; which latter symptoms are present in cases of
vertebral caries from their very commencement, but only exist in very

* The above cut is sketched from a preparation of Mr. W. Fergusson's, in the
King's College Museum.

severe degrees of curvature from debility. *Treatment.*—(1) *Rest* in the horizontal posture is absolutely necessary. A water-bed or fracture-bed may be used, if easy or convenient. But the patient must not be taught to lie on his back, nor must any means be used with a view of straightening the spine, as they would merely impede the natural process of recovery, by preventing the remains of the diseased vertebræ from falling together. A bandage, containing strips of whalebone, and reaching from the head to the hips, is of use in keeping the trunk at perfect rest. 2. *Issues* should be made and be kept open with caustic on each side of the spinous processes of the diseased vertebræ. At the same time, steel, iodine, or other tonics or alteratives, may be given if required. These measures should be continued till pain and tenderness cease.

III. LUMBAR AND PSOAS ABSCESS.—These are abscesses, arising from that diseased condition of the spine which has just been described. Sometimes they point in the back, (constituting *lumbar abscess* if low down,)—sometimes the matter makes its way between the abdominal muscles,—sometimes it enters the sheath of the psoas muscle, (constituting *psoas abscess*,) causes absorption of that muscle, and points below Poupart's ligament;—forming a tumour which diminishes or disappears when the patient lies down, and receives an impulse on coughing. Its diagnosis is alluded to in the chapters on Aneurism and Hernia. If these abscesses enlarge in spite of the issues and other measures directed against the vertebral disease, they must be treated in the manner directed for *large chronic abscess*, p. 80.

IV. DISLOCATION AND FRACTURE.—Dislocation of the spine is rare except in the cervical vertebræ, but it occasionally does occur even in the lumbar and dorsal without any accompanying fracture. When fracture occurs, it generally passes transversely across the body and arch of a vertebra. The ill consequences of these accidents will of course be proportioned to the amount of injury inflicted on the spinal cord; and if that escapes compression, the consequences may not be serious. Thus it may happen that the cervical vertebræ may be twisted round, and be replaced successfully;—and the last dorsal and first lumbar vertebræ have been displaced backwards, the patient recovering with permanent deformity, but nothing worse.*

But it more frequently happens in fracture and dislocation of the spine, that the part of the trunk above the injury is thrown forwards so as to compress or lacerate the spinal cord. Then the results will be as follow:

If the injury affect one of the lumbar or lower dorsal vertebræ, the legs and lower part of the trunk are palsied and insensible,—the penis is erect,—the fæces are discharged involuntarily, owing to palsy of the

† Guerin, L'Expérience, Dec. 3, 1840; Shaw, Med. Gaz. vol. xvii. p. 936.

sphincter ani,—and the urine cannot be voided voluntarily, owing to palsy of the muscular coat of the bladder. Immediately after the injury, the secretion of urine is diminished, but in a few days it becomes copious, ammoniacal, and offensive, and the mucous coat of the bladder inflames and secretes a quantity of viscid adhesive mucus. The bowels are distended with wind, and obstinately costive;—in protracted cases the evacuations become black, treacly, and extremely offensive. The temperature of the palsied parts at first rises,—in one case so high as 111° F.

If the fracture or dislocation be high in the back, or at the lower part of the neck, there will, in addition to the above symptoms, be palsy of one or both arms, and great difficulty of breathing, especially of *expiration*, because the intercostal and abdominal muscles are palsied, and the diaphragm has no antagonist.

If the injury be above the origin of the phrenic nerve, (fourth or fifth cervical,) the diaphragm is palsied, and death instantaneous. The most frequent example of this is the dislocation of the odontoid process, which is sometimes caused by ulceration of its transverse ligament, sometimes by blows on the back of the head, or by lifting a child up by the head.

V. VIOLENT BLOWS, not causing fracture, may produce *concussion* of the spinal cord, so as to annihilate its functions; the symptoms being precisely those which have been just described. If palsy of the legs and the other symptoms of compression of the spinal cord come on *gradually* after a blow, it may be conjectured that they are caused by extravasation of blood.

VI. SOFTENING is a frequent consequence of concussion or laceration. The affected part of the cord becomes pulpy and diffluent, without, however, any traces of inflammation.

VII. ACUTE INFLAMMATION of the spinal cord is a very rare consequence of injuries, except penetrating wounds, which generally prove speedily fatal in consequence. It is known by rigours, delirium, opisthotonos, or general convulsions, followed by palsy and coma.

*Prognosis.*—If a fracture be high up, so as to affect the respiration, the patient rarely survives more than a day or two. If fracture be in the lower part of the back or loins, he may live two or three weeks or a month, and in some rare cases recovery has occurred, with, of course, permanent paraplegia. The prognosis is very uncertain after severe blows; sometimes the patient has recovered the use of his limbs even after complete paraplegia,—sometimes recovery occurs with permanent paraplegia,—sometimes, on the other hand, the patient having appeared to recover from the ill effects of the injury, most unexpectedly becomes paralytic, and dies from slow disorganization of the cord.

*Treatment.*—1. If there be any displacement, an attempt may be made to reduce it by extension and pressure. In dislocations of the neck, however, the attempt should be very cautious indeed, or it may produce instant death. 2. The patient must be kept at perfect rest in the horizontal posture, and the greatest care must be taken to prevent or delay *gangrene from pressure*, by arranging pillows, &c. Nothing can be better than Macintosh's air-cushions, half filled with water. 3. The urine must be drawn off by the catheter, and the bowels be kept open by powerful purgatives, to which Sir B. Brodie recommends ammonia to be added. Tonics and the muriatic acid may be given to support the strength, and obviate the derangement of the urine. 4. Bleeding must be employed if the pulse is firm, and there is great pain. But in the majority of cases, if fracture has occurred and the cord is injured, bleeding is contra-indicated by the pulse, and would hasten a fatal issue. 5. If the patient recover with his life, any remaining weakness or palsy may perhaps be attempted to be removed by the cautious use of blisters or issues, friction, warm bathing, and the internal use of strychnine, but they will very rarely do any good.*

VIII. Spina Bifida or, *hydrorachitis*, is an affection depending on want of development of the spinous processes and laminæ of some of the vertebræ, generally the lower dorsal or lumbar. The spinal membranes, deprived of their ordinary support, yield to the pressure of the fluid which they contain, (which also is secreted in unusual quantity,) and bulge out, forming a fluctuating tumour in the middle line of the back. The legs are often palsied. The ordinary course of the case is, that the tumour enlarges, the skin becomes distended, inflames, and ulcerates,— the fluid is discharged,—the spinal membranes inflame, and the patient dies. Sometimes, however, when it happens that the skin and membranes are strong enough to support the distention, the patient may live out his threescore years and ten. *Treatment.*—Moderate support by properly-adjusted trusses and bandages, and occasional punctures with a grooved needle when the tumour is much distended, are the only remedies.†

* Vide Cooper on Dislocations, and Brodie on Injuries of the Spinal Cord, in Med. Chir. Trans., vol. xxi.

† Two or three cases of persons who have lived to maturity with spina bifida, are given in Cooper's Surgical Dictionary, and one has come under the author's observation.

# CHAPTER XII.

## OF THE INJURIES AND DISEASES OF THE EYE.

SECTION I.—OF WOUNDS AND FOREIGN BODIES.

I. Wounds of the eyelids or eyebrows should be most carefully adjusted by means of small silk sutures, introduced with a very fine sewing needle. A linen rag wetted with cold water should then be laid on the part,—inflammation should be counteracted, and the patient be kept at rest till the wounds are healed. Wounds of the forehead are liable to be followed by amaurosis, in consequence of injury to the frontal nerve.

II. Blows on the eye are generally followed by a disreputable looking ecchymosis, which is inconvenient enough. But sometimes a blow on the naked eyeball causes permanent blindness from concussion of the retina. Antiphlogistic measures are the only resource.

III. When a patient complains of a *foreign body* in the eye, the surgeon should first examine the inside of the lower eyelid and lower part of the globe, telling the patient to look up. If nothing is discovered there, the eye should be turned downwards, so as to expose the upper part of the globe, whilst the upper eyelid should be turned inside out, which may easily be done by taking the eyelashes between a finger and thumb, and turning them upwards over a probe. If any substance stick into the cornea, so that it cannot be removed by a probe, or silver toothpick, or fine forceps, the point of a cataract needle or lancet should be carefully passed under it so as to lift it out. If, however, the removal cannot be effected without considerable difficulty, it is better to leave it to be detached by ulceration. Every means must be taken to obviate inflammation, and if the wound in the cornea is painful or irritable, it should be touched with nitrate of silver. To remove particles of lime or mortar, the eye should be well syringed or sponged with weak vinegar and water, or with oil, or with pure water if neither be at hand.

IV. Prolapse of the Iris, in consequence of penetrating wounds of the cornea, may be attempted to be reduced (provided the pupillary margin is not prolapsed) by closing the eye, and very gently rubbing the lid against the cornea, or by exposing it to a strong light, so as to cause the pupil to contract. But if the pupil is prolapsed, belladonna should be applied to cause dilatation.

SECTION II.—DISEASES OF THE EYELIDS.

I. HORDEOLUM, or sty, is a small painful boil at the edge of the eyelid. *Treatment.*—Leeches, poultices, and early puncture, (which will perhaps permit some concreted sebaceous matter to be squeezed from an obstructed meibomian follicle—a frequent cause of the complaint;) subsequently ung. hydr. nitrat. dilut., to remove any remaining hardness. The health must be treated as in cases of boils.

II. OPHTHALMIA TARSI is an inflammation of the edge of the eyelids, with disordered secretion of the meibomian glands—so that the eyelids stick together and become encrusted with inspissated mucus during sleep. It may be *acute;*—attended with great pain and soreness, and requiring leeches or even bleeding—but in general it is chronic and obstinate, and attended with violent itching. It occurs to weakly persons with disordered digestive organs. It may lead to ulceration of the eyelids, loss of the lashes, and subsequent thickening or inversion of the edge of the lids. *Treatment.*—The bowels must be opened, the biliary secretion regulated, and the general health improved, according to the directions for chronic inflammation and scrofula. Whilst there is heat or swelling, poppy fomentations should be applied, and the edges be smeared with lard—subsequently an astringent collyrium (F. 36, 97) should be often used during the day, and the lids should be touched at night with weak ung. hydr. nitric oxyd. (gr v. ad ℥ss,) or ung. hydr. nitrat. (ʒi *cum* ol. amygdal. fʒiii.) The lashes should be plucked out if there is any ulceration, F. 73.

III. SYLPHILITIC ULCERS of the eyelids, if primary, will be known by their sudden appearance and rapid progress in a patient otherwise healthy, and by their not having been preceded by a wart or tubercle like malignant ulcers. Secondary ulcers will be known by their copery colour. *Tratment.*—Mercury and the treatment of syphilis generally.

IV. TRICHIASIS signifies a growing inwards of the eyelashes. The misplaced hairs must be perpetually plucked out, or if that do not suffice, their bulbs must be extirpated with a fine knife.

V. ENTROPION, permanent inversion of the eyelid, may (1) be caused by contraction of the ciliary margin of the lid, after protracted ophthalmia tarsi—the remedies for which are either to make two perpendicular cuts with scissors quite through the lid, near each angle—or rather to dissect off the edge of the lid with the lashes and their bulbs. (2) If there is no disease of the margin of the lid, and the patient is old, with the skin of the cheek loose and flabby, a flap of the loose skin, and of the orbicularis beneath, should be cut out of the eyelid, in order that the inversion may be counteracted by the contraction of the cicatrix.

VI. ECTROPION, or eversion of the eyelid, may be caused by a fleshy thickening of the conjunctiva, owing to long-continued inflammation. The weak ung. hydr. nitric. oxyd., or lotion of arg. nit. (gr. ii. ad ℥i) may be tried first in order to bring the conjunctiva into a healthy state—but if they do not succeed, a portion of the thickened conjunctiva must be removed by scissors.   This failing, it may be necessary to cut out a triangular slip from the tarsus.   If caused by a cicatrix on the cheek, the cicatrix must, if possible, be dissected out.   *Lagophthalmus*, (hare eye,) a shrinking of the eyelid, so that it cannot cover the eye, may be produced by the same cause, and must be treated in the same manner.

VII. PTOSIS signifies a falling of the upper eyelid from palsy of its levator muscle.   It may be a precusor of apoplexy, and may be attended with headach, giddiness, and other signs of conjestion in the head, which should be treated by bleeding, purgatives, mercury, blisters, &c.   If it occur without any assignable cause, and persists notwithstanding the employment of every measure calculated to improve the health, a portion of skin must be snipped out from under the eyebrow, so that the lid may be attached to the occipito-frontalis, and be elevated by it.

VIII. ANCYLOPLEPHARON.—Union of the edges of the lids, when complete and congenital, (which is very rare,) may be removed by an incision; when partial, and consisting of a junction of the lids near one angle, which is sometimes caused by cicatrizing ulcers, it is incurable.

IX. SYMBLEPHARON signifies a union of the lid to the globe, following some accident that has caused ulceration of both—the introduction of lime, for instance.   It is irremediable, if the adhering surfaces are extensive.   Very slight adhesions (fræna) may be divided.

X. TUMOURS, vascular or encysted, occurring outside the eyelids, are to be treated the same as elsewhere.   Sometimes thin cysts, or hydatids, containing a watery fluid, grow beneath the loose fold of conjunctiva which passes from the lid to the globe.   If that fold be divided longitudinally, they may be extracted by a hook or forceps.   Small encysted tumours sometimes grow from the surface, or within the substance of the tarsal cartilage.   They should be punctured from within.

## SECTION III.—DISEASES OF THE LACHRYMAL APPARATUS.

I. THE LACHRYMAL GLAND is very rarely the seat of disease.   It is, nevertheless, occasionally subject to acute and chronic inflammation,—(the symptoms and treatment of which will be obvious.)   It is also liable to morbid growths, for which it has occasionally been extirpated.

II. XEROPHTHALMIA signifies a dryness of the eye from deficiency of the tears.   It is a consequence of disorders of the lachrymal gland, and may be palliated by frequently bathing the eye with tepid water by means of an eye-cup.

III. Epiphora signifies a redundancy of tears, so that they run over the cheeks. It may depend on general irritability of the eye, and is not unfrequent in scrofulous children. When arising from this cause, it should be treated by aperients and alteratives, with tonics and antacids, (F. 28, or quina, with small doses of sodæ carb.) An emetic may be given if the stomach is foul. The same local applications may be used that are prescribed for scrofulous ophthalmia. Search should be made for foreign bodies or inverted eyelashes.

IV. Closure of the Puncta Lachrymalia is another cause of epi-phora. The openings must be restored by a fine gold pin, and one of Anel's gold probes should be frequently passed through them. It must be introduced first perpendicularly, then horizontally towards the nose.

V. Obstruction of the Nasal Duct is known by watering of the eye, dryness of the corresponding nostril, and distention of the lachrymal sac, which forms a small tumour by the side of the nose, from which tears can be squeezed upwards through the puncta, or downwards in the nose, if the obstruction be not quite complete. It mostly leads to,

VI. Chronic Inflammation of the Lachrymal Sac—tenderness of the sac, perhaps redness of the superjacent skin; irritability and constant tendency to inflammation of the conjunctiva;—and if the sac be squeezed, glairy mucus escapes with the tears.

VII.—Acute Inflammation of the sac is known by great redness, swelling, pain, and tenderness at the inner side of the nose, implicating the eye, and attended with fever and headach. If it be not soon relieved, the sac may suppurate and burst.

VIII. Fistula Lachrymalis signifies an ugly fistulous aperture at the inner corner of the eye, communicating with the lachrymal sac. It is the ordinary consequence of the three preceding affections if unrelieved. Tears escape from the aperture, which is generally crowded with fungous granulations, and the skin around is red and thickened.

*Treatment.*—Acute inflammation of the sac must be treated by leeches, (or bleeding,) purgatives, and cold lotions or poultices. If the pain increase in severity, and become throbbing, the sac should be opened. Chronic inflammation of the sac should be got rid of by an occasional leech, and attention to the digestive organs. When the sac becomes distended, the patient should press its contents down into the nose; and he should also frequently draw in his breath strongly whilst his mouth and nostrils are closed, so as to draw the tears down the duct. The secretions of the eyelids should be corrected with the ointments above mentioned, and a few drops of some astringent collyrium (F. 36) should be put twice a day into the inner angle of the eye, so that it may be absorbed by the puncta, and carried into the sac. By these means the thickening of the duct may perhaps be removed; at all events the patient may go on pretty comfortably.

*Treatment by the style.*—But if there is constant irritability of the eye, or if there is a fistulous orifice between the sac and the cheek, measures should be adopted to restore the obstructed duct. Supposing that there is a fistulous aperture, the fungous granulations, or thickening of the skin about it, should be first removed by nitrate of silver and poultices. If there is no aperture, the sac should be opened by a lancet, introducing it just below the *tendo oculi*, and carrying it downwards and outwards for one fifth of an inch. The escape of tears and mucus shows when the sac is opened. Then a common probe should be pushed through the

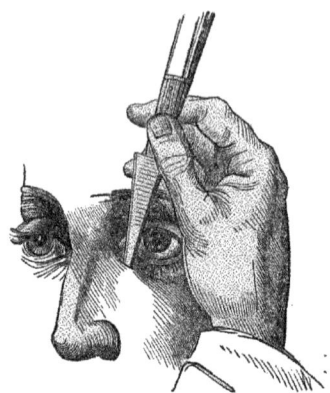

duct into the nose. It should be pushed downwards, but a little backwards and inwards. It will be known to have reached the nose by the escape of a little blood. When inflammation has subsided, a *style* should be introduced, *i. e.* a silver-gilt probe about an inch long, with a head like a nail, which lies on the cheek, where it passes unnoticed like a black patch. The constant presence of this instrument causes the duct to dilate, so that the tears flow by its side. It should be occasionally cleaned, and then be replaced; and it causes so much comfort, and the duct is so likely to close if it be left off, that it generally is worn for life.

SECTION IV.—OF INFLAMMATION OF THE EYE GENERALLY, AND OF THE DISEASE OF THE CONJUNCTIVA.

I. COMMON ACUTE OPHTHALMIA consists of inflammation of the conjunctiva. *Symptoms.*—Smarting, heat, stiffness, and dryness of the eye, with a feeling as if dust had got into it; the conjunctiva of a bright scarlet redness; the redness superficial, so that the enlarged vessels can be moved by pulling the eyelids; slight intolerance of light and flow of tears on exposure of the eye, and more or less headach and fever. *Causes.*—Slight local irritation, disorder of the digestive organs, or cold and damp.

*Catarrhal Ophthalmia* is a variety of this inflammation, caused by cold and damp, and attended with a thin mucous discharge,—which in severe cases becomes thick, purulent, and doubtless contagious.

*Treatment.*—A few leeches to the temples, an emetic if the stomach is foul, a dose of calomel, followed by a black draught;—the eye to be frequently bathed with dec. papav., or F. 97, or the weaker forms of F. 36, lukewarm or cold, according to the patient's choice;—the edges of the eyelids to be smeared at night with fresh lard, and with weak ung. hydr. nit. ox. after the first day or two;—a green shade to be worn over *both* eyes, whilst there is much intolerance of light; but the patient not to be confined to the house too long, unless the case is very severe, or the weather bad.   In the catarrhal variety, a large drop of solution.of arg. nit. (gr. ii.—iv. ad ʒi) may be put into the eye twice or thrice a day.   If the patient is plethoric, and there is much pain, headach and fever, bleeding and calomel in repeated doses will be required.   But it is a great mistake to treat common inflammation of the eye, when it occurs, to delicate subjects, by lowering measures.   After the bowels are cleared, good diet, and exposure to moderate light and cool air, will do more good than black draughts, leeches, and green shades.

II. INFLAMMATION OF THE WHOLE EYE is a rare disease.   It may be caused by severe injuries, or may be a consequence of the common ophthalmia if neglected.   The symptoms are great redness and swelling of the conjunctiva; pain, both burning, aching, and throbbing; intolerance of light, dimness of vision, and severe headach and fever.   It may lead to suppuration of the whole globe; or to opacity of the cornea and lens, adhesions of the iris, insensibility of the retina, and atrophy of the whole globe.   The treatment must be decidedly antiplogistic; and if it be clear that suppuration of the whole globe has occurred—there being rigours—the cornea yellow and distended, and excruciating pain unrelieved by farther depletion, a free incision should be made into the cornea to let the matter escape.

III. CHRONIC INFLAMMATION OF THE CONJUNCTIVA may be a sequel of the acute,—or may be caused by some local irritation, such as inverted eyelashes,—or by some derangement of the health.   *Treatment.*—(1.) All local sources of irritation should be removed.   (2.) The general health should be amended, in the same manner as directed for chronic inflammation generally, (vide p. 59.) (3.) The distended capillaries must be unloaded by occasional local bleedings, and be excited to contact by stimulants and astringents, such as the various collyria in F. 36 and 37, which should be used with an eye-cup; or the vinum opii, of which a few drops may be put into the eye daily.   The edges of the eyelids should be smeared every night with weak ung. hydr. nit., and blisters should be applied behind the ears if the case is obstinate.

IV. PURULENT OPHTHALMIA.—This is the most violent form of inflammation of the conjunctiva, and there are three varieties of it: the purulent ophthalmia of children, the common purulent ophthalmia of adults, and the gonorrhœal ophthalmia.

THE PURULENT OPHTHALMIA OF CHILDREN always begins to appear a few days after birth. *Symptoms.*—At first the edges of the lids appear red, and glued together; their internal surface is red and villous, and the eye is kept closed. Then the conjunctiva of the globe becomes intensely scarlet and much swelled, (the swelling often causing eversion of the lids;)it secretes a thick, purulent discharge, and the child is very restless and feverish. If neglected, this disease may occasion opacity or ulceration, or perhaps sloughing of the cornea; but it generally yields to early and proper treatment. *Causes.*—Exposure to cold or damp, improper food, the contact of diseased secretions from the vagina during birth, or neglect in washing the natural cheesy secretion of the skin away from the eyes. *Treatment.*—The bowels should be cleared with a grain of calomel or hydr. c. creta, followed by a little castor oil or rhubarb;—a leech should be applied to the upper eyelid;—if both eyes are affected a *small* leech may be applied to each;—the insides of the lids may be scarified; the discharge should be washed out three or four times a day with F. 37 or 36; and the nitrate of silver should be applied once a day, either in the form of solution, (gr. ii. ad ℥i,) or of ointment (gr. x. ad ℥i.) If the cornea ulcerate or slough, or if the discharge be obstinate, tonics are required, (quin. sulph. gr. ℈.—vel. ext. cinchon. gr. iii. ex lacte,) and the astringent collyria should be persevered in. It must be recollected that, in these forms of ophthalmia, the collyria must be thrown into the eye with a syringe, for it is of no use to dab them on the eyelids.

V. PURULENT OPHTHALMIA IN ADULTS—(*Contagious or Egyptian Ophthalmia.*) *Symptoms.*—This disease begins with stiffness, itching, and watering of the eye, with a sense of dust in it, and slight swelling of the lids, which stick together during sleep—and on examination of their internal surface, the palpebral conjunctiva is found to be intensely red, thick, and villous, like a fœtal stomach injected. As the disease advances, the ocular conjunctiva becomes also intensely red, swollen, and villous, and discharges a copious secretion of pus. The swelling of the ocular conjunctiva is called *chemosis.* It is produced by a secretion of blood, lymph, and serum into the cellular tissue which connects the conjunctiva to the sclerotic; and it elevates the conjunctiva into a kind of roll around the margin of the cornea. These symptoms are accompanied with severe burning pain, extending to the cheek and temple, and great headach and fever; the palpebræ also are swollen, tense and shining, so that the patient cannot open the eye. *Consequences.*—This affection may lead to ulceration or opacity, or perhaps sloughing of the cornea; or to adhesion of the iris; or to impairment of vision, from extension of inflammation to the internal parts of the globe. *Causes.*—It may be produced by severe local irritation, as the introduction of lime, for instance. It is endemic in Egypt owing to the glaring sunshine and the particles of sand with which the air is loaded; but when once produced by any cause whatever, it is most probably both *contagious* and *infectious*;—that is, capable of being propagated both by contact with the purulent secretion, and by exposure to its vapour, if many persons affected with the disease are crowded together.

VI. GONORRHŒAL OPHTHALMIA is the most violent form of purulent conjunctivitis. The *symptoms* are essentially the same as those of the last species; but the chemosis is greater, the discharge thicker and more abundant, the constitutional disturbance more severe, and the cornea much more apt to slough. *Cause.*—This disease arises without doubt from the application of gonorrhœal matter to the eye. *Prognosis.*— This is very unfavourable. The sight of the affected eye will either be lost, or excessively impaired, unless treatment be very early and efficacious. *Consequences.*—The most frequent and detrimental is *sloughing of the cornea*, which is supposed to be caused by the constriction of its vessels by the chemosis. The sloughing generally occurs quite suddenly; the cornea may be clear in the morning—cloudy and flaccid in the evening—and by the next morning it may have burst;—and this change may supervene at any time from the second day of the disease till the last. After this has occurred, the swelling of the lids subsides, the discharge diminishes and becomes thinner, and the pain greatly abated. If the slough is very small, the iris may protrude, and close the aperture, imperfect sight remaining,—but generally the major part of the cornea perishes.

*Treatment.*—The indications are, (1) to mitigate inflammation; (2) to alter the action of the inflamed part by certain stimulants.

1. A full bleeding should be performed from the arm or jugular vein;— the bowels should be well cleared;—calomel and antimony (F. 6.) should be administered in repeated doses, and Dover's powder at bed-time to allay pain. The patient must be kept in bed in a darkened room, with the head elevated, and on low diet. But if these measures do not arrest the disease, and the chemosis is evidently extending round the cornea, and the cornea is becoming hazy, Mr. Tyrrell's plan of dividing the chemosis should be put in practice; that is to say, six or eight incisions should be made completely through the swollen conjunctiva, beginning at the margin of the cornea, and radiating towards the circumference of the eye. By this means, Mr. Tyrrell believes that the tension of the conjunctiva will be relieved without cutting through the vessels that supply the cornea. The incisions should be fomented with warm water, that they may bleed. *Leeches* should be repeatedly applied; the forenoon is the best time, in order to anticipate the exacerbation of pain which generally supervenes in the evening. The eye may be covered with a poultice, or with poppy fomentation, or with any warm or cold

application that is agreeable. *Cold affusion* of the head has been much recommended when it is heavy and painful. *Blisters* should be applied to the neck, or behind the ears, after the abstraction of blood.

2. From the beginning of the disease, the eye should be frequently but gently syringed with warm water, or poppy decoction, containing a grain of alum to an ounce, in order to get rid of the secretion. But as soon as the chemosis is lessened—(or as soon as the cornea has perished) —the proportion of alum should be increased, or F. 37, or the weaker preparations of F. 36, may be used instead. The diet also should be improved; and the edges of the lids should be smeared at night with weak ung. hyd. nit. ox. If the strength becomes impaired, and the cornea has given way, tonics (especially F. 1) or sarsaparilla should be administered; which, with repeated blisters, and a continuance of the astringent applications, are the measures for removing the relics of the disease.

We have given precedence to Mr. Tyrrell's plan of treatment,[*] because it is the most recent, and apparently the most successful; but before it was introduced, it was the custom to attempt to check the inflammation by the application of powerful stimulants and astringents. Some persons employed liq. plumbi acet. undiluted, or the ol. terebinth, but a strong solution or ointment of nitrate of silver (gr. iv—x—ad $\tilde{3}$i aquæ) was generally preferred. Mr. Guthrie in particular recommended an ointment of arg. nit. gr. x. liq. plumbi ℳ xv. adipis ʒi, the nitrate to be very finely powdered, and the lard well washed. A piece of ointment the size of a pea, or a large drop of the solution on a hair pencil, to be thoroughly diffused between the lids and globe twice a day at least. The ointment should turn the membrane white.

VII. Scrofulous Ophthalmia (*phlyctenular ophthalmia*) generally attacks children under eight years of age.

*Symptoms.*—Extreme intolerance of light,—the lids spasmodically closed,—the head turned obstinately away from the light,—no general vascularity of the conjunctiva, but one or two enlarged vessels running towards the cornea, and terminating at one or more *phlyctenulæ*, or small opaque pimples, (or sometimes pustules,) on the cornea, either of which may lead to opacity or ulceration of that part. *Treatment.*—The first and chief point is to look after the general health. The alimentary canal, therefore, should be cleared by an emetic and dose of calomel and jalap, and, after feverishness has subsided, recourse must be had to steel, sarsaparilla, and alkalis, and to the various combinations of tonics, aperients, and antacids, and to the other general remedies directed for scrofula, (p. 118.) Quinine is particularly recommended by Mackenzie. *Secondly,* the distressing intolerance of light must be relieved. This is sometimes effected by cold lotions applied to the outside of the eye, and to the forehead and temples; such as poppy decoction with a little spirit, or water

---

[*] Med. Chir. Trans., vol. xxi., part 2; and Tyrrell on the Eye, vol. i. p. 73.

to which a little vinegar, or spirit, or nitric æther, has been added, or the white of egg curdled with alum. But warm poultices, or dec. papav. vel anthemid., or exposing the eye to the vapour of warm water, or of laudanum or sp. camph., which may be put into a tea-cup and be held in warm water—or warm lotions of ext. belladon. vel hyoscyami ($\ominus$ i. ad$\mathfrak{Z}$j aquæ,) or those extracts smeared on the brow, are of more efficacy. Small doses of extract of conium are also of service. Moreover, *both* eyes should be protected by a shade. *Thirdly*, if the insides of the lids are turgid, they may be scarified;—any enlarged vessels running from the conjunctiva to the cornea may also be scarified across; and blisters or the tartar emetic ointment may be applied behind the ears, or to the nape of the neck. Lastly, in the advanced stage of the disease, benefit will be derived from droping in a few drops of vin. opii, or lotion of nitrate of silver (gr. i. ad $\mathfrak{Z}$i) once a day.

VIII. Granular Conjunctiva signifies a thick, rough, fleshy state of that membrane, (especially of that part of it which lines the eyelids,) and is a frequent consequence of severe and long-continued ophthalmia. It causes great pain and disturbance to the motions of the eye, and, if it continues, will render the cornea opaque by its friction. *Treatment.*— In the first place, the thickened part should be scarified, then (waiting a day) it should be touched with lunar caustic or sulphate of copper, or be washed with strong astringent collyria every day or two,—the ung. hyd. nit. oxyd. should be smeared at night on the edges of the lids,—blisters should be applied behind the ears, and the general health be attended to. But if these measures prove fruitless, the granular surface must be shaved off with a fine knife or scissors.

IX. Pterygium is a peculiar alteration of the conjunctiva, a triangular portion of which, with the apex towards the cornea, becomes thickened and elevated,—sometimes transparent, sometimes red and fleshy. It may spread over the cornea and obstruct vision. *Treatment.*—If it does not disappear under the use of vin. opii or caustic lotion, it must be completely scarified across, and if that fail, it must be seized with a hook and be extirpated.

SECTION V.—OF THE DISEASES OF THE CORNEA.

I. Acute Inflammation of the Cornea is generally a consequence of neglected injury. The part becomes red and opaque,—the sclerotic around highly vascular,—and ulceration of the cornea, or suppuration between its layers, or abscess of the anterior chamber, may ensue. Local and general bleeding, mercury and antimony, and fomentations, are the remedies. Stimulating applications are prejudicial.

II. Scrofulous Corneitis most frequently occurs between the ages of eight and eighteen. *Symptoms.*—The cornea opaque, rough and red, and unusually prominent,—the surrounding sclerotic also red,—pain and

intolerance of light are generally trivial,—there is considerable tendency
to inflammation of the iris and retina,—the pulse is frequent, and the
skin dry.  *Treatment.*—For the acute, leeches, emetics, purgatives,
calomel and antimony, fomentations, and belladonna smeared on the eyebrow.  For the chronic, quinine should be perseveringly administered;
blisters should be repeatedly applied to the nape of the neck, and behind
the ears, and the health should be treated after the manner directed for
scrofula.  The vin. opii and ung. hydr. nit. ox. to the eyelids are almost
the only local applications admissible.

III.  OPACITY of the cornea may be a consequence of the ADHESIVE
INFLAMMATION, and of effusion of fibrine between its layers, or between
it and the conjunctiva.  When the opacity is slight and diffused, it is
called *nebula;*—when denser and of a firmer aspect, *albugo.*  Sometimes
the albugo becomes vascular, and one or more vessels run to it from the
circumference of the eye.  These affections may be a result of any form
of ophthalmia, but most frequently of the scrofulous.  *Treatment.*—(1)
All sorts of irritation about the eye or lids, (inverted hairs, granular conjunctiva, &c.) must be removed, and any existing degree of inflammation be counteracted by proper measures.  Then (2) absorption of the
lymph may be promoted by counter-irritants; such as blisters and the
tartar emetic ointment—by alteratives and measures calculated to improve
the health;—and by the application of stimulants to the eye.  The ordinary applications are caustic lotion (gr. ii—x ad ℥j) or hydr. bichlor.
gr. i—ii ad aq. ℥j;—vin. opii;—ung. hydr. nit. ox.;—or a powder composed of hydr. nit. ox. ℈j, sacchari ℈j, very finely powdered, a little of it
to be blown into the eye.  Whichever is selected should be applied regularly, and should not excite long-continued pain or active inflammation.
Any enlarged vessels running from the circumference of the eye to the
opacity should be divided.  Gooch used to cure opacity of the cornea,
even of long standing, and, in fact, other forms of chronic inflammation
of the eye, by the administration of corrosive sublimate, in doses that
would now be considered hazardous.  He gave gr. $\frac{1}{4}$ twice a day; and
in a few days time increased the dose to gr. $\frac{1}{2}$, and then to gr. i.  It
caused feverishness, purging, slight sweating, and headach.

IV.  LEUCOMA signifies an opaque cicatrix of the cornea.  If recent, it
may be partially removed by the measures just indicated for the cure of
the adhesive inflammation.  If of long standing, it is irremediable.

V.  ONYX signifies a suppuration between the layers of the cornea, and
is a result of acute ophthalmia.  It derives its name from its resemblance
in shape to the white spot at the root of the finger nail.  It mostly disappears with proper antiphlogistic treatment.  If it extend very fast, it
may be necessary to puncture the external layers of the cornea to relieve
the great pain, but the sight will be lost.

VI.  ULCERS of the cornea are most frequently the results of the
*phlyctenulæ* of scrofulous ophthalmia, in which case they are deep, and

tend to perforate the cornea, or they may arise from mechanical injury, or any form of conjunctival inflammation.

These ulcers may, as Mr. Tyrrell observes, exist in three states. " *First,* that which we may term healthy, when its surface and circumference exhibit a degree of haziness or opacity of a whitish or gray aspect, which is owing to the effusion of adhesive matter on the surface, and in the surrounding texture, which is essential to the healing of the part." In this state, the case merely requires to be watched, to prevent injurious increase of action.

*Secondly,* an ulcer may be inflamed—when its hazy circumference will be observed to be highly vascular. Leeches and counter-irritation, with soothing applications, are the remedies.

*Thirdly,* an ulcer may be indolent, without any vascularity, or effusion of lymph. This state requires stimulating applications, (arg. nit. gr. i. ad aq. ℨi.)

Again, ulcers may form on a surface that is already rendered opaque and nebulous by scrofulous inflammation. However, in any case, counter-irritation—and measures to improve the health—together with weak caustic lotion or vin. opii used twice a day, are the chief remedies. If an ulcer is very irritable, it should be touched with a fine pencil of nitrate of silver.

VII. STAPHYLOMA signifies a protrusion on the anterior surface of the eye. 1. *Staphyloma iridis* is a protrusion of the iris, which occurs when the cornea is perforated by ulcers or wounds. The protruded part should be punctured, or be snipped off if large, and be subsequently touched with arg. nit.

2. Staphyloma of the cornea is said to exist when a portion or the whole of the cornea is opaque, white, and prominent, the iris adhering to it—a consequence of severe inflammation. If *partial,* the nitrate of silver or butter of antimony may be applied to the apex of the staphyloma, so that the inflammation excited may thicken the cornea, and enable it to resist farther protrusion. The caustic should be well washed off with milk before the lids are closed. If *general,* the staphyloma should be shaved off, for, as it is not covered by the eyelids, it is a source of constant irritation and pain.

VIII. CONICAL CORNEA—the part gradually becoming thin and exceeding convex, but transparent—causes almost total deprivation of vision, (which, however, can be partially aided by looking through a minute aperture in a piece of blackened wood.) It is incurable, although its progress may be retarded by tonics, counter-irritants, and mild stimulating applications. *Vide* Artificial Pupil, p. **339.**

CAUTION.—If the *acetate of lead* is used as a collyrium when there is any abrasion of the conjunctiva or cornea, a white precipitate is formed, which may become fixed in the cicatrix as a dense white spot. The film may, however, sometimes be removed by a needle. The *nitrate of silver*, if applied too long, is apt to turn the conjunctiva to a deep olive hue.

## SECTION VI.—DISEASES OF THE SCLEROTIC.

I. ACUTE INFLAMMATION OF THE SCLEROTIC (*rheumatic ophthalmia*) is known by redness of the sclerotic, no great intolerance of light, severe stinging pain of the eye, and aching of the bones around which is greatly aggravated at night, and fever. It may be caused by cold. Sometimes, like other rheumatic inflammations, it is a sequel of gonorrhœa. It may lead to opacity of the cornea, or to iritis. *Diagnosis.*—It is known from inflammation of the conjunctiva, by the aching rheumatic character of the pain;—and by the redness being deeper seated, and of a pale pink colour, and by the vessels running in *straight* lines on the sclerotic, and terminating at a red circle around the cornea,—whereas the vessels of the conjunctiva are scarlet and superficial, and can be moved about. *Treatment.*—In severe cases, it will be necessary to bleed and purge, and administer colchicum, F. 95; or perhaps calomel and opium till the gums begin to suffer. The other measures are, friction of the forehead with extract of belladonna dissolved in warm laudanum (3j ad Ʒj,) or with mercurial ointment and opium every afternoon;—warm pediluvia, or warm bath,—blisters behind the ears,—and Dover's powder at bed-time. Subsequently tonics will be useful, especially F. 31, or a combination of dried carbonate of soda and powdered bark, five grains of each of which may be given every four hours. Dry warmth, by means of muslin bags, filled with camomile flowers and heated in a hot plate, is the most soothing local application.

II. CATARRHO-RHEUMATIC OPHTHALMIA is a combination of inflammation of the sclerotic with that of the conjunctiva. Roughness and sense of dust in the eye,—muco-purulent discharge and superficial scarlet redness, are combined with the deeper-seated, straight-lined redness, and with the zone around the cornea, and fits of nocturnal aching, that characterize inflammation of the sclerotic. This disease is very apt to lead to onyx, or to ulceration of the cornea. *Treatment.*—Nitrate of silver, astringent collyria, scarifications, ung. hydr. nit. ox., and the other topical applications for conjunctival inflammation, must be used in addition to bleeding, calomel, and opium, and the other remedies prescribed for simple inflammation of the sclerotic.

## SECTION VII.—INFLAMMATION OF THE ANTERIOR CHAMBER, OR AQUO-CAPSULITIS.

This affection is generally the consequence of some other form of ophthalmia, but it may occur by itself. *Symptoms.*—The iris dull, the cornea mottled, the eye very tense and painful, and fever. The most peculiar consequence of this disease, whether primary or consecutive of some other inflammation of the eye, is *hypopion; i. e.* an effusion of an albuminous (or perhaps purulent) fluid into the anterior chamber. It is distinguished from *onyx* by the white fluid moving in different positions of the head, and by its uper margin being straight, not convex. *Treatment.* —Calomel and opium, and belladonna, and the general treatment of iritis will remove the inflammation, and cause absorption of the hypopion.

SECTION VIII.—OF THE DISEASES OF THE IRIS.

I. IRITIS.—*Symptoms.*—Intolerance of light, dimness of sight, pink redness of the sclerotic, a red circle around the cornea, and pain; which is sometimes severe and burning, sometimes seated in the forehead and temple; and sometimes remarkably absent even in acute cases. In severe cases, the conjunctiva also becomes vascular. In the first stage, the fibrous structure of the iris appears confused, and it becomes dark and muddy, with perhaps a reddish tinge. In the next stage lymph is effused; sometimes in the form of a thin layer, causing the surface to appear rusty and villous,—sometimes in small nodules;—sometimes the pupil (which from the first is contracted and irregular) is filled with a film of it,—sometimes it is poured out in such abundance as to fill the whole cavity of the aqueous humour. *Causes.*—Iritis may be caused by injuries, or by over-exertion of the eye; but it more frequently depends on constitutional taint, syphilis, or gout. *Prognosis.*—Favourable, if the disease is recent and confined to the iris, although the impairment of vision be considerable;—but doubtful, if it be of long duration (*i. e.* more than a fortnight;)—if there be much deep-seated pain, and especially if there be great effusion of lymph behind the iris. *Varieties.*—(1) *Syphilitic iritis* is the most frequent variety. It is generally attended with effusion of lymph in little nodules of a reddish or brown colour, which cause the pupil to become angular. There is great pain at night, and but little by day, and other secondary venereal affections are usually present at the same time. (2) *Arthritic, gouty* or *rheumatic iritis* is known by the general character and previous diseases of the patient. There is generally great pain in the neighbourhood of the eye,—the vascular circle around the cornea is dull, and does not quite touch the latter, but is separated from it by a narrow white interval. (3) Scrofulous iritis is rarely a *primary* affection, but generally a consequence of neglected strumous ophthalmia. (4) Iritis may be either *acute* or *chronic*.

*Treatment.*—The indications are, 1, to subdue inflammation; 2, to arrest the effusion of lymph, and cause absorption of what is already effused; 3, to preserve the pupil entire. 1st. If the patient be strong,

43

and the disease acute, with much pain and fever, bleeding should be performed, and be repeated according to the pulse. In chronic cases, cupping will be preferable. The bowels must be well cleared, and the antiphlogistic regimen generally be observed. 2ndly. Mercury must be given so as to affect the system speedily—gr. ii—iv of calomel with gr. ¼—½ of opium being administered at intervals of from four to eight hours. And when the mouth becomes sore, the lymph will generelly be found to break up and gradually disappear. 3rdly. The pupil should be kept well dilated by means of extract of belladonna, a thick solution of which should be painted on the eyelids, or dropped into the eye. Stramonium or hyoscyamus may be substituted if preferred.

*Turpentine* is a valuable remedy in iritis. It may either be given in large doses (F. 18) to act upon the bowels during the administration of mercury, or it may be given in small doses (ʒj) three times a day, so as to act on the kidneys, if from any cause (such as great debility, or previous severe salivation) mercury is deemed inadmissible. Blisters are injurious except in chronic cases, and the only local application of any use (except the belladonna) is poppy fomentation to soothe the pain.

In *gouty iritis*, calomel is only to be used in order to evacuate the bowels and amend the secretions, and it is highly injurious if given to the extent of affecting the system. But colchicum in doses of ♏xx of the wine, (F. 95,) with turpentine purgatives, (F. 18,) must be used instead. Bleeding, local and general, must be employed as the strength permits, and pediluvia containing mustard should be used every night.

II. SYNECHIA POSTERIOR—adhesion of the *uvea* to the capsule of the lens;—SYNECHIA ANTERIOR—adhesion of the iris to the cornea;—and ATRESIA IRIDIS, or closure of the pupil—three consequences of organization of lymph from protracted iritis—may be partially removed by mercury if recent, but are irremedial except by operation if the lymph has become organized. But belladonna should always be applied; because if a very small portion of the pupil is by chance unadherent, it may be dilated so as to afford a very useful degree of vision.

III. MYOSIS—a preternaturally contracted pupil—is often met with in persons accustomed to look at minute objects. MYDRIASIS—a preternaturally dilated pupil—generally depends on insensibility of the optic nerve. But if the nerve be sound, vision may be assisted by wearing a pair of spectacles having, instead of glasses, two pieces of pasteboard blackened within, and perforated with an aperture of the natural size of the pupil. This affection, moreover, has been said to be cured by ergot of rye.

IV. TUMOURS OR CYSTS growing upon the iris must be removed if they become large, so as to interfere with vision, or to inflame the eye by their pressure. A section of the cornea must be made as for extraction of cataract, and the diseased part of the iris, having been drawn out, must be snipped off.

V. ARTIFICIAL PUPIL.—There are certain cases in which it becomes expedient to alter the shape and position of the pupil, or to form a new pupillary aperture in the iris.

1st. In cases of conical cornea, or of permanent opacity of the centre of the cornea, it is advisable to bring the pupil opposite to a transparent part of it; and Mr. Tyrrell observes, that if the position and extent of the opacity do not forbid, the pupil should always be brought downwards and outwards. This is done in the following way. A broad needle is carefully passed through the cornea, close to its junction with the sclerotic. Through the puncture thus made, Tyrrell's hook, a fine blunt hook with a long bend, is passed into the anterior chamber, with the bent limb forwards. As soon as it has reached the pupillary margin, the hook is turned backwards so as to catch it; and then the hook is withdrawn, through the corneal puncture, bringing out the iris with it, and of course rendering the pupil oblong. The piece of the iris that protrudes should be snipped off with a fine pair of scissors.

2ndly. In cases where the pupil has been nearly or altogether lost in consequence of prolapse of the iris through wounds or ulcers, or slough of the cornea;—or where vision is obscured by opacity of the cornea, with adhesion of the iris, to it;—or by partial staphyloma of the cornea with adhesion of the iris, a new pupillary aperture may be made, or the old pupil (if not quite abolished) may be extended opposite to that part of the cornea which remains transparent, by the same operation which we have just described. But if the old pupil is quite lost, it will be necessary to make a little puncture of the iris with the needle which is employed to puncture the cornea,—into which puncture of the iris the hook is to be inserted. Supposing, moreover, that after either of these operations the new pupil degenerates into a mere slit, this slit must be enlarged, by another operation of [the same kind—that is, by making another puncture of the cornea at little distance above the first, and dragging up the upper margin of the slit with the hook.

3rdly. In cases where the pupil has closed after the removal of a cataract—whether in consequence of prolapse of the iris, or of inflammation and organization of lymph, an artificial pupil may be made by making an opening at the margin of the cornea, about a quarter of an inch in extent. Through this, a small pair of scissors (Maunoir's) is introduced, and a V shaped cut is made in the iris. Or in cases where part of the cornea is opaque, a new pupil may be made with the needle and hook as above described.*

---

* This operation, when performed by means of an incision in the iris, is technically called *coretomia;* when performed by the excision of a little piece, it is called *corectomia;* and when effected by detaching the iris from the ciliary ligament, it is called *coredialysis. Κορη, pupilla.*

But before resorting to any of these operations, it must be ascertained, 1st, whether the adhesions of the iris cannot be removed by mercury or belladonna, or opacity of the cornea by external applications; 2ndly, that the retina is perfectly sound; 3rdly, that all tendency to inflammation (syphilitic or otherwise) has ceased. It is not advisable to operate if one eye be quite sound;—and supposing one eye to be irrecoverably lost, it is not advisable to form an artificial pupil in the other, provided the patient find his way about with it. Moreover, the new pupil should be made large, because it will always contract somewhat afterwards.

### SECTION IX.—INFLAMMATION OF THE CAPSULE OF THE CRYSTALLINE LENS.

This is a very rare affection, always chronic. Vision is confused,—objects looking as if they were seen through a fine gauze. On-examining the eye with a strong lens in a good light, and the pupil being well dilated with belladonna, a number of minute red vessels are seen in the pupil. If the anterior capsule be affected, the vessels form a circular wreath of vascular arches with the centre clear;—if it be the posterior capsule, they are arborescent and central. The iris is always slightly discoloured and sluggish. *Treatment.*—Local or general bleeding;—mercury, counter-irritation, change of air, and alteratives.

### SECTION X.—OF CATARACT.

DEFINITION.—An opacity of the crystalline lens or its capsule.

SYMPTOMS.—Before examining any patient with suspected cataract, the pupil should be dilated with belladonna, and then, if there be cataract, there will be seen an opaque body of a gray, bluish white, or amber colour, behind the pupil. The patient usually gives as his history, that his vision has become gradually impaired, that objects appear as if surrounded with a mist, or as if a cloud was interposed between them and the eye, and that the sight is better in the evening, or when the back is turned to the window, or after the application of belladonna,—obviously because the pupil being dilated under those circumstances, permits more light to pass through that part of the lens which is yet transparent. In the most confirmed cases, the patient is able to distinguish day from night.

CAUSES.—Cataract (especially of the capsule) is sometimes attributable to inflammation, and may be caused in a short space of time by wounds or other injuries of the lens. But the ordinary cataract of the old seems to be a mere effect of impaired nutrition.

DIAGNOSIS will be spoken of under Amaurosis.

VARIETIES.—1. *Hard* cataract. This is the form that is generally met with in elderly people. The lens is shrunk and hard, amber yellow in the centre, gray towards the circumference. There is an appreciable interval between the lens and iris. 2. *Radiated* cataract. In this form the opacity commences in streaks at the circumference, which, as the disease advances, slowly converge towards the centre. In this variety there is of course some little diversity from the ordinary symptoms. For instance, the patient sees best in a bright light, when the pupil is contracted; and, moreover, he is apt to see objects double, or distorted, in consequence of irregular reflections of light from the opaque streaks. 3. *Soft* cataract,— the lens of the consistence of soft cheese or cream, and of a gray or bluish, or pure white colour, without any amber tint. This variety is generally met with in persons under forty, and causes a greater degree of blindness than the hard variety,—moreover, the lens being swelled projects against the iris, and interferes with its motions. 4. *Capsular* cataract. Opacity of the capsule is said to occur in spots or streaks, with less opaque intervals. It is not unfrequently the result of a slow inflammation, which may be accompanied with pain in the eye, and signs of congestion in the head;—or of inflammation produced by direct injury to the lens or its capsule;—or of inflammation extending from the iris or conjunctiva. Opacity of the *anterior* portion may be seen immediately behind the iris, and has a glistening, chalky, or pearly white appearance. That of the *posterior* appears at some little distance behind the pupil, and presents a concave striated surface, of a dull yellowish appearance. 5. *Capsulo-lenticular* cataract is very common,—in fact, opacity of the capsule is always followed by opacity of the lens.

TREATMENT.—The cataract must be removed by operation. No other treatment is of any avail to get rid of the disease, although perhaps its progress may be retarded by counter-irritation, and stimulating applications to increase the flow of tears, and sternutatories, and measures calculated to lower vascular action. It is, however, a general rule not to operate till the cataract is *mature;*—that is, not whilst the degree of vision is sufficient for ordinary purposes; more particularly if the patient is very old and feeble, or if one eye is already lost;—because under these circumstances a failure of the operation would entail utter blindness. Therefore the patient should dilate the pupil by dropping into the eye one or two drops of a carefully-filtered solution of extract of belladonna ($\ominus$i. ad $\zeta$i.) in distilled water night and morning, and defer the operation till, despite of that aid, his blindness is complete.

*Prognosis.*—This will be favourable if the patient is in good health, of a spare frame, and temperate habits; if the iris move freely, and if the retina seem perfectly sensible to light. On the other hand, it will be doubtful if there are signs of vascular disturbance in the eye or head—if the iris is motionless or altered in colour, or if it is adherent to the capsule;—or if the cataract is complicated with amaurosis, synchysis, or glaucoma.

*Preparation.*—Before operating, the patient should be put into as perfect a state of health as possible. The bowels should be cleared, the secretions be regulated, and bleeding and low diet be enjoined if the habit is inflammatory. Moreover, the operation should always be performed in mild weather.

There are three methods of operating;—extraction, depression (or *couching,*) and the operation for causing absorption.

I. EXTRACTION.—This operation effectually removes the cataract, but in the event of a failure sight is almost irretrievably lost. It is best adapted for hard cataracts in elderly people. But it should not be attempted, 1st, if the patient is very old and feeble, in case the wound of the cornea might not unite. 2ndly, If the anterior chamber is very small and the cornea very flat, so that a sufficiently large opening cannot be made in it. 3rdly, If the iris adheres much to the cornea, or if the cataract is large and pushes it forwards, or if the pupil is habitually contracted. 4thly, If the eye is sunken, or if the fissure of the lids is preternaturally small. 5thly, If the eyes are very unsteady, or if the patient is subject to habitual cough or asthma, or is unmanageable in consequence of infancy or idiocy. One eye only should be operated on at a time, the other being kept as a reserve.

*Preliminaries.*—The patient should be seated in a low chair with a high back, opposite a window that admits a good clear light, but no sunshine, and should be placed somewhat obliquely, so that the operator may not see the image of the window on the cornea. The surgeon should sit immediately before him on a higher chair; and should have a stool, so as to raise one knee to a proper height for steadying the elbow of the operating hand upon it. Behind the patient an assistant should stand, whose duties are, 1st, to steady the head against the back of the chair, or against his own breast. 2ndly, To elevate the upper eyelid, and fix it against the margin of the orbit, with one forefinger. 3rdly, To drop it at a preconcerted signal from the surgeon.

*Operation.*—The surgeon, 1st, depresses the lower eyelid, and steadies the globe with the fore and middle fingers of one hand, but without exerting any pressure on it. He particularly endeavours to prevent it from rolling inwards during the operation. 2ndly, holding the *cornea-knife*\*

---

\* The knife called Beer's is most used. It has a triangular blade :—the point sharp :—the back straight and blunt, the edge slanting obliquely, and the blade increasing in breadth and thickness as it approaches the handle. The advantages of this shape are, that it fills up the incision which it makes, and prevents the escape of the aqueous humour; and that the flap of the cornea is made by one simple motion, that is, by pushing the knife inwards.

like a pen, (in the right hand for the left eye, and *vice versâ*,) and rest-ing the other fingers on the patient's cheek, he touches the cornea once or twice with the flat part of the blade, in order to take off the patient's alarm. 3rdly, He *punctures the cornea* close to its outer margin, push-ing the point of the blade perpendicularly towards the iris, and not obliquely; otherwise it would pass between the laminæ of the cornea instead of entering the anterior chamber. 4thly, He must push it steadily across parallel to the iris, till it cuts its way out, making a semi-circular flap of the lower half of the cornea; immediately upon which the eyelid should be dropped. 5thly, Waiting a few seconds, the surgeon takes a *curette*,—introduces the pointed end with the convexity upwards, and freely lacerates the capsule with it;—and then withdraws it with the convexity downwards. 6thly, He makes *very gentle* pressure on the under part of the globe, and on the upper eyelid, till the lens rises through the pupil and escapes. Lastly, The eye should be opened after a minute or two, to see that the flap of the cornea is rightly adjusted, and that the iris is not prolapsed:—if it is, the eyes should be exposed to a bright light, so as to make the pupil contract, and the prolapsed portion should be gently pressed upon with the spoon of the curette. Then the opera-tion is finished.

VARIETIES.—Some persons make a flap of the upper instead of the lower half of the cornea. The patient lies on a couch; the surgeon sits behind him, and elevates the lid and fixes the globe with one hand. "The advantages of this operation," says Mr. Lawrence, "are, that the operator has a more complete control over the globe; he can fix it very perfectly; that the aqueous humour does not escape so readily, and con-sequently that the section of the cornea is more readily accomplished; that there is less chance of prolapsus iridis; and that the upper lid keeps the flap of the cornea in exact apposition."

*Complications.*—(1.) If the point of the knife should be completely entangled in the iris, the best plan is, to withdraw the instrument, heal the wound, and repeat the operation afterwards. If, however, a little bit of it should get under the edge of the knife, when the section is nearly complete, the operation may be finished with a small curved knife. (2.) If the opening of the cornea is not large enough, it must be enlarged with a similar knife. (3.) If a portion of the lens remain behind, it should be left to be absorbed—unless it has passed into the anterior chamber, and can be removed very easily indeed. (4.) If the vitreous humour seem disposed to escape, the cataract should be hooked out with the curette. But the escape of a little is of no consequence.

*After Treatment.*—The patient should be put to bed, with the shoulders raised, the room darkened, and with a very soft dry linen rag over both eyes. No food should be allowed which requires mastication, the bowels should be kept open, and every thing be avoided which is likely to provoke coughing, sneezing, or vomiting.  If he goes on comfortably, the eyelid may be raised on the fifth day, and then if there be no prolapse of the iris, and the cornea be united, he may get up occasionally, wearing a shade, sitting in a darkened room, and walking about a little.  After a fortnight the eye may be opened in a weak light, and be gradually brought into use.  But inasmuch as it remains weak and irritable, the patient must take the greatest care to avoid exposure to cold, excess in diet, over-exertion of the eye, or exposure of it to too strong a light.  Gray spectacles are the best protectors against wind, or too glaring a light. The patient will require convex spectacles for exact vision, but they must be used very sparingly at first.  He should have two pairs, one with a short focus for near objects, and another of longer focus for distant objects.

The inflammation which may come on after the operation may be of two kinds.  If the eyelids are swollen, and florid, and tender, and there is a thick yellow secretion about the lids, and the conjunctiva is red, and swollen, and chemosed, the inflammation is acute, and requires to be treated by bleeding and purging.  But if, as Mr. Tyrrell shows, the palpebræ are not much discoloured, and are rather œdematous than tinged with blood;—and if the secretion is light coloured, and the conjunctiva œdematous, the patient will be benefited by good broth, carbonate of ammonia, and opium.

II. DEPRESSION is adapted to those cases of hard cataract, of which the extraction would be unadvisable, for reasons mentioned in a preceding page, (342.)  The preparation of the patient, his position during the operation, as well as that of the surgeon, and the duties of the assistant, are the same as required for the operation of extraction.  The pupil should be dilated with belladonna.  There are four ways of operating.

*Operations.*—(1.)  A couching-needle is passed through the outer side of the sclerotic, about two lines behind the margin of the cornea, and a little below the transverse diameter of the eye, so as to avoid the long ciliary artery.  It is carried upwards and forwards behind the iris, and in front of the cataract, and then is steadily and gently pressed upon it till it has carried it downwards and backwards out of sight.  It should be held for a few moments to fix it, then should be lifted up, and if the lens rise also, it must be again depressed for a short time.  Then the needle is withdrawn.

(2.)  According to *Scarpa's plan*, a curved needle is used instead of a straight one.  It is to be introduced with its convexity forwards, and the lens is to be depressed in the manner just described—but before withdrawing the needle, its point is to be turned forwards, and made to lacerate the capsule freely.

(3.)  *King's Operation.*—A curved needle is passed perpendicularly through the sclerotic, as low down as possible; and if the patient's eye is directed upwards and inwards, it can be made to enter almost perpendicularly below the centre of the cornea, and one-eighth of an inch from its margin. It should then be passed onwards with a slight rotatory motion to the pupil, having its convexity forwards, i. e. towards the back of the iris. When it reaches the pupil, these rotations are to be increased, so that the point may cut the anterior capsule into small pieces. The needle is then slowly withdrawn, and the lens follows it, so that it is left at the bottom of the eye close to the puncture made by the needle. If the lens should not immediately follow the needle downwards, the latter is to be stuck into it again.*

(4.) The method of *reclination*, which consists of turning the lens backwards from an upright to a horizontal position, is not much in vogue, although some surgeons recline the cataract before they depress it.

The disadvantages of depression, compared with extraction, are, that the pressure of the lens on the ciliary process and retina is liable to be followed by protracted inflammation, or amaurosis; and that the lens may rise again to its old place, and obstruct vision as before.

III. The Operation for producing Absorption is very easily performed, and excites very little inflammation. Its disadvantages are, that it requires to be repeated, and that the cure is very slow, occupying several weeks or months. It is well adapted for soft cataracts, especially the congenital.

*Operations.*—(1.) The needle may be introduced behind the iris in the same manner as for depression. Then the anterior layer of the capsule is to be freely divided, and the needle, having been passed once or twice through the substance of the lens, is to be withdrawn. Care must be taken not to dislocate the lens in this first operation. The cataract will be more or less dissolved by the aqueous humour, and be absorbed. After the lapse of a few weeks, the operation may be repeated, the capsule may be lacerated more extensively, and the lens be cut up into fragments, which, if perfectly *soft*, may be pushed through the pupil into the anterior chamber, where absorption is more brisk. This operation may be repeated again and again if necessary. But if a hard fragment be pushed into the anterior chamber, it may probably excite great inflammation, and require to be removed by operation; so that the surgeon had better avoid attempting to do too much at once.

(2.) Some recommend the needle to be introduced through the cornea, an operation styled *keratonyxis*. The pupil must be well dilated. Then the needle is passed through the cornea about an eighth of an inch from its margin, and is made to lacerate the capsule to the extent of the pupil. It should be of such a shape as to prevent the escape of the aqueous humour. This method is liable to induce iritis, and does not enable

---

* Lond. Med. Gaz., vol. xxii. pp. 701 and 1009.

the surgeon to act upon the body of the lens. It should therefore be merely employed as a *first* operation, to divide the capsule.

(3.) There is a third modification of this operation, which Mr. Tyrrell terms the operation by *drilling*. It is particularly adapted for cases of capsular or capsulo-lenticular cataract which have been caused by extension of inflammation from the iris. It is performed by introducing a fine straight needle through the cornea near its margin, and passing it through the pupil to the lens. It is then to be made to enter the substance of the lens to the depth of about one sixteenth of an inch, and to be freely rotated. This operation may be repeated at intervals of three, four, or five weeks; and if the puncture be made in a fresh place at each operation, that portion of the capsule which is behind the pupil will become loosened and detached, and the lens absorbed. This operation may also be occasionally resorted to in order to diminish the size of the lens, previously to depression or extraction.

OPERATIONS ON INFANTS.—Congenital cataracts should be operated on early—within four months if possible, lest the eye, which when born blind habitually oscillates from side to side, may never acquire the power of being directed to any particular object. The pupil being well dilated, the child should be placed on a table—the head on a pillow, and rather hanging over it—one assistant holding the legs and trunk, a second the arms and chest, a third fixing the head between his two hands, and a fourth, depressing the *lower* eyelid with one hand, and steadying the chin with the other. The operator then, seated behind the patient, performs the operation for absorption as before described; at the same time elevates the upper lid, and fixes the globe with an *elevator*. Care must be taken not to dislocate the lens, and not to wound the posterior capsule or vitreous humour. This operation on children, and in fact on persons under twenty, generally excites so little inflammation, that both eyes may be operated on at once; but the bowels must be kept open, and leeches should be applied if there be pain.

CAPSULAR CATARACT.—When congenital cataract is left to itself, the lens becomes absorbed, and the capsule remains tough and opaque. And it sometimes happens that an opaque capsule is left, or that it becomes opaque after one of the operations for cataract. There are three plans of treatment. (1.) A needle with cutting edges may be introduced, as for depression; and then may be made to cut crucially through the opaque capsule, which then may shrink and leave the pupil clear. (2.) The upper part of the capsule, for four-fifths of its circumference, may be detached by the needle from the ciliary processes, and then be pushed down below the pupil. (3.) If no other plan succeed in removing a detached piece of capsule, an opening may be made in the cornea, through which it may be extracted by means of a small hook or forceps. Mr.

Middlemore has recently proposed a plan for removing such bodies through the sclerotic.*

I. GLAUCOMA is a slow inflammatory affection of the vitreous humour and deep-seated tunics of the eye, generally occurring to the gouty and intemperate. *Symptoms.*—Severe pain in the head and eyebrow—gradually increasing dimness of vision—and a greenish deep-seated discoloration of the pupil; it sometimes appearing as though there were a piece of metal at the bottom of the eye. The pupil is mostly dilated, and moves sluggishly—and the lens after a time becomes opaque. *Diagnosis.*—Glaucoma is known from cataract by the greenish tint of the pupil, and by the disappearance of the discoloration when the pupil is viewed laterally or obliquely. The loss of vision is not proportionate to the discoloration;—and the sight is best in a strong light. *Treatment.*—Cupping, purging, low or moderate diet, a course of mercury, or a course of colchicum if the pain be severe, and rest of the eye, will, if persevered in, remove the headach and other signs of congestion, and will retard the disease, although they may not cure it.

II. SYNCHYSIS is an unnatural fluidity of the vitreous humour, which may or may not be also discoloured. The eye feels soft and flaccid, the iris is peculiarly tremulous, shaking backwards and forwards like a rag in a bottle of water, the retina becomes insensible, and the lens opaque. This affection is sometimes the result of wounds, and sometimes comes on without obvious cause, it is supposed to depend on a slow inflammation. It is irremediable.

III. DROPSY of the vitreous humour causes enlargement of the globe, with loss of sight and constant excruciating pain, only to be relieved by puncturing the sclerotic with a needle.

I. INFLAMMATION OF THE CHOROID commences with more or less intolerance of light and dimness of vision, together with pain in the eye, eyebrow, and forehead, and lachrymation. The conjunctiva is not uniformly red, but one or more enlarged vessels are seen to proceed from the back of the eye, and to terminate in a vascular zone partially surrounding the cornea. The pupil is often displaced, and brought towards the affected side of the choroid. If it proceed, the sclerotic becomes thin and blue, showing the choroid through it—a watery fluid is effused be-

* Med. Gaz., April 7, 1838.

tween the choroid and retina, causing the thinned part of the sclerotic to bulge out, (*staphyloma scleroticæ*) and finally the cornea may become opaque, the eye protrude from the socket, and the whole globe suppurate. The digestive organs are generally much deranged from the first, and hectic and emaciation come on when the eye becomes much distended and painful. *Treatment.*—1. Repeated and profuse local bleeding, by cupping on the temples, and afterwards by many leeches to the eye;—purgatives of calomel and black draught, followed by daily doses of blue pill (gr. v.) and aloes (gr. iv.) the tartar emetic ointment to the nape of the neck, and the vapour bath to excite the secretion of the skin, are the remedies for the first stage. *Ptyalism* is not considered useful. Afterwards tonics, such as the oxide of iron and quinine, but especially the liq. arsenicalis, in doses of ♏. iv. ter. die, are of service. When the sclerotic becomes much distended, it should be punctured with a needle—the instrument being introduced for one eighth of an inch towards the centre of the eye so as not to wound the lens.

II. INFLAMMATION OF THE RETINA (*retinitis*) may occur in three forms; acute, subacute, and chronic. 1. In the *acute* form the symptoms are severe, deep-seated, and throbbing pain in the eye, extending to the temples and head; vision rapidly impaired, or even altogether lost, frequent sensations of flashes of light, with great fever and delirium. The pupil gradually closes—the iris loses its brilliancy, and the sclerotic is highly vascular and rose-red. If unrelieved the whole globe may suppurate. 2. *Subacute.*—Dimness of sight, headach, or giddiness, flushed countenance and fever, the pupil soon becoming motionless, and the iris turbid. 3. *Chronic.*—Gradually increasing dimness of sight—visions of black spots or flashes of light—irritability of the eye, and intolerance of light—but the patient, though he may shade the eye, does not always shut it. These affections are distinguished by the circumstance that dimness of sight and intolerance of light occur before redness, or any external sign of inflammation. *Causes.*—Exposure to vivid light, flashes of lightning, strong fires, the reflection of the sun from snow, and the like—or habitual exertion of the eye on minute objects, together with neglect of exercise, confinement of the bowels, and over-indulgence in food and spirituous liquors. *Prognosis.*—If, in the acute or subacute form, vision is not much impaired, nor the iris altered, nor the pupil much contracted, the prognosis may be favourable. *Treatment.*—General and local bleeding, purgatives, mercury administered so as to affect the mouth—belladonna, and the antiphlogistic treatment generally, according to the urgency of the symptoms and the strength of the patient.

### SECTION XIII.—OF AMAUROSIS.

DEFINITION.—Imperfection of vision, depending on some change in the retina, optic nerve, or brain.

SYMPTOMS.—1. The first and chief symptom is impairment of vision, which is sometimes sudden and complete, but more frequently slow and progressive. At the commencement of the disease, it usually occurs at occasional intervals—perhaps in the form of night-blindness, or day-blindness—or after the eye has been fatigued by writing or other exertion. Sometimes it commences as indistinct vision, (*diplopia*,) objects appearing doubled—or as *hemiopia*, one half only of the objects looked at being seen;—or objects may appear crooked, disfigured, or discoloured; or they may be seen covered with patches; or the affection may commence as near-sightedness or far sightedness. The flame of a candle generally appears split, lengthened, or broken into an iridescent halo.

2. *Ocular spectra*, sometimes in the form of floating black spots, (*muscæ volitantes*,) sometimes as flashes of light, or as a coloured cloud or network.

3. Sometimes incipient amaurosis is attended with great intolerance of light—sometimes, on the contrary, with a constant *thirst for light*, or feeling as if objects were not illuminated enough.

4. The patient walks with a peculiar uncertain gait, and his eyes have a vacant stare;—the eyelids move imperfectly and seldom—the pupil is generally dilated, (unless it be an incipient case, attended with intolerance of light;)—the iris moves sluggishly, and in confirmed cases is totally motionless. But if one eye be sound, and be exposed to light during the examination, the iris of the affected eye will often move in sympathy with that of the sound one.

DIAGNOSIS.—Amaurosis may be distinguished from cataract by noticing, 1. that in cataract, an opaque body can be seen behind the pupil, and that the impairment of vision is in proportion to the extent of that opacity: whereas, in pure amaurosis, the pupil either shows its natural colour, or else a deep-seated greenish discolouration. 2. That, in cataract, (with the exception of the radiating variety,) vision is simply *clouded*, and that a lighted candle appears as if enveloped in a mist; whereas, in amaurosis, objects are seen *dis*coloured or perverted in shape; and that a lighted candle seems split, or lengthened, or iridescent; and the *muscæ volitantes*, and flashes of fire when the eyes are shut, are not present in pure cataract. 3. That in cataract vision is better in a dull light, whereas it is generally the reverse in amaurosis. 4. That a patient with cataract is always able to discern light from darkness, and that he looks about him and moves his eyes as though conscious that vision still exists, although he may be unable to discern particular objects; whereas in confirmed amaurosis there is a peculiar fixed vacant stare, and the eyeball is protruded and motionless.

PROGNOSIS.—This is generally unfavourable—unless the disease depends on some palpable cause which admits of removal, and unless the remedial measures employed very soon produce good effects.

VARIETIES.—Amaurosis has been divided into the *functional* and *organic:* the former depending on some sympathetic or other disorder which does not primarily affect the structure of the nervous apparatus of the eye.

CAUSES.—The usual causes of amaurosis are circumstances that over-stimulate and exhaust the retina;—such as long-continued exertion of the eye on minute objects;—or exposure to glaring light, especially if combined with heat—and these exciting causes are particularly aided by intemperance, stooping, tight neckcloths, too much sleep in bed, and any other circumstances capable of producing determination of blood to the head. Amaurosis may also be a consequence of organic change, inflammation, concussion, compression from extravasated blood, fractured bone, morbid effusions, tumours or aneurisms—whether affecting the brain, optic nerves, or eye.

TREATMENT.—The indications in every case are, 1. To rectify any palpable disorder—inflammation or plethora by depletion;—debility by tonics. 2. To neutralize determination of blood to the eye or head by counter-irritation. 3. To stimulate and restore the excitability of the retina. For practical purposes, it will be convenient to classify the disease under the five following heads.

1. *Inflammatory.*—(*a*) If amaurosis be attended with any of the symptoms of retinitis that have been before enumerated;—(*b*) or if it suddenly follow some injury to the eye, such as a punctured wound, or blow on the naked eyeball, or exposure to a flash of lightning; or if the patient be engaged in occupations that necessarily tax the eye severely; (*c*) or if there be plethora, headach, giddiness, red turgid countenance, with a hot skin and a hard pulse,—and if there are frequent flashes of light, or streams of red-hot balls seen before the eyes, (especially when stooping, or undergoing some active exertion;) (*d*) or if the complaint have followed a suppression of any accustomed evacuation, such as bleeding from piles, or the translation of erysipelas or gout; bleeding or cupping on the temple or mastoid process should be performed at intervals. The bowels should be well cleared, the diet should be low, and all employment of the affected organ and all violent bodily exertion should be desisted from. Mercury should be administered—rapidly if the case be sudden in its attack, and present urgent inflammatory symptoms—but more slowly if it present a more chronic aspect—but in either case it should be given so as to bring the system under its influence, and its effects should be kept up for some time. Small doses of tartarized antimony may sometimes be conveniently combined with the mercury, (calomel gr. ii. ant. tart. gr. ⅓,) or may be given according to F. 34 and 35, but it is scarcely advisable to cause vomiting whilst there are signs of active congestion. Counter-irritants of all sorts are beneficial; blisters, or the tartar-emetic ointment applied behind the ears, or to the nape of the neck—immersion

of the feet in hot water and mustard—or an issue in the arms in chronic cases.

2. *Atonic* amaurosis may come on at the close of some long and exhausting illness, or may be produced by great loss of blood, menorrhagia, immoderate suckling, leucorrhœa, excessive venery, or other debilitating circumstances. It is attended with general debility, pallid lips, frequent trembling pulse, and dilated pupils;—and the patient generally sees best after a meal or a few glasses of wine, and in a strong light. The practitioner must carefully examine into the causes of debility—whether they consist in some disorder of the system, or in depraved and unhealthy habits of life. The *treatment* consists, first, in suppressing any habitual discharge, or other source of exhaustion. Secondly, in strengthening the system by change of air, tonics, quinine, steel and zinc, and especially by good living. At the same time the abdominal secretions should be well regulated by aperients, (such as aloes and rhubarb,) that act copiously, but not drastically; and the cutaneous and general circulation be promoted by exercise and bathing, especially the shower-bath. Camphor, or arnica,* assafœtida, and other fetid stimulants, or strychnine in very small doses (gr $\frac{1}{12}$) may be of service. It is in this form, if in any, that local stimulants are applicable—such as exposing the eye to the vapour of æther, or sal volatile, (a tea-spoonful of either being held in the hand,)—taking electric sparks from the eye; stimulating snuff, (F. 32, 33,) cataplasms of capsicum to the temples; strychnine applied to the temples after the skin has been denuded by a blister, beginning with gr. $\frac{1}{8}$, and gradually increasing it to gr. i;—friction of the forehead with cajeput or croton oil, or with an alcoholic solution of veratria.

3. *Sympathetic.*—(*a*) Amaurosis not unfrequently supervenes on an attack of jaundice. If there be evidence of congestion in the head, as there frequently will be, blood should be taken by cupping, whilst the abdominal disorder should be removed by appropriate measures. (*b*) If there be foul tongue, disagreeable eructations, tumid belly, and other evidence of abdominal congestion and disorder, emetics, repeated once or twice a-week, blue pill or hyd. c. creta., in small doses every night; and purgatives, such as senna, aloes, and rheubarb, with soda, magnesia, and ipecacuanha, till the secretions are set to rights, followed by tonics and counter-irritants, are the requisite measures. In similar cases, some foreign authors recommend the use of Schmucker's or Richter's *resolvent pills*, F. 34, 35. Turpentine should be given both as a purgative and enema, if there be signs of worms. (*c*) Amaurosis sometimes arises from irritation of the fifth pair of nerves. If it follow a wound on the fore-

---

* Dose, f℥i of an infusion, made with ℥ss of the dried leaves, to Oj of boiling water. It should be combined with aromatics.

head, the latter should be dilated, or if it have healed, the cicatrix should be cut out. Tumours of all sorts near the eye, or carious teeth, should be removed.

4. *From Poisons.*—Amaurosis is liable to be induced by certain poisons, such as lead, belladonna, hyoscyamus, and especially by tobacco, that great patron of undertakers and bailiffs, whether administered in large doses, or applied slowly and frequently. After the removal of the immediate effects of the poison, the various local stimulants and counter-irritants mentioned above are most likely to be useful.

5. *Organic.*—These cases are the most hopeless. If the disease has followed an injury of the head, or fit of apoplexy, or syphilis, or if there be reason to suspect tumours,—a moderate course of mercury, with alkalis and sarsaparilla, and with counter-irritants, and attention to the general health, should be tried, and sometimes may effect a cure. For other forms of organic disease, especially if there be fixed pain in the head, palsy, or epilepsy, or idiocy, the best thing that the surgeon can do will be to prevent congestion in the head by occasional depletion, and counter-irritation;—to maintain the secretions of the liver and bowels; to keep up the strength by a nutritious but not stimulating diet, and to guard the patient from every excess or exertion, mental or bodily, that is capable of accelerating the cerebral circulation.

## SECTION XIV.—OF SHORT AND LONG SIGHT.

I. SHORT SIGHT (*myopia*) most probably depends on some vice of conformation—such as a too great thickness, density, or convexity, of the lenses and humours of the eye, whereby the rays of light are brought to a focus before they reach the retina. It is most frequently congenital, and is perceived in early childhood; but doubtless it may be induced by habits of study, and of looking at minute objects, which, by irritating the eye, cause the secretion of aqueous humour to be increased, and render the cornea more convex. It is a popular error to imagine that the sight improves as the individual grows older. *Treatment.*—The eyes should be exercised and accustomed to look at distant objects. When children display any tendency to short sight, their studies should be abridged, and they should have plenty of exercise in the open air. Shooting, archery, cricket, and field sports in general, are highly beneficial. It is worth while also to try a plan of treatment invented by Berthold, and consisting in the use of an instrument which has received the sesquipedalian title of *myopodiorthoticon.* This is really nothing more than a support for the chin, to prevent the patient stooping forwards ; whilst he reads from a book with large print. And the book is every day to be placed at a slightly greater distance from the eyes, till the patient has acquired the faculty of reading at the ordinary focal distance—that is to say, at about fifteen inches. *Concave glasses* should be avoided if the patient can go on pretty comfortable without them; or at all events should only be worn when required to prevent unseemly stooping in reading or playing music. But if the myopia is very decided, or if the eyes feel fatigued after any ordinary use of them, it will be better to wear the glasses continually. Spectacles should always be used in preference to a single glass. The patient should choose a pair that enables him to see objects within forty feet as distinctly as other people,—the names on the corners of the street for instnnce; but the glasses are too concave if they make objects appear dazzling, or smaller than usual.

II. PRESBYOPIA, or longsightedness, depends on diminished density of the humours, and is one of the earliest signs of impaired nutrition in old age. The patient's sight must be remedied by *convex glasses;* but he should not resort to them at first—nor change those first selected for stronger ones before he is absolutely compelled; and the sight should be spared by candle light as much as possible. The glasses should cause minute objects near the eye to appear bright and distinct, but not larger than natural. If they do, they are too convex.*

### SECTION XV.—OF SQUINTING.

SQUINTING, or STRABISMUS, may be defined to be a want of parallelism in the position and motions of the eyes.

The essential cause of the affection appears, in most instances, to be some weakness of sight, or some want of adjustment in the visual axis of the affected eye, in consequence of which it is involuntarily turned aside, in order to avoid the double or distorted vision that would result from looking at objects with two eyes of different powers. The immediate mechanism by which the squint is produced, is most probably a relaxed or inactive state of the external rectus muscle, so that its antagonist muscle, the internal rectus, preponderates in force, and draws the eye inwards.† Sometimes, although more rarely, it may be supposed that the affection commences by an original spasm of the internal rectus.

The ordinary form of squint is the *convergent*, or that in which the

---

* Presbyopia in an elderly gentleman has been cured by a vio'ent fall and contusion of the eyes; which doubtless produced an increased secretion of aqueous humour. Presbyopia occurring in young persons generally arises from intestinal irritation, and may be a precursor of amaurosis.

† This is shown by the results of the operation of dividing the internal rectus, after which the eye is merely drawn by the external rectus into its natural position; whereas, when (in various accidents) one of the recti of a sound eye has been severed, its antagonist has drawn it completely over to its *own* side. Vide Sir. C. Bell, Practical Essays, 1841.

45

eye is turned inwards; the *divergent*, or that in which the eye is everted, is more rare. It occasionally happens that both eyes squint; but it must be remarked that they do not both squint at the same time, but alternately. When one eye is distorted and *fixed*, the affection is called *lusitas*.

CAUSES.—1. Squinting may be caused by congenital malformation. 2. It may be induced by bad habits; such as the imitation of parents, nurses, or schoolfellows, if they happen to squint;—or by constantly looking at specks or pimples on the nose; or it may follow affections (such as hordeolum) which render motion of the eye painful; and during which the patient turns the eye inwards, and keeps it motionless. 3. It may be caused by using one eye constantly to the neglect of the other. It may be observed, that all short sighted persons have more or less tendency to squint, for the following reason. They never use both eyes whilst they are reading or examining small objects near the eye; but sometimes use the right eye, and sometimes the left. If, however, they were by accident to persist in using one only, it would become stronger by use, and the other weaker by disuse; and the weaker eye might squint. In this manner, squinting has been known to occur after one eye has been for a long time shaded in consequence of an inflammatory attack; which shows the expediency of always covering both eyes when a shade is necessary. 4. If there happens to be an opacity on the cornea of one eye, and that eye is the best, it will sometimes happen, that the patient will continue to use it for ordinary vision, but for that purpose is obliged to distort it so as to remove the corneal opacity from the visual axis. 5. Squinting like almost every other conceivable consequence of defect of nervous influence, is sometimes a relic of fevers and the exanthemata. 6. It may be. induced by irritation or disorder of the stomach and bowels, teething, worms, constipation, and so forth;—it may, moreover, be caused by fright or violent fits of passion; and in some children it always appears when the health is out of order, and disappears again when it is restored. Lastly, it may be caused by some disorder of the circulation in the brain. Thus it is pretty frequently the precursor of acute hydrocephalus or convulsions in children; and when it is associated with dropping of one or both eyelids, and with unusual sleepiness, or torpor of the intellect, or faltering in the gait, some mischief within the head may fairly be anticipated.

TREATMENT.—If the affection be recent, it may perhaps be removed by judicious medical treatment. The patient should be secluded from the society of every squinting person who might be imitated. Any disorder in the stomach or bowels should be removed by purgatives, antacids, and tonics, and if the patient is a weakly child, and if the squinting has followed a severe illness, a course of steel wine, or small doses of sulphate of zinc, may be of service. An endeavour should be made to strengthen and exercise the squinting eye, by covering the sound one with a light shade for one or two hours every day; but this must be done with moderation; because it has happened, that whilst a squinting eye has been cured by this means, the sound one has been weakened by seclusion, and has been made to squint instead. It is a useful plan to make the patient exercise his eye before a glass in the following manner. He should be told to close the sound eye, and look at a particular point with the squinting one. Then let him open the sound eye. Upon this, the squinting one will immediately diverge; but by perseverance the patient may educate it, till he can command it, and keep it parallel with the other. If a child is beginning to squint, it should be carefully watched, and be told to endeavour to correct it; close application to study should be interdicted; plenty of exercise should be taken in the open air; and if the sight is short, a pair of shallow concave spectacles should be used. Lastly, cases are related of recent squinting cured by very small doses of strychnia, and by taking electric sparks from the eye, or by passing slight galvanic currents between the frontal and infraorbital nerves.

But if the squint is of long standing and is habitual, very little good can be done unless the internal rectus muscle is divided; or the external rectus, if the squint is divergent. This operation (the rationale of which will be alluded to in the chapter on Club Foot,) will be of equal efficacy, whether the squint is produced by spasm of one muscle or by weakness of its antagonist. It is easily performed in the following manner. The patient, if an adult and manageable, sits in a low chair;—if an unruly child, he should be rolled up in a sheet, and be placed on a table with the head supported by a pillow. The sound eye should of course be ban-

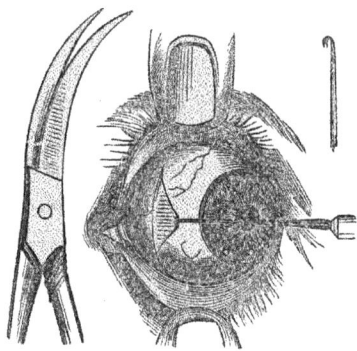

daged, and an assistant should place two fingers on it to keep it steady during the operation. Then the upper lid of the squinting eye being held up by the assistant's finger, or by a wire speculum, and the lower lid being held down by another assistant's finger, or by a small catch or *bulldog* forceps, (which may be made to seize the conjunctiva inside the lid, and will hold it down by its weight,)—these preliminaries being arranged the surgeon introduces the fine double hook into the conjunctiva just inside the cornea, and having drawn the eye outwards, gives it to an assistant to hold steadily. Then he raises the conjunctiva on the inner side of the eyeball with a forceps, and divides it perpendicularly with the curved scissors. Next, he raises some reddish cellular tissue, and cuts through it in the same manner; and thirdly, he cuts through the muscle; which being divided will expose the clear white sclerotic. He should be careful to divide perpendicularly every fibre which covers the sclerotic for the extent of half an inch; and if he does so, he will find that the patient can move the eye more freely than before in all other directions, but that he *cannot move it directly inwards*. This is a sign that the operation is complete.

After the operation the eye should be protected from cold and light, and any inflammatory symptoms be checked by appropriate measures. But it is very rarely succeeded by any untoward symptoms, although the author knows one case in which the eyeball suppurated and burst.

This operation may be performed for two purposes. The first is, to get rid of the deformity of the squint. And this purpose is generally answered effectually; although it must be confessed that the inner side of the eyeball is apt to project somewhat, and the eye to look large and goggled. But the patient must make his own choice between this and the squint.

The second purpose is that of strengthening the eye, and enabling the patient to bring it into use. And this purpose is no doubt answered in some measure, so that both eyes are used for the vision of remote objects, and the patient says that the eye feels stronger and clearer; but it is not likely to be useful in near vision till after a long time, if at all. Moreover, after the operation, it is very common for some degree of double vision to be complained of. This will be perfectly intelligible when it is considered that objects are viewed by two eyes of different powers and adjustments. But this inconvenience soon passes off, because the patient learns to neglect the image presented by the weaker eye.

### SECTION XVI.—OF MALIGNANT DISEASES OF THE EYE.

I. SCIRRHUS.—After years of supposed inflammation, the eye becomes shrunk and hard, and the conjunctiva tuberculated, thickened, and red. The eye is exquisitely tender; there is much burning or lancinating pain, and severe hemicrania. After a time, ulceration occurs, and spreads to the neighbouring parts, and the patient sinks. *Treatment.*—Extirpation,

if it can be adopted before the lids are affected; if not, the local and general employment of narcotics.

II. FUNGUS MEDULLARIS is not unfrequent, especially in children. Its
most frequent seat is the termination of the optic nerve. The eye is accidentally discovered to be blind, and a small tumour of a peculiar metallic lustre can be detected very deep behind the pupil. This gradually
advances, and generally appears whitish or yellowish, and lobulated, and
more or less streaked with blood-vessels. In a space of time, varying
from a few months to two or three years, the cornea bursts before the
enlarging tumour, a bleeding fungous protrudes, the cervical glands enlarge and the patient perishes. There is not usually much pain before
the cornea begins to be distended. Melanosis is sometimes combined
with this disease. *Treatment.*—Much may be hoped from a light nutritious diet, fresh air, occasional leechings, and a gentle course of mercury, which should be kept up for some weeks. By these means the
disease, if malignant, may be checked; if not malignant, may be cured.
Extirpation is scarcely ever deemed advisable in children, (1) because the
disease if really malignant is sure to return; (2) because there are sundry scrofulous tumours which cannot be distinguished from the malignant, and which either disappear, or give no trouble. The diagnosis may
be considered doubtful, if such tumours follow an evident wound or injury; if there be scrofulous disease in other parts, and if the eye shrink
and become atrophic.

III. EXTIRPATION OF THE EYE.—The operator first passes a ligature
through the anterior part of the globe in order to steady it, and slits up
the external commissure of the lids. Then he raises the upper eyelid,
cuts through the fold of conjunctiva reflected from it to the eye, and dissects backwards, so as to separate all the soft parts from the roof of the
orbit. The same process is repeated below and on the sides—taking
care to cut close to the bone, and to remove the lachrymal gland. Then
a curved knife is introduced on the outer side to cut through the optic
nerve and origin of the muscles, and so the eye is detached. The patient must then be put to bed, with a cloth dipped in cold water laid over
the face. If there is a very great hæmorrhage from the ophthalmic artery, it may be restrained by pressure with a piece of lint,—which should
be removed as soon as it is suppressed; and the orbit must by no means
be stuffed with that substance.

After staphyloma or any other disease which has rendered the eyeball
shrunken and sightless, if the patient objects to the trouble and expense
of an artificial eye, it may be convenient to divide the levator palpebræ.
in order that the lids may remain permanently closed. This may be effected by making a transverse incision in the upper eyelid just below the
orbit, and seizing the belly of the muscle as far back as possible. Then
a piece should be snipped out of it with scissors.

IV. ENCANTHIS is an enlargement of the caruncula lachrymalis, and semilunar fold of the conjunctiva, which may be easily extirpated by curved scissors. Sometimes, however, it assumes a malignant action, becoming dull red, very hard, and subject to lancinating pain; and finally it degenerates into a cancerous ulcer. Sir A. Cooper thinks that in this case extirpation is inadmissible.*

---

# CHAPTER XIII.

## OF THE DISAESES AND INJURIES OF THE EAR.

I. FOREIGN BODIES may be removed from the ear by syringing it violently with warm water—or by a pair of small forceps—or by a small scoop, or curette, or bent probe, which may be introduced behind the intruding substance, so as to draw it forwards. Insects may be removed by similar means, or by introducing a piece of cotton fastened to the end of a probe, and smeared with honey, or some other viscid substance.

II. OTITIS. ACUTE INFLAMMATION of the *external* ear is known by violent pain in the part, which is increased by pressure, and by noise, as well as by the motions of the head and of the lower jaw, and by exposure to cold air. Hearing is confused, and there are noises in the ear, (*tinnitus.*) The meatus is swelled, and highly vascular, and secretes a thin serous fluid. Inflammation of the *internal* ear is attended with much severer pain, and constant ringing, throbbing sounds. Both are accompanied with severe headach and fever, and may prove fatal. They are generally *caused* by cold, or foreign bodies, or by gastric derangement, and are most frequent in children. *Treatment.*—Leeches behind the ear, or bleeding if the patient is old enough to bear it, and if it is demanded by violent fever and delirium;—subsequently, an emetic followed by a dose of calomel with antimony, purgatives, and salines. The ear may be very gently syringed with poppy decoction, or milk and water, or may be poulticed. All foreign bodies, or hardened wax, should be gently removed.

---

* Vide Lectures by Professor Green, in Sir A. Cooper's Lectures, Renshaw's edit.; Lawrence on Diseases and on Venereal Diseases of the Eye; Copland Dict., Art. Eye, Amaurosis, &c.; Middlemore on Diseases of the Eye; Guthrie on the Operative Surgery of the Eye, and in Lond. Med. and Surg. Journal; Littell's compendium; Foot's Ophthalmic Memoranda; Morgan on the Eye, Lond., 1839; Tyrrell on the Eye, Lond., 1840; and especially Mackenzie on Diseases of the Eye, 3rd edit., Lond., 1640, a work of the greatest erudition and practical utility.

Blisters should be applied to the nape of the neck, or behind the ear, when the acute stage is subsiding. If the cavity of the tympanum have suppurated, which will be known by an aggravation of the throbbing pain, and headach, and by a sense of weight and bursting in the ear, and by the membrana tympani* appearing white and convex externally, it should be opened with a long slender knife, to save the pain and delay of its ulcerating or bursting. But this operation should not be hastily performed; and if early and free antiphlogistic measures are employed, it will rarely be required.

III. CHRONIC INFLAMMATION—(*otorrhæa*)—producing a mucous or muco-purulent discharge from the ear, is very common in scrofulous children, and may last for a long term of years. *Treatment.*—Mild aperients should be given frequently, together with tonics; such as iron, bark, and iodine, in the manner directed for scrofula. *Sulphur* is much praised as a laxative in these cases. Blisters may be applied behind the ear, or to the nape of the neck, and may be repeated, or be kept discharging by cerat. sabinæ. It is well known that sundry dangerous affections of the brain, or disorders of the eye, or of other parts, are liable to supervene upon the suppression of this discharge. Therefore, till the constitution is set to rights, no other local applications should be used save mild injections to cleanse away the discharge; such as warm milk and water, or dec. papav.;—avoiding oily matters, lest they become rancid and irritating. If, under the employment of these measures, the discharge diminishes, without any ill consequences, mild astringent injections may be tried, beginning with lime-water, or inf. rosæ, and afterwards the different lotions in F. 36, 37, 21, 22, taking care to increase their strength very cautiously, especially if the membrana tympani have been perforated by previous ulceration or suppuration. If the discharge cease, and there be pain in the ear or head, hot poultices or fomentations, and the remedies for acute inflammation, should be adopted.

IV. CARIES of the temporal bone, especially of the mastoid process, may be a consequence of extension of inflammation from the mucous membrane of the ear, particularly if the cavity of the tympanum has suppurated, and matter has lodged and become putrid, after the membrana tympani has burst, or has been opened. There is constant *otorrhæa*, and the discharge is sanious and fetid, and stains silver probes. This is a most serious disease. Death may be caused by extension of the caries to the cranial cavity and suppuration on the dura mater, or by inflammation of the brain or its membranes, through contiguous irritation,—or the side of the face may be palsied through compression of the portio dura. Sometimes an abscess bursts behind the ear, or burrows amongst the

---

* In order to bring this' part into view, the auricle requires to be drawn outwards, upwards, and forwards; if necessary, the meatus must be dilated with a speculum.

muscles of the neck and points low down. *Treatment.*—Tonics altera-tives, counter-irritants, and mild astringent injections, frequently repeated, to wash away the fetid discharge. Abscesses near the ear should be opened as soon as possible. Injections of weak nitric acid lotion (F. 17) may be employed to correct the disease of the bone, provided there is no fear that it may have reached the dura mater. If the patient be labour-ing under secondary venereal symptoms, sarsaparilla may be given with advantage. If inflammation, or symptoms of compression of the brain supervene, they must be treated as was detailed in Chapter X., recollect-ing that depletion and mercury must be used with the greatest modera-tion, as they cannot remove the exciting cause.

V. EARACH—(*otalgia*)—(1.) Genuine *neuralgia* of the ear,—occur-ring in fits of excruciating pain, shooting over the head and face,—may be distinguished from *otitis* by the sudden intensity of the pain, which is not throbbing,—does not increase in severity,—is not attended with fever,—and comes and goes capriciously. Its *causes* are the same as of neuralgia generally, (p. 304) but particularly caries of the teeth ; and its *treatment* principally consists in removing carious teeth, or stopping them, and giving large doses of carbonate of iron.

(2.) *Common earach*, which is frequently produced (in children espe-cially) by decay of the posterior teeth, or by cold, although a sympathe-tic affection, is generally somewhat inflammatory. *Treatment.*—An emetic and purgative will mostly be of service. Carious teeth should be extracted, and gum-boils be opened. The pain may be relieved by filling the meatus with a warm mixture of ol. oliv. 3i, tinct. opii 3i, the concha being plugged with cotton, to keep it in; or by exposing the ear to the vapour of sp. æther. c. 3iii aq. f3iv, which may be put into a phial, im-mersed in hot water,—or by the crumb of a hot loaf applied to the head;—or by sponging the head with hot water, and wrapping it up in an oil silk cap, together with pediluvia and enemata, and in obstinate cases, blisters. An examination for hardened wax, or foreign bodies, in the meatus, should never be omitted.

VI. WARTS and excrescences in the meatus are not uncommon in chronic inflammation, and may be snipped off, if they are not removed by various injections before mentioned.

VII. DEAFNESS may be a consequence of very many pathological conditions. (1) It may be caused by *chronic inflammation* of the exter-nal meatus, or membrana tympani, with thickening, or excrescences of the membrane, and purulent discharge. These cases must be treated by blisters behind the ear, attention to the health, and the cautious use of injections. If the cuticle of the meatus and membrana tympani is much thickened, injections of arg. nit. or of ung. hydr. nit. 3j, ol. oliv. 3iii, are much recommended. The internal ear may have suppurated, and the *ossicula* may have sloughed away, but still deafness is not total unless the *stapes* has perished,—the loss of which lays open the *fenestra ovalis*, and permits the escape of the fluid in the *labyrinth*.

(2.) *Accumulations of hardened wax* depend on a diseased state of the meatus. They should be frequently removed with the syringe; and combinations of oxgall ʒii vel ol. terebinth fʒj with ol. oliv. fʒvii, or tinct. castorei, may be occasionally dropped into the ear. Similar applications are sometimes used when it is conceived that there is a deficiency of wax. In syringing the ear, the water mostly requires to be rather hot, and a little wool should be introduced afterwards to prevent cold.*

(3.) Deafness is frequently caused by *tumours of the tonsils* obstructing the eustachian tubes, or by relaxation of the mucous membrane of the throat, with secretion of viscid mucus in the tubes—or by contraction, or by obliteration of the tubes consequent upon ulcers,—a thing not uncommon after scarlet fever or venereal sore throat. These cases will be known by the patient's history, and by examination of the throat. *Treatment.*—Chronic sore throat, or swelling of the tonsils, must be removed by stimulating and astringent gargles, or by touching the parts with a hair pencil dipped into a strong solution of nitrate of silver;—as well as by the use of iodine, tonics, counter-irritants, and attention to the general health. If these measures fail, the enlarged tonsils must be abridged by the knife. The eustachian tubes may be known to be pervious if the shock of air can be heard against the membrana tympani, by means of the stethoscope applied to the mastoid process, whilst the patient closes his mouth and nostrils and makes a strong expiration. These tubes or the cavity of the tympanum may be known to be clogged with mucus, when loud crackling or gurgling noises are heard by the patient, (or by the surgeon with the stethoscope,) when he expires strongly with the mouth and nose closed. For this state, it is useful to wash out the tube and tympanum with warm water. A bent silver catheter (of the size of a common probe) is introduced along the floor of the inferior meatus of the nostril into the pharynx. It should be introduced with its convexity uppermost; and when it has reached the pharynx, if its point be turned upwards and outwards, it will slip into the tube. Warm water may then be gently injected by a syringe, and if the tube be pervious, it will be heard and felt to strike against the membrana tympani. If the tube be not pervious, a catgut bougie (made of the small E string of a harp) may be very gently passed through the catheter to dilate it. But this bougie should never be introduced more than an inch and a half into the tube, and should on no account be passed into the tympanum. Moreover it is quite fruitless to perform this operation if the patient cannot hear a watch tick when it is put between his teeth. *Perforation of the membrana tympani* may be resorted to when the eustachian tube

---

* It is never justifiable to put wool or cotton *into the meatus;* it should be put merely into the cavity of the concha.

46

is known to be quite impervious. It is best accomplished by means of an instrument that cuts out a little circular piece.

(4.) Deafness is often caused by *blows* on the head, which either produce concussion or rupture of the auditory nerve, or extravasation of blood into the tympanum or labyrinth. Depletion, if any inflammatory symptoms are present, with alteratives and counter-irritants afterwards, are the only remedies; but if deafness immediately succeed the injury, they will scarcely relieve it.

(5.) It may be produced by *organic* alterations in the brain, tumours or the like, and may be attended with epilepsy or idiocy, or may be a consequence of apoplexy or convulsions. The *treatment* must be the same as for amaurosis arising from similar causes (p. 352.)

(6.) It is sometimes connected with general plethora, or with suppressed menstrual or hæmorrhoidal discharge, and attended with giddiness, tinnitus, and flushings of the countenance. To be treated antiphlogistically.

(7.) Deafness is said to be *nervous* when it depends on general torpor and debility, and is better at some times than at others, especially in fine weather, and when the patient is cheerful or excited, and the stomach in good order. *Treatment.*—Aperients and alteratives, with diffusible stimulants, especially ammonia, æther, and valerian, taken occasionally, and the employment of excitants locally; such as stimulating gargles, (tinct. capsisi f℥ß ad inf. rosæ Oß,) *masticatories* of pellitory, snuffs, (F. 32,) the introduction of oxgall or turpentine, or the vapour of æther or of sp. am. ar. into the meatus, and the application of garlic, mustard, and other counter-irritants behind the ear. *Electricity* may be mischievous.*

# CHAPTER XIV.

## OF THE DISEASES AND INJURIES OF THE FACE AND NOSE.

I. Salivary Fistula is formed when a wound or an ulcer has made a communication between the *stenonian* duct and the skin, so that the saliva dribbles out on the cheek. *Treatment.*—In the first place, a good pas-

---

* Vide Copland Dict., art. Ear and Hearing: Kramer on Diseases of the Ear, translated by Bennett; Pilcher on the Structure and Diseases of the Ear, Lond. 1838; and Essay on the Ear, by Joseph Williams, M. D. Lond. 1840.

sage must be established from the duct into the mouth. This may be done by puncturing the mouth through the fistula in two places, passing a small skein of silk, or, still better, a piece of very flexible wire, through the apertures, and securing the two ends in the mouth by a knot. After a few days the edges of the fistula must be pared, and be brought into contact by sutures, in order that they may unite by adhesion. When there has been a loss of substance it may be necessary to apply the actual cautery to the margin of the aperture, in order that the fungus granulations succeeding the burn may supply the deficiency; or to cover it with a flap of skin raised from the adjoining parts.

II. LIFOMA, a hypertrophy or sarcomatous tumour, sometimes affects the cellular tissue and skin of the nose, especially of persons who have been addicted to the pleasures of the table. These tumours are very inconvenient and unsightly, but not malignant. They grow slowly—are indolent and painless—the sebaceous follicles are much enlarged, and secrete profusely, and the skin is more or less mottled with veins. *Treatment.—* *If the patient desires it,* the tumour may be removed with the knife; but he must observe rigid abstemiousness, and have his bowels well cleared for a fortnight previously. An incision may be made in the median line nearly down to the cartilage. Then an assistant distends the nostrils with his forefinger, whilst the surgeon seizes the morbid growth, and shaves it clean off, close to the cartilage. After the operation, there will be considerable hæmorrhage from numerous vessels. Some of these may be tied, some may be pinched with a forceps, some may be tied with a very fine cambric needle and thread; and any general oozing may be restrained by the application of a cloth dipped in cold water, or if it be obstinate, by plugging the nostrils, and making pressure with strips of plaster.

III. FOREIGN BODIES may be removed from the nose by a small curette, or scoop, or bent probe. If they cannot be brought through the nostrils, they may be pushed back into the throat. The removal should be effected as early as possible.

IV. EPISTAXIS or hæmorrhage from the nose, may, like other hæmorrhages, be produced, 1st, by injury; 2ndly, by an *active* exhalation of arterial blood from the capillaries, owing to general excitement and plethora, or determination of blood to the head, or to the suppression of some other discharge; 3rdly, by a *passive* draining of blood, (principally venous,) owing to obstruction of the circulation by disease of the heart or liver, or to a morbidly thin state of the blood, together with relaxation of the vessels, as happens in scurvy, purpura, and the last stage of fevers. *Treatment.—*(1.) If the patient be redfaced, plethoric, and subject to headach and giddiness, the hæmorrhage should be regarded as salutary, and should not be restrained too suddenly. If it be very profuse, and attended with much headach, venesection may be performed, and at all events purgatives and low diet should be prescribed. (2.) But the hæmorrhage requires to be stopped, either if it have continued so long that the patient will be injuriously weakened—or if it arise from injury,—or if it be a *passive* hæmorrhage depending on visceral disease, or general cachexy. If an upright posture, cold applied to the head, and a piece of cold metal to the back, with a draught of any cold liquid, and compression of the nostril, do not stop it; the patient may snuff up powdered gum, or gall nuts; and, that failing, the nostril must be plugged with lint, or with putty. In very urgent cases, the posterior orifice of the nostril must be plugged also. This is easily done by passing a bougie, with a long piece of silk fastened to its end, through the nostril into the pharynx. The end of the silk in the pharynx is brought through the mouth with a pair of forceps, and a piece of soft sponge, less than an inch in diameter, is tied to it. Then, by pulling the silk back through the nose, the sponge is drawn into the posterior opening of the nostril. The plugs, or coagula, in severe cases, should not be disturbed for three days. Nitre and other salines: or pills of plumbi acet., with draughts containing vinegar, F. 60, 61, may be given with advantage in inflammatory cases—and the nitric or sulphuric acids, opium, alum, quinine, small doses of turpentine, (m xv,) and the ergot of rye, in those of atony and debility.

V. Nasal Polypus.—There are four varieties of this affection, (1) The common *gelatinous* polypus is a tumour of the consistence of jelly, pear-shaped, yellowish, slightly streaked with blood-vessels, attached by a narrow neck to the mucous membrane, especially that on the turbinated bones, and apparently consisting of organized lymph. The patient has a constant feeling of *stuffing* and cold in the head, which is increased in

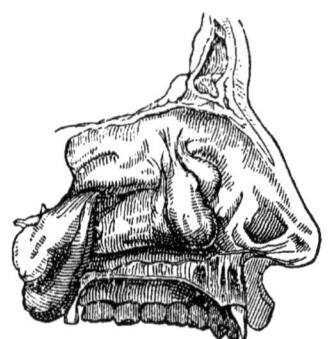

damp weather. If he force his breath strongly through the affected nostril, whilst he closes the other, the polypus may be brought into view. There are very often more than one of these tumours, and they are very liable to return when removed. If polypus be permitted to remain, it continually increases in size, blocks up the nostril, displaces the septum, and obstructs the other nostril, causes prodigious deformity of the cheek, prevents the passage of the tears, and may even cause death by pressure on the brain.* *Treatment.*—A probe should be introduced to feel for the neck of the polypus, which should then be seized with forceps, and be gently twisted off. If, as sometimes happens, it projects backwards into the pharynx, it must be extracted through the mouth with curved forceps. After the operation, the nostril should be plugged to restrain bleeding.

2. The *hydatid polypus* is a rare species, consisting of a number of thin vesicles filled with a watery fluid, and attached by a peduncle. The vesicles burst upon the slightest pressure, and their reproduction may be prevented by touching the peduncle frequently with a hair-pencil dipped in butter of antimony.

3. The *carcinomatous polypus* is nothing more than a scirrhous tumour in the nose. It may be known by its occurring to elderly persons—by the cancerous cachexia, the hardness of the tumour, and lancinating pain.

4. The *fungoid polypus* is a soft red tumour, growing with great rapidity, frequently bleeding, and pursuing the ordinary course of fungus hæmatodes. This, like the last, admits only of palliative treatment.

VI. CHRONIC INFLAMMATION, and tumefaction of the Schneiderian membrane, produces a constant feeling of weight and stuffing, as from a bad cold in the head, and more or less discharge, which is very apt to be fœtid. It is very common in young persons of scrofulous constitutions, and if neglected may lead to an obstinate ozæna. It is to be treated, by applying one or two leeches to the inside of the nostrils, once or twice a week;—by keeping the bowels open with mild purgatives, and occasional doses of hyd. c. creta; and by administering sarsaparilla with alkalis, F. 56, 57. Sometimes in young children, the membrane swells into little red fleshy eminences, which may be touched with nitrate of silver, but must not be mistaken for polypi, nor be meddled with by the forceps.

VII. OZÆNA signifies an obstinate fetid discharge from one or both nostrils, depending on ulceration of the membrane, with or without disease of the bones. It is most frequently a venereal affection, and when so, must be treated accordingly, (p. 214.) But it sometimes occurs in scrofulous children, and in others who are perfectly free from venereal taint. Astringent injections—of nitrate of silver, sulphate of copper, &c.—and of the chlorides of soda and lime, to correct the fœtor, with attention to the health, are the only remedies.

VIII. The nostrils are sometimes *imperforate*, owing to congenital malformation. The passage may (if the parents wish it) be restored by a cautious incision, and must be kept open with bougies. If, however, the obstruction be seated far back, it ought not to be meddled with.

* This cut is taken from Liston's Practical Surgery.

DISEASES OF THE ANTRUM.

IX. ABSCESS OF THE ANTRUM may be caused by blows on the cheek, but it more frequently results from the irritation of decayed teeth. The *symptoms* are permanent aching and uneasiness of the cheek, preceded probably by acute inflammatory pain and fever, and followed by a slow, general enlargement of the cheek, and loosening of the subjacent teeth. The parietes of the cavity sometimes become so thin from distention that they crackle on pressure like parchment. Sometimes (though rarely) the matter makes its way into the nostril; and sometimes the abscess points externally, or bursts into the mouth. *Treatment.*—A free aperture must be made into the cavity. If either of the molar teeth is loose or carious, it should be extracted; and a trocar be pushed through the empty socket into the antrum. But if the teeth are all sound, or if they have been all extracted before, an incision should be made through the membrane of the mouth above the alveoli of the molar teeth, and the bone be pierced by a strong pair of scissors or trocar. The instruments should not be made of too highly tempered steel, lest they might break. The cavity should be frequently syringed with warm water, in order to clear away the matter, which is sometimes thick and lardaceous. If the discharge continues profuse and fetid, search should be made with a probe for loose pieces of bone, which should be removed without delay, the aperture being enlarged if necessary.

X. DROPSY OF THE ANTRUM.—The antrum may become enormously distended, and its parietes thin and crackling on pressure, in consequence of an accumulation of its natural clear mucous secretion, if the aperture into the nostril has become obliterated. An opening must be made in the manner just described.

XI. FUNGUS MEDULLARIS may commence in the lining membrane of the antrum, or in the sockets of the adjoining teeth. In its first stage it forms a hard tumour in the cheek; with a constant sense of pain and uneasiness. After a time, some portion of it feels soft and pulpy, and then bleeding fungous tumours project from the cheek, or into the mouth, or into the orbit, causing horrid pain and deformity, protruding the eye from its socket, and leading to the inevitable fatal results of fungus hæmatodes. (p. 126.) *Treatment.*—The only remedy is extirpation of the superior maxillary bone; but, to be of any use, it must be performed before the diseased growth has burst from the cavity, and before the skin and lymphatic glands have become implicated.

XIII. A NON-MALIGNANT TUMOUR is sometimes developed in the antrum, or on the external surface of the superior maxillary bone. On a section, it appears a dense, homogeneous; fibrinous mass, containing spiculæ of bone. Its origin is generally ascribed to external injury, or to disease of the teeth. It may be distinguished from malignant disease by noticing that its growth is slow, that its surface is lobulated, that it feels hard and elastic, like brawn interspersed with bony particles; that although the superjacent skin may become turgid and purple with distended veins, still that it does not become incorporated with the tumour; and that although ulceration may accidentally occur on its surface, still that the ulcers are superficial, furnish no fetid discharge, and may heal on the removal of the exciting cause. These tumours may, if suffered to remain, destroy life by suffocation and starvation. *Treatment.*—The tumour must be extirpated entirely, and for this purpose it will be necessary to remove the superior maxillary and perhaps the malar bone. An incision must be made with a straight bistoury from the nasal process of the superior maxillary bone to the mouth. It must go quite down to the bone,— must detach the nasal cartilages, and cut through the lip in the median line. A second incision must be made from the external angular process of the frontal bone to the corner of the mouth; and if the malar bone is to be removed, a third, at right angles to the second, must be made along and down to the zygoma. The flap is then dissected up, the infraorbital nerve divided, the inferior oblique muscle and other parts separated from the floor of the orbit, and supported with a narrow bent copper spatula; the nasal process of the superior maxilla, and its junction with the malar, are divided with strong bone forceps, (or if the malar is to be removed, its junction with the frontal and the zygoma must be divided instead;)— a notch must be made with strong scissors in the alveolar process of the middle incisor tooth, (which should be extracted before the operation,)— then the anterior half of the roof of the mouth must be divided with a pair of strong scissors, one blade being put into the nostrils, the other into the mouth. The tumour being thus loosened is then to be forcibly moved, and its remaining attachments are to be divided with the knife, carefully preserving the velum palati. During the operation, the common carotid is to be compressed to prevent hæmorrhage. After it, arteries are to be tied, the chasm to be filled with lint, and the wound closed with sutures.

XIII. Rhino-plastic Operations.—When a portion or the whole of the nose has been destroyed by disease or accident, the deficiency may be restored by a transplantation of skin from an adjoining part. (1.) When the *whole or greater part of the nose* has perished, a triangular piece of leather should be cut into the shape which it formerly presented, and be spread out flat on the forehead, with its base uppermost, and its boundaries should be marked out on the skin with ink. Then the remains of the old nose (if any) are to be pared, and the margins of the nasal aperture are to be cut into deep narrow grooves. When the bleeding from these wounds has ceased, the flap of skin marked out on the forehead is to be dissected up, and all the cellular tissue down to the periosteum with it, so that it may hang attached, merely by a narrow strip of skin between the eyebrows. When all bleeding has ceased, the flap is to be twisted on itself, and its edges are to be fitted into the grooves made for their reception, and to be fastened with sutures. The nose thus made is to be supported, but not stuffed with oiled lint;—it should be wrapped in flannel to support its temperature, and if it become black and turgid, owing to a deficiency in the return of blood from it, a leech may be applied. When adhesion has thoroughly taken place, the twisted strip of skin, by which its connexion with the forehead was maintained, may be cut through, or a little slip may be cut out of it, so that it may be laid down smoothly. (2.) The *septum or columna nasi* is often restored by the same operation with the nose itself, by means of a flap from the forehead; but it is better as Mr. Liston proposes, to form it out of the upper lip at a subsequent operation. A strip is cut out of the centre of the upper lip, a quarter of an inch in breadth, and of its whole thickness. The fraenulum having been divided, this strip is turned up, but not twisted; and its labial surface having been pared off, and the inside of the apex having been made raw, the latter two surfaces are united by the twisted suture, and the wound of the lip is also united by the same. During the cure, the nostrils must be kept of their proper size by introducing silver tubes occasionally. (3.) When *one ala nasi alone* is destroyed, a portion of integument may be measured out on the cheek, and be raised to supply the deficiency. But if both alae are lost, or if the cheek is spare and thin, it is better to supply their place with skin brought from the forehead. The slip which connects the engrafted portion with the forehead will of course be long and thin; and in order to maintain its vitality, a groove may be made to receive it on the dorsum of the nose. But when union has occurred, this connecting slip may be raised and cut off, and the groove which contained it be united by sutures. (4.) *Depression of the apex* of the nose is to be remedied by raising the parts, dividing any adhesions that may have formed, making, if necessary, a new *columna*, in the manner described above, and supporting the parts carefully with plugs of lint, till they have acquired firmness. (5.) *Depression of the ridge*, owing to loss of the osa nasi, may be remedied by pairing the surface, and covering it with a flap of skin from the forehead; or by making a longitudinal incision, and engrafting a small portion of skin from the forehead into it; or, if the case is slight, by cutting out one or two *transverse* slips, and bringing the cut edges together by sutures, so that thus the surface may be stretched to its proper level.

XIV. HARE-LIP signifies a congenital fissure of the upper lip. It may exist only on one side, or there may be a double fissure with a small flap of skin between. Sometimes there is also a fissure in the bony palate,— sometimes in the soft palate also,—and sometimes the upper incisor teeth and their alveoli project through the fissure,—all which conditions give rise to considerable'deformity and impediment in speaking and feeding. *Treatment.*—The edges of the fissure which are red like the lip are to be pared, and then made to unite by adhesion. The operation should be performed either before the cutting of the teeth, or after it—that is, when the child is about two years and a half old;—the latter time is the safer. If the patient is a child, his body should be entirely wrapped in a cloth to prevent struggles; and the surgeon sits behind him, taking the head between his knees. Then he seizes the lip by its corner, penetrates it with a narrow straight knife above the angle of the fissure, and carries the instrument downwards so as to shave off the˘edge of the fissure. This process is repeated on the other side, and the two strips are next detached from the upper angle. When bleeding is checked, the edges are to be brought into most exact union by the twisted

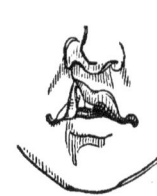

suture. Two hare-lip pins should be used, (or long slender needles with spear points, shown at p. 130, may be substituted.) The first pin should be inserted near the angles of the fissure; and if the labial artery bleed, the other should be placed so as to transfix and compress it. The pins should penetrate full two thirds of the thickness of the lip. They may be removed on the fourth or fifth day; and a slip of adhesive plaster may be drawn from one cheek to the other instead. If the hare-lip is double, both sides may be operated on at once, the middle flap being transfixed by the pins. If one or more teeth project in the fissure so as to offer any impediment to its union, they should be extracted; and if the bone project, it also should be cut off with pliers, the soft parts on it having been first divided with the knife.*

XV. FISSURE OF THE PALATE, when extending through the bones, and forming a wide aperture into the nose, cannot be cured. The parts, however, become slightly approximated during growth—and at puberty the defect may be palliated by means of a metallic or ivory plate. But when the *velum pendulum palati* alone is fissured—and the fissure not very wide, it may be remedied by the operation of *staphyloraphe*—which, however, must necessarily be deferred till puberty, or it would be defeated by the patient's struggles. The edges of the fissure are first pared—then they are united by three interrupted sutures, which may be very easily introduced by means of Mr. Beaumont's instrument described in the twentieth volume of the Med. Chir. Trans. Before the sutures are tightened, a shallow incision may be made in the velum on each side near the alveolar border, in order to diminish the tension. The patient must fast for twenty-four hours, and on the succeeding days must take very small quantities of thick fluids.

* This cut is taken from Liston's Practical Surgery.

47

XVI. Cancer of the Lip commences as a small scirrhous tumour, or wart, or as a small fissure caused by the irritation of smoking, which gradually degenerates into a foul ulcer, with hardened base and ragged surface. *Treatment.*—The disease must be extirpated by a V incision—taking care to include the whole of it—and uniting the wound afterwards like that made in the operation for hare-lip. If, however, the whole or greater part of the lip be implicated, the diseased parts should be freely removed without any attempt to unite the edges of the incision. The extirpation cannot be expected to be effectual unless performed before the glands are implicated—but it is justifiable at any stage—in order to avoid for a time the horrible pain and fœtor of the ulcerative process. It has been very clearly shown by Mr. Earle, that any ulcers, if subjected to perpetual irritation, (and especially ulcers near the outlets of the body,) may assume a malignant appearance, which ceases on the removal of the irritant. When therefore there are foul ulcers on the lips, cheeks, or tongue, the teeth should be well examined in order to remove any roughness, or collections of tartar.

XVII. Cancrum Oris—(*Phagedæna oris, gangrenous erosion of the cheek,*)—is a phagedæno-gangrenous affection of the lips and cheeks, occurring almost exclusively amongst the ill-fed squalid children of large towns. It appears to be a disease of debility, and to be induced by want of proper food and of fresh air, and by neglect of cleanliness. Like other disorders of a similar character, it is very liable to follow the measles or scarlatina, or any other severe and weakening illness.

*Symptoms.*—In the instances which have fallen under the author's observation, it has commenced as a shallow ulcer on the lip, or inside of the cheek; with a peculiarly dirty gray or ash-coloured surface, and black edges. Sometimes it is said to commence with an exudation of a pale yellow, fibrinous matter like that which is exuded in croup, and some forms of putrid sore-throat. At the same time the face is swollen, the breath exceedingly fetid, and there is a dribbling of fetid saliva mixed with blood. If the disease proceeds, the ulcer becomes gangrenous, and destroys the cheek and gums; the teeth drop out, typhoid symptoms supervene, and the patient dies exhausted. The swelling which accompanies this disease, shows nothing like active or healthy inflammation. It is moderately firm, or what may be called semi-œdematous, and is either pale, or else of a faint pink colour. In the most rapid form of the disease, it commences at once as a black spot of gangrene, which slowly spreads, and is not accompanied by any inflammation whatever; all the parts around being quite pale and wax-like. The constitutional symptoms are at first those of weakness, and disorder of the stomach and bowels, and afterwards the rapid feeble pulse, and stupor of typhus.

*Diagnosis.*—The diagnosis of this affection is of some importance, because, when a child has died of it, the parents, through ignorance or malice, are liable to bring the surgeon into trouble, by accusing him of having caused death through profuse mercurial salivation. The chief points of distinction are, that in this disease the ulceration or gangrene is *circumscribed*, and is generally confined to one side; and that it commences usually in the cheek, and that it only affects that part of the gums which is in close contiguity, and that the tongue is untouched. Whereas in severe mercurial salivation, the ulceration is diffused, the whole of the gums, and the lining membrane of the cheeks, and the tongue, as well as the palate, being affected from the first.

*Treatment.*—The indications are threefold. 1st, To evacuate and correct the secretions of the stomach and bowels by mild but efficient purgatives—especially rhubarb and magnesia, which should be administered daily. The author believes that one or two grains of calomel may be advantageously added to the first dose. 2ndly, To keep up the strength by wine, beef-tea, and other nutritious articles, and by bark or quinine in sufficient doses. 3rdly, To excite a healthy action in the diseased part by stimulating lotions—especially solution of nitrate of silver, alum, sulphate of copper, or the chloride of lime; and lastly, if these means fail to arrest the disease, the strong nitric acid should be applied so as to destroy the whole of the diseased part, in the same manner as was directed for hospital gangrene.*

XVIII. SMALL TUMOURS containing a glairy matter, and probably consisting of obstructed mucous follicles, are often met with on the inner surface of the cheeks and lips.

XIX. RANULA is a tumour of the same nature, situated under the tongue. It may either consist of one of the Whartonian ducts, or of a follicle obstructed. This and the foregoing tumours are best treated by snipping out a small piece of the sac, and rubbing the interior with lunar caustic;—or by passing a small seton through the sac.

XX. TONGUE-TIE—a prolongation of the frænum linguæ, confining the apex of the organ—is by no means so common as is often supposed. If it does really exist, the frænum may easily be divided with a blunt-pointed pair of scissors—taking care to direct their points downwards, so as to avoid the lingual artery.

XXI. WOUNDS of the tongue are liable to be attended with severe hæmorrhage from the lingual artery. If the bleeding orifice cannot be tied, one or more ligatures must be introduced with curved needles, so as to include and constrict the bleeding parts—or a heated iron may be applied through a tube.

XXII. INFLAMMATION of the tongue—known by great swelling, tenderness, and difficulty of speaking and deglutition, must be treated by

* Vide James on Inflammation, p. 527; Marshall Hall in Lancet for 1839-40, p. 409 ; P. H. Green, *ibid.;* and also in Cycl. Prac. Surg. Art. *Concrum Oris;* and Willis on Cutaneous Disease.

bleeding and leeches, purgatives, slight incisions, and the antiphlogistic regimen generally. Inquiry should be made whether the patient has been taking mercury. If abscess form, the fluctuating part should be opened.*

XXIII. HYPERTROPHY.—Slow enlargement, without tenderness or structural disease, sometimes affects the tongue, causing it to protrude permanently from the mouth. The superfluous portion may be removed by ligature—a needle armed with a strong double ligature being passed through the centre of the tongue, and one thread being then tied very tightly round each half. But if it be not very considerable, a A shaped portion may be cut out from its anterior extremity—the cut surfaces being united by suture after the bleeding vessels are tied, and oozing has ceased.

XXIV. CANCER.—A foul excavated ulcer, with extremely hardened base, prominent edges, burning and lancinating pain, and preceded by nodular scirrhous enlargement. The constitutional symptoms are those of the cancerous cachexia, (p. 123.) *Treatment.*—The diseased part should be early extirpated with the knife—or if extensive, with ligatures, in the manner before described.

XXV. ULCERS ON THE TONGUE, presenting very formidable characters, are often attributable to local irritation, (from diseased teeth, &c.,) or to some derangement of the health—perhaps a venereal taint.—The obvious indications are, to remove irritation from rough teeth—to keep up the secretions of the liver and bowels—to regulate the diet—and support the strength. Plummer's pill—sarsaparilla—or F. 29 and 30— hyoscyamus and conium—perhaps iodine—and the local and general treatment of *irritable* ulcers will be of service.

XXVI. STAMMERING.—This affection requires to be noticed here, because of two operations which have been recently introduced for the cure of it. The first operation, which is intended to divide the muscles of the tongue, is performed by drawing the tongue as far as possible out of the mouth, and then making a very deep incision completely across the base of it. In addition to this, a triangular notch is cut out from the anterior edge of the transverse incision. This operation is necessarily attended with so much hæmorrhage, and danger to life, that the author believes it to be utterly unjustifiable for the relief of a mere inconvenience. It may truly be styled muscle-cutting gone mad. The other operation, which is also of quite recent invention, is performed on the supposition that stammering may be caused by an obstruction to the passage of air from the pharynx into the mouth, in consequence of an enlargement of the tonsils, or a contraction of the arch of the palate. This latter operation consists in cutting off the uvula, and in removing part or the whole of the tonsils,

* Vide a curious case of fatal enlargement of the tongue by Mr. Lyford of Winchester, Lancet for 1828, p. 16.

so as to enlarge the passage from the mouth into the fauces.   There are many doubts as to the success of this plan; but as the author has yet had no experience of it, he will pronounce no opinion.   It has long been known to be useful in some cases of deafness.   At all events, it is not liable to the objections that may be urged against the former, on the score of danger, and there is good reason for believing that the kind of obstruction which it is intended to remove may possibly exist in some cases; whereas there is certainly never such a state of organic rigidity of the tongue, as to render the division of its muscles even probably expedient.*

XXVII. LANCING THE GUMS.—If at any time during dentition a child be feverish and restless, with its stools slimy and clay-coloured, or if there be any symptoms of disorder in the head or chest, the gums should be examined; and if any part, especially where a tooth is soon expected, appear red and swollen,—a free incision should be made with a gum lancet quite down to the tooth.   This affords instant relief by removing the tension and pain.   The edge of the lancet should be turned outwards, so as to avoid the sacs of the permanent teeth.

XXVIII. IRREGULARITY OF THE PERMANENT TEETH is a frequent consequence of injudicious haste in extracting the temporary set—an operation which not only permits the arch of the jaw to become contracted, but disturbs the nutrition of the permanent teeth, hurries their appearance, and ensures their early decay.   The temporary set should therefore always be suffered to remain as long as possible. ˊThe only ones that there need be any haste in extracting, are the uppei incisors, in order to prevent there successors from growing behind their natural position, which would render the mouth underhung.   If either of the canine teeth, or of the incisors of the jaw, project much, the patient should be taught perpetually to endeavour to push it back into its proper situation with his fingers.   But if at the age of fourteen or fifteen this method has not succeeded, and the teeth are much crowded, the projecting tooth may be removed—although in many cases it is better to sacrifice one of the bicuspides to make room for it.   If one or more of the superior incisors project backwards, it must be drawn forwards by means of ligatures attached to a gold bar worn in front of the teeth—for the manner of applying which the reader is referred to Bell on the Teeth.

XXIX. FRACTURE AND DISLOCATION OF TEETH.—If a portion of a tooth is broken off, the exposed surface should be filed smooth, and then no immediate inconvenience will probably follow.   If, however, the greater part of the tooth is lost, and considerable pain and swelling should arise, extraction should be performed—but if a useful portion remain, leeches, &c. should first be tried in order if possible, to remove inflam-

---

* These operations are described in the Med. Gaz. March 12th, and the Athenæum March 13th, 1841; and the Med. Gaz. for March 19th, 1841.   Mr. Brain of Manchester speaks of an operation for dividing the frænum epiglottidis.

mation.  If a tooth is loosened by a blow, it should be fastened by silk
to its neighbours.  If a tooth is entirely driven out, it should be replaced
as soon as bleeding has ceased, and be fastened in by silk; no food should
be allowed that requires mastication, and inflammation should be combated by repeatedly leeching the gum.

XXX.  CARIES OF TEETH signifies a successive softening and decay;—
strictly corresponding to ulceration.  It generally begins at the surface
of the bone of the tooth, and appears as a dark spot underneath the enamel, which after a time gives way and exposes a cavity.  The disease
gradually spreads and reaches the central cavity of the tooth, which from
that time is subject to fits of toothach.  This disease may be caused, (1)
by original weakness of the teeth, which is often hereditary, and appears
to be connected with the strumous diathesis—the teeth being remarkably
white and pearly.  The profuse administration of mercury during early
childhood is justly conceived to be another predisposing cause.  (2) Injuries to the teeth—the abrasion of their enamel—the use of very hot or
very cold drinks—and especially of ices, are exciting causes.  *Treatment.*—If the caries be slight and recent, the whole of the decayed portion should be removed by proper instruments, and the cavity be filled
up with gold.  This operation should not be performed indiscriminately,
however, if the decay has advanced so far as to lay open the central cavity
of the tooth,—or if the introduction of an instrument causes the peculiar
pain arising from pressure on the nervous membrane.  Such a proceeding might very probably cause excruciating agony, and induce suppuration in the centre of the tooth and in its socket.  Under these circumstances, the indications are to remove the diseased substance, and to protect the surface of the tooth from the irritation of contact with food and saliva, and to diminish its sensibility.  For these purposes the best plan is,
to fill the cavity with a composition of powdered chalk, with a very little
tannin, mixed up into a paste, with a solution of mastic in alcohol; or frequently to introduce a drop of some narcotic or stimulating solution;—such
as a solution of acetate of morphia, or of tannin; or of alcohol, or sp. camph.,
or nitrate of silver, (gr. x. ad $\zeta$i.)—and to wear in the cavity a little piece
of lint or cotton, dipped in a strong solution of mastic.  By these means
the tooth may very probably be brought into a state to bear stopping with
gold.  The patient should avoid exposure to cold—or drinking very hot,
or cold, or sweet, or acid fluids—and should be careful not to induce
feverishness by any errors in diet.  A peculiar fungous excrescence occasionally grows from the lining membrane when exposed by caries.
Sometimes it is indolent—sometimes acutely sensible; but it always gives
more or less annoyance in mastication.  A strong solution of nitrate of
silver is the best application.

XXXI. TOOTHACH.—This disagreeable infliction may be caused by four
circumstances.  (1.) The most common form is that which arises from

*caries*—the lining membrane being rendered irritable by exposure, and being liable to nervous or inflammatory pain from local irritation or disorder of the health. *Treatment.*—We may arrange the multifarious remedies for this form of toothach in the following order. (*a.*) *Purgatives* and low diet are indicated if the pain followed exposure to cold or excess at table, and if it is attended with foul tongue, hot skin, and headach. (*b.*) *Scarification* of the gums, or leeches to them or to the cheek, will be useful if the tooth is tender and the gums swollen. (*c.*) *Derivatives.*—Pediluvia of hot water and mustard—and rubefacients to the cheeks—especially ammonia and ether applied in the palm of the hand, or mustard poultices, are generally of service; and (*d.*) *Sialagogues,* especially ginger, cloves, and pellitory, or steaming the mouth with hot water, are equally so. (*e.*) *Anodynes.*—A small quantity of laudanum, or of a solution of morphia, or a paste made with opii gr. j, camph. gr. iv—or of morphia, chalk, and solution of mastic;—or a drop of tincture of aconite—inserted into the tooth, are often of great benefit; but it is of no use to administer large doses of opium internally—they disorder the system without adequately relieving the pain. A drop of the hydrocyanic acid inserted into the hollow of the tooth, and two minims of the same, given every four hours in a saline draught, are the best remedies of this class. (*f.*) *Stimulants*—such as the essential oils of cinnamon, origanum, cloves, and the like, creosote,—solution of the nitrate of silver,—alcohol,—diluted hydrochloric acid (ℨß ad ℨii aquæ)—solution of alum in nitric ether (ℨß ad f$\frac{z}{3}$ß,) very hot or very cold water,—are popular remedies, whose efficacy is supposed to depend on their exhausting the sensibility of the nerve. Perhaps the best plan, when the lining membrane is exposed, and there is severe toothach, is to introduce either a drop of a strong solution of nitrate of silver, or else a little fragment of it, and to stop up the cavity with wax, or diachylon plaster, softened between the fingers. Mr. Tomes has found that great relief is often obtained from tannin, especially if the tooth looks soft. A little piece of wax may be softened and formed into a roll by the fingers, and some of the powdered tannin may be taken up on the end of the wax and be inserted into the tooth. He believes that much more good is to be effected in general by the repeated application of mild stimulants, than by using them in too concentrated a form. (*g.*) *Alkalis.*—It sometimes happens that toothach arises from disorder of the stomach, and an acid state of the secretions of the mouth; and may be relieved almost immediately by rinsing the mouth with a solution of carbonate of soda. (*h.*) *Cauterants.*—It has been proposed to introduce the concentrated sulphuric or nitric acids, or a red hot wire, into the carious cavity, in order to disorganize the nervous pulp. One author has recommended it to be broken up by a sharp steel punch. But these remedies can scarcely ever be applied with a certainty of accomplishing their object—if they do not

cure the toothach, they will be sure to aggravate it,—and in the hands of a
bungler they might be productive of very great mischief.  The chloride
of zinc is the most useful of this class of substances.  It was recommended by Mr. James, and has been extensively used by Mr. Tomes, in
the following manner.  He dilutes it with ten parts of powdered plaster
of Paris, and then dips the end of a little roll of softened wax in this
powder, and stops it into the cavity.

(2.) *Inflammation* of the lining membrane sometimes affects a tooth
that is apparently sound.  It occasions severe, heavy, throbbing pain
extending to the head, and considerable tenderness of the tooth and of
the gum around.  It may lead to suppuration of the pulp, or to abscess
in the alveolus, and death of the tooth in consequence.  *Treatment.*—
Leeches, low diet, and purgatives.

(3.) *Neuralgic* toothach, whether it occurs in teeth that are entirely
sound or partially carious, is to be distinguished by its occurring in
paroxysms which come and go suddenly, in more or less regular intervals.  It is very common in the earlier months of pregnancy.  *Treatment.*—Quinine or the carbonate of iron in large doses, together with
aperients and alteratives, are the most successful remedies.

(4.) *Exostosis*, a deposite of bone of the root of a tooth, occasions
severe pain that can hardly be distinguished from that of neuralgia.  It
sometimes occurs on teeth that are perfectly sound, but more generally
on carious teeth, or stumps.  The excessive pain of this affection is in
general only to be relieved by extraction.

XXXII. NECROSIS OF TEETH.—A tooth is said to be necrosed when
it has become black and unsightly, and loose in its socket.  This affection may be caused by blows which have torn across the nutrient vessels,—
or by inflammation of the pulp, (perhaps from the abuse of mercury.)
Extraction must be performed, if the tooth cause inflammation or other
inconvenience.

XXXIII. EXTRACTION OF TEETH.—The instruments for extracting
teeth, are the forceps, the elevator, and the key.

The forceps is the instrument that is now generally employed by dentists.  It should be made with sharp edges, so that it may be pushed up
between the tooth and the gum, and should seize the tooth by its neck,
close to the alveolus.  For this purpose also, the jaws of the instrument
should be made to incline towards each other in such a way, that they
may slip up and embrace the neck of the tooth accurately when the han-
dles are pressed together.  The surgeon will require eight sets of forceps,
and should have two or three sizes of each set.  Four sets will be required
for the molars, and should be ground so as to fit accurately the necks of
the teeth on each side of both jaws.  One set will be necessary for
the bicuspides and canines of the upper jaw, and another for those of the
lower jaw; and two sets will be necessary for the incisors of either jaw.

In extracting teeth by the forceps, there are two things to be done; first to loosen the tooth, and then to pull it straight out. In extracting the incisors and canines of the upper jaw, they may first be loosened by giving them a gentle twist, and then may be pulled down perpendicularly. The incisors and canines of the lower jaw are to be loosened by giving them a firm but gentle motion backwards and forwards, and then may be pulled straight up; and the bicuspides and molars are to be loosened by moving them from side to side, so as to make the alveolar process yield a little, and then may be pulled perpendicularly, upwards or downwards, as the case may be.

The elevator is highly useful for stumps, and for old straggling teeth. The point is to be thrust firmly down between the tooth and its socket, and then by bringing the instrument into a horizontal position, and making a fulcrum of the edge of the alveolar process, or of the adjoining tooth, or of the operator's fingers, the tooth may be lifted out.

The key is an instrument that is very generally employed for the extraction of the bicuspides and molares; but it is more painful than the forceps, and apt to injure the gum and periosteum. Care should be taken to select an instrument of proper size, and to place it neither too high nor too low. If the key is too small, and the fulcrum too high, (as in Fig. 1,) very probably the crown of the tooth will be snapped off. If the key is too large, and the fulcrum too low, (as in Fig. 2,) either the claw of the instrument may be snapped across, or the alveolar process be extensively splintered. Fig. 3, is intended to show the right position, which will draw the tooth more or less perpendicularly from its socket. The fulcrum ought to be placed on the *inner* side, for the bicuspides of the lower jaw, and molars of the upper; and on the outer side for the molares of the lower jaw. The *dentes sapientiæ* of the upper jaw should never, according to Bell, be extracted with the key, because of the delicate texture of the bone on which the fulcrum must rest.

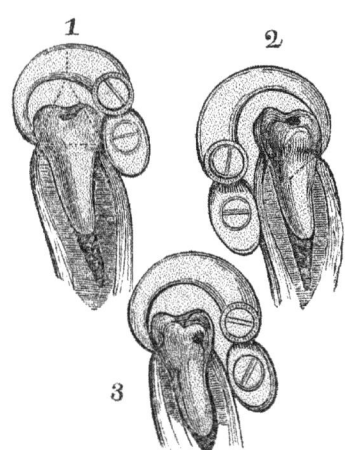

Before extracting teeth with the key, it is usual to cut away the gum from their necks by means of a gum lancet;—a practice which some authorities consider unnecessary. It certainly is unnecessary in the majority of cases, especially for the extraction of the temporary teeth, and of the teeth of old persons;—but it should be performed, 1st, if the gum has been subject to repeated inflammation—which renders it adherent to the tooth, and liable to be lacerated on its removal; 2ndly, to afford room for the claw, if the tooth has decayed down to the gum. Some persons, instead of using a lancet, separate the gum by means of a small tenaculum, and it certainly is less painful and equally efficacious.

This operation is sometimes followed by very severe and dangerous hæmorrhage. A strong solution of nitrate of silver may be tried first; but if that does not suppress it, the alveolus must be plugged in the following way. It is first to be cleansed from coagulum,—then one end of a long thin strip of lint is to be firmly pressed into it, so as to come into contact with its very bottom, and the remainder in successive portions is to be forced in till the socket is filled up to the level of the gum. A compress should then be placed on the part, thick enough to be pressed upon by the antagonist teeth, and the mouth should be kept firmly closed by a bandage passing from under the chin to the vertex.

XXXIV. TARTAR, or *salivary calculus*, is an earthy matter deposited on the teeth from the saliva. It is found most abundantly on the superior molares and inferior incisors—obviously because those teeth are nearest the orifices of the salivary ducts. If suffered to accumulate, it causes inflammation and absorption of the gums, and gradual loosening of the teeth. *Treatment.*—The deposite of this substance is to be prevented by taking care not to disorder the stomach, and by the strictest cleanliness. The teeth should be cleaned at least twice a day, and a soft toothpowder (camphorated chalk is the best) with a little soap should be used twice a week. The hairs of a toothbrush should be soft, and not too closely set;—so that they may penetrate the better into the interstices of the teeth. When any quantity of the tartar has accumulated, it should be removed by the *scaling instruments*. The edge or point of the instrument is to be introduced between the concretion and the gum, so as to detach the former in flakes,—in the meanwhile a finger or thumb, guarded with a towel, should be pressed firmly on the cutting edges of the teeth, so that they may not be loosened by the force necessarily employed. Sometimes a small portion of this substance is found sticking in the orifice of one of the salivary ducts, and creating great discomfort by its irritation. It may be easily removed.

XXXV. INFLAMMATORY ABSORPTION, vulgarly called *scurvy* of the gums, generally affects middle-aged or elderly people, and may be a consequence of the accumulation of tartar, but more frequently depends on a congested state of the liver and bowels. The gums are swollen, spongy, exceedingly tender and subject to constant aching pain, and they bleed on the slightest touch. If the disease proceeds, they separate from the teeth;—the alveoli gradually become absorbed, and the teeth loosen, and at last fall out. These consequences are sometimes speedy, and are attended with suppuration in the alveoli, but more frequently they are slow—the teeth dropping out one by one in the course of years. *Treatment.*—The gums should be unloaded by deep and free scarifications and repeated leechings,—the bowels should be well cleared by a course of purgatives and mercurials,—and gargles should be employed to correct the secretions of the mouth, and excite the vessels to contract. Whilst there is much pain and soreness, dec. papav. vel anthemid., or three drachms of nitre dissolved in a pint of barley-water, will answer best. Subsequently, recourse may be had to F. 39, or to gargles of dec. cinchon. with alum or dilute sulphuric acid and tinct. myrrhæ, or of liq. calcis chlorid. f3j to half a pint of brandy and water.

XXXVI. Gum Boil (*alveolar abscess, parulis*) ,is a small abscess commencing in the socket of a tooth, and bursting through the gum, rarely through the cheek. It is usually caused by the irritation of a dead or carious tooth. *Treatment.*—Leeches and fomentations,—removal of the tooth,—and a puncture as soon as matter can be detected. If the tooth is extracted soon, the sac of the abscess very often comes away with it.

XXXVII.—Epulis is a tumour formed by the growth of the gum, without any apparent alteration in its structure. It generally commences between two teeth, which it gradually separates, then loosens, and finally displaces,—and may spread so as to involve several of them. This tumour is indolent, painless, and of slow growth. *Treatment.*—The tooth on either side must be extracted, and the tumour entirely cut out.

A portion of the alveolar process must be removed likewise, if necessary, in order to render the extirpation complete.

A similar tumour is sometimes formed when a dead portion of the root of a tooth remains in its socket, and the gum has healed over it. The tumour should be entirely removed with the knife, and the extraneous body should be sought for, and be extracted if possible. *Malignant tumours* of the gums are exceedingly rare; they will, however, be recognised by their rapid growth and tendency to hæmorrhage.

XXXVIII. Tumours of the Lower Jaw may, like those of the upper, be either simple or malignant. Their distinctive character have been before alluded to (p. 366.) Free extirpation is the only remedy. A tooth must be extracted on each side of the tumour,—the soft parts within and without are to be detached, and then the bone may be sawn through on either side of it. But if the tumour is not very extensive, it may be possible to leave a little rim of the basis of the jaw,—sawing the bone nearly through on both sides of the tumour, and then cutting out the intermediate portion with forceps. If a central portion is extirpated, including the attachments of the genio-hyoidei and digastric muscles, great care must be taken to counteract the retraction of those muscles and of the tongue, which might cause suffocation. In removing a lateral portion of this bone, an incision should be made beneath its basis;—this will afford a perfect view of the tumour, and the cicatrix will not be obvious afterwards. Dis-articulation of either half of the bone is performed by making a curved incision from beneath the ear, along the basis of the jaw, to the chin. The flap so formed is to be dissected up, and the masseter with it;—a tooth is to be removed, and the bone to be sawn vertically through;—the end is then seized and depressed, and the temporal muscle dissected from the coronoid process,—the pterygoid muscles and other internal attachments are then to be divided, and finally the ligaments of the joint. After bleeding has been restrained, the wound is to be closed by sutures, excepting at the middle, where an aperture should be left for the ligatures, and to permit the escape of discharge.*

# CHAPTER XV:

## OF THE SURGICAL DISEASES AND INJURIES OF THE NECK.

I. Acute inflammation of the Tonsil is known by rapid swelling of the part, great pain in deglutition, and fever. It must be treated by leeches or bleeding, purgatives, gargles calculated to promote the secretions of saliva, (F. 39,) and the ordinary antiphlogistic routine. If the gland continue to swell, or if it occasion any embarrassment to the breathing, an incision should be made into it, to unload the vessels, and give exit to matter. The tongue should be depressed with one forefinger, whilst a straight bistoury, wrapped round with lint, except an inch and a half of its point, is plunged directly into the tumour, and made to cut its way out towards the median line.

* Vide Liston's Elements of Surgery, and Practical Surgery, 2nd ed.; Copland's Dict. art. Hæmorrhage; Sir A. Cooper's and Lawrence's Lectures; Guthrie in Med. Gaz. vol. xvii.; Brodie, ibid. vol. xv.; Liston on Tumours of the Face, in Med. Chir. Trans., vol xx.; Bell on the Teeth; and Jobson on the Teeth. Disease of the lower jaw requiring amputation has been caused by a projection anteriorly of the coronoid process, which hindered the evolution of the wisdom tooth. Forbe's Rev., vol. viii.

II. Chronic Enlargement of the Tonsil is a frequent sequel of repeated inflammation of the tonsils, especially in scrofulous children. It causes sundry inconveniences. The parts are liable to repeated inflammation—deglutition is impeded—the voice is rendered hoarse—respiration is noisy and laborious, especially during sleep—there is more or less deafness from the obstruction of the eustachian tubes—and suffocation has even been caused by viscid mucus entangled between the swollen glands. *Treatment.*—In the first place, the system must be strengthened, and the secretions be kept up by proper tonics and alteratives. The iodide of iron, the combination of corrosive sublimate with tinct. cinchonæ, and other remedies mentioned at p. 116, may often be administered with benefit. At the same time absorption of the tumour must be promoted by astringent gargles (of dec. cinchon. with alum, or F. 92.)—by washing it once a day with strong lotions of arg. nit., or cupri sulph. on a hair pencil—by applying stimulating, or mercurial, or ioduretted liniments and ointments to the skin;—and by lancing the gums over the wisdom teeth if tumid, and removing any decayed teeth that cause irritation. But if these measures fail, part of the gland should be removed with the knife—a much more expeditious and cleanly method than the ligature. The surgeon seizes the tumour with a hook or *vulsellum*, (depressing the tongue with its handle,) then introduces a blunt-pointed curved knife, and shaves it off—cutting upwards, parallel to the isthmus faucium. There are certain other instruments occasionally used for this operation, such as a kind of guillotine instrument, consisting of a ring with which the tonsil is encircled, and a blade moving in a groove; but the simple knife and forceps answer every purpose.

III. Enlargement of the Uvula produces tickling cough and expectoration by irritating the larynx. If it does not yield to the treatment directed for enlarged tonsil, it should be stretched and steadied with forceps, and be cut through in the middle with a pair of long scissors.

IV. Polypus growing from the Epiglottis has been known to produce fits of suffocative spasm of the muscles of the glottis, which have proved fatal. Any such tumour, if ascertained to exist, must be removed.

V. Spasm of the Œsophagus (*spasmodic stricture*) is known by its generally occurring in sudden fits—the patient at a meal finding himself altogether incapable of swallowing—and the attempt to do so producing spasmodic pain and a sense of choking. The *diagnosis* between this and the *organic* or *permanent stricture* is founded on the suddenness of its accession; it being much better at some times than at others; and the fact that the bougie, if passed, either meets with no obstruction, or with one that very easily yields. *Treatment.*—This affection always depends on a weakened or hysterical state of the system, or on the pressure of some other disorder, as has been mentioned whilst treating of neuralgia.

Brodie relates a case that ceased on the removal of bleeding piles; and Mayo, another that was cured by relieving chronic disease of the liver. Tonics, anti-spasmodics, and alteratives—especially the carbonate of iron, thrice a day, with pills of aloes and galbanum at bed-time—exercise in the open air, the shower-bath, and other forms of warm and cold bathing —great attention to the diet—care not to swallow any thing imperfectly masticated or too hot, and the occasional passage of a bougie, are the remedies.

VI. Palsy of the Œsophagus occasions inability of swallowing, but without pain or other symptoms of spasm; and a bougie, when passed, meets with no obstruction. It generally depends or organic disease of the brain or spinal cord, which must be examined into and cured if possible. The patient should be fed by the stomach-pump, by nutrient enemata, and by pushing soft food occasionally down the œsophagus with a probang. The palsy has sometimes been temporarily relieved by electrifying the patient on an insulating stool. Nutrient enemata should be composed of very strong beef or mutton broth, without salt or spice, and with ten to twenty drops of laudanum. The quantity injected at one time should not exceed four ounces.

VII. Dilatation and Sacculation.—The œsophagus has been found after death exceedingly dilated. The symptoms during life were, great *dysphagia*,—food when swallowed never seemed to reach the stomach, and was vomited in a few minutes. If this condition should be ascertained during life, the patient should be fed as in palsy. Sometimes a blind pouch is connected with the œsophagus, and occasions great distress in swallowing by intercepting the food. It may be formed either by a protrusion of the mucous membrane through the muscular fibres, or by the sac of an abscess which has burst into the tube. The only remedy is, to feed the patient constantly with the stomach-pump, so that the pouch may be allowed to close.

VIII. Permanent Stricture of the œsophagus signifies a narrowing produced by an inflammatory thickening of its mucous and submucous coats, which form a firm ring, encroaching on the canal. It is generally found just below the termination of the pharynx; that is, opposite the carocoid cartilage;—and is most frequent in females. The *Symptoms* are, difficulty of swallowing—noticed probably for years—gradually increasing—never absent—and occasionally aggravated by fits of spasm. The act of swallowing frequently produces pain in the chest, which shoots between the shoulders, and up to the head. When a bougie is passed, it meets with an obstruction, and displays the impression of the stricture on its extremity. The *causes* of this affection are generally unknown—sometimes, however, it appears to be a sequel of repeated quinsy, or to be caused by swallowing boiling or corrosive liquids;—in one case it appeared to be induced by violent retching in sea-sickness. If unrelieved its *consequences* will be ulceration of the œsophagus, either above or below the stricture, with salivation, vomiting of purulent matter, and impossibility of deglutition—which in no long time will be followed by death. The fatal termination may be owing either to sheer starvation, or to the irritation of the local disease, or the extension of ulceration to the lungs. *Treatment.*—A mild course of mercury, so as just to affect the gums,—combined with hyoscyamus or conium, if there be much irritability—a seton between the scapulæ—and the occasional passage of a bougie, or of a *ball probang*—an ivory ball attached to a piece of whale-bone or flexible wire—or of a piece of sponge moistened with a weak solution of nitrate of silver, and attached to a stout copper wire, as recommended by Sir C. Bell, are the remedies. The method of introducing the bougie is as follows. The patient sits upright, with the head thrown back, and the mouth wide open. The bougie, which should be previously warmed in the hand and oiled, and gently curved, is passed down into the pharynx in such a manner that its point may slide along the vertebræ. In order that it may not excite cough by interfering with the epiglottis, the patient should be directed to protrude the tongue from the mouth as far as possible;—or to perform the act of deglutition just when the bougie is entering the pharynx. If it meets with an obstruction to its descent, the surgeon should slightly withdraw it,—then again press it gently against the obstruction, increasing the pressure for a few minutes if it gives no pain. If it fail to pass, it should be taken out, and its point be examined; and if it bear the impress of a stricture, a smaller one should be tried.

IX. SCHIRRHUS of the œsophagus produces the same symptoms as stricture, and must be treated in the same manner.

X. ULCERATION of the œsophagus is generally situated at its upper part, and on its posterior surface. It causes great *dysphagia*, and burning pain on the passage of food. If a bougie is passed it meets with one obstruction just above the ulcer, and with another just below it,—and its point returns marked with bloody pus, and presenting the ragged impression of the ulcer. *Treatment.*—Alteratives, couter-irritants, and nutrient enemata. The burning pain is sometimes relieved by swallowing small quantities of iced cream.

XI. TUMOURS pressing on the œsophagus—whether abscesses, aneurisms, bronchocele, or enlargement of the bronchial glands, will produce all the symptoms of organic stricture. Aneurisms and abscesses have been burst by the passage of bougies—with, of course, instant death in the former case, and relief in the latter. Before performing this operation, therefore, the chest ought to be well scrutinized by auscultation, to detect any unnatural pulsation or *bruit;* and any signs of embarrassed circulation or respiration should not be overlooked.*

* Vide Sir E. Home on Strictures, vols. i. and ii. Monro on Morbid Anatomy of

XII. FOREIGN BODIES, when fixed in the pharynx, of about the aperture of the larynx, or in the œsophagus, produce a sense of choking, and fits of suffocative cough. This accident may prove fatal in two manners. The patient may either be suffocated at once, by spasm of the glottis;—or if the foreign substance remains impacted, it may produce a fatal ulceration of the parts—attended with exhaustion cough and dyspnœa, and profuse fetid expectoration. *Treatment.*—the patient should be seated in a chair, with the head thrown back and the mouth wide open. The surgeon should then introduce his finger—regardless of attempts to vomit—and should pass it swiftly into the pharynx, and search the whole of it thoroughly. When the substance is felt, it may perhaps be entangled in the point of the nail—or curved forceps may be guided to it by the finger. Pins or fish-bones are often entangled about the velum, or in the folds of mucous membrane between the epiglottis and tongue.

If the body has passed into the œsophagus, and it is small and sharp, (a fish bone for instance,) it may be got rid of by making the patient swallow a good mouthful of bread. If large and soft, (as a lump of meat,) it may be pushed down into the stomach with the probang. But large hard bodies, especially if rough and angular, (such as pieces of bone or glass, &c.,) should be brought up if possible. A pair of long curved forceps, or a piece of whalebone armed with a flat blunt hook, or with a skein of thread, so as to form an infinite number of nooses, are convenient instruments. If, however, it can neither be brought up nor down, and if it be lodged in the cervical portion of the tube, it must be extracted by incision in the following manner.

XIII. ŒSOPHAGOTOMY.—This operation should be performed on the side towards which the foreign substance projects. Its situation having been ascertained, an incision of sufficient length must be made through the skin and platysma between the sterno-mastoid muscle and trachea. The cervical fascia must next be divided on a director. The surgeon must then divide the cellular membrane with a blunt knife, or lacerate it with his fingers, avoiding the carotid and thyroid arteries, and the recurrent nerve. A common silver catheter may then be passed down the throat, and be made to project in the wound, so that the œsophagus may be opened by cutting on it. This small wound in the œsophagus should be dilated with forceps, in order to avoid hæmorrhage, and the foreign body should then be extracted.* This operation has occasionally been performed for the purpose of conveying food into the stomach in cases of stricture of the œsophagus, but with no very satisfactory results.

XIV. FOREIGN BODIES IN THE LARYNX AND TRACHEA.—It sometimes

the Gullet, &c. Brodie on Local Nervous affections, (*spasmodic stricture*) Mayo's Pathology, Stokes in Cyclop. Pract. Med. vol. ii. ; and Sir C. Bell's Institutes of Surgery, vol. i.

* Vide Arnot on Œsophagotomy, Med Chir. Trans. vol. xx.

happens that a person who is busily laughing and talking during a meal,
suddenly rises from table, attempts to put his finger into his throat, speedily turns blue in the face, and then drops down dead.   This arises from
a piece of food getting into the rima glottidis.   It rarely happens that the
surgeon arrives in time to do any good; but if he should be promptly on
the spot, he ought to search the pharynx with his fingers, and to pass a
probang down the œsophagus, to see whether the obstruction can be removed;—and if not, he ought to perform laryngotomy or tracheotomy
immediately;—and to pass a probe up into the larynx through the
wound, so as to push the foreign substance up into the mouth.

When a foreign substance has passed the rima glottidis, and has got
into the trachea, it will produce different symptoms according to different
circumstances.   For, in the first place, it may become impacted in the
ventricles of the larynx or upper part of the trachea; in which case it will
probably produce violent spasmodic cough and difficulty of breathing,
together with a fixed pain referred to one particular spot—a croupy sound
during respiration, which may be heard by the stethoscope most distinctly at the seat of that pain; and loss of voice.

In the second place, the foreign substance may be loose in the trachea.
In this case, the violent coughing and sense of suffocation produced by
its first introduction generally subside for a time;—but every now and
then there are violent fits of coughing, during which the substance may
be heard or perhaps may be felt by the finger to be forcibly impelled
against the upper part of the larynx.

Thirdly, the foreign substance may have passed into one of the bronchi, (generally the right,) where perhaps it may be detected by causing
a whistling or murmuring sound.

It is sometimes difficult to distinguish the symptoms produced by a
foreign body in the larynx or trachea from those of croup or laryngitis.
But the surgeon may generally pretty confidently decide that a foreign
body is present, if the symptoms come on suddenly during a meal; or
perhaps the history will be that the patient was playing with a button,
or cherrystone, or some similar body in his mouth, and that he chanced
to fall down, when the button disappeared, and the symptoms came on
directly afterwards.   Moreover, in these cases expiration is generally
more difficult than insipiration, whereas it is usually the reverse in croup,
Besides, when there suddenly occurs a fixed pain, and a fixed whistling
sound in the larynx or bronchi, without any other symptoms of croup,
the case must almost of necessity arise form a foreign body.*

XV. Laryngotomy and Tracheotomy.—The former of these operations is most quickly and easily performed, and is to be preferred in sudden emergencies, but the latter most readily admits of the removal of

---

* Vide an interesting paper by Mr. C. Hawkins, and another by Mr. Travers, jun.
on this subject, Med. Chir. Trans. vol. xxiii.

foreign bodies, and is always to be chosen in cases of suffocation from disease.

*Laryngotomy* is performed by cutting at once, or pushing a trocar through the *crico-thyroid* membrane, which may be felt as a soft depression, an inch below the *pomum Adami*.

*Tracheotomy* is thus performed. The head being thrown back, an incision, an inch and a-half to two inches long, must be made exactly in the median line from the cricoid cartilage to the top of the sternum. The skin, superficial fascia, and fat, are then divided; the sterno-hyoid muscles are separated with the point of the knife; the loose cellular tissue and veins are cleared from the front of the trachea with the fingers or handle of the scalpel; the thyroid gland, if in the way, is pushed up; then the patient being told to swallow, the surgeon seizes the moment, and whilst the trachea is stretched, sticks in his knife at the bottom of the wound, and carries it upwards, so as to divide three or four of its rings. The foreign body is then usually expelled with

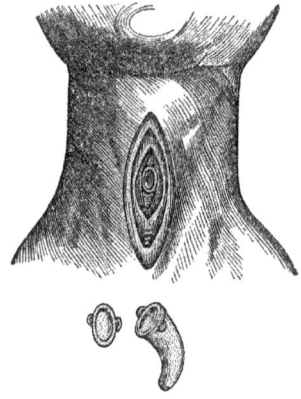

a strong gust of air; but if not, it must be searched for with a probe, and be removed by forceps, or by a blunt hook. The wound may be closed by plaster when bleeding has ceased, but not before. If the operation were performed for the relief of dyspnœa, a *conical* curved tube should be introduced for the patient to breath through. From its shape, it fits tightly into the aperture, and prevents the entrance of blood into the trachea. It should be of such a size, as Trousseau has remarked, that the air may pass through it in respiration without any whistling noise.* When the patient wishes to cough or speak, he must be taught to close its orifice with his finger. It should be frequently cleared of any mucus that may lodge in it. If any veins bleed profusely during the operation, they must be tied.

XVI. SCALDS OF THE GLOTTIS, through swallowing boiling water or corrosive fluids, produce the ordinary symptoms of laryngitis—suffocative

* Trousseau de la Tracheotomie, L' Experience, Nov. 5, 1840.

cough, and dyspnœa. *Treatment.*—Leeches, ice to the throat, calomel in large doses, so as rapidly to affect the system, and tracheotomy if required.

XVII. HANGING may destroy life in three ways. (1.) By dislocating the neck. (2.) By compressing the trachea, and suspending respiration. (3.) By compressing the jugular veins, and inducing apoplexy. *Treatment.*—Artificial respiration, bleeding from the jugular vein if the face be turgid, dashing cold water on the face and chest, and a current of galvanism passed from the nape of the neck to the pit of the stomach, so as to excite the diaphragm.

XVIII. DROWNING, *Treatment of.*—If respiration has ceased, it should instantly be commenced artificially; at the same time the body should be wiped dry, and be assiduously rubbed with hot cloths. Hot bricks and bottles of hot water should be put into the axilla, between the thighs, and to the feet; the head should be raised, the nostrils irritated with a feather, or with the fumes of hartshorn, and a warm enema of turpentine may be thrown up. It need scarcely be said that enemata of that filthy narcotic, tobacco, must not be thought of. As soon as the patient can swallow, he should have some weak wine and water; and soon afterwards an emetic of mustard, to clear the stomach of the water which he has swallowed, and to restore the circulation by the impetus of vomiting. After some hours he will suffer from severe headach and fever, which must be relieved by bleeding or leeching, purgatives, and other remedies, according to the exigencies of the case. One case is narrated in which, after every other means of exciting respiration had failed, an incision was made below the seventh rib, and a current of galvanism was applied immediately to the diaphragm, and with success.

XIX. ARTIFICIAL RESPIRATION is required in all cases of suspended animation,—whether from internal injury, noxious gases, or narcotic poisons, including alcohol. It may be performed by passing a pipe through the mouth, or a male catheter through the nostril into the glottis; or by simply putting a pipe into one nostril, and closing the mouth and the other nostril, and blowing through it. But it is a better plan to use a small pair of bellows, putting its muzzle into one nostril. The operator should be careful to force the air into the lungs with very great gentleness, and to press the larynx against the spine, so that it may not go down the œsophagus. If the larynx has been crushed by a rope, or by a violent blow, it may be necessary to perform tracheotomy, so as to impel a current of air directly into the trachea—but not otherwise.

XX. STOMACH-PUMP.—The tube of this instrument is to be introduced in the same manner as the œsophagus bougie. It is usual to place a gag in the patient's mouth, having a hole for the tube to pass through, in order that it may not be compressed by the teeth. Before pumping out the contents of the stomach, one or two pints of water should be injected into it, and care should be taken *not to withdraw quite as much* as was injected. More water should then be thrown in, and the process should be repeated till it returns colourless.

The stomach-pump is by no means so universally efficacious as is popularly supposed. It ought only to be employed in those cases of poisoning by opium, or alcohol, or other narcotics, in which the stomach and nervous system are rendered so insensible that vomiting cannot be excited. For, in the first place, the operation is not free from danger. It is a well established fact, that a tube may sometimes be passed into the trachea of a sensible person without creating any peculiar sensation, or exciting cough; but if the patient be insensible, that accident will be much more liable to happen. In fact, a case is on record in which a meddling surgeon, with more zeal than knowledge, did actually pass the tube down the trachea, and inject the lungs with chalk mixture, which he had far better have permitted his luckless patient to have swallowed quietly; and Sir C. Bell tells us, that he has seen on dissection both lungs filled with broth, which was intended to have been injected into the stomach. Again, it is known that in one case the mucous membrane of the stomach was sucked into the holes of the tube, and torn into strips,—a thing likely to happen if the stomach is pumped too empty. Besides, this artificial evacuation of the stomach is by no means so efficacious as free vomiting, assisted by plenty of diluents. Lumps of arsenic were left in the stomach, in the very case just cited, in which the mucous membrane was torn. But yet surgeons have been reprimanded by attorney-coroners and " respectable" juries for not using this instrument, even in cases in which it must have been either useless or injurious. These are the fruits of permitting the office of coroner to be filled by men who have no knowledge of the subjects that they are required to sit in judgment on.*

XXI. WOUNDS OF THE THROAT are generally made with intention of suicide, and are extremely dangerous, no less from the importance of the parts injured, than from the despondency of the patient. *Treatment.*— The general indications are, 1st, to arrest hæmorrhage; 2ndly, to obviate difficulty of breathing; 3rdly, to prevent inflammation of the trachea or chest.

In the first place, any arteries that are wounded must be tied, and hæmorrhage from large veins must be restrained by pressure with the finger, kept up as long as may be necessary. The patient should be put to bed in rather a warm room; and as soon as all oozing has ceased, but not before, his shoulders should be raised by pillows, and the head be bent forwards, and be confined by a bandage passing from each side of the nightcap to the shoulders. Plasters are inadmissible, and so are

---

* Vide an amusing Clinical Lecture on the Abuse of the Stomach-pump, by Professor Watson, in Lond. Med. Gazette, vol. xvii.; and Roupell's Illustrations of the Effects of Poisons.

sutures, except in the cases that will be alluded to presently. If the wound penetrates the trachea or larynx, it should be covered with a loose woollen comforter, or, after the first week, with one of Jeffrey's respirators, if it can be nicely adapted. The patient should not be kept too low, and if the pharynx or œsophagus is wounded, a common, large-sized, elastic catheter may be passed, through which nutritive fluids can be injected by means of an elastic bottle. But if during the inflammatory stage the attempt causes great irritation, it may be necessary to employ nutrient enemata merely. No tubes should be passed through the wound for that purpose. The great thirst and dryness of the fauces, experienced in these cases, may in some measure be mitigated by sucking a wet rag. If the patient finds great difficulty in expectorating through the wound, he must be taught to close it partially by leaning his head forwards and placing his fingers on it, so that he may expel the air with a sudden gust.

In every stage of the cure, difficulty of breathing should be viewed with suspicion. It may arise from several causes. (1) If the wound is above the larynx, it may be caused by the epiglottis being detached from the tongue, and hanging down upon or irritating the *rima glottidis*,—or by clots of blood collecting in the pharynx. (2) It may be caused by an irregular and jagged division of the larynx or trachea, so that some pieces of the cartilage hang into the tube; or supposing the trachea to have been completely cut through, it may be caused by the aperture of the lower portion being overlapped by the upper. In these cases it may be requisite to employ sutures, but they should be passed merely through the cellular tissue around the cartilage, aud neither through the cartilage nor the skin. (3) It may be caused by swelling of the mucous membrane of the larynx and trachea in the acute inflammatory stage immediately after the injury—or by chronic thickening of that membrane from the continned irritation of cold air, if the wound is very slow in closing. In the former of these cases, free antiphlogistic measures must be used;—the latter must be prevented by using a proper position, so as to promote the approximation of the wound whilst it is healing. In either case it may be necessary to make a longitudinal division of the trachea to relieve the dyspnœa. (4) Another frequent cause of dyspnœa is the passage of blood into the trachea, if the wound is prematurely closed, and especially if it is sown up or covered with plasters. Even supposing the trachea not to be opened, great danger may result from closing a wound of the throat before bleeding has ceased, for the blood may accumulate in the cellular tissue, and coagulate, and compress the trachea.

XXI. ˊBRONCHOCELE (*Goître, Derbyshire neck*) is an hypertrophy of the thyroid gland. *Symptoms.*—A soft, projecting, elastic, tumour occupies the front of the neck, in the situation and of the shape of the thyroid gland. It is rarely tender, and the skin is not discoloured. Frequently one lateral lobe is larger than the other;—and occasionally the middle lobe or isthmus is solely or principally affected. *Consequences.*—When of moderate bulk, it rarely causes any inconvenience;—except occasional headach, and difficulty of breathing in a stooping posture. But when very large, it may produce a most dangerous difficulty of swallowing and breathing, and congestion in the head by its pressure on the trachea, œsophagus, and jugular veins; or it may induce thickening and disease of the trachea, with most obstinate cough, which may end in consumption. *Diagnosis.*—It is to be distinguished from encysted and other tumours by its shape, by its want of fluctuation, and by its mostly affecting both sides. *Prognosis.*—If it be soft and recent, and occur in a young patient, it will most likely be cured; but probably not, if it be old, hard, and the patient advanced in life. *Anatomical Characters.*—The cells of the gland are found enlarged;—of various sizes from that of a pea downwards;—and filled with a viscid fluid, which becomes gelatinous if immersed in alcohol. Hence it has been presumed that the disease consists essentially of an increased secretion of the matter contained in the cells of the gland. Sometimes they are filled with blood. In old cases, the tumour becomes hard, resembling a sarcomatous formation; and may contain ossific deposites.* *Causes.*—Bronchocele is extremely prevalent in Derbyshire, Nottingham, and the chalky parts of England generally,—but, above all, in the Tyrol and valley of the Rhone. The use of water impregnated with calcareous (or, as a late writer has surmised, *magnesian*) particles, to which the inhabitants of all those places are more or less habituated, although not perhaps the invariable cause, is the most probable that can be assigned. In England it most frequently affects females about the age of puberty, and in many cases is obviously connected with the uterine derangement. Patients so often refer its origin to some twist or strain of the neck, that there is some reason for believing that such an accident may be an exciting cause. There are some persons who always have more or less enlargement of the thyroid gland, and who invariably find it increase in bulk when their health is out of order, or their strength lowered. *Treatment.*—The best remedy for this disease is iodine. The dose should not be large enough to cause pain or disorder of the stomach, or any diminution of the general health. The tincture of pure iodine is objectionable, because it is not miscible with water, and is apt to cause pain in the side. But the iodine should be combined with an alkali, or with the iodide of potassium, or with iron; and an aromatic or a little hyoscyamus often makes it sit more lightly on the stomach, (F. 41, 74.) Before administering the iodine, however, it is useful, if the complaint is of recent origin, to apply leeches, and purge the patient

* Vide Baillie's Morbid Anatomy, by Wardrop, 2nd ed. p. 84, and Turner's Art of Surgery, vol. i. p. 198.

freely. An ointment or liniment or iodine, or of the iodide of potassium, may also be rubbed into the tumour, but it must be remembered that the swelling generally enlarges, instead of decreasing, if the skin be irritated. The patient, if possible, should remove from a residence in which the malady is prevalent, and should drink boiled or distilled water. A residence on the coast and warm sea-bathing are mostly advantageous. If the iodine does not succeed, the burnt sponge, in doses of 3ß ter die, is the best substitute. Any disorder in the digestive or uterine organs should be carefully removed. Pills composed of aloes, soap, and assafœtida (āā gr. ii—iii.) may be given at bed-time with advantage. Other remedies which were in vogue before the discovery of iodine, and which may be resorted to if that fails, are as follow—mercury, iron;—potass and soda; —chlorides of barium and calcium;—digitalis, hyoscyamus, and belladonna;—and sea water.

If medicines prove ineffectual, and the tumour enlarges rapidly so as to threaten suffocation or apoplexy, surgical operations must be resorted to. There are three which have been proposed and practised:—viz. the introduction of setons;—ligature of the arteries which supply the gland;— and extirpation. The general results of these operations may be stated thus. All three of them have at different times succeeded;—all of them are hazardous to life, and have proved fatal;—and the first two have in some instances failed to remove the disease, although the patient has recovered with his life.

If a *seton* be passed, it should be of silk, and large enough to fill the wound made by the needle, so that there may be no fear of bleeding. The needle should be long and narrow. The utmost precaution must be taken, both before and after the operation, to avoid inflammation. If after the seton has remained for some time, it ceases to produce a diminution of the gland, it should be withdrawn, and be re-introduced in another place.

*Extirpation* of the gland is performed by making an incision in the mesial line of the neck;—the skin and muscles must then be dissected from the tumour;—and every artery be tied as soon as it is divided. Then (as it is mostly enlargement of the isthmus, or middle lobe, that requires this operation) a strong double ligature should be passed through it, and should be firmly tied on each side of it before it is cut out.

Sometimes *cysts* are formed in this gland, which contain a glairy matter or blood. If necessary, they may be punctured;—when they will most likely inflame, suppurate, and contract. If bleeding prove troublesome, the wound must be filled with lint.

This gland may farther be affected with acute or chronic *inflammation*, and tubercular deposite; either of which may lead to abscess. Their *treatment* must be conducted on general principles.

XXIII. HERNIA BRONCHALIS (*Bronchocele vera, Goître aerien*) is a very rare tumour, formed by a protrusion of the mucous membrane through the cartilages of the larynx, or the rings of the trachea, and caused by violent exertions of the voice. Larrey met with sundry instances of it in French officers, and in the muezzin or priests that call the people to prayer from the top of the minarets in Mohammedan countries. The tumour is soft and elastic,—can often be made to disappear by pressure—and is increased by any exertion. The only available treatment is moderate support.*

XXIV. PAROTID TUMOURS.—The parotid gland is occasionally, although rarely, the seat of malignant disease, and perhaps of sarcomatous enlargement. But the tumours behind the ramus of the jaw (commonly called *parotid tumours*) generally depend on disease of the lymphatic glands, which are embedded in the parotid, and which cause the natural texture of the latter to be displaced or absorbed, so that they may extend inwards to the pterygoid and styloid processes, and be intimately connected with the branches of the *portio dura*. "If there be reason to suspect," says Mr. Liston, "that the disease is of malignant nature, and not thoroughly limited by a cellular cyst, no interference is admissible. If, on the contrary, it be at all moveable, has advanced slowly, possesses a smooth surface, and is firm, (neither of stony hardness, nor pulpy,) then an operation may be contemplated."

XXV. TUMOURS IN THE SIDE OF THE NECK, if subjacent to the skin merely, may be readily removed,—but if they lie deeply, and are bound down by the platysma and fascia, they require some consideration. If a tumour be of slow growth, defined in its outline, and moveable, so that it is probably not malignant,—or if it interferes with deglutition or respiration, its extirpation may be attempted. The patient should always be warned of the probability of facial palsy after removal of a parotid tumour. See the remarks on the removal of tumours in Part V.

XXVI. WRYNECK is a peculiar distortion in which the head is bent down towards one shoulder, (generally the right,) and the face is turned to the opposite. The right eyebrow and right corner of the mouth generally become elevated, so as to preserve their horizontal position, notwithstanding the distortion of the neck.

*Varieties.*—This affection presents many varieties. It may perhaps be only a part of general lateral curvature of the spine. Or (2) it may depend on caries of the cervical vertebræ. (3) It may be caused by contraction of the cicatrix of a burn or ulcer; or (4) by glandular enlargement on one side of the neck;—the treatment of which cases requires no observation in this place.

But the genuine wryneck is produced by permanent contraction of one

* Larrey, Clinique Chirurgicale, tom. ii. p. 81. Paris, 1829.

sterno-mastoid muscle,—which may depend (1) on *inflammatory spasm* of that muscle, with or without subacute inflammation of the cervical fascia. This form generally occurs somewhat suddenly to weakly children with disordered digestive organs. The skin over the muscle is often hot and tender, and any motion causes pain. *Treatment.*—Perfect rest in the horizontal posture,—leeches,—and poultices or hot fomentations, so as to keep the skin constantly moist and perspirable,—with purgatives and alteratives.*

(2) It may depend on *rigid atrophy* of the muscle, which may be a sequel of the state of inflammatory spasm last described,—or may be congenital. (Vide p. 223.) *Treatment.*—Long-continued friction with mercurial ointment, or with lin. hydrargyri,—or Scott's ointment (F. 25) worn as a plaster,—with blisters behind the ears, and to the nape of the neck,—and the use of a machine to keep up extension,† may be of service in cases that are of no very long duration. If they fail, or if the case is congenital, division of the sternal (or perhaps of both) origins of the muscle is the last resource. It is best performed thus: The skin covering the muscle at about an inch from the sternum is to be pinched up between the left forefinger and thumb. A narrow curved bistoury is then to be thrust under the muscle, and is to be made to divide it as it is being withdrawn,—but the wound in the skin must only be large enough to admit the instrument. The aperture may be made at the anterior border of the right muscle, and between the sternal and clavicular portions of the left. As soon as the division is complete, the ends of the muscle retract with a dull snap, and the thumb should be pressed on the part, to prevent effusion of blood under the skin. When the wound has healed, but not before, an apparatus should be applied to elongate the callus, and restore the neck to its proper position. · A stiff collar to the diseased side is the simplest and best apparatus.

(3) Lastly, this distortion may be caused by *palsy* of one sterno-mastoid muscle, in consequence of which the other muscle, being uncontrolled, drags the neck permanently to its own side. If the administration of remedies calculated to remove any existing disease in the head or back, and to improve the health,—and if strychnine, blisters, issues, and electricity fail, division of the sound muscle has been recommended.‡

* For farther information respecting this form of wryneck, consult Abernethy, Lect. xxxii., Renshaw's ed.; James on Inflam., 2nd ed., p. 484; and Brodie on Local Nervous Affections.

† See a plate in Cooper's First Lines.

‡ Vide Cases of Wryneck, &c, by Dieffenbach, in the Lancet for Sept. 1838. Gooch gives a case of wryneck and distortion of the jaw caused by contraction of the platysma myoides, and cured by division of that muscle, in the year 1759.

50

# CHAPTER XVI.

## OF THE SURGICAL DISEASES AND INJURIES OF THE CHEST.

I. Pneumothorax signifies a distention of the cavity of the pleura with air, and collapse of the lung. It is known by the following symptoms. On the affected side there is an absence of the respiratory murmur, with an exceedingly clear sound on percussion, and immobility of the ribs—and there is *puerile respiration* on the other side. It may be caused (1) by a fractured rib which has lacerated the lung—and in this case it is attended with emphysema—as has been detailed at page 253. (2.) It may be caused by the bursting of an abscess of the lung into the cavity of the pleura. This case will be indicated by *succussion*, and by *metallic tinkling*, in addition to the signs mentioned above. *Succussion* simply consists in making the patient shake himself, when (inasmuch as both air and fluid have escaped from the lung into the pleural cavity) the fluid will be heard to splash, if the ear is applied to the chest. The *metallic tinkling* is a clear sound, like the dropping of water into a cask. It is produced when the patient coughs,—by which means a drop of fluid is shaken from the orifice in the lung, and made to fall to the bottom of the chest. *Treatment.*—If the breathing become very difficult from pneumothorax, a grooved needle or small trocar should be introduced between the fifth and sixth ribs, to let the air escape.

II. Hæmothorax, which signifies the presence of blood in the pleural cavity, may be suspected if great dyspnœa and dulness on percussion follow a fractured rib. The blood may proceed either from the intercostal artery, or from the lung. *Treatment.*—If the difficulty of breathing be very urgent, *paracentesis* must be performed to let the blood escape.

III. Hydrothorax, or water in the chest, is indicated by great difficulty of breathing, especially when lying down—livid countenance—disturbed sleep—dulness on percussion—and if the effusion be confined to one side of the chest, there is very great difficulty in lying upon the other. *Treatment.*—If the hydrothorax were merely an inflammatory effusion from pleurisy, a local affection, *paracentesis* might be advisable for the relief of dyspnœa; but if (as it is generally) it is a mere effect of organic disease of the heart or lungs, the operation would do no good. At all events, both sides of the chest must not be punctured.

It has been suggested to the author by Dr. Ferguson, that it might be advantageous to employ the needle for the cure of serous effusion into the pleura, in the same manner that it is employed for the cure of hydrocele and ganglion. That is to say, half a dozen punctures might be made with an acupuncture needle or grooved needle through one of the intercostal spaces; and thus the serum might pass through the punctures into the cellular tissue outside the pleura, whence it might be absorbed. The same plan might also be adopted in cases of hydrops pericardii and ascites.

IV. EMPYEMA signifies abscess of the chest, or suppuration of the pleura. It is an effect of acute inflammation, whether idiopathic or caused by injury. It is known by dulness on percussion—gradually increasing enlargement of the side of the chest—separation of the ribs—dyspnœa—difficulty of lying on the sound side—and more or less œdema of the parietes of the chest. If left to itself, the abscess may point and burst between the ribs. *Paracentesis* is decidedly required, if the case be clear;—if it be not, two or three punctures may be made with a grooved or cataract needle, and a cupping-glass be applied over them to extract some fluid.

V. PARACENTESIS THORACIS is performed by making an incision an inch and a half long on the upper edge of the sixth rib, at or a little behind its middle. The intercostal muscles are then to be cautiously divided, and the point of the bistoury to be passed through the pleura. If fluid escapes from this puncture, it may be slightly enlarged. This operation is liable to be followed by many of the mischiefs that result from the opening of large chronic abscesses. (p. 77.) The pleural cavity is incapable of contracting as the fluid escapes;—air consequently enters to supply its place, and causes irritation of the cyst, and putrefaction of its contents. The discharge becomes profuse and fetid, and the patient suffers severely from irritative fever, under which he may sink. It is therefore advisable to place the patient on the diseased side immediately after the puncture, so that the matter may flow out without the ingress of air—to close the wound with lint and plaster before too much has escaped—to bandage the chest—and to repeat the operation in a few days if necessary, instead of leaving the wound open.

VI. HYDROPS PERICARDII may occur under the same pathological conditions as hydrothorax, and may be combined with it. Its diagnosis is obscure. It may be suspected to exist if the patient complain of constant weight in the præcordia, great dyspnœa, especially when lying on the back, and faintness upon exertion;—if there is great dulness on percussion, and manifest fulness over the region of the heart—if its pulsations are tremulous—and the circulation embarrassed. The operation of *paracentesis pericardii* has been practised, although it can rarely be of much benefit. It has been attempted in sundry cases of hydrothorax, which were mistaken for hydrops pericardii; but by a second lucky mistake the pleura was opened instead. It may (if thought advisable) be performed, either by making an incision opposite the heart's apex, and dividing the muscles and pericardium with the same precautions as in paracentesis thoracis—or by first making an opening into the pleura, opposite the junction of the fifth or sixth rib with its cartilage—and then introducing the finger, feeling for the distended pericardium, and cutting into it with curved scissors.

VII. WOUNDS AND CONTUSIONS OF THE PARIETES of the chest require the same treatment, whether the ribs are fractured or not. A firm bandage (having an aperture to admit of the dressing of any wounds) must be applied to prevent motion of the ribs. Free venesection must be employed to prevent inflammation;—the bowels must be opened, the diet low, and cough and irritation be allayed by opiates.

VIII. PENETRATING WOUNDS of the thorax, unattended with wound of the lungs, are exceedingly rare. In some cases, when the chest is laid open the lung collapses, just as it would in a dead body; in others, on the contrary, it does not recede from, or it even may protrude out of the wound. If so, it must be immediately returned by gentle pressure. *Treatment.*—Bleeding must be restrained; foreign bodies if any, removed, and the wound be closed; then the surgeon must employ free bleeding, and the other measures spoken of above. The *intercostal artery*, if wounded, must if possible, be tied, the wound being enlarged for that purpose if necessary. If this cannot be done, pressure must be kept up on the bleeding orifice by the finger.

IX. WOUNDS OF THE LUNG are known by the following symptoms. There is great dyspnœa and sense of suffocation; the countenance is pallid and extremely anxious—and there is an expectoration of blood;— which is coughed up in florid arterial mouthfuls, mixed with occasional clots. The dangers of these wounds are threefold. 1st, The great *hæmorrhage*, which may destroy the patient by inanition, or may fill up the air-passages and induce suffocation. 2ndly, *Inflammation*, which is sure to supervene from the injury, and may be aggravated by the irritation of clots of blood, or of other extraneous bodies. 3rdly, Profuse and exhausting *suppuration*, with cough, debility, hectic, and all the symptoms of phthisis. *Prognosis.*—This of course must be extremely guarded. But there may be good hopes of recovery after the day is passed. Death is seldom caused after the first forty hours. *Treatment.*—The first indication is to check the hæmorrhage. This can only be done by abstracting a large quantity of blood from the arm, provided the patient be not already faint. Then the wound should be examined, and if it be of large size, or a gunshot wound, the finger should be introduced into it, to remove clots of blood, splinters of bone or any other foreign substances that it may find. If it is not sufficiently large for this purpose it may be dilated by a probe-pointed bistoury. At the same time, an intercostal artery, if wounded should be secured. The wound should then be accurately closed with lint and plaster, and the patient should be suffered to lie as quiet as possible. He should have plenty of cool air, and a very light covering. It is a general rule, in all injuries of the thorax and abdomen, to place him on the wounded side. In the course of a few hours the pulse will probably rise, and the pain, and cough, and spitting of blood return. Upon the first appearance of such symptoms, venæsection must be repeated, and it must, without hesitation, be resorted to again and again if they recur. The diet must be rigorously low; nothing but cold acidulated drinks—lemonade, or barley-water with lemon-juice—can be allowed for several days; the bowels must be opened and opiates be given to allay cough and pain.

*Secondary hæmorrhage*, after wounds of the lung, may (1) be caused by inflammatory excitement; or (2) (if the wound be gunshot) by the separation of the sloughs from the lung; or (3) by the sloughing of an intercostal artery that may have been brushed by the ball. Venæsection is the remedy for the first two cases, and the ligature, or pressure, for the third.

If, after the primary dangers of hæmorrhage and inflammation have ceased, and the wound has closed, there are rigours, dyspnœa, and other signs of *empyema paracentesis* is requisite. And if these symptoms come on soon after the injury, the paracentesis should be performed at the site of the wound; but if they come on at a distant period, the paracentesis should be done at the usual place, in order to avoid the adhesions that are sure to be formed near the wound.

*Foreign bodies* in the chest add greatly to the danger of exhausting suppuration, although patients have recovered for years with balls, or pieces of cloth, encysted in the lung or pleural cavity. In some cases, a ball has remained rolling loosely about in the plural cavity. If any foreign body is detected, it should if possible, be removed, and part of the upper border of a rib may be sawn away with Hey's saw, if necessary, in order to get at it.

Some surgeons direct penetrating wounds of the chest not to be closed; or they even recommend tents or canulæ to be inserted, to provide for the escape of blood or matter. But it must be evident that there will be much less liability to severe inflammation if the wound is closed,—just as in wounds of joints and compound fractures. Besides, "if the patient," says Hennen, "is placed with the wound in a dependent posture, the exit of effused fluids is not necessarily impeded. If they exist in large quantity, the wound is effectually prevented from closing; if the flow is so minute as to admit of the union of the wound, the quantity effused is within the power of the absorbents to remove."

After wounds of the chest, there is a constant susceptibility of inflammation from slight causes, so that the patient should be cautious to avoid over-fatigue, intemperance, and atmospheric vicissitudes.

X. WOUNDS OF THE HEART generally prove fatal from hæmorrhage. Numerous instances, however, are on record, in which stabs or musket wounds of this organ healed, both in man and animals, without any remaining ill effects.   The diagnosis and prognosis will of course be extremely doubtful.   The only available *treatment* is free depletion and opiates, in order to prevent hæmorrhage, and keep the circulation as quiet as possible, so that the blood may coagulate in the wound, and the coagulum become adherent and organized.

# CHAPTER XVII.

## OF THE SURGICAL DISEASES AND INJURIES OF THE ABDOMEN.

I. PARACENTESIS ABDOMINIS is required in *ascites* and *ovarian dropsy,* when the abdomen is so distended that the breathing and the circulation of the lower extremities are seriously impeded.   *Ascites* is known by the abdomen being *equably* enlarged and fluctuating—not feeling harder at one part than another—and by the clear tympanitic sound produced by percussion of the anterior surface of its parietes, whilst the patient lies on his back.   In *ovarian dropsy,* the swelling fluctuates less distinctly,—is evidently composed of distinct cysts, some of which feel more distended than others,—and a dull sound is emitted on percussion of the abdomen whilst the patient lies on her back.   *Operation.*—The patient must be seated in a chair.   A broad towel must then be passed round the lower part of the abdomen, and its ends be crossed behind and entrusted to two assistants, who are to be instructed to draw it tight and support the belly as the fluid escapes; otherwise, the removal of the compression to which the abdominal veins have been habituated would cause the blood to gravitate into them from the heart, and induce syncope,—or perhaps they might burst, and occasion a fatal hæmorrhage. A piece of flannel broad enough to cover the whole abdomen, and having a notch cut out of it above and below, (and the edges sewn together afterwards,) is a good substitute for the towel.   The surgeon then plunges a trocar and canula through the linea alba, two inches below the umbilicus, (or perhaps it is better to make a cautious puncture with a lancet, and introduce a *blunt* trocar and canula,)—then he draws out the trocar, and receives the fluid into a proper vessel—the assistants drawing the towel tight as it escapes. The aperture is afterwards to be closed with lint and plaster,—and the patient to be put to bed, with the towel fastened round the loins. A broad flannel roller should be substituted for it before she rises. If a patient with ascites happens also to have an old irreducible hernia, and the sac is much distended, and preserves a free communication with the abdomen, it is a good plan to puncture the sac instead of the linea alba.

II. OVARIAN DROPSY.—This disease consists apparently in the conversion of the ovary into a large tumour, composed of one or many cysts, filled with a serous or glairy fluid. Its diagnosis from ascites has been spoken of in the preceding paragraph. It need scarcely be said, that this form of dropsy is very little if at all under the influence of medicine, and that it generally continues to increase, and fill up the abdomen, till it proves fatal by interfering with the functions of the stomach, and exhausting the powers of life;—a termination which is never very far postponed by the ordinary operation of paracentesis. Several other operations have therefore been proposed at different times. *Extirpation* of the entire tumour, by means of a large incision through the abdominal parietes, has been of late years practised by Mr. Lizars;—but with how little success will be evident, when it is considered, that in some cases the patient died from the operation;—in some others, after the abdomen was opened, it was found that the tumour could not be removed, and the wound was closed again;—and lastly, in some cases in which the tumour was extirpated, and the patient survived, the disease returned again afterwards. *Injection* of the cyst with weak wine and water has been proposed repeatedly, and especially by Majendie, but it appears to be dangerous and inefficacious.* The latest operation, however, and one that is certainly more promising than any other, is that which was first practised by Mr. Jeaffreson. It is performed by making an incision into the abdomen, an inch and a half long, below the umbilicus. As soon as the ovarian cyst is exposed, it is to be punctured, and the edges of the puncture being seized with forceps, the whole of the cyst may be dragged out of the wound, as the fluid escapes;—then the pedicle of the cyst is to be tied tightly with a single silk ligature, and cut off. An estimate may be formed whether the tumour consists of one cyst or many, by the quantity of fluid which escapes when the puncture is made; and if a second cyst is discovered, it may be punctured and dragged out as well. Of the instances in which this operation has been performed, about half have proved successful.†

III. VIOLENT BLOWS ON THE ABDOMEN from obtuse substances—the

* Magendie, Leçons sur les Phénoménes Physiques de la Vie, Paris, 1836.

† Vide Jeaffreson, Lancet, 7th January, 1839 : King, Lancet, 21st January, 1837; West, Lancet, 25th November, 1837 ; also Med. Gaz., November 24th, 1838; and case by Mr. B. Phillips, which proved fatal, Med. Gaz., October 10th, 1840.

passage of cartwheels, spent shot, and so forth, may produce various results. (1) They may cause severe *concussion* and collapse, which may
either speedily prove fatal,—or may pass off without farther ill consequences, or may be succeeded by inflammation, (p. 17.) (2) They may
produce *laceration* of the bowels, or of the solid viscera;—with effusion
of blood or of their secretions into the peritonæal cavity. This may be
suspected if the patient complains of excruciating pain radiating over the
whole belly;—if the features are pinched, the belly, soon swells, and the
pulse is very small and tremulous. *Treatment.*—The patient must be
suffered to lie quietly during the stage of collapse, without any officious
administration of stimulants: and as soon as pain or vomiting comes on,
he should be bled. Subsequently bleeding, leeches, and fomentations to
the belly, to abate inflammation; and large doses of opium to support the
system under the irritation, are the only available remedies. The
bowels should not be disturbed either with purgatives or enemata for the
first three days,—nor should any nutriment be taken, save very small
quantities of the mildest fluids at intervals.

IV. Abscesses between the abdominal parietes occasionally result from
contusions or punctured wounds, and sometimes occur idiopathically.
According to the principles laid down in a preceding page, (76,) they
should be opened early, both because of the tendinous structures by
which they are covered, and of the possibility that they might burst into
the peritonæum.

V. Penetrating Wounds of the abdomen may be divided into four
species; namely, 1st, simple wounds of the parietes; 2ndly, wounds of
the viscera; 3rdly, wounds of the parietes with protrusion of the viscera;
and 4thly, wounds in which some of the viscera are protruded and wounded likewise.

(1.) In the case of a *simple wound of the parietes*, the surgeon must
first (if it be large enough) gently introduce his finger, to ascertain that
no part of the intestines is beginning to protrude:—then the wound must
be closed by sticking-plaster; or by suture if it is extensive. If the epigastric artery is divided, it must be cut down upon and tied.

(2.) *Wounds of the viscera.*—In the case of small wounds of the abdomen without protrusion, it will be often impossible to say whether the
bowels are wounded or not, but the treatment must be altogether the same,
whether they are or not. (*a*) Wounds of the *stomach* may be known
by the situation and depth of the wound,—by vomiting of blood,—by the
very great depression and collapse,—and by the nature of the matters (if
any) that escape from the wound. (*b*) Wounds of the *bowels* may *perhaps* be known by the passage of blood with the stools,—or by fæcal
matter escaping from the wound,—or by the symptoms of extravasation
of their contents into the abdominal cavity—that is to say, excruciating
pain, radiating over the whole belly from the seat of the injury, and at-

tended with signs of great collapse.   Fortunately, however, as Mr. Travers has shown, wounds of the stomach and intestines, unless very large, are not so liable to be attended with extravasation as was formerly thought. For, in the first place, the mucous membrane protrudes through the muscular, so as to fill up a small aperture; and secondly, any tendency to extravasation is counteracted by the constant equable pressure of all the abdominal viscera against each other.   Lymph is soon effused, and glues the neighbouring parts together, and thus the aperture is circumscribed, and any future extravasation is prevented.   (c) Wounds of the *liver*, if extensive are, from its great vascularity, nearly as fatal as those of the heart. Small wounds may be recovered from.   There will at first be symptoms of great collapse, which, if the patient survive, will be succeeded by severe sickness, pain in the liver, yellowness of the skin and urine, great itching, and a glairy, bilious discharge from the wound.   (d) Wounds or rupture of the *gall bladder* are almost invariably fatal, although there are one or two instances of recovery on record.   (e) Wounds of the *spleen*, if deep, are also fatal from the great hæmorrhage that follows, although the whole organ has been removed from animals (and it is said from man) without much consequent evil.   (f) Wounds of the *kidneys* are attended with bloody urine.   They are exceedingly dangerous, first from hæmorrhage, next from violent inflammation with excessive vomiting; and lastly, from profuse suppuration, kept up by the passage of urine through the wound.   Venæsection, very mild laxatives, the warm bath, avoidance of too much drink, very light dressings so as to admit of the flow of urine through the wound, and some unctuous application to prevent excoriation of the surrounding skin, are necessary measures. (g) Wounds of the *bladder*, if communicating with the peritonæum, are extremely dangerous, owing to extravasation of urine.   In fact, unless there is an external wound through which it can escape, they are almost uniformly mortal.   The catheter must be worn constantly.

(3.) *If the intestines protrude*, and are neither wounded nor gangrenous, they should first be freed from any foreign particles that stick to them, and then be returned as soon as possible.   The patient should be placed on his back, with his shoulders raised, and his knees drawn up. If absolutely necessary, the wound must be a little dilated with a probe-pointed bistoury.   Then the surgeon should return the bowel portion by portion, passing it back with his right forefinger and thumb, and keeping his left forefinger on that which is already replaced, to prevent it from protruding again.   He should be careful to replace intestine before omentum, and the part that protruded last should be returned first.

(4.) If the stomach and intestines, when *protruded, are found to be wounded*, the wound should be sewn carefully up with a fine needle and silk by the *continuous* or *glover's suture*, (p. 131,) in such a manner as to bring the edges into apposition, and prevent all extravasation between

51

them. Then the part should be replaced, and the external wound be closed. The aperture in the bowel will be united, as in other cases, by the adhesion of contiguous surfaces; and the silk employed in the suture will be detached by ulceration, and fall into its cavity. If, however, any part of the bowel that is protruded be much bruised or lacerated; or be gangrenous, it should not be returned, but be left hanging out, that an *artificial anus* may be formed.

The *after treatment* of all these cases is the same. The patient must be kept at perfect rest, and should lie on the wounded part, if such a posture be easy. Venæsection and leeches must be sedulously employed to avert hæmorrhage and inflammation, and the indication for bleeding must be taken rather from the stomach than from the pulse. The pulse, will from the nature of the parts inflamed, be small and perhaps weak—but if there be vomiting, bleeding may be performed without fear. After the bleeding, large doses of opium should be given, and should be repeated so as to keep the system under its influence. Nothing but water, or thin arrowroot, should be given for three days, when the stomach or intestines are probably wounded.

The author hopes that it is unnecessary to warn his readers against the fatal and abominable custom of giving purgatives in cases of inflammation of the bowels arising from wounds of the abdomen. It is quite true that the bowels will be obstinately costive; but this costiveness arises from their being inflamed and unable to propel their contents onwards; and the proper remedies for it, are such as will relieve the inflammation—that is, bleeding, leeches, fomentations, and calomel and opium. But if, in spite of common sense, the surgeon attempts to overcome the costiveness by colocynth pills and black draughts, he will soon induce an obstinate vomiting, that will render all other remedies nugatory. If in any case of inflammation of the bowels it is probable that they are loaded with fæces, the proper remedy is the repeated injection of warm water as an enema.*

VI. ARTIFICIAL ANUS signifies a preternatural communication between the intestine and skin. It may be a consequence of penetrating wounds— of abscess or ulceration of the intestines—or of mortification of intestine in strangulated hernia. The external opening is irregular, everted, and red—and the surrounding skin excoriated. The aperture in the intestine adheres by its margin to the peritonæum, so that extravasation into the abdomen is prevented. That portion of intestine which is immediately above the aperture, and that portion which is immediately below it, meet at the artificial anus at a more or less acute angle—and present

---

* Vide Travers on Wounds of the Intestines, Lond. 1812; Hennen's Military Surgery; the observations on the treatment of enteritis in Ferguson on Puerperal Fever; Griffin's Medical Problems, and Dr. Holland's Notes and Reflections.

two orifices—one by which matters descend from the stomach, and another leading down the rectum. These two orifices are separated by a sort of crescent-shaped septum, formed by a projection of the mesenteric side of the bowel opposite to the aperture. Now it may readily be understood, that the greater the aperture in the bowel, the more acute will be the angle at which the upper and lower portions meet—and the greater will the septum also be—and that if the septum is large, it will act as a valve, and close up the orifice of the lower portion of bowel—causing any matters that come down through the upper portion to escape externally, instead of passing into the lower.*

The *consequences* of this affection may be, 1st, that the patient may suffer from inanition, if the aperture is near the duodenum. 2ndly, that a portion of intestine may protrude and form a hernia;—besides the constant disgusting annoyance occasioned by the escape of fæcal matters and flatus.

*Treatment.*—If the affection is of recent origin, and especially if it is consequent upon strangulated hernia, the patient should remain in bed, and great care should be taken to keep the parts clean; and then, perhaps, the external aperture may contract and cicatrize. If the latter is very small, and if the passage between it and the bowel is of some length,—(a state of parts termed *fæcal fistula*,) something may perhaps be done by compression; and by engrafting a piece of skin over the aperture.

But if the loss of substance in the bowel is considerable, and the projecting septum large, the chance of recovery is not great. A pad of simple linen or lint may be worn to compress the aperture and prevent discharge from it—or sometimes a hollow truss with a leathern or horn receptacle may be used with advantage. Enemata are useful in all cases. Moreover, a tent may be thrust into both internal orifices in order to enlarge the lower one, and repress the septum, as proposed by Dessault. As a last resource, a small portion of the septum may be nipped and strangulated by the forceps invented by Dupuytren for that purpose.

* Vide the chapter on Artificial Anus in Lawrence on Hernia, and Dupuytren in Dict. de Med. tom. iii.

# CHAPTER XVIII.

## OF HERNIA.

SECTION I.—OF THE NATURE AND TREATMENT OF HERNIA GENERALLY.

DEFINITION.—Hernia signifies a protrusion of any viscus from its natural cavity. But the term, employed singly, is restricted to signify protrusion of the abdominal viscera.

CAUSES.—The formation of hernia may be readily understood by considering that the abdominal viscera are subject to frequent and violent pressure from the diaphragm and other surrounding muscles—a pressure which tends to force them outwardly against the parietes of the abdomen. Consequently, if any point of the parietes be not strong enough to resist this pressure, some portion of the viscera may be forced through it, and form a hernial tumour externally.

The *predisposing* cause of hernia, therefore, is a weakness of the parietes of the abdomen, which may be produced by various circumstances. Thus (1) some parts of the parietes are naturally weaker than others; especially the inguinal and crural rings, and the umbilicus: and it is at these parts that hernia most frequently occurs. (2) The abdominal parietes may be weak from malformation, or congenital deficiency. (3) They may be weakened by injury or diseases, such as abscesses, wounds, and bruises—or by distention by the pregnant uterus, or by dropsy. The *exciting* cause is compression of the viscera, by the action of the muscles that surround them. Hence hernia is so frequent a result of violent bodily exertion—lifting heavy weights and the like—especially if the patient have been previously weakened by illness. Moreover it is not uncommon in persons afflicted with stone or stricture, from the immoderate straining that they employ in passing their urine.

The viscera most liable to hernial protrusion are the small intestines, omentum, and arch of the colon. But every one of them has occasionally been found protruded, partially or entirely—especially in cases of congenital deficiency of the abdominal parietes.

THE SAC of a hernia is a portion of the *parietal* or *reflected* layer of peritonæum which the protruding viscera push before them in their escape, and which forms a pouch containing them. It very soon contracts adhesion to the surrounding cellular tissue, and is consequently incapable of being replaced. As the hernia increases in size, the sac also increases;—partly by growth; partly by distention, and slight laceration or unravelling; partly by fresh protrusion of peritonænm. Sometimes it diminishes in thickness whilst increasing in capacity—sometimes, on the contrary, it becomes thick, indurated, and divisible into layers. Its *neck* (the narrow part which communicates with the abdomen) always becomes thickened, rigid, and more or less puckered, in consequence of the pressure of the muscular or ligamentous fibres which surround it. Sometimes the sac has two necks—either because (as in oblique inguinal hernia) it passes through two tendinous apertures—(the external and internal abdominal rings)—or because the original neck has been pushed down by a fresh protrusion. Some herniæ, however, are destitute of a sac—or at least of a complete one. This may happen, (1) if the protruded viscus is not naturally covered by peritonæum; as the cœcum. (2.) If the hernia occur in consequence of a penetrating wound. (3.) In some cases of congenital umbilical hernia. (4.) Hernia may be considered virtually without a sac, if the sac has been burst by a blow, or if it has become entirely adherent to its contents.

DIVISION.—Hernia is divided into several species (1st) according to its *situation*—as the inguinal, femoral, and so forth; (2ndly) according to the *condition of the protruded viscera;*—which may be (*a*) *reducible,* (or returnable into the abdomen;) (*b*) *irreducible; (c) strangulated;* that is, subject to some constriction which not only prevents their return into the abdomen, but interferes with the passage of their contents, and with their circulation.

I. REDUCIBLE HERNIA.—*Symptoms.*—A soft compressible swelling appears at some part of the abdominal parietes. It increases in size when the patient stands up;—if grasped, it is found to dilate when he coughs or makes any exertion—and it diminishes or disappears when he lies down, or when properly directed pressure is made upon it. If the sac contains intestine, (*entero-cele,*) the tumour is smooth, rounded, and elastic;—*borborygmi* (or flatulate croakings) are occasionally heard in it,—and when pressed upon, the bowel returns in the abdomen with a sudden jerk and gurgling noise. If, however, it contains omentum, (*epiplocele,*) the tumour is flattened, inelastic, flabby and unequal to the touch, and when pressed, it returns without noise, and very slowly,—the pressure requiring to be continued till it has entirely disappeared. But very often one hernia contain both intestines and omentum, (entero-epiplocele.)

*Treatment.*—The indications for the treatment of reducible hernia are, to replace the hernia, and to prevent its return. The latter object is to be accomplished by the use of a *truss;* an instrument consisting of a pad placed on the seat of protrusion—and of a steel spring which passes round the body, and causes the pad to press with a requisite degree of force. In order to take the measure for a truss, the patient should lie down, and the hernia should be replaced—then he should stand up and be told to cough—whilst the surgeon ascertains with his fingers the exact spot at which the protrusion commences. The distance from this spot round the hip to an inch on the other side of the spine gives the required ad-measurement. If the hips are very flat, or peculiarly formed, the measure should be taken with a piece of wire, stiff enough to keep its shape, so that it may be taken to the instrument-maker's for a pattern. The pad should not be too large, nor the spring too weak, or the instrument will be loose and inefficient;—nor should the spring be too forcible, or the pad too small, otherwise it will cause pain. But the patient must expect to find it rather irksome for the first week. The truss should be con-stantly worn by day; and if the patient will submit to wear it at night also, so much the better. If he will not do this, he should at all events apply it in the morning before he rises from the recumbent posture. Thousands of trusses, with every possible complication and variety of spring and pad, are daily advertised by their inventors; but any one who has had much practical knowledge of the subject, will not fail to agree with Mr. Liston, that " the simple truss well constructed, made for and fitted to the particular individual, with or without a thigh-strap, is to be preferred."

*Radical cure.*—If the patient is below the age of puberty, or not much above it, and if the hernia has not existed very long, it is probable that the truss, if constantly worn, may effect a permanent cure. The her-uiary aperture, no longer subject to distention, may become firmly closed, and the neck of the sac obliterated. This cure may perhaps occur in two or three years. but as a measure of precaution, the truss should be worn for two or three years more. As for the old-fashioned attempts to obtain a radical cure by cutting out the sac—or by including its neck in a wire or other ligature—or by making a large slough of the superjacent skin —or the modern American plan of making forcible pressure on the neck of the sac by means of a truss with a strong spring and a wooden or ivory pad, so as to excite the adhesive inflammation there—or M. Bel-mas's scheme of poking little bladders of goldbeater's skin upon sticks of gelatin into the neck of the sac for the same purpose*—the less that is said about them the better. One or two measures for the radical cure of inguinal hernia will be mentioned in their proper place.†

* Vide Lancet, 1829–30, vol. ii. p. 390.

† In this paragraph, Mr. Druitt has done great injustice to what he styles " the modern American plan " for the radical cure of Hernia.

The truss of Stagner, with the various modifications it has received from Dr. Chase and others, has been thoroughly tested by the most competent surgeons in the country, and, on all hands, pronounced one of the most valuable contributions of mechanical, to the healing art.

When fitted and applied by a person of adequate professional knowledge and skill— and no others are entrusted with these duties, by the proprietors, who are themselves

II. IRREDUCIBLE HERNIA.—Hernia is said to be *irreducible* when the protruded viscera cannot be returned into the abdomen, although there is no impediment to the passage of their contents, or to their circulation.

*Causes.*—Hernia may be rendered irreducible, (1) by an adhesion of the sac to its contents, or of the latter to each other, or by membranous bands formed across the sac. (2.) By enlargement of the omentum or mesentery—whether from simple deposition of fat, or from sarcomatous or other organic change. (3.) Omental hernia may be rendered irreducible by a contraction of that portion which lies in the neck of the sac, so that it is not stiff enough to stand against the pressure intended to push it back into the abdomen, but doubles up under it.

*Consequences.*—Irreducible hernia may produce sundry inconveniences. In the first place, the patient is often liable to dragging pains in the abdomen, and vomiting after food, or when he assumes the erect posture—because the protruded omentum or intestines, being fixed, resist all distention or upward movement of the stomach. These inconveniences will be greatly aggravated, if the patient increase in corpulency, or become pregnant. Moreover, the protruded bowels being deprived of their natural support, their fæculent contents are apt to lodge in them, and frequently cause colic or constipation. Lastly, the bowel is greatly exposed to external injury, and in constant hazard of strangulation.

*Treatment.*—This may be either palliative or radical. (1.) The *palliative* treatment consists in applying a hollow bag truss, or else a truss with a hollow pad that shall firmly embrace the hernia, and prohibit any additional protrusion. The patient should avoid all violent exertion or excess in diet, and should never let his bowels be confined.

(2.) *Radical Cure.*—It has occasionally happened, after confinement to bed for several weeks with fever or some other emaciating ailment, that a hernia, irreducible before, has been replaced with ease, owing to an absorption of the fat of the omentum or mesentery, and relaxation of the abdominal apertures. The same result has also in some cases been effected by art—by keeping the patient in the recumbent posture and on very low diet for six weeks or two months, and by the frequent use of glysters and laxatives. This plan is very uncertain as to its results, and will be effectually defeated if there are any adhesions; and besides, there

eminent medical men,—these instruments are harmless and comfortable supports, and, in a large proportion of cases, favour the contraction of the ring, or promote adhesions about it—which result in a permanent cure of the complaint. It would seem that Mr. D. does not fully understand the principles on which this result is supposed to depend—Dr. Chase would do well to send him a copy of his exposé.

Dr. Dodson, of this city, deserves to be mentioned among those who have contributed to the perfection of these instruments, by important improvements in their construction. F.

are not many patients who will submit to it. It will be more likely to succeed if the hernia is omental, than if it contains intestine. Any surgical operation with the view of opening the sac, dividing adhesions, and returning the parts into the abdomen, is scarcely justifiable, as it would be exposing life to too great a hazard for the removal of a mere inconvenience.

III. STRANGULATED HERNIA.—Hernia is said to be strangulated, when it is constricted in such a way, that the contents of the protruded bowel cannot be propelled onwards, and the return of its venous blood is impeded.

The *causes* of strangulation may be (1) A sudden protrusion of bowel or omentum through a narrow aperture, in consequence of violent exertion,—(a thing not unlikely to happen if a truss has been worn for some time, and then is carelessly left off.) (2) Swelling of the neck of the sac, or spasm of the muscular fibres around it. (3) Distention of the protruded intestines by flatus or fæces, or congestion of the omentum or mesentery.

The *seat of stricture* is generally at the neck of the sac, but in some rare cases the bowel has been constricted by membranous bands, or by apertures in the omentum, or in the sac itself.

The *symptoms* of strangulated hernia are, *first*, those of obstruction of the bowels;—*secondly*, those of inflammation. The patient first complains of flatulence, colicky pains, a sense of tightness across the belly, desire to go to stool, and inability to evacuate. (It is true that stools may be passed if there be any fæcal matter in the bowel below the hernia, or if the hernia be entirely omental, but with very transient relief.) To these symptoms succeed vomiting of the contents of the stomach,—then of mucus and bile,—and lastly, of matters which have acquired a *stercoraceous* smell by being delayed in the small intestines. Meanwhile the tumour is uneasy, tense, and incompressible. If this state of things continue, the inflammatory stage comes on. The neck of the sac becomes tender, and tenderness diffuses itself over the tumour and over the abdomen, both of which become very painful and much more swelled. The countenance is anxious;—the vomiting constant;—the patient restless and despondent;—and the pulse small, hard, and wiry. After a variable time, the constricted parts begin to mortify. The skin becomes cold,—the pulse very rapid and tremulous,—and the tumour dusky red and emphysematous, but the pain ceases, and the patient, having perhaps expressed himself altogether relieved, soon afterwards dies.

*Varieties.*—There is often considerable diversity in the rapidity and violence of these symptoms. If the patient be a strong adult, and the strangulation has commenced suddenly with a fresh protrusion during strong exertion, the inflammatory stage may come on instantly, and be followed by death in a very few hours. On the other hand, if the patient is old,—if the hernia has been long irreducible, and has a large neck,—and if the strangulation is produced by distention of the protruded bowel with flatus or fæces—the symptoms of mere obstruction may last many days before those of inflammation come on. To this latter class of cases the term *incarcerated* is applicable. Again, if the hernia be omental, the symptoms will be less acute than if it be intestinal.

*Diagnosis.*—If a patient with irreducible hernia be attacked by colic, or enteritis, or peritonitis, the case will present many of the features of strangulation. Yet it may perhaps be distinguished by noticing that the pain and tenderness did not begin at the neck of the sac, and are not more intense there than elsewhere. The diagnosis will be very obscure if the inflammation commences on the omentum or intestine in the sac. But the general rule is, *when in doubt, operate.* In every case of sudden and violent vomiting and colic, the bend of the thigh should be well examined, and inquiry should be made for any tumours about the abdomen—because the patient may have been labouring under hernia for years, and yet from ignorance or *mauvaise honte* may not mention it.

*Morbid Appearances.*—After death from strangulated hernia, the bowels are found reddened,—the upper portion of them much distended,—and there are effusions of turbid serum and lymph. Around the sac, the tissues are œdematous or emphysematous. The strangulated intestine is dark, claret-coloured, and turgid with blood,—roughened in patches by a coating of lymph,—and displaying patches of gangrene, *i. e.* greenish or ash-coloured spots, which break down under the finger. The omentum is dark red—if gangrenous, it feels crispy and emphysematous, and the blood in its veins is coagulated. The sac also contains bloody turbid serum.

*Treatment.*—The indications are, 1st, to return the intestine, or any portion of it that may not be irreducible; 2ndly, to divide any constricting part, if necessary; 3rdly, to obviate inflammation.

In the first place, an attempt should be made to return the protrusion by a manual operation—technically called *taxis.*\* The bladder having been emptied, the patient should lie down, with his shoulders raised; and both his thighs should be bent towards the belly and be placed close to each other, so that every muscle and ligament connected with the abdomen may be relaxed. He should be engaged in conversation to prevent him from straining with his respiratory muscles. Then the surgeon, if the tumour be large, grasps it with the palms of both hands,—gently compresses it in order if possible to squeeze a little of the flatus into the abdomen—pushes it *in the axis of the neck of the sac*, and at the same time with his fingers gently kneads and *sways* the parts at the neck of

---

\* From τασσω, I set in order.

the tumour, so as if possible to dislodge them. This operation may be continued for a quarter or half an hour—longer if the tumour is indolent, but not so long if it is tender,—and at last, perhaps, the surgeon will be delighted to hear a gurgling sound accompanying the return of a portion of intestine. The operator should recollect that too much force may bruise or rupture the viscera, or drive sac and all into the abdomen,—and that he must not be satisfied with a partial reduction of the volume and tension of the tumour, if the vomiting remains unrelieved,—because, as Mr. Mayo has shown, such a diminution might be caused by merely forcing the serum contained in the sac into the abdominal cavity.

If the taxis do not succeed, certain auxillary measures may be resorted to, in order to relax the muscles, reduce the heart's action, and diminish the size of the tumour. *Bleeding* to the approach of faintness, and the *hot bath*, are the most important, and may be used *before the taxis*, if the belly is tender, and the patient pretty robust. But it must be recollected that a delicate person will not be very likely to bear the shock of an operation; if bled or boiled to death's door first of all. The *tobacco enema* (3j ad Oj aq. ferv. allowed to stand ten minutes, and half to be used at a time) has certainly been successful in many cases, especially of inguinal hernia,—but it requires great caution. It has proved immediately fatal to some patients, and has rendered others incapable of surviving the shock of the operation. *Cold* applied to the tumour by means of pounded ice or a freezing mixture (F. 12) in a bladder, is useful by reducing inflammation, condensing flatus, and constringing the skin. It is most applicable to large scrotal herniæ. It, too, is not without its hazards, for it may cause gangrene of the skin if applied too long, or if hot applications are incautiously used after it. *Opium* is sometimes of service after bleeding, especially if vomiting is violent. *Tartar emetic*, given as in dislocation, is said to have been employed with benefit, but it is a most hazardous remedy. *Purgatives and enemata* are irritating and mischievous in sudden acute strangulation, but vastly beneficial if the patient is aged, the hernia large and long irreducible, and if the attack has been preceded and caused by constipation. Large doses of calomel and colocynth are the best purgatives, and the enemata should consist of as much salt and water as can be injected without causing very much pain or distention. They should be injected with a pumping syringe, and not with those filthy, inefficient, and now obsolete instruments, the bladder and pipe, or old-fashioned pewter syringe. Moreover, Dr. O'Beirne has fully shown that greater benefit is to be derived in cases of incarcerated hernia and obstinate constipation from passing up a long tube—(the tube of a stomach pump answers very well)—into the colon, than from the use of the ordinary short enema pipe. The long tube relieves the bowels of their flatus; and of course by diminishing the bulk of the contents of the abdomen, renders the return of the hernia more easy.* But finally, if the taxis, bleeding, and warm-bath do not succeed, it is the safest plan, on the average, to perform an operation for dividing the stricture without delay,—using the other remedies only if the patient will not consent to the operation—except of course in the class of cases in which purgatives are likely to give relief.

The *operation* generally performed consists in opening the sac, dividing the stricture, and returning the intestine. Some surgeons, however, recommend the sac not to be opened,—but that the stricture should be released by dividing the parts surrounding its neck, and then that the intestine should be returned by the taxis. The advantage of this plan (which is advocated by Mr. Key) is supposed to be, that it lessens the danger of peritoneal inflammation, by not opening the cavity. This practice *may* be adopted if the hernia is small and quite recent,—but as a general rule it is unsafe, (1) because the seat of stricture may be in the sac itself, particularly at its thickened neck,—and (2) because it is always desirable to examine the state of the intestine before returning it. When the sac is opened, the intestine should be well examined, and especially that part of it which has been actually compressed by the stricture, and which should be gently drawn down for that purpose. If it be merely dark claret-coloured from congestion,—or slightly roughened with lymph, —or if it exhibit a few black patches of ecchymosis, it should be returned; the operator being careful to replace it bit by bit—intestine before omentum—and those parts first which protruded last. The wound may then be closed with one or two sutures, and a firm compress be placed upon it.

If the hernia were irreducible long before it was strangulated, and if its contents are united to the sac by firm broad adhesions, they should not be disturbed. But if adhesions are recent, or very thin and slight, they may be divided and the bowel be returned.

If the intestine is mortified, which will be known by the softened green or ashy spots, the mortified part should be slit open, the stricture be divided, and the patient left to recover with an artificial anus. Again, if a large portion of the intestine, which has been long irreducible in an elderly person, appear extremely dark and advanced towards sphacelus, so as to render it doubtful whether it would be capable of performing its functions when returned,—the safest plan is to make an opening into it, and so afford an outlet for its contents, although the inconvenience of an artificial anus must of course be considered.

If the omentum is gangrenous, or if it is thickened and indurated, it would, if returned, excite dangerous irritation of the peritoneum. In this case, some surgeons advise it to be left to granulate in the sac,—or to cut it off close to the neck of the sac, and leave it there as a plug to pre-

---

* Vide Lancet, July 6 and 27, 1839; also James's Retrospective Address, in Prov. Med. Trans., 1840; and O'Beirne on Defæcation.

vent farther protrusion.   Macfarlane and others, on the contrary, recommend it to be cut cleanly off, and all the vessels to be tied with fine silk
ligatures, and the end to be then passed quite into the abdomen—breaking up any adhesions about the neck of the sac, if necessary;—thus
avoiding the dragging pains and colic which are liable to occur if a portion of the omentum or intestine is fixed.

*After Treatment.*—After the hernia has been returned, whether by
taxis or operation, the patient should be put to bed—all exertion being
strictly forbidden.   Vomiting must be treated by large doses of calomel
and opium, and by effervescing draughts containing one or two drops of
prussic acid,—tenderness and pain by bleeding, leeching, calomel and
opium, and fomentations.   If the bowels do not act in six or eight hours,
they may be solicited by injections; but salts and other acrid purgatives
administered by the mouth can scarcely fail to be mischievous; for as
the intestine that was constricted remains for some time inflamed,
weakened, and incapable of propelling its contents, they will but irritate
it uselessly.   Mr. Travers has very satisfactorily shown, that the great
danger after the return of the hernia, arises from palsy, and not from
inflammation of the bowels.*   Castor oil, or rhubarb and magnesia, may
be resorted to after twelve hours.   A truss should be applied be'ore the
patient gets up again.


SECTION II.—OF INGUINAL HERNIA.

DEFINITION.—Inguinal hernia is that which protrudes through one or
both abdominal rings.

VARIETIES.—There are four varieties.   The oblique,—direct,—congenital,—and encysted.

(1.) The *oblique* inguinal hernia is the most common.   It takes precisely the same route as the testicle in its passage from the abdomen into
the scrotum.   It commences as a fulness or swelling at the situation of
the internal abdominal ring, that is to say, a little above the centre of
Poupart's ligament,—next passes into the inguinal canal,—(and in this
stage is called *bubonocele*,)—and if the protrusion increase, it projects
through the external ring, and descends into the scrotum of the male, or
labium of the female.   The *coverings* of this hernia are, 1, Skin.   2, A
strong layer of condensed cellular tissue, derived from *superficial fascia*
of the abdomen, in which the *external epigastric artery* ramifies.   With
this is mostly incorporated, 3, the *fascia spermatica*—a tendinous layer,
derived from the margin of the external ring.   Under this lies, 4, the
*cremaster muscle*—sometimes called *tunica communis.*   5. Next comes
the *fascia propria*, a cellular layer continuous with the *fascia transver-*

* Travers, case of Hernia, &c., Med. Chir. Trans., vol. xxiii.

*salis* of the abdomen; and lastly, 6, the sac. The *internal epigastric artery* is always internal to the neck of the sac. The *spermatic cord* is generally behind the sac; but, in some old eases, the tumour has passed backwards between the vas deferens and spermatie artery, so as to place them in front of it.

The *direct* inguinal hernia bursts through the *conjoined tendon* of the internal oblique and transversalis muscles, just behind the external ring. Its coverings are the same as those of the oblique variety, except the cremaster, for it has no connexion with the cord. The epigastric artery runs external to the neck of the sac.

3. The *congenital* hernia is a sub-variety of the oblique, and is so called because that state of parts which permits of it, only exists at or soon after birth. A portion of omentum or intestine accompanies the

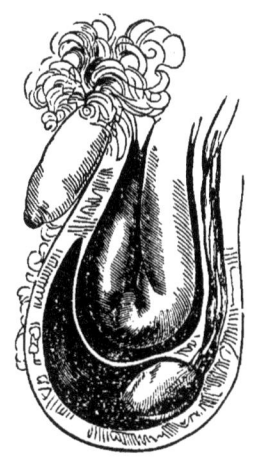

testicle in its descent, and passes down with it into the very pouch of peritoneum which forms the *tunica vaginalis reflexa*, before its communication with the general peritoneal cavity has become obliterated. The sac of this hernia is consequently formed by the tunica vaginalis,—its coverings in other respects are the same as of the oblique variety—and the protruded bowel lies in immediate contact with the testicle, and if not replaced, generally adheres to it.

4. The *encysted* (or *hernia infantalis*) is a sub-variety of the congenital. The protruding bowel pushes before it a sac of peritoneum either into or close behind the tunica vaginalis, and this tunic and the sac adhere very closely together. This hernia, therefore, (as may be seen in the adjoining diagram of Mr. Liston's) has, as it were, two sacs, viz. one proper sac, and another anterior, composed of the tunica vaginalis, which in these cases is very liable to be the seat of hydrocele.*

DIAGNOSIS.—(1.) The difference between the *oblique and direct inguinal herniæ*, and their relations to the epigastric artery, are shown in the accompanying figure. In the oblique, the neck of the tumour inclines

---

* This form of hernia was first described by Hey of Leeds, in a letter to Gooch, (Vide Gooch's Chir. Works, vol. ii. p. 217.) He says, "The intestine in this case had forced its way into the scrotum before the tunica vaginalis had formed its adhesion to the cord, but after its abdominal orifice was closed; under which circumstance it brought the peritoneum down with it, forming the hernial sac : contrary to what happens in the hernia congenita, where the intestine descends before the orifice in the tunica vaginalis has closed and consequently has no hernial sac but that tunic."

upwards and outwards, and causes a fulness extending up to the middle
of Poupart's ligament.    In the direct, it inclines (if at all) rather inwards;
and when the hernia is reduced, the finger, carrying integument before

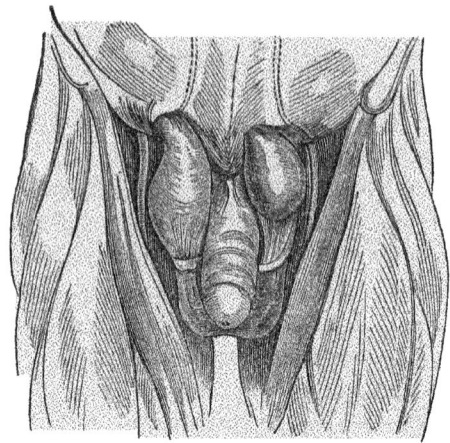

it, can be passed straight back into the abdominal cavity.    But in old
cases of oblique hernia, the neck of the sack is dragged down towards
the mesial line, so that all distinction is lost.

(2.) *Hydrocele* may be distinguished from hernia by its beginning at
the bottom of the scrotum—by its being semi-transparent and fluctuating,
and preventing the testicle from being clearly felt, (whilst the cord can
be distinctly felt above it,) and by not dilating on coughing.    Whereas
hernia begins at the top of the scrotum; it is not transparent; does not
fluctuate; does not prevent the testicle from being clearly felt, although
it obscures the cord; and dilates on coughing.    But hernia may and does
often co-exist with hydrocele, the former beginning from above, the latter from below.

(3.) *Hydrocele of the cord*, if low down, may be distinguished by its
transparency and fluctuation; but if high up, it may extend into the abdominal ring, and receive an impulse on coughing, and the diagnosis be
very difficult.    But as a hernia may be concealed behind this kind of
tumour, the rule, *when in doubt, operate*, should be acted upon in case
of symptoms of strangulation.

(4.) *Varicocele*, (or *cirsocele*,) which signifies a varicose enlargement
of the spermatie veins, resembles hernia, inasmuch as it increases in the
erect posture, and perhaps dilates on coughing; but it may be distinguished
from hernia by its feeling like a bag of worms; and although, like hernia,
it disappears when the patient lies down, and the scrotum is raised, still
it quickly appears again, if pressure be made upon the external ring,
though that pressure would effectually prevent a hernia from coming

down again. Lastly, it needs scarcely be said that an imperfectly descended testicle must not be mistaken for bubonocele.

*Treatment.*—(1.) Inguinal hernia, if *reducible*, must be kept up with a truss, of which the pad generally requires to press on the internal abdominal ring, and the spring should pass round midway between the trochanter and ilium. Care must be taken not to let the pad slip down, and bear against the spinous process of the pubes. In fact, it should be made to press accurately against the internal ring, where the protrusion begins, and not be permitted to slip down so as to bear against the spermatic cord. Malgaigne found that out of two hundred cases in which a common truss was applied, there was disease of the cord or testicle in sixty-five.*

Two plans have been proposed for the radical cure of this hernia. One (which is useless) consists of transfixing the root of the scrotum with a number of pins, and making pressure at the same time with corks, (through which pins are passed,) so as to create the adhesive inflammation in the sac.

A second plan, which is more feasible, consists in pushing a fold of integument as far up as possible into the neck of the sac, securing it in this inverted or invaginated position by means of two sutures, (both ends of a ligature being passed from within the invaginated skin,) and then denuding the pouch of invaginated skin of its cuticle by means of liquor ammoniæ; so that the surfaces of skin and peritoneum thus opposed to each other may adhere, and the neck of the sac be effectually plugged.

This operation, which was proposed by M. Gerdy, has been practised by Mr. Bransby Cooper, and with some benefit. For the herniary aperture was so large before the operation, that it was impossible that the bowel could be kept up by a truss; whereas after the operation, a common truss enabled the patient to pursue a laborious occupation with safety and comfort.†

(2.) The *irreducible* must be supported with a bag truss. If it only contain *omentum*, a common truss may perhaps be applied in the usual manner, so as to make it adhere to and plug the neck of the sac. But this cannot often be borne, and is liable to induce swelled testicle.

(3.) In performing the taxis for the relief of strangulated oblique inguinal-hernia, the patient should be placed in the position described in a foregoing page (409,) with his thighs as close together as possible (although the surgeon must put one arm between them,) and the pressure must be made upwards and outwards.

The *operation* for this hernia is performed thus—The parts being shaved, and the skin made tense, an incision three or four inches long must be

* Malgaigne, Bulb. Gen. de Therap. 1839
† Bransby Cooper, Guy's Hosp. Rep., October 1843.

made through the skin, along the axis of the tumour, beginning from above its neck. This will be quite long enough even for the largest herniæ; because the object is to bring the seat of stricture fully into view, without exposing too much of the sac. Then the successive coverings before enumerated are to be divided in the following manner—a little bit of each is to be pinched up with forceps, and to be cut into with the knife held horizontally; a director is to be passed into this little aperture, and the layer is then to be divided on it to the extent of the incision in the skin. Cautious operators will find (or make) many more layers than those usually enumerated—which are, in fact, easily subdivisible, especially in old herniæ. When at last the sac is reached, which will be known by its bluish transparency—it is to be opened to the like extent —a little bit of it being first pinched up and cut through so as to admit the director. If possible, it should be done at a part where there is some serum, or omentum, between it and the bowel. Then the left forefinger should be passed up into the neck of the sac to seek for the stricture, which will generally be at the internal ring. It may be at the external ring, (or at both,) but wherever it may be, it must be dilated so as to allow the finger to pass into the abdomen. A curved blunt-pointed bistoury—not cutting quite up to the point—should be passed up flat on the finger through the stricture, and its edge be then turned up so as to divide it; and in every case the division should be made DIRECTLY UPWARDS —parallel to the linea alba; and then, whether the hernia be direct or oblique, the epigastric artery will not be wounded. If no stricture be discovered in the neck, it must be sought for in the body of the sac.

The subsequent proceedings—the return or otherwise of the intestine, and the after treatment—are detailed in the preceding section.

### SECTION III.—OF FEMORAL OR CRURAL HERNIA.

*Definition.*—Femoral hernia is that which escapes behind Poupart's ligament.

It passes first through the *crural ring*—an aperture bounded internally by *Gimbernat's ligament*—externally by the femoral vein—before, by Poupart's ligament—and behind by the bone. It next descends behind the *falciform process* of the fascia lata—thirdly, it comes forwards through the *saphenic opening* of that fascia—and, lastly, as its size increases, it does not descend down on the thigh, but turns up over the falciform process, and lies on the anterior surface of Poupart's ligament. The *coverings* of this hernia are—1. Skin. 2. The *superficial fascia* of the thigh—loaded with fat, and divisible into an uncertain number of layers. 3. *Fascia propria,* a layer of cellular tissue derived from the sheath of the femoral vessels—or, according to others, from the *fascia cribriformis* which closes the saphenic aperture. It is in general pretty dense about the neck of the hernia, but thin, or even deficient on its fundus. 4. The sac. Between the last two there is often found a considerable layer of fat which might be mistaken for omentum. This hernia rarely attains a very large size. It is much more frequent in the female than the male—obviously from the greater breadth of the pelvis.

DIAGNOSIS.—(1.) Femoral hernia may be distinguished *from the inguinal* by observing that Poupart's ligament can be traced over the neck of the sac, and that the spinous process of the pubes lies internal to it; whereas it is the reverse in the inguinal hernia. Besides, the femoral is generally much smaller and is more frequent in women.

2. *Psoas abscess* resembles this hernia in its situation—in dilating on coughing, and diminishing when the patient lies down. The points of distinction are, that it is generally more external, that it fluctuates, but does not feel tympanitic, and that it is attended with symptoms of disease of the spine.

3. *Varix of the femoral vein* also resembles this hernia, inasmuch as it dilates somewhat on coughing, and diminishes when the patient lies down; but then, if pressure be made below Poupart's ligament, the swelling quickly reappears, although it must be evident that under such circumstances a hernia could not come down.

4. *Bubo and other tumours of the groin* may in most cases be recognised by their general character and history, and by their being unattended with adominal disorder. But if there be any such swelling, and symptoms of strangulation as well, an incision should certainly be made to examine it. The very best surgeons have been known to fail in their diagnosis of these cases.

TREATMENT.—(1.) The reducible femoral hernia should be supported by a truss; the pad of which requires to be bent downwards at an angle with the spring. Its pressure should tell against the hollow which is just inferior and external to the spinous process of the pubes. This hernia is very seldom, if ever, cured radically.

(2.) The irreducible should be supported by a truss with a hollow pad, or perhaps (if it be omental) the pressure of a common pad may be borne.

(3.) The femoral hernia, when strangulated, gives rise to much severer symptoms than the inguinal does, because of the denser and more unyielding nature of the parts which surround the neck of the sac. In performing the taxis, the patient should be placed in the usual position, with the thigh of the affected side much rolled inwards, and crossed over towards the other side. The tumour should first be drawn downwards, from the anterior surface of Poupart's ligament, and then be pressed with the points of the fingers backwards and upwards. If, however, the taxis (with bleeding and the warm bath if the tumour is tender) does not soon

53

succeed, the operation should be resorted to.   No good will be done by
any other measures.

*Operation.*—In the first place, the skin must be divided." Some surgeons make one simple perpendicular incision.   Sir A. Cooper directs
one like an inverted ⅃; and Mr. Liston prefers making one along Poupart's ligament, and another falling perpendicularly from its centre over
the tumour, thus, (for the right ⟍        side.)   The skin may be very
safely and expeditiously divided     ⟋⟍    by pinching it up into a fold,
and running the knife through      |      it with its back towards the sac.
Then the different cellular layers down to the sac must be divided by
the bistoury and director, as in the inguinal hernia, and the sac must be
opened with very great care, because it is generally very small, and embraces the bowel tightly, and seldom contains any serum or omentum.
Then the finger should be passed up to seek for the stricture, which, according to Sir A. Cooper, Mr. Liston, and the other best authorities, will
be found to be the *inner edge of the falciform process.*   This must be
gently divided for a line or two, the incision being directed UPWARDS AND
A LITTLE INWARDS, towards the spinous process of the pubes.   It must
be recollected, that if this incision were carried too far, the spermatic cord
in the male, or round ligament in the female would be injured.   The division of Gimbernat's ligament (which is recommended by some) is considered by the above-named authorities to be much less efficacious;—and
it is rather hazardous, inasmuch as the obturatrix artery not unfrequently
runs round behind that ligament, and would be infallibly divided.


SECTION IV.—OF THE UMBILICAL, VENTRAL, AND OTHER REMAINING
SPECIES OF HERNIA.


I. UMBILICAL HERNIA—(*exomphalos*)—is, for obvious reasons, most
frequent in children soon after birth.   It is also not uncommon in women
who have been frequently pregnant, although, in many of the so called
umbilical herniæ in adults, the hernial aperture is really not at the umbilicus, but a little on one side of it.   The coverings of this hernia are skin,
superficial fascia, and sac; they are always very thin, and not unfrequently
the sac is adherent to its contents.   *Treatment.*—If *reducible,* and the
patient an infant, the best plan is to place a hemisphere of ivory with its
convex surface on the aperture, and retain it there with cross strips of
plaster, and a bandage round the belly.   A pad of linen, covered with
sheet lead, will do as well.   But the belly should by no means be bound
up too tightly, otherwise there will be danger of producing inguinal hernia.   An adult should wear a truss or broad belt, with some contrivance
to prevent it from slipping down below its proper level.   For the irreducible umbilical hernia, a large hollow pad should be worn.   The reduc-

tion of this hernia is affected by the ordinary manual taxis; but if it be very large, Sir A. Cooper recommends it to be compressed by a wooden platter. If it become strangulated, and the patient is aged, and the strangulation was preceded by constipation, purgatives and copious enemata should have a fair trial. If the operation is necessary, an incision three inches in length should be made at the upper part of the tumour through the skin, fascia, and sac, in succession. The stricture should then be dilated directly upwards in the linea alba with the knife recommended in other cases. But perhaps it is better to make the incision so as to divide the under side of the neck of the sac, as advised by Mr. Liston.

II. VENTRAL HERNIA is that which protrudes through the *lineæ semi-lunares* or *transversæ*, or in fact through any other parts of the abdominal parietes, save those which are the ordinary seats of hernia. Its treatment requires no distinct observations; but if it should ever be necessary to operate for the relief of strangulation, care must be taken to avoid the epigastric artery.

III. PERINÆAL HERNIA descends between the bladder and rectum, forcing its way through the pelvic fascia and levator ani, and forming a tumour in the perinæum.

IV. VAGINAL HERNIA is a variety of the preceding;—in which the tumour projects into and blocks up the vagina, instead of descending to the perinæum.

V. LABIAL or PUDENDAL HERNIA descends between the vagina and ramus of the ischium, and forms a tumour in one of the labia. It is to be distinguished from inguinal hernia by the absence of swelling at the abdominal rings. These three herniæ must be replaced by pressure with the fingers, and be kept up by pads made to bear against the perinæum, and by hollow caoutchouc pessaries worn in the vagina.

VI. OBTURATOR or THYROID HERNIA projects through the aperture in the obturator ligament which gives exit to the artery and nerve.

VII. ISCHIATIC HERNIA protrudes through the sciatic notch. This and the preceding are exceedingly rare;—and the tumours are of necessity small. If discovered to exist during life, they must be returned and supported by proper apparatus—and if strangulated, the stricture must be divided by operation.

VIII. DIAPHRAGMATIC HERNIA is generally a result of congenital deficiency, or accidental separation of the fibres of the diaphragm. But it may also be caused by violent falls on the abdomen, or by violent pressure of any kind, capable of lacerating the diaphragm, and driving some of the bowels into the thorax.* This form of hernia, if strangulated, will produce the ordinary symptoms—vomiting, constipation, and pain;—

* Ried on Diaphragmatic Hernia, Ed. Med. and Surg. Journ.; Jan. and July, 1840.

which are not in any manner to be distinguished from the symptoms of ileus or intus-susception—or from those produced when a fold of bowel is entangled in a rent in the omentum, or mesentery; or when the bowel is constricted by membranous bands resulting from previous inflammation of the peritoneum.

# CHAPTER XIX.

## OF THE SURGICAL DISEASES AND INJURIES OF THE RECTUM AND ANUS.*

I. Foreign Bodies in the rectum sometimes require to be removed by surgical art. They may either consist of small bones or the like that have descended from above, or of pins, glyster-pipes, or other bodies introduced from below. Substances of very extraordinary dimensions (a blacking-bottle, for instance) have been forced into the anus. The grand point is

* Nothing has been more remarkable, in my surgical experience in the west, than the disproportioned frequency of diseases of the rectum and adjacent textures—fistula, piles, prolapsus, &c., and I advert to the fact chiefly for the purpose of adding a cautioning remark respecting the causes of it. Doubtless it is partly to be referred to the chafing and contusions incident to horse-back riding which is a much more common mode of travelling here, than at the east; but it is mainly attributable to the habit of indiscriminate and excessive purgation, so prevalent both as a remedial and prophylactic measure.

A large portion of the practitioners of the valley of the Mississippi have been educated under a system of medicine whose theory, regards portal congestion and hepatic derangement as the essential elements of all disease, and whose practice consists, almost exclusively, in the exhibition of drastic purgatives.

It is natural that the people should imitate the therapeutics of their medical advisers, when so simple and easily applied, and accordingly they are very much in the habit of drenching themselves, and teasing the alimentary canal on every occasion of illness, with some concentrated purgative, in the form of pills.

Under one of the most constant laws of irritation in mucous canals, the terminating portions of the apparatus of defecation, is thus perpetually suffering under propagated as well as direct stimulation, and reacts in the various forms of disease under notice.

Besides these direct mischiefs, and others involving the health in other ways, occasioned by the pernicious doctrines referred to—which are, indeed, themselves essentially empyrical—they encourage the greatest species of quackery, by promoting the consumption of vast quantities of patent pills and other purgative nostrums.

In proportion as a more rational pathology shall prevail among physicians, the habits of the population will undergo a corresponding change, and the preponderance of diseases of the rectum in the duties of the surgeon, may be expected to disappear accordingly. F.

first to dilate the bowel well, by passing in several fingers (oiled) or by means of a speculum;—and then a proper forceps, or a lithotomy scoop, may generally be used with success.

II. IMPERFORATE ANUS (*atresia ani*) signifies a congenital closure of the rectum, and may occur in various degrees. The gut may terminate in a blind pouch at any point from the sigmoid flexure downwards, and the anal aperture be altogether wanting—or the anus may be opened for an inch or two, with an obstruction beyond. *Treatment.*—If the end of the intestine can be felt protruding when the child cries, a crucial incision may be made into it without delay—if it cannot be felt, a day or two should be waited, so that it may become distended with meconium, and then a cautious incision should be made with a double-edged bistoury, in the direction of the curve of the sacrum. If it succeed in reaching the bowel, the aperture should be kept open by tents.

But if this operation should fail in reaching the bowel, or if the rectum appears to be altogether deficient, so that it is useless to attempt it, the only resource is the *formation of an artificial anus*; a measure which it is the surgeon's duty to propose to the parents, and to perform if they wish it; although it really appears more humane to let the child die quietly, than to subject it to the pain of the operation, and the perpetual misery and filth of an artificial anus if it survives. The best operation for this purpose is one that has been twice performed successfully by Amussat in cases of obstruction of the rectum by disease. A transverse incision is made in the left lumbar region, just above the crista of the ilium, so as to come upon the descending colon where it is not covered by peritonæum. As soon as the gut is reached, a loop of thread should be passed through it to fix it, and then it may be opened with a bistoury. The constant prolapsus, which is such a source of distress when artificial anus is situated in the groin, is not so likely to occur when an aperture is made in this situation.*

III. SPASM OF THE SPHINCTER ANI is known by violent pain of the anus, with difficulty of evacuating the fæces. On examination, the muscle feels hard, and resists the introduction of the finger. This affection may be caused by constipation of the bowels, or disorder of the health. It may occur in sudden paroxysms which soon go off,—or may last permanently, and lead to organic thickening and stricture of the anus. *Treatment.*—In recent cases, a dose of calomel and Dover's powder, followed by castor oil, and by enemata of warm water with a little laudanum will relieve the paroxysm. In more obstinate cases, a bougie or mould candle should be passed daily,—alteratives and enemata of warm water should also be administered daily; but if they fail, the sphincter must be divided and made to heal by granulation. *Division of the*

* Forbes, Brit. and For. Rev., Jan. 1840.

*Sphincter* is easily performed by introducing the forefinger into the anus, and a straight, narrow, blunt-pointed bistoury by its side—and then making an incision of sufficient extent towards the tuberosity of the ischium.

IV. HÆMORRHOIDS, or PILES, are small tumours situated near the anus, consisting *anatomically* of hypertrophied cellular tissue, containing a number of dilated varicose veins. The *predisposing causes* are any circumstances that produce fulness of the abdominal vessels, or that impede the return of blood from the rectum—such as luxurious and sedentary habits of life—pregnancy, constipation, disease of the liver or lungs, retarding the passage of blood through them, and tight stays. The *exciting causes* may be any thing that irritates the lower bowels,—particularly large doses of aloes—ascarides—horse exercise, or the application of cold and damp to the posteriors. Piles are most frequent in women, and are rare under puberty. They are divided into *internal* and *external*, according as they are situated within the rectum or around the anus. They may be met with in two states—*indolent* or *inflamed*. When indolent, they merely produce the inconveniences that necessarily result from their bulk and situation.

When piles are inflamed, they occasion the following *symptoms*. Pain, heat, itching, fulness and tension about the anus—pain and straining in passing evacuations—with perhaps more or less bleeding. These symptoms may, in violent cases, be complicated with irritation of the bladder, frequency of micturition, pain in the back, pain and aching down the thighs. The young surgeon should be aware, that a patient with piles may not be aware of the nature of his complaint, or through delicacy may abstain from mentioning it. Whenever, therefore, a patient complains of unusual irritation of the bladder, or of symptoms of dysentery— that is to say, frequent, painful, and unsatisfactory efforts to pass motions, the surgeon should always make inquiries after piles.

*Internal Piles* are generally firm tumours, varying in size from that of a pea to that of a walnut, of a pale or reddish-brown colour when indolent, but dark or bright red when congested or inflamed. They are exceedingly liable to hæmorrhage, and generally cause great inconvenience by protruding at each motion.

*External piles* may be met with (1) in the form of round hard tumours just at the margin of the anus, and covered half with skin and half with mucous membrane; or (2) of oblong ridges of skin external to the sphincter. These are commonly called *mariscæ*, or blind piles, because they do not bleed.

*General Treatment.*—The grand objects are to remove the predisposing and exciting causes. The patient, if stout, plethoric, and of sedentary habits, ought to live abstemiously, and take plenty of exercise. The bowels should be regulated by some mild aperient, capable of producing daily copious soft evacuations without straining or griping. Senna, sulphur, castor oil, cream of tartar, and magnesia, in the form of electuaries (F. 42) are the best; and blue pill, or hydr. c. creta should be added if the liver is inactive. It is worth knowing that the nauseous greasy taste of castor oil is pretty effectually disguised by mixing it with milk, and adding a little nitric æther, and oil of cinnamon. In cases of long standing, the confect. piperis comp. may be given with great benefit in doses of 3j ter die. In similar cases, especially if the patient is advanced in years, and the piles are attended with a flow of mucus, copaiba may be given in the dose of thirty or forty drops every morning in milk; and a scruple of common pitch may be taken in pills every night at bed-time. Old people rarely dislike the taste of copaiba. The bowels should act once daily—and Dr. Burne says, that the evening is a much better time for that purpose than the morning. The seat of the water-closet should shelve inwards at its margin.

If the *piles are inflamed,* leeches to the anus, or cupping on the sacrum, a dose of calomel and opium at bed-time, followed by castor-oil in the morning; low diet, rest in bed, warm fomentations and poultices; and enemata of warm water, if the anus is not too tender to bear the introduction of the pipe, are the requisite measures. Cold lotions of lead (with a little tinc. opii) may be substituted for the warm applications, if more comfortable. If there is a ·tense bluish solid tumour, evidently containing coagulated blood, it may be punctured.

*Local Treatment.*—(1.) The first and most essential measure is *perfect cleanliness.* Mr. Mayo directs the anus to be well washed with *yellow soap* and water after each motion—and if the piles are internal, and protrude during evacuations, they should be washed before they are returned. Moreover, great comfort will often be derived from the custom of washing out the rectum with an enema of cold or tepid water after each injection. (2.) *Astringents*—the zinc lotion (F. 15) or unguentum gallæ, to which latter a little of the liq. plumbi diac. may be advantageously added, (F. 43,) are generally of benefit. Dr. Burne recommends an ointment composed of pulv. hellebori nigri 3j adipis $\tilde{3}$j, which he says never fails of affording great relief, although exceedingly painful for a time. (3.) *Pressure* by means of a bougie introduced occasionally—or of a pad of ivory with or without a spring, made to bear against the anus with a T bandage, are often of service. There is an instrument consisting of a short egg-shaped ivory bougie, which is introduced into the anus, and which is attached by a slender neck to an ivory pad—so that pressure is thus made both internally and externally, that is extremely useful in cases of internal piles with prolapse.

(4.) *Extirpation* is the last resource, if the preceding constitutional and local measures fail. But the surgeon must bear in mind that it is highly dangerous to operate upon internal piles if the health is broken, or if there is any organic disease of the liver and kidneys; and the ope-ration must be both preceded and followed by a course of most abste-mions diet, and medicines to maintain the secretions. External piles may be removed by *excision* with the knife or scissors.

Internal piles must be removed by ligature, for excision of them might occasion a fatal hæmorrhage. The operation is performed as follows. The bowels having been previously well cleared, the patient must be told to protrude the piles; and if he cannot do it easily, he should sit over a vessel of warm water, or have an enema of warm water. Then the piles should be drawn out with a tenaculum, and a ligature (not too fine) be tied as tightly as possible round the base of each. If one of the tumours is large, a double ligature may be passed through its base with a needle, and either half be tied separately. Before finally tightening the ligatures, the piles should be slightly punctured. After the operation, the ends of the thread should be cut short, and be returned into the rectum. The patient should remain in bed, and the bowels should not be disturbed for forty-eight hours after the operation. Pain is to be relieved by an opiate, or by leeches; and if it persist, the piles should be examined to see whether the ligatures remain as tight as possible, and if not, they should be reapplied.

V. WARTS, CONDYLOMATA, and other excrescences around the anus, that arise from local irritation, are to be removed with the knife, and the surface from which they grew should, during the granulating stage, be treated with astringent lotions.

VI. HÆMORRHAGE from the rectum—an exhalation of blood from the mucous membrane in consequence of congestion or of determination of blood—is a very frequent concomitant of piles—from the surface of which, in fact, the discharge may proceed. The blood is generally of a florid hue, it is exuded copiously during the passage of an evacuation, and covers the fæces, but is not intimately mixed with them. *Treat-ment.*—(1.) If the hæmorrhage is moderate in quantity—if it has been of habitual or periodic occurrence—if it induces no weakness—and if it brings relief to pain in the head, or any other feeling of disorder—the only justifiable means of suppressing it are exercise, temperance, and alterative and aperient medicines, with the view of removing the state of plethora that occasions it. (2.) But if the patient is weak and ema-ciated; if the lips are pale, and the pulse feeble, the bleeding should be at once suppressed. (We may observe here, that whenever a patient applies for relief in consequence of violent palpitations and shortness of breathing; or giddiness and swimming in the head, if the lips are pale, and the extremities tend to swell, the surgeon should always inquire for piles, because, as we before observed, some patients, through false deli-cacy, will not mention them.) Or if the bleeding, as sometimes hap-pens, instead of relieving symptoms of heat and fulness in the rectum, aggravates them, the bleeding should also be stopped, whatever the patient's complexion may be; and if he is of a full habit, he should live abstemiously, and keep the bowels open with Seidlitz powders. The means of checking hæmorrhage from the rectum are, (1.) That piles, if any exist, should be tied. (2.) Astringent applications, such as injections of dec. quercus, or infus. catechu, used cold. (3.) The salts of iron, or bark with sulphuric acid, or the balsams of copaiba and Peru, or oil of turpentine (in the dose of $\mathfrak{m}$ xx in mucilage.) F. 60, 61, 69.

VII. DISCHARGE OF MUCUS—clear and viscid—without faecal odour, may be caused by piles, ascarides, the use of aloes, or any other causes of irritation to the rectum. To be treated by mild aperients, astringent injections, and copaiba. F. 8, 9, 42, 20.

VIII. ABSCESSES near the rectum may be caused by the irritation of foreign bodies, or by caries of an adjacent bone, but they are much more frequently the result of the various causes of disordered circulation in the hæmorrhoidal vessels that were mentioned as producing piles, and especially of tubercles in the lungs. They may either be large and deep-seated, or small and superficial. (1.) Deep-seated abscesses are attended with great aching and throbbing,—difficulty and pain in evacuating the fæces,—and fever,—and on internal examination a fulness or fluctuation may be felt. If these abscesses are left to themselves, a vast quantity of matter may accumulate in the loose cellular tissue of the pelvis, and severe irritative fever result from its confinement. (2.) Superficial abscesses are attended with more or less pain, tenderness, and throbbing, and swelling around the anus. They are often chronic, and often occur in the consumptive. *Treatment.*—Leeches and fomentations may be tried at first—but if they do not very soon remove the pain and tenderness, or if there is the least suspicion that matter is forming, a bistoury should be pushed home into the inflamed part,—and if it be at all extensive, two or three punctures should be made.

IX. FISTULA IN ANO signifies a fistulous track by the side of the sphincter ani. It is extremely difficult to heal, both because the constant contractions of the sphincter and levator ani interfere with the union of its sides, and because of the passage of faecal matter into it from the bowel. There are three kinds spoken of in books. (1.) The *complete fistula*, which has one external opening near the anus, and another into the bowel above the sphincter. (2.) The *blind external fistula*, which has no opening into the bowel, although it mostly reaches its outer coat. (3.) The *blind internal fistula*, which opens into the bowel, but not externally, although its situation is indicated by a redness and hardness near the anus. This affection is a common result of abscess by the side of the rectum. Sir B. Brodie's opinion is, that it always commences with an ulceration of the mucous membrane of the rectum, and an escape of faecal matter into the cellular tissue; which gives rise to abscess, and

.54

the abscess to fistula. This opinion is corroborated by the circumstance that fistula is so common in consumptive persons, who are also very sub-jcet to ulceration of the bowels. It also accounts for the fœtor of the discharge.*

*Treatment.*—The grand remedy for this affection is division of the sphincter ani, so as to prevent contraction of that muscle for a time, and cause the fistula to heal from the bottom. The digestive organs and secretions must first be put in good order, and the bowels be well cleared by castor-oil and an injection, so that they may not want to be disturbed for two or three days. *Operation.*—The patient being placed on his knees and elbows on a bed, or being made to kneel on a chair and lean over the back of it, and the nates being kept asunder by an assistant, the surgeon introduces his left forefinger into the anus, and at the same time explores with a probe the whole extent and ramifications of the fistula. If it is of the *blind internal* kind, its situation must be ascer-tained, and a puncture be made into it by the side of the anus. Perhaps a probe bent at an acute angle may be passed into it from the bowel, and serve as a guide for the puncture. Then, one forefinger being still in the anus, the surgeon passes a strong curved probe-pointed bistoury up to the farther end of the fistula. Next (if the internal opening cannot be found) he pushes it through the coats of the bowel, so that its point may come in contact with his forefinger. Then he puts the end of his fore-finger on the point of the bistoury, and draws it down out of the anus; and as soon as it is fairly emerged, he pushes the handle towards the orifice of the fistula, so as to divide skin, sphincter, and bowel at one sweep. Sir B. Brodie recommends that the bistoury should always be passed through the internal opening of the fistula, and says that the affection will very likely return if it is not divided;—he also condemns the practice of cutting through the bowel higher up than this opening. A few threads of oiled lint are then to be placed in the wound, and the patient to be kept in bed for three days. The subsequent treatment consists in the use of perfect cleanliness, and the daily introduction of a very little slip of lint (which may be dipped in some stimulating lotion if necessary) between the edges of the wound for the first few days, so as to prevent its premature union, and cause it to granulate from the bottom. If hæmorrhage prove violent after this operation, and does not yield to the application of cold, the anus must be well dilated with a speculum, so as to expose the bleeding surface to the air,—and any artery discern-ible may be tied.

If the patient will not submit to this operation, or if he is labouring under disease of the lungs or liver in an advanced stage, so that it would be

* This was also the opinion of M. Ribes, who held that the internal orifice of this stricture might always be found at about an inch and a quarter from the anus.

unsafe,—the confect. piperis, or copaiba and tonics, may be administered internally, and stimulating injections and ointments be applied to the fistula; but they will rarely be of any avail.

X. RHAGADES—fissures and excoriations about the anus—produce the utmost pain during the passage of evacuations, and if neglected may lead to spasm and permanent stricture of the sphincter. *Treatment.*— Aperients and alteratives,—regular diet,—astringent applications, such as decoction of rhatany, zinc lotion, borax and honey,—or mercurial ointment, or ung. hydr. nitrat. dilut., to which a little ext. belladon. should be added if there be much pain or spasm of the sphincter, and the strictest cleanliness. But if a fair trial of these measures is unavailing, the sphincter must be divided.

XI. PROLAPSUS ANI consists in an eversion of the lower portion of the rectum, and its protrusion through the anus. This affection is most common in infancy and old age. It may depend on a natural laxity and delicacy of structure, or be caused by violent straining, in consequence of costiveness, or of the existence of stone or stricture. *Treatment.*— Whenever the protrusion occurs, the parts should be carefully washed, and then be replaced by pressure with the hand. If there is any difficulty in doing so, the forefinger oiled should be pushed up into the anus, and it will carry the protruded part with it. If, however, as sometimes happens, a larger portion than usual has come down, and it is so swelled and tender from the constriction of the sphincter, and from being irritated by the clothes, that it cannot be returned, leeches, fomentations, a dose of opium, and rest in the horizontal posture for some hours, will remove the difficulty. To cure this affection, the bowels must be regulated by gentle aperients, (F. 42,) so as to prevent costiveness and straining,— the stools should be passed whilst the patient is in the horizontal posture,—injections of dec. quercus—dashing cold water on the part— tonics, especially steel wine—the occasional passage of a bougie, and support by pads and T bandages, may be used to give tone and firmness to the parts—and piles or any other source of irritation must be removed by appropriate remedies. But if the diligent employment of these measures is of no avail, certain operations may be resorted to. (1.) The mildest consists in pinching up two or three folds of mucous membrane on the protruded bowel with forceps, and tying them tightly with ligatures. (2.) Or ligatures may be passed by needles through several folds of skin just at the margin of the anus, which are then to be tied up tightly. Either of these operations may be repeated as often as necessary. Their effect in producing adhesion and consolidation of the relaxed tissues must be obvious. There is a new French operation, which consists in excising a portion of the sphincter ani; but when this operation used to be performed (as it commonly was sixty years ago) for fistula, it was often followed by inability to retain the faeces.

XII. INTERNAL PROLAPSUS.—Sometimes the upper part of the rectum becomes prolapsed and invaginated within the lower, giving rise to most of the symptoms of stricture. On examination with the finger, the canal of the rectum is found obstructed by a tumour with a capacious *cul de sac* around it, and with the natural passage of the bowel in its centre. *Treatment.*—Aperients, mild astringent injections, and the bougie, the point of which should be carefully guided into the orifice in the centre of the prolapsed portion.

XIII. SPASMODIC STRICTURE of the rectum—known by great difficulty in evacuating the bowels, with spasmodic pain on doing so—is an affection about which but little is known. "It generally depends," says Mr. Mayo, "on a vitiated state of the secretions; and is more frequently relieved by a regulated diet and alterative medicines, and the use of injections, than by the employment of the bougie."

XIV. PERMANENT STRICTURE.—In this affection there is a chronic thickening and contraction of the mucous coat of the rectum, so as to form a ring encroaching on its canal. It is generally situated at from two inches and a half to four inches from the anus. More rarely it is met with higher up, or even in various parts of the colon. The *symptoms* are great pain, straining and difficulty in voiding the fæces, which are passed in small, narrow flattened fragments;—and on examination the stricture may in ordinary cases be readily felt. Irritation of the bladder and uterus, and pains or cramps in the leg, with headach and dyspepsia, are occasional additional symptoms. If this affection be unrelieved, it leads to ulceration of the rectum above the stricture, with a consequent aggravation of all the symptoms, and death from irritation. *Treatment.*—The remedies are aperients and injections, so as to produce daily soft unirritating stools,—and the bougie. A soft bougie, capable of being passed with moderate facility through the stricture, should be introduced once in three or four days, and be allowed to remain fifteen or twenty minutes; and its size should be gradually increased when a larger one admits of being passed. The best bougie is a short one, made of India rubber, which may be received altogether within the sphincter; and it may be withdrawn by means of a riband at one end. Instruments of every sort introduced into the rectum should be handled with the utmost gentleness. Nothing is gained by forcing a large bougie through a stricture. The cure is to be effected by the repeated and gentle stimulus of pressure,—so as to excite absorption,—not by mere mechanical dilatation. There are numerous fatal instances on record in which the bowel has been torn by bougies, and by that most dangerous and loathsome instrument the common clyster syringe, in the hands of careless or ignorant people. For the administration of enemata, the pipe should be only an inch and a half in length, with a large bulbous extremity. Or if in cases of stricture, or of obstinate costiveness with great accumulation of fæces or of incarcerated hernia, it is desirable to introduce a tube farther, it should be quite flexible like that of a stomach pump. But the natural sharp fold at the junction of the rectum with the sigmoid flexure, and the fact shown by Mr. Earle that the bowel not unfrequently makes a horizontal curve to the right before descending into the pelvis, render the introduction of bougies into the sigmoid flexure a very blind, hazardous proceeding, and one that is not often to be justified.

XV. SIMPLE ULCER of the rectum is generally situated on its posterior surface, just above the sphincter, where it may be felt with a slightly indurated edge. It generally begins as a small crack or fissure of the mucous membrane, caused by straining to get rid of hardened fæces.

It produces great pain and difficulty of defæcation;—more or less discharge, occasionally tinged with blood, and irritation of the bladder. *Treatment.*—Laxatives, enemata of warm water, to which a little laudanum may be added when there is much pain,—and the application of mercurial ointment or solution of arg. nit. to the ulcer,—which failing, the sphincter must be divided and made to heal by granulation.

XVI. SCIRRHOUS ULCER of the rectum presents, according to Mr. Mayo, the following appearances: The mucous membrane disappears for a certain extent; and the muscular coat which is exposed is pale, hard, and gristly like cartilage. The symptoms are great pain, tenesmus, fetid discharge, and irritation of the bladder. The treatment consists in the use of aperients, astringent and opiate injections,—and the very occasional passage of a bougie.

XVII. FUNGUS MEDULLARIS occasions all the symptoms of permanent stricture. It is known by the projecting fungous masses. The bowels must be kept loose,—pain and irritation must be allayed,—and the bougie be passed occasionally, to delay contraction of the passage. It is sometimes advisable to cut through the morbid growth, to provide for a time for the passage of the fæces,—but any attempt at extirpation is hardly to be thought of.

XVIII. PRURITUS ANI, a very violent itching of the anus, is a very troublesome affection. The best plan is, to keep the bowels open with sulphur, seidlitz powders, or castor oil, with occasional doses of blue pill;—to put the stomach in proper order;—to bathe the part very frequently with water as hot as can be borne; and to apply some stimulating or astringent substance—such as nitrate of silver, weak solution of corrosive sublimate, or the citrine ointment.

# CHAPTER XX.

## OF THE DISEASES OF THE URINARY ORGANS.

### SECTION I.—OF STRICTURE OF THE MALE URETHRA.

THERE are two kinds of stricture, the *spasmodic* and *permanent;* some add a third, the *inflammatory.*

I. SPASMODIC STRICTURE is supposed to depend on spasm of the muscles (Wilson's) which surround the membranous portion of the urethra, at which point, according to most surgeons, the obstruction is invariably found. It generally affects persons who are labouring under some degree of permanent stricture,—or whose urethra has been rendered irritable by repeated attacks of gonorrhœa, or by a diseased condition of the urine, (especially a tendency to phosphatic deposites;)—these therefore are the *predisposing causes.* The usual *exciting causes* are, exposure to cold and wet,—and indulgence in punch or champagne, or similar acid liquors, which disorder the stomach and render the urine unusually irritating. Hence an attack of spasmodic stricture generally comes on about four hours after dinner. It may also be caused by cantharides, whether taken by the mouth, or absorbed from the skin.

The *symptoms* are,—sudden RETENTION OF URINE; that is to say, the patient finds himself suddenly unable to pass his water, although he makes repeated straining efforts to do so. The bladder soon becomes distended, and can be felt as a tense round tumour above the pubes, and unless relief is given, the countenance becomes anxious, the pulse quick, and the skin hot. The straining efforts at micturition also become more frequent and violent. And supposing the patient to have been subject to repeated attacks, and that relief is delayed, either the bladder may burst into the peritonæum;—or the urethra behind the stricture, (which of course becomes dilated and weakened under the pressure of the urine impelled by the whole force of the abdominal muscles,) bursts into the perinæum, and gives rise to *extravasation of urine,* as will be described in the next section.

The *inflammatory stricture* is a variety of the preceding, in which great pain and tenderness of the perinæum, and fever, are combined with spasm. It is generally caused by abuse of injections, or by exposure and intemperance during acute gonorrhœa. The treatment of this and of the spasmodic variety must be the same.

*Treatment.*—In the first place, the bladder must be relieved if possible.

A silver catheter may first be introduced. But if that fails to pass, a small gum catheter, which has been kept for some time on a curved wire, so that it retains its curve when the wire is withdrawn, or a catgut bougie, or a common bougie, may be tried in succession. In introducing either of these instruments, the surgeon should be careful, 1st, to draw the penis well forwards on it, so as to stretch the urethra, and prevent the instrument from becoming entangled. 2ndly, To make the point slide along the upper surface of the urethra. 3rdly, On meeting with the obstruction, to press against it steadily, but very gently. And by one or other of these means, used with delicacy and perseverance for five or ten minutes, the stricture will in most cases be made to yield. The instruments used should not be too small.

If, however, they all fail, certain remedies for relaxing the spasm must next be resorted to.

(a) Venæsection, or cupping from the perinæum—if the patient is of an inflammatory habit, or complains of much pain; (b) An enema, or some purgative of speedy operation—if the attack is caused by excess at table;—followed by (c) an enema of solution of starch f℥iii with tinct. opii f℥i,—or by repeated doses of opium or Dover's powder;—together with (d) immersion of the whole body in a hot bath (104° F.) till faintness supervenes,—are the most useful. But there are many others that are often of very great service; especially (e) the *tinct. ferri sesquichloridi* in doses of ♏x every ten minutes—(f) affusion of cold water on the genitals—(g) large draughts of lime water—(h) and belladonna smeared on the perinæum. (i) A slight touch with the caustic bougie sometimes produces immediate relief, when there is some degree of permanent stricture, which is exceedingly irritable, and liable to frequent spasm. (k) Quinine has cured cases in which spasmodic stricture occurred periodically.

*Puncture of the bladder.*—If none of these means succeed, and the bladder has become exceedingly distended, it must be punctured. This operation may be performed in three places, viz. by the rectum,—above the pubes, — or by the perinæum. The first is to be preferred in cases of retention of urine by stricture,—the second when the prostate is enlarged,—and the third when urine is extravasated.

PUNCTURE OF THE BLADDER BY THE RECTUM is performed by placing the patient on his hands and knees,—introducing the left forefinger into the anus, and a curved trocar and canula by its side,—then feeling for the distended bladder just behind the prostate, and exactly in the middle line, and plunging the trocar into it—leaving the canula for four-and-twenty hours.

II. PERMANENT STRICTURE is a contraction of the urethra caused by chronic inflammation. Sometimes it is situated in the membranous portion, where it may be easily induced by repeated attacks of spasmodic stricture. But this form of stricture is also very commonly found in the spongy portion of the urethra, especially at the distance of four inches from the orifice. The extent of a stricture is at first only a few lines, although it may be extended to one or two inches. The *cause* is generally repeated gonorrhœa.

*Symptoms.*—In what may be called the first stage, the patient finds that he wants to make water oftener than usual, and that he has more or less uneasy sensation in the perinæum after doing so; he also notices that a few drops of the urine hang in the urethra, and dribble from him after he has buttoned up. Then he observes that the stream of water is smaller than usual, and forked, or scattered, or twisted, and that he requires a longer time and greater effort than usual to pass it. Itching of the end of the penis and gleety discharge are not unfrequent concomitants. If the disease proceeds to 'its second stage, the bladder becomes irritable,—obliging the patient to rise in the night to void his urine. He is liable to attacks of spasm with complete retention, as has been described in the preceding paragraphs. In one of these, the urethra may ulcerate or burst,—giving rise to urinary abscess, or to extravasation of urine, as will be described in the next section. Rigours occurring in paroxysms like ague fits are not uncommon. Finally if the complaint is permitted to continue, the health suffers from the constant irritation and want of sleep; the complexion becomes wan; the appetite fails; the patient complains of chill and flushes, of aching and weakness in the back, and of great langour and depression of spirits; and the urine is constantly loaded with fetid mucus. After death, the urethra behind the stricture is found greatly dilated; the bladder, with its muscular coat, enormously thickened;—the uterus dilated, and converted into subsidiary receptacles for the urine, and the kidneys either greatly dilated or disorganized.

*Treatment.*—In the first place, any disorder of the general health, or of the digestive organs, and any derangement of the urine, must be corrected by proper remedies. (Vide Gleet, Chronic Inflammation of the Bladder, and Urinary Deposites.) The patient also must avoid violent exercise, especially on horseback. But the stricture can only be cured by *mechanical means.* And these are five. 1. The bougie,—2. the catheter kept in the urethra,—3. the caustic bougie,—4. puncturation with the stilette, —and 5. division from the perinæum.

1. *The bougie.*—In order to ascertain with precision the existence of stricture, the urethra should be examined with a common plaster bougie of full size, i. e. one that will readily enter the orifice, and that will fill the urethra without stretching it. The surgeon takes the cornea glandis in his left hand, and introduces the bougie (previously oiled and bent to the shape of the urethra) with his right—holding it loosely like a pen. If it meets with an obstruction, it should be slightly withdrawn,--

then tried again.  If it now seem to pass, the surgeon should relinquish his hold,—and then if it recoils, it is a sign that it has bent against the stricture;—whereas if it has entered the stricture it will be held, and will require a gentle force to dislodge it.  If after all it does not pass, a metallic sound or catheter may be tried, because a slight obstacle to the instrument at its first introduction must not be set down at once as stricture. The patient generally suffers somewhat from sickness and faintness on the first trial.  When the stricture is clearly made out, the surgeon should mark and lay by a bougie that will just pass through it.  In three or four days' time he introduces the same bougie again,—lets it remain a few minutes,—then withdraws and introduces another of a size larger, which he suffers to remain for ten or fifteen minutes.  After three more days the process is repeated,—first using the instrument that was passed on the former occasion,—then one of a size larger; and this process repeated a sufficient number of times affords in most cases an easy, painless cure.

*Metallic bougies* or sounds are to be preferred to those of the ordinary soft materials, 1st, if the stricture is old and very hard and gristly; 2ndly, in cases of very irritable urethræ, because their smooth polished surface is not so apt to cause spasm; 3rdly, in cases where a false passage has been formed, which these instruments, as they can be directed with greater precision, can be better made to avoid.  They should be eight or nine inches long, slightly curved, and mounted on a firm wooden handle. Very small ones should be avoided.

2.  If a *small catheter is retained in the bladder* for two or three days, the passage suppurates and dilates remarkably; just as the lachrymal duct does from the presence of a style.  This method of cure is extremely speedy and efficient.  It may therefore be employed, 1st, when time is of much value; 2ndly, when the stricture is very gristly and cartilaginous, 3rdly, when the urethra is irregular, or has had a false passage made in it; 4thly, when the urethra is so irritable that severe rigours and fever are occasioned by the passage of the urine after the use of the common bougie—a circumstance common enough with patients who have lived in hot climates.  The catheter should be retained by means of two strings, which may either-be fastened to the penis with sticking-plaster, or may be tied to the thighs, or may be passed backwards between the thighs, and be fastened to a band round the waist.  It should be removed in three or four days, and a larger catheter should be passed after twelve or four-and-twenty hours, and should be introduced often enough subsequently to keep up the dilatation.  In cases of stricture which will not suffer any instrument to pass, Mr. Guthrie recommends a bougie to be kept in the urethra, and to be made to press constantly against the anterior surface of the stricture.  He says that this plan " has never failed in his hands to clear the urethra, and to effect a passage into the bladder."  Mr. Liston, however, describes it as " a very futile and unsurgical proceeding," and

one " not likely to be called for in the practice of a man with hands to act and head to guide them."

3. The *caustic bougie* is a powerful agent in diminishing the irritability of strictures, and is advisable in cases where there is a perpetual tendency to spasm. It may also be applied to very firm strictures of small extent. But it should never be used till other means have failed, and never should be repeated more than three or four times about the same period,—for it is liable, if misused, to induce inflammation, abscess, spasm, hæmorrhage, or false passage. The manner of using it is this:— the distance of the stricture is measured by a common bougie,—then the caustic bougie is passed down to the same distance, and is to be pressed firmly and heavily against the stricture for a quarter or half a minute. The process should not be repeated in less than three days.

4. *Puncturation*, or division of the stricture by means of the *lanceted stilettes* invented by Mr. Stafford, may be resorted to with advantage in some cases of old stricture, especially if at the anterior part of the urethra. But if the stricture is far back, it is a blind, dangerous proceeding; and if any instrument whatever can be passed, it is unnecessary.

5. The operation of OPENING THE URETHRA or PUNCTURE OF THE BLADDER BY THE PERINÆUM is absolutely requisite in all cases of rupture of the urethra with extravasation of urine,—and it may also be expedient in cases of very old stricture with extensive urinary fistulæ. It is performed thus:—the patient is placed in the lithotomy position; a grooved staff is passed down to the stricture, and the left forefinger, introduced into the rectum, is to feel for the urethra, and serve as a guide to the incisions. Then a straight bistoury is to be plunged in just above the anus to the depth of an inch, and made to cut its way out upwards in the middle line of the perinæum. The end of the sound should next be felt for and cut upon,—and the knife is then to be carried backwards through the stricture into the urethra beyond it, which is always more or less dilated. A gum catheter should then be passed into the bladder, and be retained there, so that the wound may heal over it, and form a new passage. It should, however, be changed once in three or four days.

There is a modification of this operation which Sir B. Brodie sometimes adopts in cases of old stricture that are so hard, narrow, and extensive, that no instrument can be passed through them, or that are complicated with extensive false passages or urinary fistulæ. He cuts down through the perinæum into the dilated part of the urethra behind the stricture. Then, having introduced the finger, he presses with it against the back part of the stricture, and passes down one of Mr. Stafford's instruments, and makes the lancet cut through the stricture. A gum catheter is then passed into the bladder, and retained for a few days.

In whatever manner a stricture has been cured, the bougie should still be used at intervals, to prevent a fresh contraction.

CONTRACTION OF THE ORIFICE of the urethra may be a congenital affection, or may be caused by the cicatrization of ulcers. It must be counteracted by the daily passage of a short bougie, otherwise it may produce all the evil consequences of stricture farther back. If the contraction is very great, the orifice must be dilated by a slight incision downwards—and any subsequent contraction be obviated by the bougie.

SECTION II.— OF CERTAIN CONSEQUENCES OF STRICTURE, AND OTHER AFFECTIONS OF THE MALE URETHRA.

I. URINARY ABSCESS is one frequent consequence of stricture. It signifies an abscess in the cellular tissue of the perinæum, and is caused in the following way. One or two drops of urine escape into the cellular tissue, in consequence of a slight ulceration or laceration of the weakened and dilated part of the urethra behind the stricture; and this small quantity of urine inflames the cellular tissue, and an abscess forms filled with dark-coloured putrid pus.* *Symptoms.*—A patient with old stricture complains of rather more difficulty of micturition than usual—he is seized with shivering, the skin becomes hot, the tongue brown, and the pulse faltering;—and on examination, a deep, hard, and painful but not prominent swelling will be detected in the perinæum. *Treatment.*— The abscess should be opened immediately, and the patient will soon be brought from the gates of death to comparative health. It will also be expedient to cut through the stricture as directed above.

II. RUPTURE OF THE URETHRA and EXTRAVASATION OF URINE.—This is another consequence of old stricture, and it generally happens in the following way. The patient, who has long been labouring under difficulty of micturition, has a fit of spasmodic retention more obstinate than usual. He is repeatedly getting out of bed, and straining with all his might to pass his water. At last, during one violent effort, he plainly feels that something has given way;—his painful sense of distention becomes immediately less, and he is very well pleased, and thinks himself better. And perhaps he is now able to make a little water by the natural passage, because the stricture generally relaxes, when, by any means whatever, it is relieved from the former pressure. But at the time when something seemed to yield, the urethra burst;—the urine was forced by the whole power of the abdominal muscles into the cellular tis-

---

* In the same manner, a little urine may escape from a minute aperture in the bladder, and give rise to abscess above the pubes.

sue of the scrotum, perinæum, and groins;—the patient soon complains of a smarting or tingling about the anus and perinæum;—the urine, which has become putrid and concentrated by long confinement in the bladder, speedily causes inflammation and sloughing;—the skin over the infiltrated parts displays a reddish blush, which is soon succeeded by black spots of gangrene,—low typhoid symptoms come on; the tongue is black, the pulse begins to falter, the skin is clammy, and there are low delirium and hiccup;—and the patient soon departs this life, unless proper measures are taken for his relief. A black spot on the glans penis, indicating that the urine has penetrated the corpus spongiosum, is a very fatal sign.

*Treatment.*—A staff or catheter must be passed as far as possible, and (as a stricture generally relaxes after the bladder is unloaded by any means) it may sometimes be passed into the bladder. Then the urethra must be opened and the stricture be divided in the manner described in the last page, and a catheter be passed through the wound into the bladder, and be allowed to remain several days. At the same time free incisions must be made into any parts that are swelled or emphysematous—showing that they have been pervaded by the urine.

The urethra may also be ruptured by blows or kicks on the perinæum, or by accidents that fracture the bones of the pelvis. The symptoms will be pretty evident. The patient will be unable to make water; or if he attempts it, the urine will be extravasated into the perinæum and scrotum. The treatment consists in retaining a catheter in the urethra, and incising the perinæum if urine has been extravasated.

III. Fistula in Perinæo, or *Urinary Fistula,* signifies an opening from the perinæum into the urethra, through which the urine dribbles. It is a frequent consequence of the two preceding affections. *Treatment.*—The first and most essential measure is, to restore the urethra to a healthy state, and to dilate any strictures that may happen to exist, by the bougie. When this has been done, the fistula should be stimulated to granulate by injection of arg. nit., or by passing a heated wire into it;— and the external orifice should be occasionally touched with potass, so as not to allow it to heal before the whole track is closed—otherwise fresh abscess will form.

Sometimes a fistulous communication forms between the urethra and rectum. This may be known by air passing through the urethra. It is to be treated by dilating the urethra, and then perhaps a heated wire may be introduced into the fistula.

IV. False Passage.—This may be produced by using too small a sound, and pushing it out of the urethra, or by the misuse of caustic bougies. There is nothing to be done for the false passage, but the stricture which was the origin of it must be treated either with the metallic sound, or by keeping in a small catheter. When the surgeon suspects that he has pushed an instrument out of the right passage, he ought to leave the urethra untouched, for at least a week.

V. HÆMORRHAGE FROM THE URETHRA may be caused by the rude introduction of bougies, or by injuries from without, or by the separation of a slough formed by the caustic bougie;—or, lastly, by a rupture of blood-vessels during acute chordee. If the application of cold does not check it, pressure may be tried. A flat piece of cork should be pressed by the patient against the perinæum far back, and be gradually moved forward till it lights on the right spot, and the dripping of blood ceases.

VI. SOLID TUMOURS in the course of the urethra, composed of indurated follicles, must be treated in the same manner as the scirrhous state of the corpus spongiosum, p. 200.

VII. ACUTE AND CHRONIC INFLAMMATION of the urethra, from whatever cause arising, differ in no respect, in their symptoms, consequences, or treatment from gonorrhœa and gleet.

VIII. FOREIGN BODIES in the urethra may consist of calculi, or of small bodies introduced from without. They may, perhaps, be pushed forward by means of the fingers, aided by the patient's strainings,—or may be seized by forceps, and be brought out through the orifice, which must be slightly dilated if necessary. Or, it is a very good plan to press the thumb on the urethra behind the foreign body, and then to inject a good stream of water from a large syringe, so as to dilate the passage. But if these means fail, the substance must be pushed back into the membranous portion, (if not there already,) and be extracted by an incision in the perinæum. Incisions in front of the scrotum should be avoided, for they are apt to leave irremediable fistulæ.

SECTION III.—OF THE DISEASES OF THE PROSTATE.

I. ACUTE INFLAMMATION of the prostate is generally a consequence of acute gonorrhœa. The *Symptoms* are, great weight, pain, and throbbing at the neck of the bladder—and tenderness of the perinæum;—the gland feels swelled and tender on examination by the rectum—and these are frequent, violent, and exceedingly painful efforts to make water. *Treatment.*—Rest in bed—cupping or leeches to the perinæum—or general bleeding if the patient is strong—hip-baths and enemata of starch ℥ii, laudanum ʒss every night. If the urine cannot be passed without it, a a very small gum catheter may be introduced;—but it should be avoided if possible.

II. ABSCESS of the prostate may be suspected if rigours, and obscure swelling, or fluctuation in the perinæum, follow the symptoms of acute inflammation. In any such case, the swelling should be freely punctured with a bistoury. If left to itself, the abscess may burst into the rectum or the urethra, which latter circumstance will be indicated by a sudden discharge of pus with the urine. If the abscess should burst into the urethra, the catheter should be used every time the patient passes his urine, in order to prevent it from entering and irritating the cyst. If the case is chronic and the habit scrofulous, quinine and tonics, and small doses of cubebs, to act as a gentle stimulus on the parts, will be of service.

III. CHRONIC ENLARGEMENT of the prostate is extremely frequent in advanced life, and seems to depend on the decay of age rather than on any disease. It generally commences, as Sir B. Brodie observes, about the time that the hair turns gray, and when earthy specks begin to be deposited in the coats of the arteries. The gland increases to and from two to fourteen times its natural bulk, and becomes hardened. The middle lobe generally forms a projecting tumour at the neck of the bladder, and, in consequence of the alteration of the shape and size of the gland, the prostatic portion of the urethra becomes lengthened, and curved abruptly upwards. The first *symptoms* are slowness and difficulty of making water, sense of weight in the perinæum, and tenesmus. In the next place, the bladder becomes irritable, and the calls to make water are oftener than before. Then, as the patient cannot empty the organ completely, in consequence of the projection formed by the tumour, a portion of urine always remains behind, and decomposes, and becomes ammoniacal. Sometimes a fit of complete retention ensues, and it may be brought on by exposure to cold or excess in venery. Next, the mucous coat of the bladder, irritated by the frequent strainings,.and by the alkaline urine, inflames and secretes a viscid mucus. Finally, the obstacle continuing to increase, the bladder is constantly distended—the urine perpetually dribbles away—the ureters become dilated into subsidiary receptacles; the kidneys become disorganized, the patient's little remaining strength is exhausted, and he dies.

*Treatment.*—Medicines are of no avail to remove the enlargement of the prostate, although they may very likely be required for accompanying disease of the bladder or kidneys. The only thing to be done is to introduce the catheter two or three times a-day, so that the bladder may be completely emptied. The instrument will meet with an obstruction just at the entrance of the bladder, occasioned partly by irregularity of the urethra, partly by the projection of the third lobe. To avoid the latter, the instrument (commonly called *prostate catheter*) should be long, and have its point well turned up. In introducing it, the point should be made to glide as close as possible round the pubes, and the handle should be well depressed as it is entering the bladder, in order that the point may ride over the projection. The finger also should be introduced into rectum to guide it. The best catheter, if it can be used, is a small gum, which has been kept for a long while on an iron wire of considerable curve; but a silver one of proper shape is more easy of introduction.

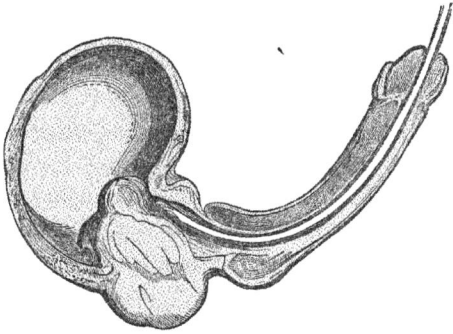

If the bladder has been long distended to the utmost, and the kidneys have become organically diseased in consequence, the sudden withdrawal of all the urine will be likely to be followed by irretrievable sinking. The urine should therefore be drawn off in small quantities at a time, and the strength be well supported with tonics, wine, and plenty of nutriment.

IV. COMPLETE RETENTION OF URINE from enlargement of the prostate. In this case, if there are inflammatory symptoms, cupping from the perinæum and the hip-bath are indicated. The catheter should be passed if possible, and when passed, it should be retained, because the bladder does not regain its contractility for two or three days, and the frequent introduction of the instrument would be irritating. If, however, the catheter cannot be passed by the natural route, it should be thrust through the projecting part of the gland, so as to make a new passage into the bladder—(or perhaps one of Stafford's *lanceted stilettes* may be advantageously employed for that purpose.) But if this cannot be done, the last resource is

PUNCTURE OF THE BLADDER ABOVE THE PUBES. This is easily performed by making a small incision through the linea alba just above the pubes, and then thrusting a long trocar and canula downwards and backwards into the bladder, where it is uncovered by the peritonæum. The canula must be retained, and the patient be kept on his back to prevent extravasation;—and no time should be lost in restoring the natural passage.

V. CALCULI of the prostate are small reddish-brown concretions of phosphate of lime formed in the ducts of the gland. They cause obscure irritation of the neck of the bladder and difficulty of micturition. They may perhaps be felt by the finger in the rectum. Sometimes it may be possible to remove some of them with the urethral forceps—or if there are many contained in one cyst, to cut upon them from the perinæum; but in general the only thing to be done is, to keep the urethra well dilated with bougies, so as to favour their spontaneous escape.

SECTION IV.—OF THE DISEASES OF THE BLADDER.

I. ACUTE INFLAMMATION of the bladder (or *cystitis*) is rarely a primary idiopathic affection. Most frequently it is a consequence of neglected or ill-treated gonorrhœa, or else an aggravation of the chronic inflammation. The *symptoms* are pain, referred to the perinæum and sacrum—tenderness of the lower part of the abdomen—micturition exceedingly frequent, attended with great straining, and followed by an aggravation of the pain—a mucous or muco-purulent sediment in the urine, and fever. *Treatment.*—Bleeding—leeches or cupping on the lower part of the abdomen or perinæum—hip-bath and warm fomentations—castor oil, so as to keep the bowels open without much straining—opiate glysters at night. If, moreover, the urine is acid, (turning blue litmus paper red,) and if the sediment in it is yellowish and not adhesive, F. 6 may be given three or four times a-day, with saline draughts containing excess of alkali (or F. 19,) in the intervals. But if the urine be alkaline, (turning red litmus paper blue,) and if it deposite a dark-coloured adhesive mucus, vın colchici ℥xx—xxx should be given three or four times a day instead of the calomel and alkalis.

II.—CHRONIC INFLAMMATION of the bladder (*catarrhus vesicæ*) is a very frequent consequence of irritation from stricture, diseased prostate, or stone. *Symptoms.*—The bladder irritable—micturition very frequent and painful—the urine loaded with mucus—which is sometimes tinged with blood, sometimes yellowish and puriform, but more generally grayish, highly alkaline, and excessively viscid, so as to stick to the bottom of the chamber-pot when turned upside down. In the early stages there is but little mucus, and the urine may remain acid; but as the disease advances the quantity of mucus becomes enormous, and the urine is voided of a brownish hue, and of a most offensive ammoniacal odour. Moreover it may clog the urethra, and cause retention of urine;—a kind of retention difficult to manage, because the mucus clogs up the eyes of the catheter. In this stage there is very frequent desire to make water, and constant pain above the pubes. In general, the mucus contains *phosphate of lime,* which may be seen in it in white streaks, and which is apt to collect and form a stone in the bladder. Perhaps the mucus membrane of the bladder may ulcerate, and after death it may be found as cleanly dissected from the muscular coat, as if it had been done with a knife. This will be attended with an intense aggravation of the pain in micturition, and with a dark colour of the urine;—owing to the admixture of a little blood which exudes from the ulcerating surface, and which, after the urine is passed, sinks to the bottom like coffee grounds. But more frequently the bladder throws out flakes of lymph, which become encrusted with patches of phosphate of lime. Moreover, the bladder, by the constant exercise of its muscles in straining, becomes hypertrophied and exceedingly thick,—and portions of its mucous membrane are apt to be forced between the intervals of its muscular fibres, and form pouches which are soon filled with mucus, or with phosphatic calculi. Finally the mucus becomes purulent, disease of the kidneys ensues, and the patient dies. Dr. Prout says that in the last stage of all kinds of bladder disease, the urine not unfrequently becomes acid suddenly, and the mucus and pus disappear, immediately before death.

*Treatment.*—In the first place, if there is a stricture, or enlarged prostate, or stone in the bladder, proper measures should be taken for their removal or relief. In the next place, if the symptoms are at all severe, the patient should keep himself in the recumbent position as much as possible, with the pelvis elevated. Thirdly, if there is at any time a great aggravation of pain, and the strength is pretty good, a few ounces of blood may be taken by cupping on the sacrum or perinæum; but, as a general rule all lowering measures are injurious. Stimulating or opiate plasters to the sacrum are sometimes of use. Pain and irritation are to be allayed by the hip-bath, and by enemata or suppositories of opium— (F. 48,) or by the internal administration of opium. The bowels should be kept properly open by mild aperients, such as castor oil or rhubarb; but griping and purging are inexpedient. The diet should consist of boiled mutton, white fish, rice, arrow-root, and other substances that are nutritious, easily digestible, and not apt to turn sour;—with cold weak brandy and water, or gin and water, or sound cherry. Mercury and alkalis are of course, as a general rule, inexpedient; yet, if the urine is still acid (not being yet made alkaline by the mucus) and the strength is good, small doses may be given, if required for the state of the stomach;—as will be shown when treating of the *phosphatic diathesis.*

Besides these remedies, the bladder may be acted on by certain medicaments, and by injections. Of medicines, the most useful, according to Brodie, is the root of the *pareira brava*, an ounce of which should be boiled in three pints of water down to a pint, and the decoction be administered in doses of $\mathfrak{Z}$iv ter die—or the extract of pareira in doses of gr. xxx ter die may be substituted. *Uva ursi*, or *buchu*, in doses of an ounce or two of a strong infusion or decoction, F. 91; or *oil of turpentine,* ($\mathfrak{m}$ xv,) or *chian turpentine,* (gr. ii.) or *cubebs* (gr. xv.,) or *copaiba,* ($\mathfrak{m}$ xx,) or *tinct. ferri mur.* ($\mathfrak{m}$ xv)—in small doses three times a day, are also remedies of similar virtues. Hyoscyamus or opium, and small. doses of mineral acids, if the urine is highly alkaline, may be added to any of them, F. 98. The sulphate of zinc may also be highly useful, F. 53.

*Injections into the bladder* are not to be thought of when there is acute inflammation of the bladder and blood mixed with the mucus, but they are highly serviceable in chronic cases, by relieving the irritability of the bladder, and washing out the organ, getting rid of the decomposed stink-ing urine and mucus. Injections of simple warm water are very useful, the best way of effecting them is that employed by Mr. W. Fergusson; it is to have a catheter with a double passage, and to throw in the water in a continuous stream by means of a small syringe like that of a stomach pump. Three or four pints of water may thus be passed through the bladder daily. Decoction of poppies or laudanum may be added in some cases. Moreover, injections of very dilute nitric acid ($\mathfrak{m}$ i—ii—ad $\zbar$iss aq. destil.) thrown into the bladder not oftener than once a day, through a double gold catheter, and allowed to remain thirty seconds, are of great service when the urine is highly ammoniacal.

III. Irritable Bladder.—Many cases described under this title are cases of chronic inflammation. Simple irritability,—that is, a frequent disposition to pass the urine without any disease,—may be caused by an irritating state of the urine; or it may be the effect of mere nervousness, which is not uncommon in elderly people; or it may be sympathetic of disease of the kidney, or of irritation in the rectum.

IV. Paralysis of the bladder may occur under many circumstances. It may be caused by injury or disease of the head or spine—it is often present in typhus fever—it may be caused for a time by any severe in-jury, especially of the legs—it generally remains for a few days after great distention of the bladder from prostatic disease or stricture—and it some-times occurs suddenly to nervous sedentary people, who, if they let their bladder get filled beyond a certain point, find that they cannot empty it. The symptoms of it are, either retention of urine;—i. e. that the patient cannot make water;—or else incontinence of urine; that is, the water dribbles away without his being able to hold it. The diagnosis of reten-tion through palsy, from retention from stricture, is easy. The retention from palsy comes on suddenly, and there is no obstacle to the introduc-tion of a catheter.

A strong decoction of *parietaria officinalis;* cantharides, and tinct. ferri mur., are the remedies for simple palsy.

V. Incontinence and Dribbling of Urine.—This is a symptom that requires particular notice; because in nine cases out of ten it happens, not because the patient cannot hold his water, but because he has retention of urine, either from stricture, or enlarged prostate, or palsy of the blad-der. For it must be noticed, that in either of these cases, as soon as the bladder becomes full, a little urine begins to dribble away through the urethra—and besides, the patient may perhaps be able to squeeze out a little by straining with his abdominal muscles, and may believe his blad-der to be empty, although all the while it is enormously distended. No surgeon will fail to put his hand on the pubes when he sees the urine dribbling away. The obvious remedy is the catheter.

VI.—Hysterical Retention of Urine.—There is one form of palsy of the bladder which is not unfrequent in hysterical women, and which consists in a deficiency of volition rather than of power. They are not unable to empty the bladder if they try—but they are unable to try. These cases must be treated with purgatives, stimulating enemata, and fetid medicines. If the catheter is not employed, the patient will generally begin to make water as soon as she suffers much from distention; but the bladder must not be allowed to go unrelieved too long.

SECT. V.——OF DISEASE OF THE KIDNEYS, HÆMATURIA, AND SUPPRESSION OF URINE.

I. ACUTE INFLAMMATION OF THE KIDNEY (*Acute Nephritis*) is sometimes caused by blows on the loins, or by the irritation of renal calculi, but is very rarely an idiopathic primary affection. The *symptoms* are, burning pain and tenderness in the loins; colicky pains in the belly; the urine scanty and high coloured, and the bladder irritable, so that there are constant attempts at micturition;—fever and great thirst, and violent vomiting. The remedies are—bleeding, cupping, and leeches—castor oil—repeated doses of calomel, opium, and antimony, with colchicum if the habit is gouty;—warm baths, or warm fomentations to the loins, and barley water and other demulcent drinks.

II. CHRONIC DISEASE OF THE KIDNEYS, when it comes under the surgeon's care, is generally a consequence of long standing disease of the urethra or bladder. When the bladder has been subject to frequent distention through stricture or enlarged prostrate, and its mucous membrane inflamed, the ureters are liable to become distended and converted as it were into subsidiary receptacles for the urine, so that all the violent strainings to evacuate it tell upon the kidneys; and these become diseased, partly from the mechanical irritation, partly from sympathy, partly from an extension of inflammation from the bladder, and partly through participating in that general degeneration of the functions and structures of the body, which is sure to ensue when any one important function is long and seriously impeded. *Symptoms.*—A person, with some chronic affection of the bladder, complains of general weakness and languor, both bodily and mental. The sleep is unrefreshing, and the appetite impaired. There is frequent pain of a weak aching character in one or both loins; occasionally shooting down to the testicles or groins. The urine is almost invariably *albuminous*,* it is generally pale-coloured and opaqueish

* Urine may be known to contain albumen if it becomes cloudy and opaque when exposed to a heat of 170 degrees or upwards, a little nitric acid being also added. Heat alone, without the acid, might cause a white deposition of the phosphates that might be mistaken for albumen;—and the corrosive sublimate, that is sometimes recommended as a test, might produce a deceptive precipitate of the lithate of mercury.

when passed; sometimes it is tinged with blood, and sometimes it displays shreds or flakes of lymph, moulded probably into the shape of the ureters. As the disease proceeds, it becomes yellowish and purulent, and deposites a quantity of pus after standing, the globules of which may be detected by examination with the microscope. These cases are almost sure to end fatally. Sometimes the patient dies of exhaustion and obstinate vomiting; sometimes of suppression of urine and coma; sometimes in a sudden fit of severe shivering; and sometimes of a rapid attack of acute inflammation. The kidneys are found after death to be soft and disorganized; readily separating from their capsule, which however adheres firmly to the fat and cellular tissue of the loins; and most likely they are dilated into cysts; the secreting tissue being spread out over the dilated pelvis and infundibula.

*Strumous Disease of the Kidneys.*—There is one form of disorganization of the kidney which is apt to be unsuspected for some time, because it is principally manifested by great irritability of the bladder. The patient is of a pale unhealthy, scrofulous appearance; he complains of very frequent and urgent desire to pass his water, and the act of micturition is followed by considerable burning pain at the neck of the bladder and in the perinæum. "The urine," says Dr. Prout, "is generally acid; of a pale-greenish, whey-like colour, opalescent from the presence of minute flocculi, or diseased particles of epithelium or mucus; of low specific gravity, (that is below 1.020;) often albuminous, but rarely bloody." The patient complains of weakness and loss of flesh and strength; of occasional pain and swelling of the testicles, and of irritation or gleet from the prepuce or the orifice of the urethra (male or female;) and also occasionally of pain in the back. But the principal symptoms are referred to the bladder, so that the surgeon might be led to suspect the existence of stone. But if in any such case the urine is albuminous, but free from the *ropy mucus* of chronic cystitis, the origin of the mischief may fairly be referred to the kidneys.

*Pyelitis.*—This is the name given by M. Rayer to inflammation of the mucous lining of the pelvis and infundibula of the kidneys. It may accompany the *catarrhus vesicæ*, or mismanaged gonorrhœa, or may be caused by renal calculus. The *symptoms* are low fever, heat and pain in the back, irritation of the stomach and testicles, and the presence of flakes of epithelium, and of mucus in the urine.

*Abscess in the Kidney.*—This may be suspected if dull pain in the loins and repeated shivering follow the symptoms of nephritis. Sometimes the abscess bursts into the ureter, and an immense quantity of pus is discharged with the urine. Abscess of the kidney also in a few cases bursts on the loins, and the patient has been known to recover.

*Treatment.*—In treating chronic disease of the kidney, the diet should be made a matter of chief importance;—all acescent and indigestible substances, acid wines, and hard water, being carefully avoided. Blisters or issues to the loins, or plasters of the emp. ammoniaci cum hydrargyro, with extract of belladonna, may be of service if the pain is severe. The skin should be kept warm, and flannel should be constantly worn. The infusions of buchu, with carrot seed or uva ursi, are sometimes beneficial. If there is a calculus in the kidney, proper measures should be taken for removing the state of urine which gave rise to it.

III.—Hæmaturia, or *Bloody Urine.*—(1.) Hæmorrhage from the kidney is generally caused by the irritation of renal calculi, or by blows on the loins; but it may also depend on a diseased state of the whole system, as in typhus fever or scurvy. The blood is rarely in large quantity, and it is equally diffused through the urine; although, perhaps, there may be some long shreds of coagulum formed in the ureter. If the urine is boiled, the blood will coagulate, and leave the fluid of its natural colour. (2.) Hæmorrhage from the *prostate* or bladder may be caused by the rude introduction of instruments, or by the irritation of stone; or by the existence of an ulcer or fungoid tumour, of which in fact it is often the earliest manifestation. When the blood is derived from the bladder, some portion of it often flows pure after the urine is discharged, and it is in much greater quantity than when derived from the kidneys; moreover the pain in the back, and other signs of renal irritation that aecompany bleeding from the kidney, will not be present.

*Treatment.*—When hæmorrhage from the kidneys is attended with inflammatory symptoms, bleeding and the acetate of lead are indicated;— when with symptoms of debility, the dilute sulphuric acid, alum, tinc. feari muriatis, or pulvis gallæ; and when with symptoms of gout, alkalis and colchicum are indicated. In hæmorrhage from the bladder, a catheter should be passed and be retained, in order to prevent both accumulation of blood in the bladder, and straining efforts at micturition. If the hæmorrhage is obstinate, the bladder may be injected with cold water containing a scruple of alum to each pint;—and if much blood have coagulated in the bladder, it will be necessary to break it down by repeated injections of water.

IV.—Suppression of Urine, *ischuria renalis.*—When the kidneys have been long abused by inordinate indulgence in strong drink, and are falling into disease, they are liable suddenly to lose their function of secreting the urine. The consequence of this is, that the urea and other elements of the urine accumulate in the blood; the patient complains of great uneasiness in the head and loins; he becomes first drowsy, and then comatose, and dies in four or five days, of effusion into the brain. This affection is alluded to here, in order to hint at the diagnosis between it and retention of urine. In suppression, if the catheter is in-

troduced, the bladder will be found empty; whereas in retention, whether
from stricture, or from diseased prostate, or from palsy of the bladder, it
may be felt full and distended above the pubes.*

SECTION VI.—OF URINARY DEPOSITES, GRAVEL, AND STONE ; AND OF THE DIA-
   THESIS, OR STATES OF CONSTITUTION WHICH GIVE RISE TO THEM.

Under particular diseased conditions of the system, certain substances
are precipitated from the urine.   If they are not precipitated from it till
it has cooled, they are commonly called *sediments;*—if they are precipitated whilst the urine is yet in the bladder, they constitute *gravel;*—and
lastly, they may lodge in some part of the urinary apparatus, and concrete into *stone.*   They may be divided into three classes; the lithic;
the oxalic; and the phosphatic.†

I. LITHIC DEPOSITES.—The lithic or *uric* acid, is an animal substance,
which is supposed by Dr. Prout to be formed out of the effete albuminous tissues of the body.   It is by itself insoluble, unless conbined with
an alkali; and in the urine, it is combined with ammonia, with which it
forms a salt, the superlithate of ammonia, the acid being in excess.  This
salt is held in perfect solution in the healthy urine; but if it is secreted in
unnatural quantity, it will be thrown down in the form of an impalpable
powder, constituting the *amorphous lithic sediment;*—and if there is an
unnatural quantity of acid in the urine, the lithic acid will be separated
from its ammonia, and will be thrown down into a crystalline form, constituting *lithic* or *red gravel.*

1. *Amorphous Lithic Sediments* may appear in three forms.  (*a*)
The first is that *yellowish sediment,* which appears in the urine of almost
every person, when the digestive organs are out of order.   It consists almost entirely of the lithate of ammonia (which Dr. Prout‡ sup-
poses to be formed of imperfect chyle) mixed with the colouring matter
of the urine, and a little of the phosphates, whose quantity will be proportioned to the whiteness of the sediment.   This form of sediment is
so common and well known, that little more need be said about it.   The
urine is always acid, and clear when passed.   The sediment is deposited
when it cools; but it may be dissolved again by adding hot water.

(*b*) A second variety is the *red* or *lateritious sediment,* which is
deposited in fever, and especially in gout and rheumatism.   This is
composed of the lithate of ammonia, combined with the colouring matter of the urine, and with a little of the *pupurate of ammonia.*

---

* See retention from stricture, p. 430; retention from enlarged prostate, p. 439;
† The chemical tests for these deposites will be shown when speaking of stone.
and retention from palsy of the bladder. p. 442.
‡ On Stomach and Urinary Diseases, Lond. 1840.

(c) A third variety is the *pink sediment*, which is very rare, and is deposited in some cases of organic disease and hectic. It consists of the lithate and purpurate of ammonia, without any of the colouring matter of the urine. Of these three sediments, and the states of constitution that give rise to them, it does not fall within the scope of this chapter to speak farther.

2. *Crystallized Lithic Deposites.*—The most common form of these is the *red gravel;* which consists of minute crystals of lithic acid like cayenne pepper. The urine from which it is precipitated is generally acid, high-coloured, and scanty, but clear. Sometimes the lithic acid is secreted in a semi-fluid state, which soon concretes into stone in the kidney. The symptoms attending the deposite of it, constitute what is called a *fit of the gravel.* They are, feverishness; pain in the loins, shooting down to the bladder; aching of the testicles and hips; and micturition exceedingly frequent, and attended with severe scalding.

*Causes.*—The *diathesis* or state of constitution in which lithic acid gravel is precipitated from the urine, is very frequently hereditary. It is intimately connected with the gout, (of which it will be recollected that deposites of the lithate of soda are highly characteristic,) and with the sanguine variety of scrofula. It may also be induced by errors in diet, and especially by inordinate indulgence in animal food, wine, and malt liquors. It is therefore in general a sign of a vigorous inflammatory habit. The ages at which it is most strongly marked, are before puberty, and between forty and sixty.

*Treatment.*—In the *first* place, the *diet* should be plain and temperate —consisting of meat once a day, and well dressed vegetables, but moderation in quantity is quite as important as attention to quality. Fermented liquors should be taken very sparingly—a little good sherry is the best. All acescent substances, such as malt liquors, pastry, and sweat wines, should be avoided. But ripe fruits, especially strawberries, are rather beneficial; the natural acids that they contain not being injurious like vinegar. *Secondly*, the action of the *skin* must be promoted by plenty of exercise—and by baths of hot water, hot air, or of the vapour of sulphur, if there is any difficulty in procuring perspiration, or if the skin is diseased. For it must be recollected that the skin naturally eliminates a considerable quantity of acid. *Thirdly*, the liver and bowels should be freely acted on by mercurials and purgatives, to which colchicum (F. 95, 99, 9, 42,) may be added if there is a gouty tendency. *Fourthly*, the superabundance of acid in the system must be counteracted by alkalis. Some prefer potass, some soda, some magnesia. About two hours after a meal is the best time for taking them. The objection to soda is, that it forms an insoluble salt with the lithic acid—and to magnesia, that it is apt to concrete into hardened masses in the intestines —so that the *bicarbonate* of potass, in doses of fifteen or twenty grains, appears the most useful. The liquor potassæ, although valuable as an alterative in skin disease, does not appear to be so efficacious in these cases as the carbonate. Lastly, benefit is generally obtained from diuretics. Dr. Prout recommends five grains of nitre to be added to each dose of alkali;—and soda water, and alkalis combined with vegetable acids, such as soda and seidiltz powders, are highly useful, for the vegetable acid is digested in the stomach, and the alkali passes to the kidneys.

II. OXALIC DEPOSITES.—The oxalic acid, when present in the system, is supposed by Dr. Prout to be derived either from the imperfect assimilation of vegetable matter in the stomach, or from an abnormal change in the gelatinous tissues of the body. Hence individuals who possess the *oxalic acid diathesis*, have generally a dry irritable skin, are exceedingly liable to boils, and in advanced age to carbuncles, and often suffer from dyspepsia, with flatulence and palpitations. But the train of constitutional symptoms belonging to this diathesis are of an irritable or nervous, rather than of a congestive or inflammatory character, as in the lithic diathesis. The urine is generally transparent, of a pale greenish yellow, or citron hue; and of moderate specific gravity. It is also remarkably free from sediments; so that individuals with this diathesis cannot be said to suffer from *gravel*. Moreover, it is very seldom (in proportion to the great number of individuals in whom this diathesis prevails) that stone is formed, and when this is the case it appears to be owing to an accidental secretion of unusual quantities of phosphate or carbonate of lime from the urinary organs; which, combining with the oxalic acid, form the *oxalate of lime*, or *mulberry* calculus.

*Causes.*—The oxalic diathesis, according to Dr. Prout, is exceedingly common; although, as it rarely leads to stone and never produces gravel, it is apt to pass unnoticed, amidst the dyspepsia hypochrondriasis, and skin disease, with which it is associated. It may be caused by residence in damp malarious situations, and by a diet of unwholesome saccharine or farinaceous matters. It may also be supposed to be induced or aggravated by partaking too freely of vegetables in which the oxalic acid exists; such as rhubarb stalks, and sorrel; although these substances in moderate quantity are readily digested by the healthy stomach.

*Treatment.*—All that can be said on this subject is, that the patient must be kept in as good a state of health as possible, by the strictest attention to diet and regimen. The diet should consist of plain animal food, with bread or other farinaceous matters, avoiding sugar, and all acescent substances, and hard water. The skin should be kept in order by flannel clothing, exercise, and occasional baths. If there are acidity and flatulence, *small* doses of alkalis with ammonia, F. 54, may be given after meals, whilst it may be advisable to fortify the stomach with bitters and small doses of mineral acids, F. 1, an hour or two before meals.

III. Phosphatic Deposites, *white gravel.* Of these there are three varieties; viz. 1. the *triple phosphate,* or *phosphate of ammonia and magnesia;* or *ammoniaco-magnesian phosphate;* 2. the *phosphate of lime;* and 3. the *mixed* or *fusible phosphates,* consisting of the first two varieties combined.

1. *Triple Phosphate.*—This salt is developed in the following manner. The phosphate of magnesia exists naturally in the urine as a highly soluble salt with its acid in excess. But it sometimes happens that it is secreted in preternatural quantity, and that at the same time the *urea* (a peculiar principle contained in the urine) is exceedingly prone to decomposition, and becomes converted into ammonia.* The ammonia, uniting with the phosphate of magnesia, forms an insoluble triple salt, the phosphate of ammonia and magnesia; which is precipitated in the form of minute brilliant white crystals, constituting the *white gravel.* The urine in these cases is always pale, more copious than natural, and of low specific gravity;—sometimes it is slightly opaque when passed;—it is very feebly acid, and scarcely, if at all, reddens litmus paper;—it has a faint nauseous smell, which soon becomes ammoniacal and offensive;—and it exhibits the peculiar crystals of the triple phosphate, which often float on the surface and look like an iridescent film of grease.

2. *Phosphate of Lime.*—This salt is deposited from the urine in the form of an impalpable powder, which is generally white, but is occasionally tinged with the colouring matter of the urine. The general characters of the urine are the same as those of the last variety. This salt is not strictly speaking, deposited *from the urine,* but is secreted by the mucous membrane of the kidneys and bladder when chronically inflamed or otherwise degenerated. We have shown in a preceding section, that it is contained in the viscid mucus of cystirrhæa (p. 440;) in fact, it is sure to be secreted if the urinary organs are subjected to long-continued irritation, whether from the too long retention of a catheter, or from a stone or other foreign body in the bladder, or from diseased urine.

3. *Mixed Phosphates.*—The phosphates of lime is very seldom deposited alone, but in by far the greater number of cases is associated with the triple phosphate;—an association that is easily accounted for;—for if the triple phosphate exist first in the urine, it is sure after a time, by irritating the urinary receptacles, to give rise to a secretion of phosphate of lime;—or, on the other hand, if the phosphate of lime is first secreted by the urinary mucous membrane, the state of constitution will be rendered such as speedily to induce an evolution of the triple phosphate from the kidneys. The urine in these cases is copious, pale, and stink-

* Urea is a *cyanate of ammonia;* and by a transposition of its elements is convertible into carbonate of ammonia.

57

ing, and deposites a thick mortar-like sediment, mixed with more or less of the crystallized triple phosphate.

*Causes.*—The *phosphatic diathesis* offers a remarkable contrast to the lithic, both in the qualities of the urine, and in the characters of the constitution, and in the causes which engender it. Persons whose urine deposites the triple phosphate, are of a pale, bloodless appearance, and complain of exhaustion and debility, and of an aching weak pain in the loins;—and Dr. Prout has very ingeniously attempted to show, that the great consumption of phosphorus, which is an essential constituent of all the nervous tissues, may be a cause of the great nervous irritability and exhaustion which accompany phosphatic deposites from the urine. This diathesis may be induced by insufficient and unwholesome food; inordinate bodily fatigue, or mental anxiety; hard study; night watching, and by lowering medicines, and especially by mercury, alkalis, and saline purgatives, (especially seidlitz powders, and others containing vegetable acid,) given in excess. Injuries of the spine also produce phosphatic urine, (vide p. 321;) and we need not again mention stricture, cystirrhæa, and other local causes.

*Treatment.*—The diet should be generous, but plain, and should include sound malt liquor, or port, or sherry.* The importance of good air and exercise needs scarcely be hinted at. The other remedies are tonics, acids, and opium. Bark, quinine, or steel, may be given in combination with the mineral acids, F. 3, 98, 26, 1, 69, and with opium; which in confirmed cases of phosphatic deposites in adults agrees remarkably well; allaying pain and nervous irritation without impairing the appetite or inducing costiveness. Buchu and uva ursi, F. 91, are also of service. If the mucous membrane of the bladder is diseased, recourse must be had to the remedies mentioned at p. 440. All diuretics are as a general rule injurious; and mercury and alkalis are unadvisable, except perhaps in small occasional doses when required by the state of the stomach. It must be observed in conclusion, that although phosphatic deposites are attended with an alkalescent state of the urine, and although they are as a general rule to be treated by acids, still that *acescent substances*, sugar, pastry, hard beer or cider, and especially the thin acid French wines which are sometimes recommended, are highly injurious. The author has had constant opportunities of observing the urine loaded with triple phosphate and highly ammoniacal, when the stomach has abounded in acidity; the simple fact being, that when the health is disordered by any means whatever, whether acidity in the stomach or not, the phosphates will be deposited if the diathesis exists. On this ac-

---

* Soda water is injurious if it contains soda, which as a mere article of luxury it ought not to do. But simple water impregnated with carbonic acid is grateful to the stomach and wholesome.

count, *small* doses of alkalis, F. 54, may occasionally be given in these cases with the greatest benefit *after meals,* if the stomach is disordered; whilst the tonics and acids may be given an hour or two before meals.

STONE.—The preceding deposites may, as we have observed, concrete into the stone, of which there are eleven species;—two lithic; three phosphatic; one oxalic; and five others, which are exceedingly rare.

I. LITHIC ACID calculi are generally oval, flattened, fawn or mahogany coloured, and on a section are seen to be composed of concentric laminæ. *Tests.*—This acid may be dissolved by boiling in *liquor potassæ;*—it burns away almost entirely before the blow-pipe, and if digested in nitric acid and evaporated, leaves a scarlet residue (*purpuric acid*) which becomes purple on the addition of ammonia.

II. LITHATE OF AMMONIA rarely forms a calculus, because it is tolerably soluble in warm urine. *Tests.*—It may be known by the same tests as the preceding—and besides it evolves ammonia when treated by liq. potassæ.

III. PHOSPHATE OF LIME or *bone earth* calculi are rare. They are pale brown, friable, and laminated. *Tests.*—Soluble in nitric or muriatic acids, and precipitated by liq. ammoniæ—infusible except at a very intense heat.

IV. TRIPLE PHOSPHATE (*of ammonia and magnesia*) forms white or pale gray calculi, composed of small brilliant crystals. *Tests.*— Soluble in acetic or muriatic acid—evolves ammonia when treated with liq. potassæ.

V. THE FUSIBLE CALCULUS is formed of the phosphate of lime and triple phosphate mixed. It forms a white friable mass like mortar, and is very fusible.

VI. THE MULBERRY CALCULUS is composed of oxalate of lime. It is dark red, rough, and tuberculated. *Tests.*—Soluble in nitric acid, and if exposed to the blow-pipe, the acid is burned off, and quick-lime is left, which, if moistened, reddens turmeric paper.

VIII. Besides the above, calculi are sometimes composed of *lithate of soda, carbonate of lime, cystic oxyde,* (a peculiar animal substance,) *fibrine* of the blood, and *silica.*

SECTION VII.—OF STONE IN THE KIDNEY AND URETER.

*Symptoms.*—The symptoms of stone in the kidney are, pain in one or both loins;—irritation and retraction of the testicles;—the urine bloody after violent jolting exercise;—and occasional fits of inflammation of the kidney. Stones in the kidney are most frequently composed of lithic acid; which will be known by the deposite of red sand from the urine.

The mulberry calculus is more rare; it may be suspected, if the urine is free from sediment either lithic or phosphatic, and if dark-coloured blood is frequently mixed with it. Phosphatic stone in the kidney is still more rare. When it does exist, it is generally composed of the phosphate of lime, and indicates incipient disease of the organ.

*Treatment.*—When a stone is ascertained or suspected to exist in the kidney, the indications are, *first*, to determine the peculiar diathesis, and take measures for counteracting it, as detailed in the last section;— *secondly*, to endeavour to expedite its expulsion through the ureter, by diluents and diuretics; and by the *cautious* use of exercise so as to dislodge it; and *thirdly*, to remove inflammation and pain by cupping on the loins, (if the habit is inflammatory,) by mild aperients, and copious enemata of warm water—by opium or henbane; and by warm baths or fomentations. Pounded ice applied to the loins gives great relief when much burning pain is complained of; but it must be used with caution.

The ordinary and most favourable event of renal calculus is, that it descends through the ureter into the bladder. In some cases, however, it remains in the kidney, increases in size, completely fills up the pelvis and infundibula, and causes the organ either to waste away or to suppurate;—the abscess bursting either into the colon, or on the loins.

THE PASSAGE OF A STONE THROUGH THE URETER causes the following symptoms. The patient complains of sudden and most severe pain, first in the loins and groin, subsequently in the testicle and inside of the thigh. The testicle is also retracted spasmodically. At the same time there are violent sickness, faintness, and collapse, which may last two or three days, and are only relieved when the stone reaches the bladder. *Treatment.*—The warm bath, large doses of opium, emollient enemata, and plenty of diluents, are the obvious remedies,—and an active purgative may perhaps be tried if the process is slow.

SECTION VIII.—OF STONE IN THE BLADDER.

STONE IN THE BLADDER produces the following *symptoms* —1. Irritability of the bladder,—frequent irresistible desire to make water. 2. Occasional sudden stoppage of the stream of water during micturition, from the stone falling on the orifice of the urethra;—the stream probably flowing again if the patient throws himself on his hands and knees. 3. Occasional pain at the neck of the bladder—always severest after micturition. 4. Pain in the glans penis. If the patient be a child, he is always attempting to alleviate this pain by pulling at the frænum, which becomes extremely elongated. 5. *Sounding.* But none of the above symptoms must be depended on alone. The existence of the stone must be made sensible to the ear and fingers by means of the sound—a solid iron rod like a catheter, but not so curved, and with a polished handle. This should be introduced—the patient lying on his back, the pelvis raised on a pillow, and the bladder nearly, but not quite, full. It should be carefully moved about to examine every part of the bladder, and if there is a stone of any size it will most probably be heard to strike and felt to grate upon it. If nothing, however, is discovered, the patient may be made to sit upright, or the finger may be passed into the rectum; or a catheter may be introduced, and the stone may perhaps be felt to strike against it as the urine flows away. But if the symptoms are well marked, the surgeon must not be contented with one unsuccessful examination. On the other hand, the rubbing of the sound on the bladder, or on gravel entangled in mucus, must not be too hastily set down as signs of stone.

The symptoms of stone vary in their severity, 1, according to its size and roughness; 2, according to the state of the urine; 3, according to the condition of the bladder, whether healthy or inflamed. They may be very slight for years,—in fact, a little pain in micturition and bloody urine after riding may be the only inconveniences. But after a certain period the bladder suffers just as it does from any other cause of irritation,—the urine deposites a slight cloud of mucus,—the bladder becomes more and more irritable and finally inflamed,—the urine becomes alkaline, and loaded with viscid mucus, and of course with the triple phosphate and phosphate of lime,—the strength fails, and finally, after years of suffering, the patient sinks under the irritation. Sir B. Brodie, however, has observed, that if the prostate become enlarged, the sufferings from stone are often mitigated; because it is prevented from falling on the neck of the bladder.

The sources of vesical calculi are two.—1, from the urine; 2, from the mucus of the bladder; and calculi are exceedingly liable to form from the latter source, if the prostate is diseased, or if foreign bodies are introduced into the bladder, so as to serve for a nucleus. In these cases, the stone is invariably phosphatic. And all calculi, whatever their original composition, are sure to become coated with the phosphates if they remain till the patient becomes old and the bladder diseased.

The *composition* of a calculus will be determined by the state of the urine. Its *size* may be appreciated, 1, by its composition—for the phosphatic are always the largest; 2, by the time it has existed; 3, by observing the force required to dislodge it from its situation; 4, it may be measured by passing the sound across its surface, or by the urethra forceps. Calculi have been known to vary in weight from a few grains to forty-four ounces, and in number from one to one hundred and forty-two. The largest that was ever extracted entire weighed sixteen ounces, but the patient died; Sir. A. Cooper was the operator. Gooch tells us that Mr. Harmer, of Norwich, in the year 1746, extracted one entire which weighed nearly fifteen ounces, and the patient lived five years.

And Mr. C. Mayo, of Winchester, extracted one weighing fourteen ounces and a half, but it was broken, and the patient lived several years.

*Treatment.*—The indications are, 1, to get rid of the diseased state of the urine; 2, to allay pain and irritation; 3, to remove the stone. The first and second are to be accomplished by measures which have been already spoken of when treating of gravel and of chronic inflammation of the bladder. The third may be executed in four ways, viz. by extraction of the stone through the urethra,—solution of it by injections,—lithotrity,—and lithotomy.

1. *Extraction by the Urethra.*—When a stone is known to have recently escaped from the ureter into the bladder, the first point is to remove all irritability of the bladder by sedatives, and by restoring the proper condition of the urine, so that there may be no spasm to obstruct its passage into the urethra. The patient also should drink plentifully, so that the bladder may be quite filled. Then, when he is going to make water, he should be instructed to lie on his face, and to grasp the penis so that the urethra may become distended with urine; and thus very probably, the sudden gush that will come, when he relinquishes his grasp of the penis, will bring the stone with it—or perhaps the urethra may be dilated by passing bougies. But should this plan not succeed after some days, Weiss's urethral forceps should be tried. The patient being placed on his back with his pelvis raised, a catheter is to be introduced to draw off the urine, and five or six ounces of tepid water, are to be injected afterwards. Next the forceps, being introduced, is to be made to feel for the stone, and the blades are to be cautiously opened over it and made to seize it. An index on the handle of the forceps will now show the size of the stone. If small, it may be extracted at once,—if very large, it must be left where it is,—if of a doubtful size, it may perhaps be brought into the membranous portion of the urethra, whence it can be extracted by incision.

2. *Solution by injections.*—Sir. B. Brodie has satisfactorily shown that *phosphatic* calculi may sometimes be dissolved altogether, and sometimes be so disintegrated or reduced in size that they may escape through the urethra by means of injections of very dilute nitric acid passed through a double gold catheter in the manner directed for chronic cystitis. At the same time, these injections diminish the secretion of mucus, which is the source of the phosphate of lime. There is no doubt also but that *lithic calculi* have been dissolved by means of mineral waters holding large quantities of carbonic acid in solution—especially the waters of Vichy; and that they have even been spontaneously disintegrated by the urine when it has been restored to its healthy condition. But the chance of such an event is so small, and the process so tedious, that it cannot at present be offered to a patient as even probable. Alkaline injections into the bladder are inexpedient.

SECTION IX.—OF LITHOTRITY.*

It need scarcely be said, that the object of this operation is to reduce stones in the bladder into fragments of so small a size, that they may be readily expelled through the urethra.

The apparatus by which this object was first accomplished by Civiale and Leroy was, as Sir. C. Bell rightly called it, villanous and dangerous enough. A straight cylindrical canula was introduced into the bladder, containing three or four branches which could be protruded from its extremity. These were made to grasp the stonè and hold it tightly, whilst it was bored, and scooped, and excavated by drills and other contrivances contained in the centre of the canula, and worked by a bow. When the stone was sufficiently excavated, its shell was crushed by a most complex piece of mechanism called the *brise coque*, or shell-breaker.

* Notwithstanding the frequency of calculous affections in the valley of the Mississippi, this operation has never been successfully performed, so far as I can learn, on this side of the mountains. ˙ On account of the deserved celebrity of Dr. Dudley, as a lithotomist, most of the cases have fallen into his hands, and his confidence is so much greater in the old operation, that he has never attempted the new one.

When Lithotrity was first exhibited in the operations of Civiale and Heurteloup, I participated in the apprehensions, entertained by most prudent surgeons, on account of the complex and dangerous machinery employed—apprehensions which were but too well justified by experience.

But often witnessing the beautiful and bloodless operations of Civiale and Leroy, during a visit to Paris in 1838, I was forced to dismiss my fears, and became persuaded that they were practising an improved method of removing vesical calculus, which every surgeon should prepare himself to imitate. The original formidable apparatus is now dispensed with—Mr. Civiale himself has hung up his drill-bow over his operating table, and now uses only the safe and simple instrument, partially figured in the text, which the combined ingenuity of an English artist and French surgeons, has furnished. This instrument may be introduced into the bladder with as much ease as a common catheter, and is no more likely to inflict injury upon that organ, if employed with ordinary intelligence and address, than the forceps that are used in Lithotomy.

Lithotrity, when employed only in suitable cases, is certainly less dangerous than lithotomy,—it is generally less painful, and far less revolting in its proceedings.

There are of course, certain conditions for its application, which do not obtain in every case of urinary calculus. It must not be offered as a universal substitute for lithotomy: but only as an alternative in a certain class of cases, and that, as I believe, the smaller class. Lithotomy must yet be the general method—lithotrity the exception. It is an exception, however, which those, in whose behalf it can be applied, are entitled to at the hands of their surgical adviser.

If practitioners would generally hold themselves prepared to employ this milder method of cure, and let the community be informed of this fact, patients would not postpone operative proceedings for relief, as they too frequently do at present from a dread of the knife, until the calculus becomes so large as to enhance extremely the danger attending the severer process which must then be employed for its removal. F.

"For sometime," says Mr. Liston, "it was maintained that almost every case of stone could be satisfactorily disposed of by this boring and grinding process. It was tried extensively," but, "after many miserable and painful failures, utterly disappointed the hopes of its advocates." Nor will these failures be wondered at, when we consider the difficulty sometimes of seizing the stone, sometimes of disentangling the instrument from it*—the extremely slow and inefficient means of disintegrating it, and the great number of times the operation was consequently obliged to be repeated;—not to mention the pain caused by the stretching of the urethra with a large straight instrument—the risk of entangling the coats of the bladder, and of seriously bruising the parts about the neck—and the most incomprehensible perplexity of the instruments employed—the nomenclature, structure, and use of which required not a little study.

The next method which was employed, and which was first practised by Heurteloup,† consisted in hammering the stone to pieces. The patient was confined to a bed of peculiar construction, called the *lit rectangulaire;* and the *percuteur courbe à marteau*—an instrument composed, like that represented in the next page, of two blades sliding on each other, was made to seize the stone. It was then broken by repeated blows with a hammer on the other extremity of the instrument, which was fixed securely to a vice. But this plan was fraught with many inconveniences. The instrument was liable to be bent or broken; its blades were apt to become so clogged with pulverized fragments, that they were withdrawn with difficulty, or perhaps not until the orifice of the urethra had been slit up;—and the bladder was exposed to injury from percussion communicated from the instrument, and from the violent splitting of the calculus.

The instrument which has now superseded the foregoing, is the *screw lithotrite* of Mr. Weiss; which is composed of two sliding blades, between which the stone is seized, and then is crushed by gradual pressure with a screw. This instrument was, in fact, originally invented in 1824, (although it was laid aside at the recommendation of Sir B. Brodie, who thought it liable to some objections, and was superseded for a time by the straight drills of Civiale and the *percuteur* of Heurteloup;)—and it was from this that Heurteloup took the idea of the *percuteur; disimproving* it, however, by substituting the hammer for the screw. It will be seen from the figure, that in order to prevent any clogging of the blades by the lodgment of fragments, the anterior blade is made open to receive

---

* In fact, in one case, the branches could not be returned into the canula; and the instrument was obliged to be dragged out open through the neck of the bladder, and urethra.

† In the year 1830.

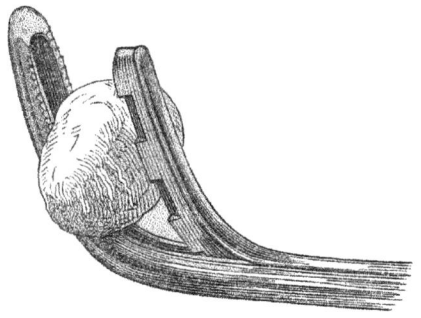

the other within it. The operation is performed as follows. The patient is placed on a couch with his pelvis well raised, and his shoulders comfortably supported;—the bladder is then emptied, and five or six ounces of tepid water injected with a proper catheter and syringe. The instrument, previously warmed and oiled, is introduced and placed upon the stone—its blades are opened and made to grasp it between them—the handle is moved from side to side, to ascertain that no part of the bladder is entangled—and then it is depressed so as to lift the stone towards the neck of the bladder. The screw is then slowly and cautiously turned backwards and forwards till the stone is crushed by its repeated impulses. The next thing is to seize and comminute the fragments either with the same instrument, or with one that has not the aperture in the anterior blade. Sometimes they may be removed with sundry scoops. But whether this can be done at one sitting or at many, must depend on the size of the stone, and the degree of inconvenience suffered by the patient.

No fair numerical estimate can yet be made of the proportion of cases in which lithotrity has been successful or otherwise. In its present improved form, and practised on patients calculated for it, it may be considered easy, safe, and effectual. But practised indiscriminately, as it formerly was, on all kinds of cases, and with imperfect instruments, the mortality was frightful—equal, as Dr. Willis says, to that of a pestilence—certainly one in four, but much more probably one in two. Whereas the statistics of lithotomy give only one unfavourable case in seven or eight. The results in the hands even of scientific surgeons have been far from favourable. Of twelve cases narrated by Mr. Key, three were cured by it—in three it was either inapplicable or unavailing, and lithotomy was resorted to—and the remaining six perished—one with abscess in the prostate soon after the operation—four with protracted sufferings from irritation of the bladder by the fragments which were retained—and one with disease of the bladder brought on or aggravated by the operation. Mr. W. Fergusson gave the results of eighteen cases; of which six were cured; seven were not cured, (and four of these underwent lithotomy afterwards;) and five died.* The source of danger is the substitution of many irregular fragments for one smooth stone, and the number of times the operation must be repeated. The preparatory treatment consists in the use of measures for removing the diseased condition of the urine, and any irritability of the bladder. In the after treatment, diluents should be employed to increase the secretion of urine, and injections of warm water to accelerate the passage of the fragments—and hip-baths, opiates, and leeches, or cupping on the perinæum, for the relief of pain or inflammation. Sometimes the fragments stick in the urethra, and require to be removed by incision in the perinæum, and sometimes it is requisite, after all, to extract them from the bladder by a regular lithotomy operation.

### SECTION X.—OF LITHOTOMY.

Supposing that a patient with stone in the bladder is an adult, that the stone is under the size of a chestnut, and that the bladder and urethra are healthy, as shown by the power of retaining the water, and making it in a good stream, the operation of *lithotrity* may be recommended. But if the stone is very large or very hard—or if there are more than one, or if the urethra is strictured, or the prostate enlarged (which would prevent the *débris* of the stone from coming away)—or the coats of the bladder diseased—or the stone adherent, or contained in pouches or sacculi of the bladder—or if the patient is very old or very young, it will be safer to extract the stone by lithotomy.

The surgeon must, however, in the first place, ascertain that the patient is free from serious organic disease—which would render him liable to sink under either operation. Languor, depression, loss of strength and flesh and appetite, irregular shiverings, pain and tenderness in the loins, purulent or highly albuminous or bloody urine, indicating organic disease of the kidneys;—excessively frequent and painful micturition, with the urine constantly bloody and purulent, indicating serious organic disease or ulceration of the prostate or bladder—the existence of hectic or pulmonary consumption, or of any other extensive disease, require the surgeon to decline the operation—or at least to perform it only at the urgent and repeated request of the patient, who should be informed of its probable result. In the second place, the patient must be well prepared by measures calculated to improve the general health, and to remove all disorder of the urine and irritability of congestion of the bladder. He should not even be sounded whilst labouring under any local or general vascular excitement.

* Ed. Med. and Surg. Journ. Oct. 1838.

There are four methods in which lithotomy may be performed, viz. the lateral operation of the perinæum—the bilateral—the recto-vesicle— and the high operation. The lateral is that which common consent has decided to be the best, except in a few rare instances. There are sundry varieties in the manner of performing it, and in the instruments employed by different surgeons. The author will first describe the method recommended by Mr. Liston, not only on account of its simplicity, but because he is enabled, by that gentleman's kindness, to make use of the same admirable wood engraving which illustrates the subject in his Practical Surgery.

*Lateral Operation.*—It is advisable that the bowels should be cleared on the morning of the operation with a simple enema. The bladder should be moderately full, and if the patient has recently emptied it, a few ounces of water may be injected. It is also desirable that the existence of the stone should be clearly demonstrated with the sound or staff, immediately before the operation.—Then the proceedings may commence by introducing the *staff*—a solid steel rod like a sound, with a deep groove, either on its convex border, or, as some surgeons prefer it, a little on its left side. It should be as large as can be conveniently introduced.

The next point is to fix the patient in a convenient posture. He should be placed on his back, on a table two feet and a-half high, with his shoulders resting in the lap of an assistant, who sits astride behind him. Then in order to expose the perinæum thoroughly, he must be made to raise and separate his thighs; and to grasp the outside of each foot with the hand of the same side; and the hand and foot are to be firmly bound together by a broad garter;—meanwhile, if not done before, the perinæum should be shaved. Every thing being now prepared,—an assistant on each side holding the thighs firmly asunder—another being at hand to give the surgeon his instruments—and a third stationed on the left side holding the staff perpendicularly, and well hooked against the symphysis pubis—in which position he is to hold steadily from first to last;—the surgeon commences by passing his knife to the depth of an inch on the left side of the raphe, about an inch before the anus, and cut downwards and outwards to the bottom of the perinæum, midway between the anus and tuberosity of the ischium. " The forefinger of the left hand," says Mr. Liston, " is then placed in the bottom of the wound about its middle, and directed upwards and forwards; any fibres of the transverse muscle, or of the levator of the anus, that offer resistance, are divided by the knife, its edge turned downwards;—the finger passes readily through the loose cellular tissue, but is resisted by the deep fascia, immediately anterior to which, the groove of the staff can be felt not thickly covered. The point of the instrument is slipped along the nail of the finger, and, guided by it, is entered, the back still directed upwards, into the groove, at this point.*   The finger all along is placed so as to depress and protect as much as possible the coats of the rectum, and the same knife, pushed forwards, is made to divide the deep fascia, the muscular fibres within its layers, a very small portion—not more than two lines—of the urethra anterior to the apex of the prostate, together with the prostatic portion of

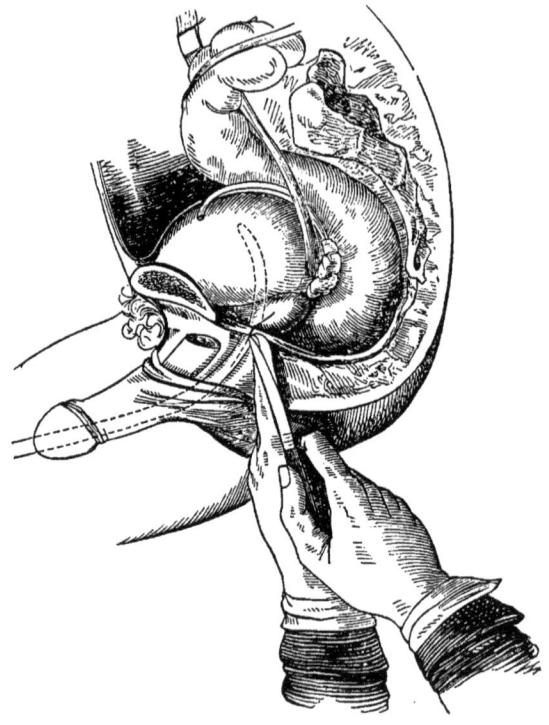

the canal and the gland to a very limited extent."   The direction of this incision through the prostate should be downwards and outwards—corresponding of course to that of the whole wound—and its extent should not

---

* Most operators at the present day, in performing Lithotomy, employ the knife in some one of its modifications for the prostatic section—indeed I know but a single exception to this practice, among distinguished lithotomists. My neighbour and friend Prof. Dudley of Lexington, who has cut more frequently than any living surgeon, and with better success than any man who ever lived and has furnished authentic reports of his operations, invariably uses the gorget, and all who have witnessed this gentleman's operations admire the dexterity, precision and despatch with which he opens the bladder with this instrument, which, in most other hands, seems clumsy and unsafe beyond any that has been invented, for the same purpose.   Dr. Dudley's extraordinary success is principally due to his judicious management of his cases previous and subsequent to the operation—an attribute which should entitle him to more credit, as a good surgeon, than the most imposing use of the best-continued apparatus, in the performance of it.

Prof. Dudley has now operated for stone in the bladder *one hundred and seventy*

be greater than seven lines. The next thing is to withdraw the knife, and pass the finger along the staff into the bladder, to ascertain the position and size of the stone. If the patient is young and thin, the forceps may now be at once introduced: but if he is an adult, and especially if the prostate is large and rigid, it will be proper to use the *blunt gorget* previously, in order to dilate the aperture in the gland. The surgeon takes it in his right hand, with the concave surface uppermost, places its *beak* in the groove of the staff, and pushes it gently into the bladder. Then the staff being removed, a forceps suited to the size of the stone is to be very gently introduced into the bladder. If the gorget was used, it may be passed along its concave surface before it is withdrawn. It must be introduced closed, and brought into contact with the stone—then the blades are opened over it and made to grasp it;—if the stone is seized awkwardly, it is relinquished and seized again—then it is extracted by slow, cautious, undulating movements.

*times*, and he is confident that a fatal termination, occurring as the effect of the operation, has taken place *in a single instance only*. A few years ago, when the number of his cases amounted to *one hundred and thirty-five*, he published a statement which exhibited such unprecedented success as to excite the astonishment of surgeons in all countries, and in some quartersto provoke expressions of incredulity and even suspicion of misrepresentation, injurious towards Dr. Dudley and unworthy of those who promulgated them. Yielding, even the four unsuccessful cases which M. Civiale has inferred from Dr. B's own account of his operations, a triumphant success must still be conceded to him in this department of our art, which should rebuke the spirit of envy, and will secure from all magnanimous cotemporaries an acknowledgment of his title to be regarded as the greatest Lithotomist of his day.

In my own operations I have used the knife recommended, and I believe, invented by Mr. Liston—an elongated scalpel with a cutting edge extending from the point to about midway of the blade. With this instrument, having a long and stout handle, the surgeon may accomplish all his incisions from the integument through, with the utmost convenience and precision, and, if sufficiently sure of his anatomy to justify an attempt at such an operation, may avoid all parts which should remain intact, with more certainty than in the employment of any one of the various instruments and apparatus which ancient or modern invention has supplied.

The directions in the text, respecting the staff, are pertinent and important. It should be held perpendicularly, and firmly in one position until the incisions are completed, as our author directs. Nothing savours more of discomfort and embarrassment in such proceedings, than to hear the operator calling to his staff holder to " bulge the staff into the perineum." If he cannot find the staff, when he has approached the membranous portion of the urethra, it is either because his anatomy fails him at the most critical point in his undertaking, or because he is bewildered by his devious and unskilful progress through the textures already divided.

In observing the direction to have the staff well hooked against the symphysis pubis, the operator should be careful not to drag upwards the portions of urethra which are to be divided, so that when suffered to resume their natural relations upon the withdrawal of the staff, the continuity of the external and internal incisions shall be interrupted. F.

The general maxims to be borne in mind during the performance of this operation are, (1) to make a free external aperture, and to bring it low enough down, so that the urine may subsequently escape freely without infiltrating the cellular tissue; (2) not to cut too high up, or to open the urethra too much in front, for fear of wounding the bulb or its artery; (3) not to wound the rectum, or pudic artery, by carrying the incisions too much inwards or outwards; (4) and above all, not to cut *completely through* the prostate, beyond its fibrous envelope, otherwise the urine will find a ready passage into the loose cellular tissue of the pelvis, and the patient will almost surely die.

The varieties of this operation before alluded to are as follow. Most surgeons direct the assistant to hold the staff so that it may project in the perinæum, and incline a little to the left side of it,—and when they have opened the urethra, and are about to incise the neck of the bladder, they take its handle in their own left hand, and bring it down horizontally. Some surgeons use a straight staff; but it renders the artery of the bulb more likely to be wounded. Again, there are great diversities' in the manner of cutting into the bladder. Many use a *beaked knife;* some a *bistouri cachée,* an instrument containing a blade that protrudes to a certain extent on touching a spring—and not a few use the *cutting gorget;* the beak of which being put into the groove of the staff, held horizontally in the operator's left hand, it is pushed cautiously on, and made to cut its way into the bladder. If this instrument is employed, every precaution must be used to keep it in contact with the staff, and not to let it slip between the bladder and rectum,—an accident that has been the death of not a few. In the case of a very large stone, it will be expedient to divide both sides of the prostate. This may be done, either by cutting into the bladder with a double-edged beaked knife—or after one side is incised in the ordinary way, by cutting through a little of the other with a probe-pointed bistoury, the edge of which should be directed towards the right *tuber ischii.* Lastly, there is the method which was employed by Cheselden, and which is still practised by a very experienced and successful lithotomist, Mr. C. Mayo of Winchester. In this method, the operator, after making the usual external incisions, " cuts into the side of the prostate as far back as he can reach, and brings out the knife, along the groove of the staff, into the membranous part of the urethra;" thus making the incision into the neck of the bladder from behind forwards, instead of from before backwards, as in the other varieties.*

*After Treatment.*—When every fragment of the stone has been re-

---

* There has been very much dispute about this operation of Cheselden's; principally because of a bungling description given of it by Dr. Douglass; but whoever will consult Cheselden's Anatomy, 6th ed. London, 1741, p. 330, will see that it agrees strictly with that performed by Mr. C. Mayo, and described by him in Med. Chir. Trans. vol. xi.

moved, and the bladder has been syringed with warm water, the patient should be put to bed. He should lie on his back with his shoulders elevated; a napkin should be applied to the perinæum to soak up the urine, and the bed be protected by oilcloth. It is a good plan to introduce a large gum elastic canula through the wound into the bladder for it to flow through. If not, the surgeon should introduce his finger after a few hours, to clear the wound of coagula. Pain must be allayed by anodynes—the bowels be kept open without purging—the wound be kept perfectly clean, and then, in favourable cases, the urine begins to flow by the urethra in about a week, and the wound heals completely in four or five.

*Complications.*—(1) Severe hæmorrhage may proceed from the pudic or bulbous arteries if wounded. If the bleeding orifice cannot be secured, it must be compressed as long as may be necessary with the finger. A general venous or arterial oozing must be checked by filling the wound firmly with lint or sponge—the tube being then indispensable. (2) Tenderness of the belly and other inflammatory symptoms must be combated by leeches, fomentations, and, if necessary, venæsection. (3) Chronic inflammation of the bladder, with continued secretion of the phosphates, by the measures directed at p. 441. (4) Sloughing of the cellular tissue from urinous infiltration, a frequent result of a hasty operation, and of too freely incising the neck of the bladder, is indicated by heat of the skin and sleepiness, followed by a rapid jerking, intermittent pulse—hiccup, —the belly tympanitic, the countenance anxious, and the other signs of irritative or typhoid fever. To be treated by wine, bark, and ammonia, and by laying the wound into the rectum, so that the urine may escape.

THE BILATERAL OPERATION is performed by making a curved incision, with the convexity upwards, from one side of the perinæum to the other —carrying it between the anus and bulb of the urethra—opening the membranous portion of the urethra—and then pushing a double *bistouri cachée* into the bladder, by which both sides of the prostate may be divided.

THE RECTOÆSICAL OPERATION consists in cutting into the bladder from the rectum, in the middle line, behind the prostate.

THE HIGH OPERATION is performed by making an incision through the linea alba, and opening the bladder, (which is projected upwards on the point of a catheter,) at its fore and upper part, where it is uncovered by peritonæum. This operation may be occasionally resorted to when the stone is of great size, and the prostate much enlarged, or the space between the tuberosities of the ischia contracted.

STONE IN WOMEN is much less frequent than it is in men, and when a renal calculus reaches the bladder, it is much more easily voided. If, however, there is a calculus too large to escape, the urethra should be dilated with one of Weiss's dilators;—and if the stone is large, the process may be expedited by making a slight incision with a bistoury, or *bistouri cachée*, through the urethra towards the pubes. Some degree of lucontinence of urine is apt to follow these operations.

---

# 'CHAPTER XXI.

## OF THE DISEASES OF THE MALE GENITALS.

### SECTION I.—OF THE DISEASES OF THE PENIS.

I. PHYMOSIS signifies a preternatural constriction of the orifice of the urethra, so that the glans cannot be uncovered. It may be a congenital affection, or may be caused by the contracted cicatrices of ulcers. Besides the obstruction which it occasions to the functions of the organ, it prevents the washing away of the natural secretions of the part, and thus renders the patient liable to frequent *balanitis* and gleets, and in advanced age to cancer of the penis.

*Treatment.*—A director should be introduced as far as possible between the glans and prepuce, and a curved, narrow-pointed bistoury be passed along its groove, by which the prepuce should be slit up. It

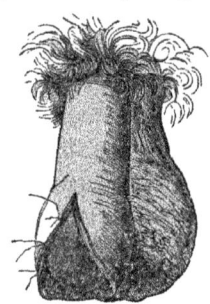

does not signify whether this is done on the upper or under surface. At the same time, if the edge of the prepuce is thickened, it should be seized between the blades of a forceps, and be shaved off. Then four or five sutures should be passed through the margin of the incision, so as to draw together the edge of the skin and that of the mucous lining of the prepuce, that they may unite by adhesion. If this is not done, the skin and mucous membrane will be separated by the swelling that follows the operation and the wound, instead of being a mere line, will be half an inch wide. For a knowledge of this operation, the author is indebted to Mr. William Fergusson.

II. PARAPHYMOSIS is said to exist when a tight prepuce is pulled back over the glans, constricting it, and causing it to swell. *Treatment.*— The surgeon first compresses the glans with the fingers of one hand, so as to squeeze the blood out of it,—then pushes it back with that hand, whilst he draws the prepuce forwards with the other. If this fails, the constricting part of the prepuce must be divided with a curved pointed bistoury.

III. CANCER of the penis may begin either on the glans or on the prepuce,—and invariably occurs to elderly persons who have had phymosis.
It forms a foul, ragged, excavated ulcer, gradually destroying the whole
organ, and contaminating the glands in the groin. *Treatment.*—The
part must be amputated before the glands are affected. The surgeon
stretches it out with one hand, and cuts it off with one sweep of a bistoury; bleeding vessels are then to be tied, and cold to be applied,—and
after three or four days a piece of bougie is to be introduced into the orifice of the urethra, and to be retained there during the cicatrization.

IV. EPISPADIAS is a congenital malformation, consisting of an imperfect closure of the urethra on its upper surface. HYPOSPADIAS is a similar deficiency of the under surface. They sometimes may be relieved by
pairing the edges of the skin on each side of the fissure, and uniting it
by suture,—provided that the urethra is pervious to the end of the penis.

V. TUMOURS.—The natives of warm climates are liable to a sarcomatous growth of the cellular tissue of the penis and scrotum, forming an
immense tumour in which those parts are completely buried. Poor Hoo
Loo, the Chinese, had a tumour of this sort. Extirpation is the only
cure,—and if the tumour is very large, no attempt can be made to save
the penis and testicles.

SECTION II.—OF THE DISEASES OF THE TESTIS AND SCROTUM.

I. ACUTE INFLAMMATION of the testis (*acute testitis, orchitis,*) may be
caused by local violence, but more frequently occurs in conjunction with
gonorrhœa, through a translation or an extension of inflammation from
the urethra. It is very liable to be induced if the patient indulges in violent exercise and fermented liquors, or neglects to use a suspensory bandage while employing injections. *Symptoms.*—The discharge from the
urethra diminishes, and the patient soon complains of aching pain in the
testis and cord, extending up to the loins, and soon followed by great
swelling, excruciating tenderness, fever, and vomiting. The epididymis
is the part chiefly affected. *Treatment.*—Bleeding if the habit is very
plethoric,—the repeated application of numerous leeches,—an emetic,
cold lotions or warm fomentations, according to the patient's feelings,—
a suspensory bandage to elevate the part,—purgatives,—and calomel,
opium, and antimony, F. 6, in repeated doses, are the requisite measures.
After the acute stage has subsided, strong astringent lotions, F. 16, may
be employed, and subsequently friction with mercurial ointment, in order
to remove the hardness and swelling which (as the patient should always
be informed) remain after the acute attack. The French surgeons are in
the habit of using *compression* immediately after the very acute stage has
subsided; and the practice is recommended by Mr. Langston Parker and
Mr. Acton. The affected testicle is grasped and separated from its fel-

low, and then is encircled with longitudinal and circular strips of adhesive plaster; which are to be applied regularly and with sufficient tightness to cause some uneasiness at first;—which, however, ought soon to
subside.*

II. Chronic Inflammation is known by more or less hardness,
swelling, tenderness, and occasional pain. Very often it commences in
the epididymis. It may be a sequel of acute inflammation,—or may be
caused by disease in the urethra, or disorder of the health. It sometimes
depends on a syphilitic taint,—which will be probable, if the patient has
the aspect of secondary syphilis, if the pain is principally severe at night,
and if there are secondary venereal affections of other parts. *Treatment.*
—The patient must be confined to his bed or sofa,—mercury be administered till it begins to touch the gums,—the bowels be kept open, the diet
moderately low. If an ordinary course of mercury seems inexpedient,
the iodide of potassium, or corrosive sublimate, with sarsaparilla, F. 29,
30, 56, 57, 93, will probably be of service. The part may be frequently
bathed with F. 11, 15, 16; or F. 25 may be applied with moderate pressure, as directed at p. 265.

III. Abscess of the testis may be a result of chronic or scrofulous inflammation—very rarely of the acute. A puncture should be made as
soon as fluctuation is clearly felt, and the skin is adherent. When an
aperture is formed, spontaneously or by art, part of the tubular texture
of the gland is apt to protrude in the form of a pink, fungous, irregular
mass. This will probably be got rid of by pressure with strips of plaster,
and by stimulating lotions and ointments,—but if not, it must be shaved
clean off.

IV. Scrofulous Inflammation commences with a deposite of tubercle in some part of the testis or epididymis, either into or between the
tubuli. A slow, painless, nodular swelling appears externally, which after a time inflames and bursts, and gives exit to the fungous protrusion
just mentioned. *Treatment.*—The health must be invigorated by tonics,
alteratives, and change of air, and the local actions be excited by stimulating lotions. When all the tubercular matter has been evacuated, the
abscess heals of itself; but before this occurs, the whole organ is often
disorganized and rendered useless.

V. Atrophy of the testicle may be a result of acute inflammation, or
of excessive venereal indulgence. The gland dwindles to the size of a
pea. There is no cure.

VI. Irritable Testis is a form of neuralgia. The testis and cord
are attacked with fits of excruciating pain, which leaves them tender and
slightly swollen. The *treatment* must be the same as that of neuralgia
generally. All the secreting and excreting organs must be set in order.

---

* Vide Acton on the Venereal Disease, Lond. 1841.

Violent purgatives in general do mischief; a few leeches,—the application of intense cold, (F. 12,)—counter-irritants, and opiate or belladonna plasters—sometimes afford relief. The internal remedies most likely to do good are, sarsaparilla, quinine, arsenic, and other tonics. But in every case, the cure is uncertain and tedious, and many patients have been compelled by the constant pain to seek relief by castration.

VII. The Hydatid Disease is very rare, and occurs almost exclusively, to adults. The testicle swells exceedingly, and its interior is filled with a number of cysts containing a watery fluid. This affection is incurable, but not malignant. When the part becomes of unsightly magnitude, it must be removed.

VIII. Malignant Disease of the testis is almost invariably medullary sarcoma, very rarely scirrhus. At first the gland swells, and becomes very hard and heavy; it is scarcely, if at all, painful or tender, and merely causes slight aching in the loins by its weight. After a time it enlarges rapidly and feels soft,—the cord swells,—there are occasional darting pains,—a fungus protrudes, the lumbar glands become affected, and cachexia, and death soon follow in the ordinary course, (P. 123.—127.) This disease is to be distinguished from hydrocele by its opacity and weight,—and from chronic inflammation or the hydatid disease by the darting pains, swelling of the cord, and cancerous cachexia. It may farther be distinguished from chronic inflammation by the fact, that neither mercury nor any other remedy produces any permanent benefit. *Treatment.*—Castration should be performed before the cord is affected.

IX. Castration is performed thus:—the scrotum being shaved, the surgeon grasps it behind to stretch the skin, and then makes an incision from the external abdominal ring to the very bottom of the scrotum. If there is any doubt as to the nature of the disease, he may next open the tunica vaginalis to examine the testis. Then he separates the cord from its attachments, and an assistant holds it between his finger and thumb, to prevent it from retracting when divided. The operator now passes his bistoury behind the cord, and divides it—and seizing the lower portion draws it forwards and dissects out the testicle. The arteries of the cord and others requiring it, are then to be tied; and the wound must not be closed till all bleeding has ceased.*

X. Hæmatocele signifies an extravasation of blood into the tunica vaginalis in consequence of injury. It is sometimes combined with ecchymosis of the scrotum. If the quantity extravasated is small, bleed-

---

* It is often more convenient to terminate the operation by the section of the cord, having previously separated the testis from the integuments. The retraction of the cord leading to irrepressible hæmorrhage, so much feared by some surgeons, may always be prevented by dissecting its cremasteric envelope from the duct and vessels well up towards the abdominal ring, and dividing these essential elements of the cord by themselves. F.

ing and cold lotions may cause it to be absorbed. If large, a puncture should be made, and a poultice be applied, for the blood to ooze into gradually.

XI. HYDROCELE signifies a collection of serum in the tunica vaginalis. *Symptoms.*—It forms a pear-shaped swelling, smooth on its surface, fluctuating if pressed, free from pain and tenderness, and causing merely a little uneasiness by its weight. The epididymis can be felt on the posterior surface of the tumour near the bottom. On placing a lighted candle on one side of the scrotum, the light can be discerned through it. *Causes.*—Hydrocele may be a sequel of inflammation of the testis, but more frequently arises without any local cause. It is often supposed to follow strains of the loins or belly. *Diagnosis.*—Solid enlargements of the testis may be distinguished from hydrocele by their weight, solidity, and greater painfulness, and by the absence of fluctuation or transparency. The diagnosis from hernia will be found at p. 413.

*Varieties.*—It sometimes happens that the tunica vaginalis preserves its communication with the abdomen, and then becomes filled with serum, forming a cylindrical tumour extending up to the abdominal ring. On raising and compressing it, the fluid is slowly squeezed into the abdomen, and slowly trickles down again afterwards. This case is liable to be complicated with a *congenital* or *encysted hernia*, to prevent which a truss should be worn. Sometimes the transparency and fluctuation of hydrocele are absent in consequence of a thickening of the tunica vaginalis, which may be known, according to Brodie, by noticing that the thickened membrane forms a projection along the epididymis,—whereas in solid enlargements of the testicle, the projection of the epididymis is lost. Sometimes the tunica vaginalis is partially adherent to the testicle. Sometimes loose cartilages are found in the sac,—they are easily removed by a slight incision.

*Treatment.*—The remedies for hydrocele are threefold. (1.) Strong discutient lotions (F. 16) which sometimes assist the cure in children, but cannot be depended on for adults. (2.) Evacuation of the serum, or the *palliative cure.* This may be accomplished by a puncture with a common lancet, or trocar; but the method most commonly adopted at present, consists in making a number of punctures with a large needle, so that the fluid may escape from the tunica vaginalis into the cellular tissue of the scrotum. There is also another plan of recent introduction. A fine curved pointed bistoury is thrust into the swelling at its lower part, and is passed up to the top of it. Then its point is to be made to divide the tunica vaginalis from top to bottom, so as to lay open the sac into the cellular tissue of the scrotum;—but it will of course be understood that the skin is merely to be punctured, and not divided farther. This *palliative treatment* is always sufficient for children, and sometimes for adults.

(3.) *Radical Cure.*—This, which is generally necessary for adults, is performed by injecting certain stimulating fluids, or by introducing setons or other foreign substances into the tunica vaginalis, in order to excite a degree of inflammation sufficient to destroy its secreting faculty. It must not be forgotten, however, that this *radical cure* is totally inadmissible, if the testis is diseased, or if the hydrocele is complicated with an irreducible hernia, or if the tunica vaginalis preserves its communication with the abdomen. Mere thickening from *previous* disease is, however, no objection. *Operation.*—The surgeon grasps the tumour behind, and introduces a trocar and canula into the sac—pointing the instrument upwards, so that it may not wound the testicle. He next withdraws the trocar, at the same time pushing the canula well into the sac, so that none of the fluid that is to be injected may pass into the cellular tissue of the scrotum. When all the serum has escaped, he injects from two to four ounces of some stimulating fluid through the canula, by means of an elastic bottle fitted with a stop-cock. Equal parts of port wine and water or zinc lotion (F. 15) are commonly used. When it has remained from three to five minutes, according to the degree of pain which it causes, it is suffered to flow out, and the canula is withdrawn. Some degree of inflammation follows, and more effusion into the sac—but the latter generally disappears in a fortnight or three weeks. If the cure is not quite perfect, the operation may be repeated after a few weeks.

XII. HYDROCELE OF THE CORD is a transparent, fluctuating, encysted tumour of slow growth, containing a clear water. If large, it must be punctured.

XIII. VARICOCELE (*Cirsocele* or *Spermatocele*) signifies a varicose state of the veins of the spermatic cord. It is caused by the ordinary causes of varix; that is to say, by obstruction to the return of blood, through corpulence, constipation, tight belts round the abdomen, and the like. It is much more common on the left side than on the right; obviously because the left spermatic vein is more liable to be pressed upon by fæcal accumulations in the sigmoid flexure of the colon, and because its course is longer and less direct than that of the right vein. *Treatment.*—In ordinary cases, sufficient relief may be obtained by keeping the bowels thoroughly open;—by frequently washing the scrotum with cold water or astringent lotions, so as to constringe the skin;—and by supporting it with a suspensory sling made of *open silk net*, and fastened up with two tapes, which are to be fastened round the abdomen and tied in front;—but it should have no tapes passing behind between the legs. But there are some cases in which this disease produces very serious inconvenience—pain in the scrotum and loins—sense of dragging at the stomach—loss of appetite and flatulence—and despondency of mind—and for these cases, something more must be done. Mr. Wormald recommends the loose skin of the scrotum to be pinched up and confined with a steel ring. Blisters and counter-irritants, so as to inflame and condense the scrotum;—division of the veins by the knife or caustic, and passing setons of thread through them, have had their advocates;—and even the barbarous operation of passing a ligature through the scrotum, and tying up all the vessels except the artery and vas deferens, and the skin of half the scrotum, so that they may be divided by ulceration, has been practised by certain Frenchmen. But the best plan is that of Sir A. Cooper, which consists in cutting away a good piece of the loose relaxed skin. " The manner of performing it is as follows;—The patient being placed in the recumbent posture, the relaxed scrotum is drawn between the fingers; the testis is to be raised to the ring by an assistant; and then the portion of the scrotum is to be removed by the knife." Any artery requiring it must be tied; and cold must be applied to check bleeding; and then the lower flap of the scrotum must be brought upwards and forwards, and be attached by sutures to the fore and upper part;—and a suspensory bag should be applied to press the testis upwards, and glue the scrotum to its surface. It is of no use to remove too little of the skin.*

XIV. Acute Œdema of the Scrotum.—The loose cellular tissue of this part is exceedingly liable to serous infiltration, from inflammation or dropsy. But there is one form of acute œdema, which has been particularly described by Mr. Liston,† and which is liable to supervene on excoriations of the parts in unhealthy persons. The scrotum becomes enormously swollen and tense, and soon sloughs unless a free incision is made in the mesial line. The case very much resembles extravasation of urine, but may be distinguished by the absence of swelling in the perinæum, and of obstruction in micturition.

XV. Chimney-sweeper's Cancer is a foul ragged ulcer of the scrotum, with the skin hardened and tuberculated around. It rarely, if ever, occurs till after the age of thirty. It commences as a small wart, and is caused by the irritation of soot. The whole of the ulcer, and of the diseased skin around it, must be extirpated—but it is rarely if ever necessary to remove either of the testicles.

### SECTION III.—OF IMPOTENCE.

Impotence in the male may depend on a variety of conditions. (1.) It may be caused by absence, or mutilation, or malformation, or original weakness and want of development of the genital organs. (2.) After

---

* Vide Sir A. Cooper, Guy's Hosp. Rep. vol. iii.; Reynaud, Journ. des Connaissances Med., Feb. 1839; and James in Prov. Med. Trans. for 1840. The diagnosis of varicocele has been spoken of at page 414.

† Med. Chir. Trans., vol. xxii.

a severe and tedious illness, the genitals may remain incapable of per-forming their functions, long after the restoration of the health and strength in other respects. Steel and other tonics, with cantharides, musk, spices, eggs, and oysters, are the remedies. Phosphorus in doses of gr. $\frac{1}{40}$ dissolved in oil, is said to be a potent *aphrodisiac* in these cases. (3.) It often happens that a young man, the first time he yields to carnal temptation—or that a newly married man on the night of his nuptials, finds himself incapable of accomplishing his wishes—through awkwardness, or timidity, or over-anxiety on his own part, or, perhaps, from something disagreeable in his bed-fellow. He straightway fancies himself impotent—and if he applies to one of the advertising scoundrels, will no doubt be told that he is so. The surgeon should cheer the patient's spirits, and should inform him that his case is by no means uncommon—that most other men feel the same incapability at times; and he should give him a little nitric æther and cinnamon water, and make him promise to sleep with the lady three nights without touching her, which will seldom fail to prove an effectual cure. (4.) Lastly, impo-tence may be produced by premature and excessive venery. Such cases frequently come under the observation of the London surgeon, who has no difficulty in distinguishing them from the last variety. The patients are generally singularly fond of talking about their ailments, and describing a number of beastly minutiæ; and they either have lost the power of erec-tion—or perhaps, a discharge of a thin fluid follows it immediately. General tonics, cold bathing, dashing cold water upon the genitals, and *perfect chastity* of thought as well as of person—so as to avoid all excite-ment of the parts—are the necessary measures, although they will not often be of much service.

# CHAPTER XXII.

## OF THE SURGICAL DISEASES OF THE FEMALE GENITALS.

I. Blennorrhœa.—Young female children are sometimes subject to mucous or purulent discharges from the parts at the entrance of the vagina; which may also perhaps be excoriated. Purgatives and tonics—perfect cleanliness, and F. 15, 36, or any mild astringent lotion, are the remedies.

II. Noma signifies a phagedænic affection of the labia pudendi of young female children, precisely resembling the *cancrum oris*, p. 370, in its causes, nature, and symptoms. After two or three days of low fever, the little patient is observed to suffer considerably whilst making water, and on examination, the labia present a livid erysipelatous redness and vesications, that are rapidly followed by phagedænic ulcers. This disease is very frequently fatal. The treatment is the same as directed for cancrum oris. The surgeon must be very careful not to mistake this or the preceding affection for the venereal disease;—an error common enough among parents.*

III. VESICO-VACINA FISTULA signifies a communication between the bladder and vagina. It generally results from sloughing of the parts after a tedious labour. As soon as it is discovered, the patient should be made to lie on her face—a catheter should be constantly worn in the urethra, and an oiled sponge in the vagina, and the bowels should be kept moderately loose. By these means the natural contraction of the parts will be aided. After some weeks, it will be expedient to pare the edges of the fissure, and unite them by suture, by means of Mr. Beaumont's instrument;—or if this fails, to touch them frequently with nitrate of silver, or a heated iron. To perform these operations, the vagina must be dilated with a speculum.

IV. RECTO-VAGINAL FISTULA must be treated by constantly wearing a sponge in the vagina, so as to prevent the passage of fæces through it, and by mild laxatives, (F. 42.) If after a time the aperture does not close, it must be treated as in the last case. *Complete laceration of the perinæum into the anus* is attended with distressing incontinence of fæces, and is prevented from healing by the action of the sphincter. Hence it is necessary to divide the sphincter on each side of the laceration, and to prevent these new wounds from uniting, by placing a few threads of lint in them, until the laceration has united.

V. A VASCULAR EXCRESCENCE, varying in size from that of a large pin's head to that of a horse-bean, is liable to grow from the female urethra. It causes great distress through its exquisite sensibility. It should be cut off, and the potassa fusa be applied to the surface to prevent its reproduction. But, immediately after the caustic, a sponge dipped in diluted vinegar should be applied, in order to prevent injury to the surrounding sound parts;—and if it is necessary to introduce the caustic within the urethra, it must be by means of a tube, which has an aperture in it corresponding to the diseased surface.

VI. UTERINE POLYPUS is a pear-shaped, tumour covered by mucous membrane, and attached by a narrow neck to some part of the uterus. The symptoms that it produces are those of uterine irritation—bearing

---

* Kinder Wood, on a fatal affection of the pudenda of female children. Med. Chir. Trans., vol. vii. p. 84.

down pains—menorrhagia—and, after a time, fetid discharges. On examination, an insensible tumour is found partially or entirely protruding through the os uteri. If it projects much into the vagina, the surgeon must carefully feel for the os uteri, and ascertain that the neck of the polypus is either attached to some part of it, or that it passes clear into the womb. Inversion or prolapsus of the womb, must not be mistaken for it. *Treatment.*—A ligature should be twisted tightly round its neck, but not too near the womb, by means of the double canula invented for that purpose by the late Dr. Gooch.

VII. IMPERFORATE HYMEN.—Sometimes this membrane completely obstructs the vagina, and causes the menstrual fluid to accumulate and distend the uterus. The impediment is easily got rid of by a crucial incision. Then all the black treacly fluid that has accumulated should be immediately syringed out with warm water, otherwise it might putrefy, and cause typhoid fever and death.

VIII. The labia may be the seat of acute inflammation, and of encysted tumours, and sarcomatous or fatty enlargements. The treatment of these cases requires no distinct comments. The clitoris and nymphæ, if they grow to an incovenient size, should be curtailed by an incision— and if they are affected with scirrhus, should be entirely extirpated at an early period.

# CHAPTER XXIII.

## OF THE DISEASES OF THE BREAST.

I. ACUTE INFLAMMATION of the breast is known by great swelling, tenderness and pain, and fever. These symptoms are soon succeeded by shivering, and formation of matter. The abscess is very slow to point. This affection may occur at any period during lactation. It may be caused by cold—by too stimulating a diet—or by neglect in suckling. *Treatment.*—The bowels should be freely kept open by saline purgatives —plenty of leeches should be applied as soon as possible, and *tepid* fomentations or poultices after them; the milk should be drawn off, if it can be done without very much pain, and Dover's powder should be given to allay restlessness. As soon as fluctuation is well established, a puneture should be made. The aperture after a time discharges a milky fluid. If it is long in healing, astringent lotions should be injected into it.

II. CHRONIC INFLAMMATION generally attacks one or two lobules only, causing them to swell into firm tumours, which on examination with the

60

finger, are felt to be composed of numerous little granules. The whole
gland may however be affected. There is very little tenderness or pain,
except at the time, of menstruation. This affection is distinguished from
malignant disease, by the circumstance that the patient is generally young,
without the leaden look of cancer, and that the tumour is more diffused,
and not so hard. *Treatment.*—The appetite and digestion—the state of
the liver and bowels, and above all, of the uterine system, must be regulated
by Plummer's pill, aloes, steel, and other alteratives, aperients, and tonics.
Occasional leechings—cold lotions—issues in the back—mercurial plasters
containing a little belladonna—and, in indolent cases, friction with weak
mercurial ointment—are the requisite local remedies. Marriage in some
cases almost a specific.

III. IRRITABLE BREAST is a neuralgic affection resembling the irritable
testis.—Extreme pain and tenderness, aggravated at the menstrual period,
with occasional heat and slight swelling, are the symptoms. This, like
the other affections of its class, (p. 304,) is extremely unmanageable, and
may remain for years. *Treatment.*—Steel, aloes, and other tonics—emmenagogues—especially the ferri ammonio-chloridum in doses of gr. ii.
ter die—with change of air, marriage, and other means for the improvement of the health,—are the chief remedies. Leeches, cold and warm
applications—mercurial, belladonna, and other plasters—issues, blisters,
and other local measures, sometimes do good, but as often the reverse.

IV. LACTEAL TUMOUR.—Sometimes a lacteal duct becomes obliterated,
and the milk accumulates in it, forming an oblong fluctuating tumour
near the nipple. If this is punctured, milk will continue to be discharged during lactation, and after the child is weaned, it will dry up
and heal.

V. SORE NIPPLES.—Excoriations and chaps about the nipples not only
cause great pain and inconvenience in suckling, but are a frequent cause
of acute inflammation, by deterring the mother from allowing the child
to suckle so freely as it ought. Borax and honey—or powdered borax
sprinkled on the part—lotions of alum, sulphate of zinc, or nitrate of silver, or arrowroot and cream, are the best applications. The nipple should
be defended from the clothes, and from the child's mouth, by a wooden
or caoutchouc shield. Women who are subject to this affection should
frequently wash the parts with salt and water or solution of alum during
pregnancy.

VI. THE HYDATID DISEASE consists in the development of a number
of cysts in the gland, filled with clear water. Sometimes the cysts are
developed by the gland—being lined with a vascular membrane, and
containing a yellow serum. Sometimes they consist of hydatids—para-
sitic animalculæ, composed of thin bladders filled with a clear water,
which are developed *in* the gland by their own vital powers, and are ca-

pable of engendering other smaller hydatids within themselves. The diagnosis of this affection is obscure. At first it occasions a hard tumour, resembling that of chronic inflammation, and unattended with pain, except at the menstrual period. Subsequently fluctuation is felt at different parts—and when any cyst has acquired a considerable magnitude, it ul-cerates, discharges its fluid, suppurates, and contracts. *Treatment.*—If there are but one or two cysts, they may be punctured, and then they will suppurate and contract. But if the whole gland is involved, it should be removed. The inconvenience arising from its bulk, and the irritation caused by the ulceration of the cysts, will thus be got rid of. At the same time, the chance that this, like other new struc-tures, may assume a malignant action, is an additional reason for the operation.

VII. The Serocystic Disease is a peculiar affection of the breast, described by Sir B. Brodie in a clinical lecture at St. George's Hospital, in January 1840. It chiefly affects the upper classes, and is rarely met with in hospitals. It consists in the development of numerous cysts, formed probably by a dilatation of the lactiferous tubes, and containing serum, which often exudes from, or may be squeezed out of, the nipple. It generally occurs to women under the age of thirty, who are unmarried, or barren. In its first stage, it appears as one or more globular tumours—the size perhaps of a marble—which seem to be moveable, because the whole breast moves with them, but are not so in reality. This disease does not affect the axillary glands, and may remain stationary for years. But in time a second stage arrives. Fibrinous matter is effused be-tween the cysts, gluing them together; and tumours are developed on their inner walls. As the disease advances, the skin ulcerates, the serum escapes, and in a few days a fungous protrudes, which ultimately causes death through bleeding and sloughing. *Treatment.*—In the early stages Sir B. Brodie recommends counter-irritation by means of blisters, or tincture of iodine, or by flannel cloths soaked in a combination of sp. camphoræ, sp. tenuioris āā f $\frac{z}{3}$ iiiss; liq. plumbi f $\frac{z}{3}$i; intermitting these applications when the skin becomes sore. Punctures are not on the whole advisable. In the latter stages the breast must be amputated, and if the whole of it is removed the disease will not return.

VIII. Schirrus generally commences as a hard, circumscribed, move-able swelling in some part of the breast. In its early stages, it is not often tender or painful. After a few weeks or months, however, it be-comes affected with paroxysms of violent lancinating pain, which are most apt to occur about the period of menstruation. Not unfrequently a little bloody fluid is discharged from the nipple. The cellular tissue and fat about the gland often become atrophied, so that the diseased breast is smaller than the sound one, and the nipple is generally drawn in, and the skin around it puckered like a cicatrix. The progress and termination of

this disease have been already described, (p. 122.) The tumour after a
time adheres to the skin, and to the muscle beneath, so as to become
fixed and immoveable. Then it ulcerates and forms a cancer. The glands
in the axilla, and sometimes those in the neck, enlarge and compress the
axillary veins, and the arm swells and becomes œdematous from the obstruction to its circulation. The ribs and pleura become scirrhous; water
is effused into the chest—the breathing becomes difficult—the patient
suffers from rheumatic pains in the bones, and at last dies. *Diagnosis.*—
In well-marked cases, this disease cannot be mistaken. The stony-hard,
moveable swelling in its early stage, or the shrunken gland and retracted
nipple subsequently,—the age about forty,—the leaden, sallow complexion,—the weakness and cachexia,—the lancinating pain,—and the circumstance (which very often happens) that the patient's mother or sis-
ters have suffered from cancer,—all distinguish it. But there are several
circumstances which may render the diagnosis doubtful. (1) In the first
place the scirrhous deposite may be attended with more or less common inflammatory pain, tenderness and swelling, so that it loses its characteristic hardness, and becomes blended in its outline with the surrounding tissues, and exactly resembles the swelling arising from chronic
inflammation. (2) It may occur in a young female between twenty and
thirty. (3) The effect of remedies may be deceitful. For although no
medicine is capable of causing absorption of a scirrhous deposite, yet it
may diminish the inflammatory swelling around, and so cause temporary
decrease of the tumour. *Treatment.*—The local and general treatment
of scirrhus of the breast must be conducted on the principles laid down in
the section of Scirrhus generally. Extirpation is the only remedy, and,
provided the diagnosis is clear, the sooner it is done the better. The
circumstances which contra-indicate an operation are also detailed in the
same section.

IX. MEDULLARY SARCOMA of the breast is generally combined with
more or less scirrhus, and rarely exists alone. It forms a large rapidly-
increasing tumour; lobulated on its surface; and the projecting parts yield
an elastic sensation. This affection may be distinguished from scirrhus
by its more rapid growth and greater softness. It is often difficult in
its early stage to distinguish it from innocent chronic tumours, more
especially as the latter may after a time degenerate into malignant action.
*Melanosis* and *gelatiniform sarcoma* (p. 128) are sometimes found in the
breast.

X. EXTIRPATION OF THE BREAST is thus performed. The patient
being placed in a convenient position, sitting or reclining, an assistant
takes the arm of the affected side and holds it out, so as to put the pectoralis on the stretch. The surgeon then makes a semi-elliptical incision
below the nipple along the lower border of the pectoralis major, and
another on the upper and inner side of the nipple, so as to include that

part between them. He next dissects out the lower and outer part of the gland, quite down to the pectoralis, (taking care not to get behind that muscle,) and then, cutting from below upwards, he separates the remainder. If an adjacent gland is enlarged, the incisions should be managed so as to include it also. When the mass is removed, its surface should be wiped and examined, and the wound should also be well examined, to ascertain that no part of the gland, and that no hardened or discoloured portions of cellular tissue or of muscular fibre are left behind. Arteries are then to be tied, and the patient to be put to bed,—and when all oozing has ceased, a few strips of adhesive plaster may be applied.

XI. Boys and girls about the age of puberty are subject to slight swelling and tenderness of the breast, which, however, may be soon got rid of by plasters of empl. ammoniaci cum hydrargyro.

XII. Men occasionally suffer from malignant disease of the breast, which manifests itself in the same manner, and requires the same treatment, as it does in the female.

# CHAPTER XXIV.

## OF CLUB FOOT, AND OTHER DEFORMITIES OF THE LIMBS.

I. CLUB FOOT (TALIPES) signifies a peculiar deformity of the foot, produced by rigidity and contraction of the muscles of the leg. (1) In the most simple variety, which is called *talipes equinus*, the heel merely is raised, so that the patient walks on the ball of the foot. (2) In the *talipes varus*, which is far more common, the distortion is much more complex. In the first place the heel is raised;—secondly, the inner edge of the foot is drawn upwards;—and thirdly, the whole foot is twisted inwards; so that the patient walks on the outer edge; and in confirmed cases, on the dorsum of the foot, and outer ankle. (3) In the *talipes valgus* the outer edge of the foot is raised up, and the patient walks on the inner ankle.

*Causes.*—This affection consists essentially in that state of shortening and rigidity of the muscles of the calf, which we have described as *rigid atrophy;* (vide p. 224.) The exciting causes are various circumstances that interfere with the supply of nervous influence, or with the proper nutrition of the muscles. Thus it may be a consequence of fevers;—of injuries of the spine;—of division of the sciatic nerve;—of long confinement and inactivity;—of repeated attacks of rheumatic or other kinds of

inflammation of the muscles of the calf;—or it may be a sympathetic
consequence of irritation of the bowels, or of some other part of the system;—and lastly, it may be *congenital*, or produced during uterine life.
As a proof of the imperfect nutrition and innervation of the distorted
limb, it is always cold and feeble; the bones are small, and the muscles
wasted.                                                                   .

*Treatment.*—If this distortion is congenital or commences in early
childhood, it may sometimes be rectified by constantly 'wearing a proper
apparatus. Slight cases in particular, occurring to children after fevers
may generally be remedied, if taken at their very commencement, by
daily extension with the hands, and friction of emollient embrocations on
the muscles, together with tonics, galvanism, change of air, and sea-
bathing. But in confirmed cases, it is better at once to resort to Stromeyer's operation of dividing the tendo Achillis. The rationale of this operation may readily be comprehended. The tendon being divided, heals
by a callus, which renders it longer, and which while recent may be
stretched to any desired length. Thus the mechanical shortening of
the muscle is neutralized. At the same time, the antagonist muscles,
which are always wasted and inert, are relieved from a constant state of
tension, and are enabled to resume their natural functions, so that the
limb rapidly increases in strength and bulk. The operation is easily performed thus. The tendon is put on the stretch; and a narrow sharp-
pointed knife is thrust through the skin on one side of it; then its edge is
turned against the tendon, and made to divide it as it is being withdrawn.
If the tendons of the tibialis posticus, or flexor policis; or in fact if any
others offer an obstacle to bringing down the heel, they may be divided
as well. Three or four days after the division, some apparatus should
be applied to extend the callus and bring the foot into its proper shape.
*Stromeyer's footboard* is recommended by Dr. Little, but *Scarpa's shoe*,
as improved by Weiss, seems to be neater and more efficient. It is admirably adapted for counteracting the threefold distortion of talipes varus.

II. WEBBED FINGERS.—This is a deformity consisting of a union of the
fingers to each other. It may be congenital, or may be caused by burns.
It is a most intractable affection. Mere division of the connecting skin
is not of any avail, for the fingers almost inevitably grow together again
when the wound heals. In order to counteract their union, a flap of skin
may either be brought from the dorsum of the hand and be engrafted between the fingers,—or ,as Mr. Liston proposes, a perforation may first of
all be made in the connecting skin near the roots of the fingers, and be
prevented from closing by keeping a piece of cord in it till the edges
have healed, and then the remainder of the connexion may be divided.

III. WEAR ANKLES.—In this affection the foot is flattened, its arch is
sunk, and the astragalus forms a projection below the internal malleolus,

rendering the internal border of the foot convex instead of concave. In bad cases the inner ankle almost touches the ground, and the patient walks with great pain and lameness. This affection depends on a weakness and relaxation of the bones and ligaments. It is sure to be brought on, if weakly children are put upon their legs too soon. It is more common amongst girls than boys—partly from their greater delicacy—partly because they are taught at an early age by ignorant governesses and dancing masters, that it is necessary for them to turn their feet out as much as possible, as the very first step towards elegance in dancing or walking. Thirty years ago it was a common practice to make school girls sit for an hour every day in a kind of stocks, with their feet turned outwards, so as to be almost in a straight line with each other. Children, however, if left to nature, stand with their toes slightly turned inwards—the position in fact which is the firmest, and most calculated to prevent this distortion whilst the bones are yet soft and yielding. *Treatment.*—The patient should wear shoes or boots with high heels, and with the inner edge of the sole much thicker than the outer. He should also be directed to turn the foot out very little, if at all. Benefit may also be derived from a well-applied bandage, such as is represented at p. 93. It shonld always be applied so as to be carried round the ankle from the inner side of the foot. In severe cases the patient should wear a tightly fitting boot, with a piece of steel or whalebone fastened to the sole, and passing perpendicularly upwards to the middle of the inner side of the leg.

IV. CONTRACTION OF THE FINGERS generally depends on shortening and rigidity of the palmar aponeuroses and tendinous sheaths—or on a ligamentous degeneration of the cellular tissue on the palmar aspect of the fingers. *Treament.*—Friction with oily liniments and extension upon splints, may be of some service. But the following operation will be of more: a longitudinal incision may be made through the skin on the palmar surface of the first phalanx, then the edges of the wound being held asunder, a curved bistoury may be passed under the contracted tissues so as to divide them. If any of the muscles in the fore-arm are rigid, their tendons may be divided by a narrow knife, as in the operation for club-foot.

V. CONTRACTION OF THE TOES.—It often happens that one of the toes is permanently elevated, and rides over its neighbours, from the habitual use of narrow boots; and the upper surface of this toe being peculiarly exposed to friction, is generally covered with corns so painful, that many persons have been compelled to have the part amputated. Division of the extensor tendon, may however, enable the toe to be brought down into its place, and prevent the necessity of its removal.

VI. SPURIOUS ANCHYLOSIS.—In cases of *spurious anchylosis,* (P. 242,) —that is to say, stiffness of joints depending on rigidity of the surrounding tissues.—or on permanent contraction of the flexor muscles owing to their having been long kept in a fixed position,—divisions of the tendons of the contracted muscles will do much towards restoring the mobility of the joint. The tendons of the hamstring muscles have been divided by Mr. Phillips with great success in case of sitffened knee from rheumatism. The pectoralis major, latissimus dorsi, teres major and teres minor muscles have been divided by Dieffenbach in order to effect the reduction of an old dislocation of the shoulder; and the pectinæus and sartorius by an American surgeon in a case of contracted hip. All these operations are of course to be performed by what is called *subcutaneous section;* that is, in the same manner in which the tendo Achillis is divided. The muscle or tendon must be put on the stretch, aud a puncture be made on one side of it. Then a curved blunt-pointed bistoury may be passed under it, and be made to divide it. In many cases it is necessary to divide the fasciæ under the knee or in the sole of the foot as well as the tendons. A few days after either of these operations some apparatus must be applied by which gradual extension may be made.

# PART V.

## OF THE OPERATIONS OF SURGERY.

---

## CHAPTER I.

### OF OPERATIONS IN GENERAL, AND OF THE EXTIRPATION OF TUMOURS.

I. THE APPARATUS necessary for operations in general comprises one or more bistouries, scalpels, or other specific cutting instruments;—a dissecting forceps, a tenaculum, and small forceps (which should have a spring or catch) to take up arteries;—plenty of well-waxed ligatures, curved needles threaded, fine sponge, water both warm and cold, and wine and hartshorn in case of faintness. There should also be a sufficient number of assistants to restrain the patient's struggles, to administer cordials, to hand the different instruments to the surgeon, or to assist him in other respects,—besides a good light, and a bed or table with pillows or cushions to make the patient's position as easy as possible.

II. INCISIONS —In making incisions, there are several points that demand attention. First of all, the manner of handling the knife,—which, as systematic writers say, may be held either like a common dinner knife,—or like a pen,—or like a fiddlestick. The first two positions are those which are employed commonly; the third is resorted to in cutting into the different layers over a hernial sac, and in sundry other delicate operations. Secondly, before commencing an incision, the skin must be gently stretched and steadied with the points of the fingers, otherwise it will be dragged along by the knife, and the incision will be ragged, and shorter than was intended. Thirdly, in cutting through the skin, the knife should be passed in at right angles to the surface, and should be at once carried down to the subcutaneous tissue—then the

61

blade should be inclined downwards, and be made to cut through the skin to the requisite extent,—and lastly, as the incision is finished, the instrument must be again brought to a right angle with the surface. By these means the whole thickness of the skin will be divided, both at the beginning and end of the incision; for nothing can be more painful than a partial division of it. Moreover, the operator should always cut the skin as speedily as possible, for it is the most painful part of every operation. He should also take care to make the incision quite as long as will be required—and rather too long than too short. To pause in the middle of an operation, and cut a little more of the skin, is most awkward on the surgeon's part, and most cruel to the sufferer. The author has not sufficient space to detail all the tedious varieties of in-cisions that are enumerated in systematic treatises. It is of little use to say that they may be made by cutting from without inwards,—or by first plunging in the instrument, and then cutting outwards (as in bleed-ing,)—or that they may be simple or compound—straight, curved, or angular. It may be noticed, however, that when two incisions are to be made to meet near their extremities, (as, for example, the two semi-ellip-tical incisions in amputation of the breast,) the second should fall into the first *nearly*, but *not quite at its extremity*, so that there may be no little isthmus of skin left undivided between them. Again, in making a V incision, the second cut should not be begun where the first termi-nated, but at its other end; that is to say, it should be made *towards* the first, and not *from* it. In making a T incision likewise, the transverse cut should be made first, and the other be directed towards it. Lastly, the angle of a V incision should if possible be always dependent.

III. THE PREPARATION of a patient for an operation is a most im-portant clement in its success. The object is to have every organ and every function in as healthy a state as possible, and vascular action a little, but not too much, below par. For the full-blooded and inflamma-tory, bleeding will be requisite, and in all cases recourse should be had to abstinence, aperients, and gentle alteratives, with or without small doses of sedatives, till the pulse has become quiet, the tongue clean, the bowels regular, the liver, kidneys, and skin in good order, and the mind cheerful. Moreover, it is best not to perform an ope-ration in very cold weather if it can be avoided, especially upon the eye. It has also been recommended, and the recommendation seems rational, that the patient should be made to keep his bed for two or three days before an operation, in order that he may become accustomed to the confinement.

IV. EXTIRPATION OF TUMOURS.—A different proceeding is to be adopted in the case of malignant and of simple growths. In the former it may be necessary to remove a portion of skin by two semi-elliptical incisions, if it appears to be contaminated by the diseased growth. But in extirpating wens or fatty or sarcomatous tumours, however large, it is a general rule not to remove any of the skin, unless it is much inflamed or ulcerated, or so entirely adherent to the tumour that its separation would be very tedious and difficult. Again, in the former case it is necessary to cut quite wide of the diseased mass, and remove plenty of the surrounding tissues,—in the latter case the incisions should be carried through the cellular cyst of the tumour. In all cases it is a better plan (unless the tumour is exceedingly large) to carry the dissection at once boldly to the deepest part where the largest vessels enter the tumour, than to tie the different branches as they are divided,—by which means some vessels may perhaps be tied more than once. Again, it is requisite in every case that the extirpation be complete, because if the smallest portion is left, it may become the nucleus of a fresh growth. If, therefore, it is found that there is any portion of a tumour which cannot be cut out without fear of dangerous hæmorrhage, a double ligature should be passed through its base, and be tied tightly on each side of it.

V. AIR IN VEINS.—The entrance of air into a vein is a most dangerous accident, that has sometimes occurred during the extirpation of tumours from the neck, or axilla. A large vein being cut across, whose coats adhere to some firm textures around so that they cannot collapse, a sort of bubbling, sucking noise is suddenly heard, the patient instantly faints, and generally dies soon afterwards. On examination the heart is found distended with air. If any such sound should be perceived during an operation, the surgeon should instantly put his fingers on the spot that it proceeds from,—and the patient, if faint, should be kept in the recumbent position with the head low; and should be well supplied with stimulants.*

---

# CHAPTER II.

## OF THE MINOR OPERATIONS.

I. VENÆSECTION at the bend of the arm should always, if possible, be performed in the median-cephalic vein. A ligature being placed a little above the elbow, (but not tight enough to stop the pulse at the wrist,)

---

* For the best account of these curious cases, refer to Sir C. Bell's Practical Essays, Lond. 1841.

See also two cases, with remarks by Prof. Warren of Harvard University, in the Medical Magazine, vol. i. p. 12.

the operator takes the fore-arm in his hand, places his thumb on the vein a little below the intended puncture,—and then (using the right hand for the right arm and *vice versâ*) pushes the lancet obliquely into the vein, and makes it cut its way directly outwards. When sufficient blood has been taken, the ligature is removed, the thumb placed on or just below the aperture to check the bleeding, and the wound is closed with a bit of lint and plaster, and secured by a small compress and figure of 8 bandage.

The jugular vein is sometimes opened in cases of apoplexy in adults, and in children if the veins at the elbow are hidden by fat. The thumb is placed on the vein a little above the clavicle, and an incision made in the ordinary way with a lancet, cutting obliquely upwards and outwards. The thumb is removed when enough blood is obtained, and the wound secured with lint and plaster. The veins in the leg, scrotum, or neighbourhood of the eye or ear, can readily be opened in the same manner instead of the ordinary venæsection, or leeching, or cupping.

Abscess in the cellular tissue, inflammation of the fascia, phlebitis, neuralgia, varicose aneurism, and aneurismal varix, are occasional ill consequences of venæsection.

II. ARTERIOTOMY.—The temporal artery should be opened above the outer angle of the eyebrow—never just above the zygoma. The surgeon feels for the largest branch, steadies it with two fingers, one placed above, the other below the intended puncture—then pushes in the lancet in the same manner as in venæsection. The incision should be directed across the vessel, and should cut it about half through. When sufficient blood has flowed, the best plan is to introduce the lancet, and cut the vessel completely across, so that its ends may retract. A firm graduated compress should then be applied, and be confined with a bandage passing round the head; and some degree of pressure should be kept up on the wound for a week or ten days. Any subsequent bleeding or spurious aneurism must be treated by completely dividing the artery, if it has not been done already, and by pressure,—but if the wound is much inflamed or ulcerated, so as not to admit of pressure, a transverse incision should be made on each side of it, and the artery be tied in both places.

III. CUPPING.—The patient being placed in a comfortable position, with towels arranged so that his clothes may not be soiled by the blood, and being moreover protected from cold, so that the flow of blood to the surface may not be checked, and the operator having this scarificator, glasses, torch, spirits of wine, lighted candle, hot water, and sponge, conveniently arranged on a table close by,—the first thing is to sponge the skin well with hot water, so as to make it somewhat vascular. The operator next dries it with a warm towel, and adapts his glasses to the part.

Their number must depend on the quantity of blood to be taken—from three to five ounces is a fair calculation for each glass. In the next place, he dips the torch in the spirit, sets it on fire, introduces it for half a second into one of the glasses, and immediately claps the latter on the skin—and the same with the other glasses in succession. As soon as the skin has become red and swollen, he charges the scarificator, and takes it between his right forefinger and thumb, at the same time holding the lighted torch between the little and ring fingers of the same hand. He then detaches one glass by insinuating the nail of his left forefinger under its edge—instantly discharges the scarificator on the swollen skin, and as expeditiously as possible introduces the torch into the glass, and applies it again. The same process is repeated with the other glasses. When they become tolerably full, or the blood begins to coagulate in them, they must be detached in succession and re-applied, if blood enough has not been taken—and when the operation is finished, the wounds should be closed with lint and plaster. There are several points connected wtth this operation that require notice. In the first place, the glasses must not be exhansted too much; if they are, the pressure of their rims will occasion severe pain—the blood will not flow—and the operations will very probably be followed by a considerable ecchymosis. Secondly, the position of the glasses must be slightly varied each time they are applied, so that their edges may not again press on the same circle of skin. Thirdly, the expediency of not burning the patient needs scarcely be hinted at. Fourthly, in taking off the glasses, the upper part of each should be detached first, so that the blood may not escape. Lastly, the length of the scarificators must be adjusted to the thickness of the skin; for if the incisions are too deep, the fat will protrude through them, and prevent the flow of blood. The direction of the incisions should correspond to the course of the muscular fibres beneath; but this is of no great consequence. For *cupping on the temples* smaller glasses and scarificators are employed. A branch of the temporal artery is generally wounded, and the flow of blood may be expedited by slightly lifting the lower part of the rim of the glass. Pressure should be kept up on the wounds for some days afterwards, in order to prevent secondary hæmorrhage or false aneurism.

IV. Acupuncture is easily performed by running in five or six needles with a rotatory motion. It is certainly very efficacious in some cases of neuralgia, but it is by no means easy to explain its operation. Acupuncture is also resorted to in anasarca, when the skin is much distended;—and we have spoken of its utility in ganglion, hydrothorax, and ascites, for the purpose of permitting the serum to exude into the cellular tissue.

V. Issues may be made by caustic or by incision. The former may be made either by rubbing a portion of skin of the requisite extent with

the potassa fusa, or by making a paste with equal parts of the potass and
soft soap, and laying it on the skin till the latter is converted into a black
slough.    The parts immediately around the issue should be protected
with several layers of sticking-plaster. After the application of the caustic,
the part should be poulticed till the slough separates, and then the sore
may be prevented from healing, either by binding several peas firmly on
its surface, or by touching it occasionally with the caustic.   The other
species of issue is made by pinching up the skin, and slitting it up with
a lancet, and then introducing some peas to prevent it from healing.    It
may be remarked that issues should never be made over projecting points
of bones, nor over the bellies of muscles; for they might degenerate into
most obstinate sores.    Thus for diseased vertebræ, the issues should be
made between the spinous and transverse process;—for diseased hip, *behind* the great trochanter, and not over it,—for diseased knee, just below
the inner tuberosity of the tibia.

VI. SETONS are introduced by pinching up a fold of the skin, and
pushing a needle through it armed with a skein of silk or cotton, or a
long flat peice of Indian-rubber.   As soon as one or two inches of the
thread are brought through, the needle is cut off.   A fresh portion of the
thread is to be pulled through the wound every day, so as to keep up a
constant irritation and discharge.   If the discharge is insufficient, the
thread may be covered with some irritating ointment before it is drawn
under the skin.

VII. THE MOXA is a peculiar method of counter-irritation long practised in the East, and occasionally employed in Europe, for the relief of
chronic nervous and rheumatic pains, or for chronic diseases of the joints.
One or more small cones, formed of the fine fibres of the artemisia
chinensis, or of some other porous vegetable substance—such as German
tinder, or linen impregnated with nitre, are placed on the skin over the
affected part, and then are set on fire, and allowed to burn away so as to
form a superficial eschar.    The surrounding skin must be protected by a
piece of wet rag, with a hole in it for the moxa.

It is convenient sometimes to use the moxa as a rubefacient or vesicant
and not as a cauteran.   A roll of German tinder ignited may be held with
dressing forceps at a little distance from the skin, the surgeon at the same
time blowing upon it with a blow-pipe till the skin become red.

VIII. THE ACTUAL CAUTERY is certainly very efficient, and it is very
far from being the most painful manner of effecting counter irritation.
It is easily effected by means of an iron rod with a knob of the size and
shape of an olive at one end of it, and a wooden handle at the other.
The knob being heated red hot, is rubbed on the skin so as to make two
or three blackened lines about half an inch wide, and an inch asunder.
Then the water dressing or a poultice may be applied till the shallow es-
chars separate;—and it appears to be better to keep the sores open by

touching them occasionally with the cautery, than by the ordinary irritating dressings.

IX. VACCINATION.—The success of this operation will depend partly on the state of health of the patient—for it will most probably be defeated if there is any cutaneous disease or disorder of the system generally—and partly on the quality of the matter which is inoculated. The matter should be taken on the eighth day, before an inflamed areola is spread around the vesicle, and it should be *lymph*, clear and transparent, not purulent. The operator should make three punctures on one arm with a fine lancet, carrying the point of the instrument obliquely under the cutiele for about ⅛ of an inch, and, if posible, without drawing blood. Then, if he has a patient to take the matter from, he ruptures a portion of the vesicle, dips the lancet in the lymph, and inserts it into each puncture. If he has the matter on *points*, he should breathe on them so as to liquefy it, and then insert one into each puncture, and allow it to remain three or four minutes.

X. ELECTRICITY AND GALVANISM.—Although these powerful agents have been by turns overrated and decried, and have lost much of their therapeutical reputation, through having been resorted to as the last desperate remedy, in cases where it was irrational to expect benefit from them, still no one who knows how to use them can doubt their efficacy. In certain cases of defective circulation and nervous influence;—when the thigh is weak and benumbed after sciatica;—in cases of atrophy of the extremities after fever;—when the extensors are paralyzed from long disuse, as after disease of joints;—in deficient menstruation;—in dyspnœa from weakness of the stomach;—in loss of voice from relaxation of the mucous membrane of the fáuces;—in hysterical neuralgia, and in other causes of nervous pain unattended with increased vascularity, they may be resorted to with every prospect of benefit. The most convenient apparatus seems to be a single battery on Smee's or Daniell's principle, with a coil, and an apparatus for giving a stream of gentle shocks.

XI. GALVANO-PUNCTURE.—In obstinate neuralgia, it is a good plan to insert two needles deeply, at two points in the course of the nerve, and to pass a galvanic current through them.

XII. BANDAGING.—The art of bandaging is not to be learned from books. Nor is it worth while to dwell upon the almost innumerable kinds of bandage that are described in the older systems of surgery. The suspensory or T bandage—the three-tailed, the four-tailed, and many-tailed —the single and double-headed, the retentive, expulsive, and uniting bandages,—many of them have fallen into oblivion, and the use and application of the others is readily acquired in a few months' attendance on hospital practice. The general rules to be observed in bandaging a limb are, to begin at the extremity, and apply the bandage most tightly there, and more loosly by degrees as it ascends—to make each successive fold overlap about one third of the preceding—to keep the bandage close to the limb, and nurol very little of it at a time—and to double it on itself on parts (such as the calf of the leg) where it would not lie smoothly other- wise.

---

# CHAPTER III.

## OF THE AMPUTATIONS.

I. AMPUTATION OF THE THIGH.—This amputation being probably the most important, and one that is very frequently practised, it will be con- venient to describe it first; and to embody in the description of it, such general precepts as are applicable to the other amputations.

In the first place, the surgeon should have his tourniquets, amputating knives, saws, forceps and tenacula, ligatures, bone-nippers, sponges, and curved needles threaded, close at hand on a tray, arranged in due order; and he should see with his own eyes that every requisite is at hand be- fore he begins.

The next point is, to place the patient in a convenient posture. For amputation of the thigh, the patient may be placed on a bed, or on a table covered with a folded blanket;—the diseased leg should project suffi- ciently over the edge, and should be supported at the knee by an assis- tant, who sits on a low stool in front;—and the sound limb should be secured to one of the legs of the table with a handkerchief.

Then measures must be adopted for compressing the main artery, and preventing too great loss of blood. This may be done, either by pres- sure with the hand, or with the tourniquet. Pressure with the hand on the main arterial trunk, if effected by a steady assistant who can be trusted, is sufficient in most cases; and if the limb is amputated so high up that the tourniquet cannot be applied, there is of course no choice;— the femoral artery must be compressed against the ramus of the pubes.

The common tourniquet consists of three parts;—a pad to compress the artery, which should be firm, narrow and flattish;—a strong band which is buckled round the limb;—and a bridge-like contrivance, over which the band passes, with a screw, by turning which the bridge is raised and the band tightened. The pad should always be placed so as to compress the artery against the bone. The advantage of this instru- ment is, that it compresses the small arteries as well as the principal trunk;—its disadvantage is, that it arrests the venous circulation, and causes a greater loss of venous blood;—wherefore, it should never be constricted tightly until the incisions are just commencing.

There is another form of tourniquet which Mr. Weiss has shown the author which produces no general constriction of the limb. It consists of a semicircular arch of steel, with a pad at each end, one of which pads is applied to the artery, and the other to the opposite side of the limb. The metallic arch has a joint in the centre, and is provided with a screw, by means of which the pads can be approximated with any requisite degree of force.

This, like other amputations, may be performed in two ways—either by the *circular incision*—that is, by cutting round the limb from without towards the bone; or by the *flap operation*—that is, by transfixing the limb, and then cutting outwards. The latter is the more fashionable at present. It certainly can be performed with greater celerity, and is said to give less pain. It should be preferred when the skin is adherent to the parts beneath, so as to be retracted with difficulty—and when the flesh on one side of the limb is destroyed by disease or injury;—for, in this latter case, the end of the stump may be covered with a flap taken almost entirely from the sound side, and a much greater length of limb may be saved. Sir C. Bell objects to it, because the nerves, being of a firm texture, are liable to be stretched out and cut longer than the surrounding parts—thus laying the foundation for subsequent neuralgic affections.[*] But, as he afterwards observes, the grand rule in all cases is, to save integument enough to cover the muscle, and muscle enough to cover the bone, and not to scrape off the periosteum. And if these things are done, it requires ingenuity to make a bad stump. It is ordinarily stated that amputation of the thigh should be performed as low down as possible—(never, however, within two inches of the patella, so as to cut into the joint)—but Mr. Liston affirms, that the thigh-bone should never be sawn lower than its middle, because there are certain difficulties in fitting an artificial limb to a long stump.

(1.) *Circular Method.*—The surgeon stands on the outer side for the left leg, and on the inner for the right; so that he may use his left hand to grasp and steady the part which he is to amputate. The artery must be compressed by one of the methods before described, and an assistant must grasp the limb with both hands, so as to draw up the skin as high as possible. Then the surgeon commences by putting his arm under the thigh, and makes an incision at one sweep completely round the limb, through the skin and fat down to the fascia. The assistant is now to

---

[*] The arteries, also, being cut obliquely, are more difficult to tie ; and it is said that the smaller arteries are unable to retract, and more liable to secondary hæmorrhage.

62

draw the skin farther up, the retraction being aided by a few touches
with the knife; and then the knife, being put close to the edge of the retracted skin, is to be made divide every thing down to the bone by
another clean circular sweep.   The next thing is, to separate the muscles
from the bone for another inch or two with the point of the knife, especially those connected with the *linea aspera*; and then the periosteum
having been divided by one more sweep—the *retractor*,—a piece of linen
with a longitudinal slit in it, is put over the face of the stump,—and the
muscles are to be drawn up with it.   Now the bone must be sawn
through.   The heel of the saw should first be put on the bone, and it
should be drawn up so as to make a groove, before working it downwards; it should be used very lightly, and the last few strokes should be
excessively short and gentle, that the bone may not be splintered.   If it
is, the irregular part must be removed with nippers.   The femoral artery
should now be tied, its orifice being seized and slightly drawn out by
forceps; and afterwards any large branches that appear in the muscular
interstices.   Then all compression should be *suddenly ceased*, so that
any arteries that are likely to bleed may do so, and be tied at once.
Hæmorrhage from large veins is to be restrained by elevating the stump,
and making compression for a short time with the finger.   If, however,
nothing else will do, they must be tied.   Any obstinate oozing from
small vessels should be restrained by sponging with cold water, or perhaps by a touch with arg. nitras.   Then a light bandage may be passed
round the limb above the stump, and the patient be removed to bed, with
the stump supported on a pillow covered with oilcloth, and having merely a
handkerchief laid over it.   After an hour or two, the edges of the skin should
be approximated with a few strips of plaster—the isinglass the best.   The
edges are to be brought together in a straight line, which may be made
either perpendicular or horizontal, the latter however being probably the
better plan.   The ligatures should be left hanging out in the interstices
of the adhesive straps.   No other application will be needed save a cloth
dipped in cold water.   Pain may be allayed by an opiate.   The stump
may remain as it is for some days, the discharge being merely wiped
occasionally from its surface.   But, after from four to six days, sooner
or later, according to the quantity of the discharge and the feelings of the
patient, the dressings should be changed, the straps being taken off and
replaced one by one, with care not to disturb the ligatures, and the hands
of an assistant being employed to support the edges, and prevent their
falling asunder.   At the subsequent dressings, the points to be attended to
are, to renew the light bandage occasionally, which was passed round
the stump soon after the operation, in order to support the muscles, and
prevent their retraction—to bring together the edges of the wound with
adhesive straps—to remove the ligatures when loose—(that on the femo-

ral artery should not be disturbed for a fortnight)—and to accelerate cicatrization by the nitrate of silver, or other stimulants, if the granulations
appear languid.

There are a few varieties in the manner of performing this circular
operation that require a brief notice. Some surgeons, after having cut
through the skin, dissect it from the fascia, and turn it back—a proceeding necessary enough if this operation is performed (which it never
should be) when the cellular tissue is condensed and adherent. Again,
if the patient is *very emaciated*, the circular incision may be carried down
to the bone at once without ceremony, because in such patients the muscles always retract greatly. Sir C. Bell recommends the skin not to be
divided quite circularly, but the knife to be inclined a little, first to one
side, then to the other, so as to make two oval flaps. The same may
be done also in dividing the muscles. He farther recommends that the
limb should be raised perpendicularly whilst the bone is being sawn, so
that the saw may be worked horizontally, by which means, he says, the
bone may be divided more evenly, and much shorter, so that its end will
be no more seen when the stump is depressed.

(2.) *Flap Operation.*—The surgeon, standing as before, grasps the
flesh on the anterior surface of the limb with his left hand, and lifts it
from the bone; then passes his knife horizontally through it—carries the
point over the bone,—pushes it through the other side of the limb, as
low as possible;—then makes it cut its way out upwards and forwards,
so as to make the anterior flap. In amputating the right leg, the knife
should be passed in behind the saphena vein. It is again entered on the
inner side a little below the top of the first incision, passed behind the

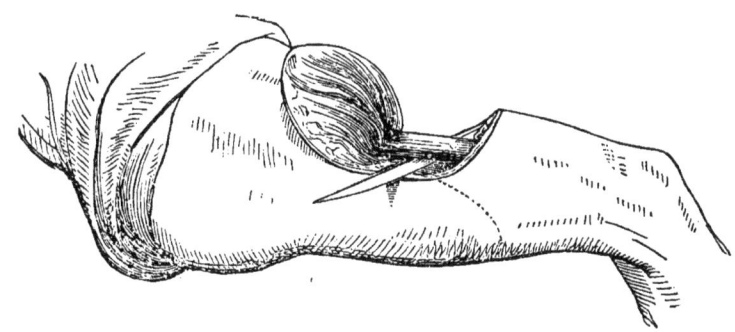

bone, brought out at the wound on the outside, and directed so as to
make a posterior flap in the direction of the dotted line, a very little
longer than the anterior. Both flaps are now drawn back; the knife is
swept round the bone to divide any remaining muscular fibres, and the
bone is sawn through. In the same manner flaps may be made from the

inner and outer sides of the limb, the surgeon first grasping the flesh, and transfixing it, and cutting a flap on one side of the bone, then passing the knife close to the bone on the other side, (without again piercing the skin,) and making another flap.

II. AMPUTATION AT THE HIP-JOINT is performed by Mr. Liston after precisely the same manner in which he amputates the thigh. The femoral artery being compressed, the knife is carried across the front of the circulation, so as to form the anterior flap. Then the anterior part of the capsular ligament being cut into, and the *ligamentum teres* and posterior part of the capsular ligament being divided, the blade of the knife is put behind the neck and trochanters of the femur, and the posterior flap is formed. The vessels on the posterior flap are tied first. But this method can hardly be preferable to that of making two lateral flaps;—first, passing the knife completely through the limb on the inner side of the joint, and carrying it forwards and inwards, so as to form a flap of the adductor muscles; then cutting into the joint, and severing the *ligamentum teres*, and the muscles attached to the digital fossa with a short strong curved knife; and lastly, putting in the knife over the trochanter, and cutting downwards and outwards, so as to make the external flap. In this manner Mr. Mayo performed this operation is less than half a minute. He previously tied the femoral artery below Poupart's ligament; but most authorities prefer compressing it during the operation, and tying its cut orifice afterwards.

III. AMPUTATION OF THE LEG, unless the patient can afford an artificial foot, should be performed as near the knee as possible;—for a long stump would be very inconvenient to a labouring man with a wooden leg.

(1.) *Circular Method.*—The artery being under command, as in amputations of the thigh, and the leg being placed horizontally, one assistant supporting it at the ankle, and another holding it at the knee and drawing up the skin,—the surgeon (standing on the inner side for the right leg, and *vice versâ*) makes a circular incision through the skin, four inches below the tuberosity of the tibia. The integuments are next to be dissected up for two inches, and turned back, and the muscles are to be divided down to the bone by a second circular incision. Then a long slender double-edged knife, called a catline, is passed between the bones to divide the interosseous ligament and muscles, and both bones are sawn through together, the flesh being protected by a retractor, which should have three tails. The spine of the tibia, if it projects much, may be removed with a fine saw or bone nippers. The anterior and posterior tibial and peronæal arteries, and any others requiring it, being tied, the stump is to be treated as directed after amputation of the thigh. The integuments should be put together, so as to make a perpendicular line of junction.

(2.) But it is agreed on all sides that the flap operation is by far the best for this situation. The surgeon passes his knife horizontally behind both bones at the level of an inch below the head of the fibula, and cuts

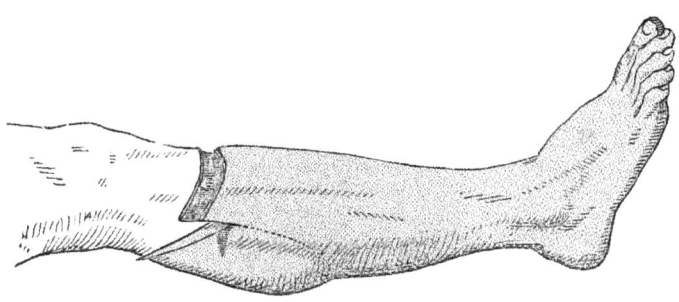

downwards and forwards, so as to make a flap of the posterior muscles about four or five inches long. A semilunar incision, with the convexity downwards, is then made across the front of the limb, the skin is slightly turned back, the parts between the bones are divided, and the bones are sawn as before. The edges are of course brought together horizontally. Mr. Liston directs this operation to be performed as follows. The knife is entered behind the fibula on the right side, and behind the inner margin of the tibia on the left, and is made to cut straight up towards the knee for one or two inches. It is next brought across the front of the limb, so as to make a semilunar division of the integument, and then, being brought to a point opposite the first incision, is made to transfix the limb, and form the posterior flap as before. When transfixing the right limb, the surgeon must take especial care not to get his knife between the two bones. In thus operating high, the poplitæal artery will be divided instead of the two tibials. The relative situation of this vessel, and the form of the flap, are shown in the following figure. The tibia, however, should never be sawn higher than its tuberosity, or the joint will be laid open. The amputation near the ankle is performed in the same manner. If low down, the *tendo Achillis* will require to be shortened after the flap is made.

IV. AMPUTATION OF THE ARM.—In amputation of the upper extremity, the flow of blood may be sufficiently commanded by compressing the artery above the clavicle, or in the arm. If it is thought proper, however, the torniquet may be applied so as to compress the artery against the humerus.

(1.) *Circular.*—The arm being held out, and an assistant drawing up the skin, one circular incision is made through the skin, which being forcibly retracted, another is made down to the bone. These incisions should be made with two slight divergences, so as to cut the

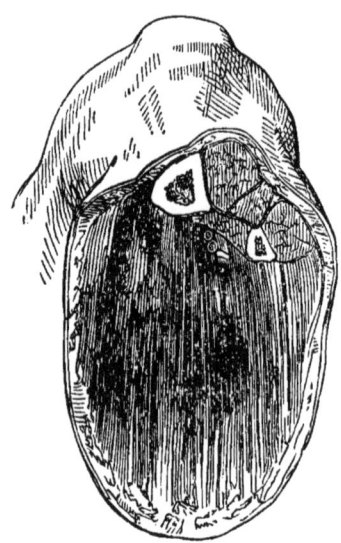

skin and muscles rather longer in front and behind than at the sides. The subsequent steps are precisely similar to those in amputating the thigh.

(2.) *Flaps.*—The knife is entered at one side, carried down to the bone, turned over it, brought out at a point opposite, (the vessels being left behind for the second flap,) and then made to cut a neat rounded anterior flap. It is next carried behind the bone, to make a posterior one of equal length; and is lastly swept round the bone, to divide any remaining fibres. The division of the bone, ligature of the arteries, and treatment of the stump, as before.

V. AMPUTATION AT THE SHOULDER may be performed in several manners. (1.) The patient being seated in a chair, and well supported, and the subclavian artery compressed, the surgeon enters a long straight knife at the anterior margin of the deltoid muscle, an inch below the acromion. From this point he thrusts it through the muscle, across the outside of the joint, and brings out the knife at the posterior margin of the axilla. If the left side is operated on, the knife must be entered at the posterior margin of the axilla, and be brought out at the anterior margin of the deltoid muscle. Then, by cutting downwards and outwards, the external flap is made. The origins of the biceps and triceps, and insertions of the infra and supra spinatus, are next cut through, and the joint is laid open. Finally the blade of the knife, being placed on the inner side of the head of the bone, must be made to cut the inner flap.

(2.) The covering for the exposed part or the scapula, in the preceding operation, was obtained from the deltoid. But it may also be obtained from the muscles in front or behind, supposing the deltoid to be implicated in the disease or injury which demands the operation. One elliptical incision may be carried from beneath the middle of the acromion to the posterior border of the axilla, and another to the anterior border. These flaps being dissected up, the head of the bone may be turned out of the socket, and the remaining soft parts be divided; or the bone may be sawn through just beneath its neck.

VI. AMPUTATION AT THE ELBOW is performed by passing the knife through the muscles in front of the joint, and cutting upwards and forwards, so as to make a flap of them. Then the operator (who stands on the inner side for the right arm, and *vice versâ*) makes a transverse incision behind the joint. He then cuts through the external lateral ligament, and enters the joint between the head of the radius and external condyle, then divides the internal lateral ligament, and lastly saws through the olecranon, the apex of which, with the triceps attached to it, is of course left in the stump.

VII. AMPUTATION OF THE FOREARM should always be performed as near to the wrist as possible.

(1.) *Circular.* The limb being supported with the thumb uppermost, and an assistant drawing up the skin, a circular incision is made through it down to the fascia. When the skin has again been retracted as much as possible, the muscles are divided by a second circular incision; the interosseous parts and the remaining fibres are next cut through with a catline; the flesh is drawn up with a three-tailed retractor, one tail of which is put between the bones, and the bones are then to be sawn through together, the saw being worked perpendicularly. The radial, ulnar, and two interosseous arteries require ligature.

(2.) *Flaps.*—The limb being placed as before, and the skin being drawn back, the surgeon grasps the wrist with his left hand, and forms one flap by cutting obliquely from the skin towards the bones, (through the extensor muscles, if he is to remove the right forearm; and the flexors, if the left.) The extremities of this incision should be made to project somewhat on the other side of the limb. The knife is then passed perpendicularly from one extremity of this incision to the other, through the muscles on the other side of the bones, and the other flap is made by cutting through them obliquely outwards; the interosseous parts are then divided, and the bones sawn as before.

VIII. AMPUTATION OF THE WRIST.—(1.) *Circular.*—The skin being pulled back, a circular incision is made a little below the level of the line that separates the fore-arm from the hand. The external lateral ligament is then cut through, and the knife carried across the joint, to divide the remaining attachments.

(2.) *Flaps.*—A semilunar incision is made across the back of the wrist, its extremities being at the styloid processes, and its centre reach-

ing down as far as the second row of carpal bones. This flap being
dissected up, the joint is opened behind, the lateral ligaments are cut
through, and the knife, being placed between the carpus and bones of the
fore-arm, is made to cut out a flap from the anterior surface of the palm.

IX. AMPUTATION OF THE HAND.—(1.)—Amputation of the *fingers or*

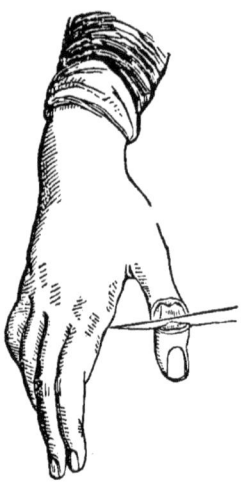

*thumb at their last joint* may be performed thus. The surgeon holds
the phalanx firmly between his finger and thumb, and bends it, so as to
give prominence to the head of the middle phalanx. He then makes a
straight incision across the head of the middle phalanx, so as to cut into
the joint, and takes care to carry it deeply enough at the sides to divide
the lateral ligaments. The joint being then held open, and the bistoury
placed as in the preceding figure, it is made to cut out a flap from the
palmar surface of the last phalanx, sufficient to cover the head of the
bone. If, however, the joint cannot be bent, this operation may be performed thus. The surgeon, holding the phalanx firmly, with its palmar
surface upwards, first passes his knife horizontally across the front of
the joint, the flat surface towards it, and cuts out the anterior flap; then
divides the lateral ligaments and the remaining attachments with one
sweep of the knife.

(2.) Amputation at the *second joint* of the fingers or thumb may be
performed in the same manner.

(3.) It is always expedient to save as much as possible of the forefinger and thumb; consequently, in cases admitting of it, the soft parts
may be divided by means of two semilunar incisions, and then being
protected with a piece of split cloth, the bone may be sawn through, or
be cut with bone-nippers. But this method is necessarily more tedious
and painful than amputation at the joints.

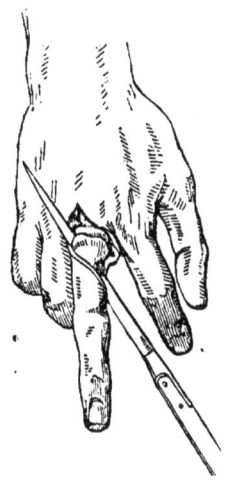

(4.) Amputation of a *finger at the metacarpel joint* may be effected by making a semilunar incision (with the convexity forwards) over one side of the prominence of the knuckle, from a quarter of an inch beyond the joint, to the middle of the digital commissure on the other side of it. The finger being then drawn to the other side, the extensor tendon is cut through, and the point of the bistoury is passed into the joint, and made to divide its ligaments. This will allow the head of the bone to be turned out, so that the bistoury being placed behind it may cut through the remaining attachments, as represented in the figure. This operation may also be performed by making an oval incision on one side of the joint, (as in the last-described method,) and then bringing it across the palmar surface, and round the other side, to terminate where it began. The tendons and ligaments are now to be divided, and the head of the bone turned out. The digital arteries must be tied, and after bleeding has ceased, the wound may be closed by confining the adjoining fingers together. It must be recollected that the situation of this joint is full half an inch above the lines that divide the fingers from the palm.

(5.) Amputation of the *metacarpal bone of the thumb* is performed thus. The thumb being separated from the fingers, an incision must be carried from the centre of the commissure between it and the forefinger, down to the articulation, with the trapezium. The incision should be inclined rather towards the metacarpal bone of the thumb. The thumb being then forcibly abducted, the blade of the bistoury is to be carried through the joint, (which, it must be recollected, lies obliquely in a line extending to the root of the little finger;) the head of the bone is to be forcibly dislocated towards the palm; the knife is then made to cut its

63

way out, so as to form a flap of the skin and muscles outside, as far as the first phalanx.

(6.) Amputation of the *metacarpal bone of the little finger*, at the joint between it and the unciform is performed thus. The flesh and integuments being grasped, and drawn away from the ulnar side of the bone, a bistoury is passed perpendicularly through them close to the joint, and made to cut its way downwards to a little beyond the articulation with the first phalanx. The skin of the hand being next strongly drawn towards the thumb side, the bistoury is placed on the other side of the bone, (without again piercing the skin,) and carried along so as to divide every thing down to the digital commissure. Then ,the ligaments of the joint are to be divided, first on the inner, and next on the dorsal aspect. It is, however, a much better plan, if it can be effected, to cut through the bone by means of the saw or bone-nippers, than to remove it at the articulation.

(7.) Amputation of the *head of a metacarpal bone* is effected by making an incision on each side of it, (as in amputation of the fingers at the joint, but extending higher up,) and then cutting through the bone with the pliers, or, if they are not at hand, with the metacarpal saw. If the part or the whole of the shaft of one of these is to be removed also, an incision should be made along its dorsum, to the point where the two former ones meet; and then the flesh being dissected away on either side, the bone may be cut through or disarticulated according to circumstances.

X. AMPUTATION OF THE FOOT.—(1.) Amputation of the *toes* at any of their joints is performed in precisely the same manner as amputation of the fingers.

(2.) Amputation of *all the toes at their metatarsal joints*—an operation which may be requisite in cases of frost-bite—is performed by first making a transverse incision along the dorsal aspect of the metatarsal bones—dividing the tendons and lateral ligaments of each joint in succession; and then, the phalanges being dislocated upwards, the knife is placed beneath their metatarsal extremities, and made to cut out a flap from the skin on the plantar surface, sufficient to cover the heads of the metatarsal bones. The arteries are to be tied and the foot laid on its outer side, so that the discharge may escape more readily.

(3.) Amputation of the *metatarsal bone of the great toe* is performed precisely like the operation for the removal of the metacarpal bone of the little finger. It is better, if circumstances permit, to cut through the bone, than to disarticulate it from the internal cuneiform bone.

(4.) Amputation of *all the metatarsal bones* is performed in the following manner. The exact situation of the articulation of the great toe to the inner cuneiform bone (to which the tendon of the tibialis anticus may serve as a guide) being ascertained, a semilunar incision, with the con-

vexity forwards, is made from a point just in front of it across the instep
to the outside of the tuberosity of the fifth metatarsal bone. The flap of
skin so formed being turned back, the bistoury is to be passed round behind the projection of the fifth metatarsal bone, so as to divide the external
ligaments which connect it with the cuboid. The dorsal ligaments are
next to be cut through, and then the remaining ones, the bone being
depressed. The fourth and third metatarsal bones are to be disarticulated
in a similar manner, dividing their ligaments with the point of the knife
and taking care not to let the instrument become locked between the bones.
The first metatarsal is next to be attacked, and lastly the second, the extremity of which, being locked in between the three cuneiform, will be
more difficult to dislodge. Perhaps it may be convenient to saw it
across. When all the five bones are detached, the surgeon completes
the division of their plantar ligaments, and slightly separates the textures
which adhere to their under surface with the point of the knife, and then,
the foot being placed horizontally, he puts the blade under the five bones,
and carries it forwards along their inferior surface, so as to form a flap
from the sole of the foot sufficient to cover the denuded tarsal bones. The
flap should be about two inches wide on the inner side, and one on the
outer.

(5.) Amputation may be performed *through the tarsus*, so as to remove
the navicular and cuboid bones, with all the parts in front of them. This
is commonly called *Chopart's operation.* In the first place, the articulation of the cuboid with the os calcis, (which lies about midway between the external malleolus and the tuberosity of the fifth metatarsal
bone,) and that of the navicular with the astragalus—(which will be found
just behind the prominence of the navicular bone in front of the inner
ankle)—must be sought for, and a semilunar incision be made from one
to the other, as in the last described operation. The flap of skin being
turned back, the internal and dorsal ligaments that connect the navicular
to the astragalus, are to be divided with the point of the bistoury—recollecting the convex shape of the head of the latter bone. The ligaments connecting the os calcis and cuboid are next divided—and lastly, a
flap is to be procured from the sole of the foot, as in the last operation.*

STUMPS, *Affections of.*—1. *Secondary hæmorrhage* may occur under
the same circumstances as after other wounds, and requires no observations distinct from those made at pages 144 and 289.

(2.) *Erysipelas* and *phlebitis* have also been fully treated of elsewhere;—

---

* For every farther information concerning amputations, the author must refer his
readers to Mr. Liston's frequently quoted Practical Surgery, (from which the wood-
cuts in this chapter are borrowed,) and to Malgaigne's Manuel de Medecine Opera-
toire.

one of them may be suspected to be coming on if the patient, a few days after amputation, is seized with a violent shivering.

(3.) It sometimes happens that the flesh shrinks away from the end of the bone, which becomes white and dry, and finally exfoliates. The nitric acid lotion is the best application.

(4.) *Protrusion of the bone* is a very awkward circumstance. It not only greatly retards the healing of the stump, but the cicatrix when formed is thin, red, constantly liable to ulcerate, and unable to bear the least pressure or friction. The cause of the *conical stump*, as it is technically called, is generally a want of skin and muscle sufficient to cover the end of the bone. Sometimes, however, it arises from spasmodic retraction of the muscles—especially if they have not been properly supported by bandages during the cure. The remedy is simple; the bone must be shortened. This may be done in slight cases by making a longitudinal incision over the bone on the side opposite the vessels, and sawing off a sufficient portion of it—removing at the same time any diseased portion of the cicatrix. But if the projection is considerable, a second amputation is necessary.

(5.) *Neuralgia* of the stump is another very untoward event. It sometimes arises, because the truncated extremities of the nerves (which after amputation always swell and become bulbous) adhere to the cicatrix, so as to be subject to constant compression and tension. Sometimes, however, it is entirely independent of any morbid state of the extremities of the nerves, but arises from some irritation in their course, or from some disease in the spinal cord at their origin. Sometimes, again, no local cause whatever is detectible; and the pain is evidently connected with an hysterical state of the system. In any case the symptoms are extreme irritability and tenderness—paroxysms of violent neuralgic pain—and spasms and twitchings of the muscles—which not unfrequently retract, and cause the bone to protrude, and the stump to become conical. *Treatment.*—(1.) Gentle friction with strong mercurial ointment—to which a little powdered camphor or extract of belladonna may be advantageously added—or Scott's ointment, F. 25, spread on lint, and worn as a plaster, or the emplastrum saponis or plumbi, combined with a little belladonna or opium—together with change of air, and the administration of remedies calculated to restore the strength, maintain the secretions, and allay irritability, such as sarsaparilla with henbane;—steel in various forms;—and aloetic pills with galbanum—sometimes suffice to remove the extreme sensitiveness of these as well as of other irregular cicatrices. (2) If the pain and tenderness are referred to one or two nerves only, their bulbous extremities should be cut down upon and removed. (3) If, however, the whole surface of the stump is implicated, or if the bone protrudes, a second amputation should be resorted to. But in the case of young hysterical women, the propriety of a second operation is extremely doubtful. The cases on record in which this practice was adopted, present no very satisfactory results; the pain was removed for a time, but returned when the wound healed. It can therefore be justifiable only when performed at the patient's urgent request, after every local and general remedy likely to be of service has been tried perseveringly, but in vain.

EXCISION OF JOINTS.—In certain cases of chronic disease or gunshot injuries of joints, an attempt may be made to save the limb, by cutting out the joint, instead of performing amputation. This operation has now been performed on most of the joints; and the results cannot be stated better than in the words of Mr. Blackburn, who says, " that excision is advisable in the shoulder and elbow;—that it is admissible, though of doubtful utility, in the ankle;—and that it is inadmissible, except under very peculiar circumstances, in the wrist, hip, and knee."*

The manner of excising the elbow joint is thus described by Mr. Liston. The patient sits in a chair; one assistant steadies him, and another holds out the hand and fore-arm. An incision about three inches long is made on the back of the joint, on the radial side of the ulnar nerve, by putting the knife through the skin and triceps, and carrying it down along the humerus and ulna. Another transverse incision, which should cut into the joint below the outer condyle, is made to fall into the middle of the first at right angles;—then " the two flaps are reverted by a few strokes of the knife, and the soft parts, along with the nerve, are turned over the inner condyle; the ends of the bones, but slightly retained by their ligaments, are turned out of the wound by flexing the fore-arm; the soft parts are detached, as much as is necessary, by cutting upon and close to the bones; the extent of ulceration or necrosis is then well ascertained, and by the application of the saw the unsound parts may be removed." A copper spatula may be used to protect the nerve and soft parts whilst the bones are sawed. The cutting bone forceps may be substituted for the saw with young patients. Any arteries that require it having been tied, the wound is closed by two or three sutures and . slips of plaster, and placed half-bent on a pillow. The ends of the bones will unite by ligament, and in many cases a very useful degree of motion will be acquired.

The shoulder joint may be exposed by making a perpendicular incision through the deltoid, three inches downwards from the acromion; and another from the extremity of the first incision to the posterior border of the deltoid. The triangular flap, thus formed, is reflected upwards and backwards; the joint may be laid open; the head of the humerus be

* Guy's Hosp. Rep., vol. i.

exposed and turned out, and sawn off; and the glenoid cavity of the scapula, if diseased, may be removed by the bone-nippers.

These operations must of course be well considered before they are
set about. They must neither be performed unnecessarily, in cases that
might get well with proper local and constitutional treatment;—nor, on
the other hand, should they be resorted to when the constitution has
become exhausted, and the limb disorganized by long suppuration;—nor
yet in cases of injury so complicated, that the patient would be liable to
sink from the ensuing irritation and discharge.

# CHAPTER IV.

## OF THE LIGATURE OF ARTERIES.

It may be as well to remind the reader, that when an artery is
wounded, the wounded part should always, if possible, be exposed, and
a ligature be placed above and below it. If the wound in the superjacent parts pass directly to the vessel, it may be enlarged in the proper
direction and to the requisite extent. If, however, the wound pass indirectly, (from the back of the thigh, for instance, to the femoral artery,)
the part of the vessel supposed to be wounded should be cut down upon
in the ordinary way. In both cases the introduction of a probe will be
a useful guide to the seat of injury. If the wounded part of the artery
cannot be tied, a ligature must be placed on the main trunk above, at the
nearest practicable point;—and perhaps it may be expedient to place another below to prevent regurgitation.

I. The Common Carotid Artery is generally tied below the spot
where it is crossed by the omo-hyoideus muscle. The patient is placed
in a recumbent position, with the head thrown back and slightly turned
towards the opposite side, and an incision three inches in length is made
along the inner margin of the sterno-mastoid muscle. This incision
should be carried through skin, platysma, and superficial fascia, and
should terminate about an inch above the sternum. The head should
now be brought a little forwards, so as to relax the sterno-mastoid
muscle, and the cellular tissue beneath is to be raised with forceps and
divided; but any veins that are found are to be turned aside with the
handle of the scalpel, and are not to be wounded if it can be avoided.
Next come the thin strong deep fascia and the omo-hyoideus muscle, to

the margins of which it adheres. It should be pinched up slightly with the forceps, just below that muscle, and be divided by cautious touches with the knife, which should be held with its flat surface towards the artery; and this division of the fascia should be made immediately over the artery, the situation of which is to be carefully ascertained with the finger. Then about half an inch of the sheath is to be opened in the same manner—avoiding the descendens noni nerve, which ramifies upon it. It should be opened rather to the inner side of the artery; so that the jugular vein may not be interfered with. Then an aneurism needle,

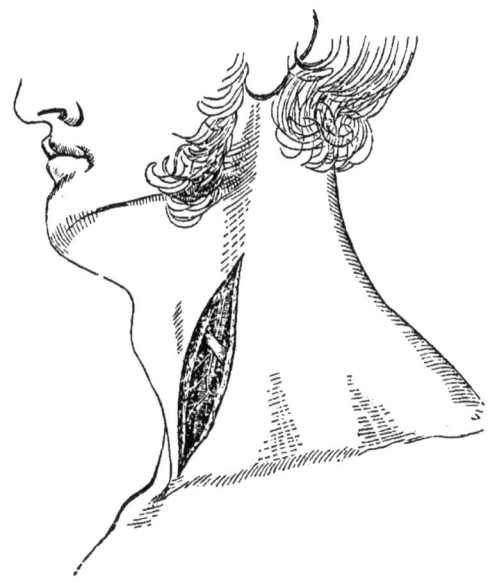

armed with a single ligature, is to be carried round the vessel. It is to be passed from the outer side, and to be kept close to the vessel, within its sheath. When its point appears on the inner side, the surgeon seizes the ligature with forceps, and withdraws the needle—ascertains that the nervus vagus is not included in the ligature—and then ties it tightly in the double knot represented at page 131. One end of the ligature may then be cut off close to the knot, and the other be left hanging out of the wound, which is to be closed with plaster when bleeding has ceased. The patient must be kept at perfect rest in bed till the ligature separates.

This artery may also be tied above the omo-hyoideus, by making an incision through the skin and platysma three inches in length, and terminating at the level of the cricoid cartilage. The fascia should next be divided on a director, in the same manner as the layers over a hernial sac, (p. 415.) The surgeon then separates the cellular tissue and veins from the sheath, and opens the sheath and passes the ligature in the manner described above.

II. The External Carotid may sometimes require a ligature, if many of its branches are wounded, *and cannot be tied*, but such an operation is very rarely, if ever, practised. An incision of the same length and direction as in the preceding two operations should be made through the skin, platysma, and sheath, so as to tie the vessel near its origin, that is, at the level of the os hyoides, and below the part where it is crossed by the digastric muscle and ninth nerve.

III. The Lingual Artery may be tied, by making a transverse incision along the os-hyoides from a little below the symphysis of the jaw to near the border of the sterno mastoid muscle. The skin, platysma, and fascia being divided, the artery must be looked for where it lies upon the greater cornu of the os hyoides, below the digastric muscle and ninth nerve. This artery has been tied in cases of tumours and wounds of the tongue; but considering the depth at which it lies from the surface, the irregularity of its origin, and the important parts in its vicinity, it is much better, as a general rule, to tie the external or common carotid.

IV. The Facial Artery may easily be tied by cutting through the skin and cellular tissue that cover it where it turns over the jaw, at the anterior border of the masseter; but such an operation can hardly ever be requisite.

V. The Arteria Innominata has been tied in cases of aneurism of the right subclavian, extending inwards as far as the scalenus. The patient being placed on his back, with the shoulders raised and head thrown back, one incision, two inches in length, is to be made along the inner margin of the sterno-mastoid muscle, terminating at the clavicle—and another across the origin of that muscle, meeting the former at a right angle. The flap of integument thus formed is to be turned up, and the sternal and part of the clavicular origin of the sterno-mastoid are to be divided on a director, which is to be passed behind the muscle, and kept as close to it as possible. The cellular tissue and fat which now appear, being turned aside, the sterno-hyoideus and sterno-thyroideus muscles must be separately divided on a director. A strong fascia, which next appears, must be cautiously scratched through, and the carotid be traced with the finger down to its origin. Then the vena innominata being depressed, a ligature may be carried from without inwards, round the artery, close to its bifurcation, taking care to avoid the vagus, recurrent, and cardiac nerves.

VI. The Right Subclavian Artery in the first part of its course, that is to say, between its origin from the innominata and the scalenus muscle, may be tied by an operation almost precisely similar to the latter. These two operations have each been performed four or five times in

cases of aneurism of the subclavian, reaching inwards as far as the scalenus, but without success.*

VII. THE SUBCLAVIAN ARTERY of either side may be readily tied external to the scalenus muscle. The patient should be laid on a table,
with the shoulder of the affected side drawn down as far as possible, and
the head slightly turned to the other side. An incision must then be
made through the skin and platysma from the margin of the sterno-mastoid to that of the trapezius. This preliminary incision may be -conve-
niently made by drawing down the skin, and cutting through it while it
is steadied on the clavicle. The superficial fascia must next be divided
to the same extent, taking care not to wound the external jugular vein.
The succeeding steps of the operation consists in cutting cautiously
through the cellular tissue and fascia down to the outer edge of the scalenus muscle. Many surgeons tear through them with a director or blunt
silver knife. The point of the finger must next be passed along the scalenus down to the rib—and in the angle between that muscle and the rib,
the artery will be found. The needle must be passed round it from below upwards. If there is much difficulty with the common needle, that
of Dr. Mott or Mr. Weiss, with a contrivance for separating the point, and
bringing it and the ligature round on the other side of the vessel, may be
used instead.

VIII. THE AXILLARY ARTERY below the clavicle may be tied by
making a semilunar incision, with its convexity upwards, from near the
sternal end of the clavicle to the anterior margin of the deltoid muscle.
The skin, superficial fascia, and clavicular fibres of the pectoralis major
muscle, are to be divided in succession—avoiding the cephalic vein and
thoracica-acromialis artery, where they pass between the pectoralis and
deltoid. The flap being turned down, a strong fascia which intervenes
between the pectoralis minor and subclavian muscles is next to be divided on a director;—the cellular tissue and veins covering the vessels are
to be turned aside;—then the axillary vein being pressed downwards, a
ligature is carried round the artery from below upwards. This operation
is exceedingly difficult, and only to be performed in case of wounds.

It is much more easy to tie this artery in the axilla. The arm being
widely separated from the trunk, and the fore-arm supinated, an incision
three inches in length is made over the head of the humerus, between
the margins of the pectoralis major and latissimus dorsi muscles, but rather
near the latter. The cellular tissue having been dissected through so as
to expose the vessel, and the vein and nerves drawn aside, the aneurism
needle should be passed from the inner side.

---

* The right subclavian was tied in the first part of its course by Mr. Partridge, in
the King's College Hospital, in February, 1841. The patient died four days afterwards, apparently from irritation of the pneumogastric nerve.

IX. The Brachial Artery is superficial in the whole of its course, and may be tied by making an incision two inches in length on the inner border of the coraco-brachialis muscle in the upper part, and of the biceps in the lower part of the limb. The incisions must be directed towards the centre of the limb—and the cellular tissue must be divided with cau⁻ tion, so as not to injure the internal cutaneous nerve, which lies super⁻ ficial to the artery in the upper part of its course. At the lower part of the limb, the basilic vein must be avoided. It must be recollected that the median nerve lies over the artery in the middle of its course—and that the vessel has two venæ comites, both of which must be carefully excluded from the ligature. Before tying the ligature, it should be ascer⁻ tained whether or not there is a *high division* of the artery, and whether the trunk that is exposed commands the circulation at the wounded or aneurismal part.

In the case of a small puncture of this artery at the bend of the elbow from carelessness in bleeding, the surgeon may either close the wound, and attempt the cure by compression—placing a graduated compress on the wound—bandaging the whole limb—and keeping the patient in bed and on low diet, so as to maintain a tranquil state of the circulation—or may at once enlarge the wound upwards and downwards to the extent of three inches—divide the fascia to the same extent, and tie the vessel above and below the wound—recollecting that the median nerve lies to its inner side. There are authorities for both practices. Supposing an aneurism to follow such an accident, it is better to cut into the tumour and tie the vessel above and below it, than to trust to one ligature at the lower part of the arm.

X. The Radial Artery in the upper third of the fore-arm may be tied by making an incision three inches in length, in a line from the bend of the elbow to the thumb, through the skin and superficial fascia, avoid⁻ ing the veins. The supinator longus and pronator teres being drawn asunder, and the deep fascia being divided to the same extent, the ar⁻ tery will be exposed, with its accompanying veins, which are to be care⁻ fully separated before the ligature is passed. The aneurism needle should be introduced from without, in order to avoid the radial nerve, which lies at a distance on the radial side.

This vessel can be readily tied in its middle third by making a similar incision through the same parts on the ulnar border of the supinator longus —and in the lower third, by making an incision on the radial side of the flexor carpi radialis. It may also be tied at the back of the carpus, just before it dips into the palm between the first and second metacarpal bones, by making an incision on the radial edge of the tendon of the ex⁻ tensor secundi internodii pollicis.

XI. Ulnar Artery.—When this vessel is wounded in its upper third, where it is covered deeply by muscles, it is an undecided point whether the wound should be dilated—cutting through or across the muscles to reach the bleeding point,—or whether the lower end of the brachial should be tied. The course of the incision for exposing the vessel in its upper third is shown in the adjoining cut. In the middle and inferior thirds of the fore-arm, this vessel may be readily exposed by cutting through the integuments and superficial fascia along the outer margin of the flexor carpi ulnaris for the extent of three inches. That muscle is then to be drawn inwards, the deep fascia to be divided, the veins to be separated from the artery, and the needle to be passed from within, so as to avoid the ulnar nerve which lies on the ulnar side.

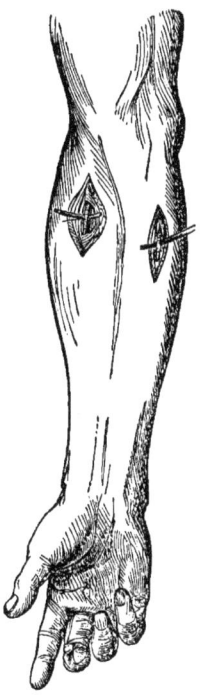

In wounds of the palm of the hand, with great hæmorrhage, the wound should be dilated, and the bleeding vessels be tied, unless they lie too deeply. If that is the case, methodical pressure should be resorted to—the wound being cleared of coagula, and filled with lint, (which may or may not be dipped in oil of turpentine,) and firm pressure being made upon it, before and behind, in the manner described at p. 288. But if hæmorrhage has recurred again and again, and the parts are inflamed or infiltrated with blood, the brachial artery should be tied just above the elbow.

XII. The Aorta, the Common Iliac, and the Internal Iliac arteries, may be tied by a similar operation. An incision from four to six inches in length must be made on the anterior surface of the abdomen.

It may either be made parallel to the outer border of the rectus, or to the epigastric artery—and it should terminate an inch above Poupart's ligament. The three layers of abdominal muscles are to be cautiously divided to the same extent—and the fascia transversalis likewise—it being first scratched through, so that the finger may be introduced be⁻ tween it and the peritonæum—to divide it upon. The peritoneum must now be detached by the fingers from the iliac fossa, as far as the brim of the pelvis, where the external iliac artery will be found beat⁻ ing—and by following this vessel upwards, the operator will come upon the internal or common iliac, or the aorta. The edges of the wound being now held asunder by copper spatulæ, the artery to be tied must be separated from its vein with the nail of the forefinger or the flat end of a probe, and the aneurism-needle be passed round between it and the vein. It will be recollected that the common iliac veins lie behind and to the right of their respective arteries—that the left internal iliac vein is behind its artery—and that the right is a little external as well as posterior. The internal iliac may require to be tied for disease or in-jury of the glutæal or other branches outside the pelvis.

XIII. The External Iliac artery may be tied, according to Sir A. Cooper's method, by making a semilunar incision (with the convexity looking downwards and outwards) from near the anterior superior spi-nous process of the ilium to the superior angle of the external abdominal ring. The skin, superficial fascia, and tendon of the external oblique having been divided, the lower margin of the internal oblique and trans-versalis muscles must be raised on the finger and be detached from Poupart's ligament,—and then if the finger is passed back under the spermatic cord, it will come in contact with the artery. The dense cellular tissue connecting the artery with the vein (which lies on its in-ternal and posterior aspect) must be scratched through, and the needle be passed between them.

XIV. The Femoral artery may be tied in any part of its course from Poupart's ligament downwards,—but the best spot for the ligature, when performed for popliteal aneurism, is just above the part where the vessel is overlapped by the sartorius—some little distance below the origin of the profunda. The patient being placed on his back, with the leg turned outwards, an incision must be made through the skin in the course of the vessel—which, it will be recollected, corresponds to a line drawn from the middle of Poupart's ligament to the inner edge of the patella. The incision may commence two inches below the groin, but its length must depend on the thickness of the parts to be divided. It is better to make it too long than too short. The cellular tissue must next be dissected down to the fascia lata—avoiding the saphenic vein. If any glands are in the way, they should be turned aside. The fascia lata is now to be

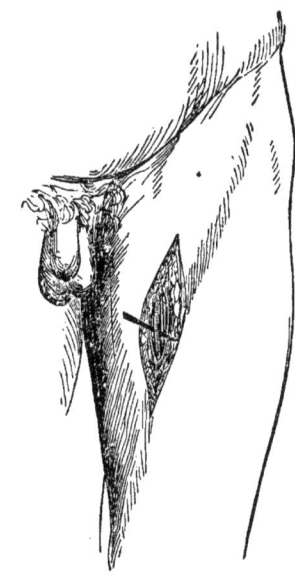

divided for about two inches, and the sartorius to be gently drawn outwards. The artery may now be felt, and when the sheath and the cellular tissue over it have been raised with the forceps and divided by cautious touches with the knife, (held with its flat surface towards the artery,)
—the point of the aneurism needle is to be gently insinuated between the
artery and the vein (which lies behind it.) The needle should be passed
from the inner side. Before finally tightening the ligature, the artery
should be compressed, to see whether the pulsation in the aneurism
ceases, in case of any irregularity in the course and distribution of the
vessel.

The FEMORAL artery may also be tied in the middle third of the thigh,
where it is covered by the sartorius, by cutting on the inner edge of that
muscle and turning it aside, and then slitting up the strong fibrous sheath
which envelopes the artery at that part; but this is a much more difficult
operation, and it has no commensurate advantages.

XV. THE GLUTÆAL artery may be tied by placing the patient on his face,
with the toes turned inwards, and making an incision from an inch below
the posterior spinous process of the ilium, and an inch from the sacrum,
towards the great trochanter. This incision should be about four inches
long. The fibres of the glutæus maximus having been cut through or
separated to the like extent, and a strong fascia beneath having been cut
through, the vessel will be found emerging from the upper part of the
sciatic notch. The SCIATIC artery may be found by making an incision
through the same parts and for the same extent, but an inch and a half
lower down. Both these operations are extremely difficult, from the
great depth to which the dissection must be carried, the unyielding na-

ture of the surrounding parts, and the hæmorrhage from the numerous blood-vessels that must necessarily be wounded. They should be attempted, however, in case of wounds—but for aneurisms of these arteries, it is necessary to tie the internal or common iliac.

XVI. The Poplitæal artery may be tied by cutting through the skin and fascia lata for the extent of. three inches on the outer border of the tendon of the semi-membranous muscle—the patient being placed on his face, with his knee straight. On pressing that tendon inwards, the artery may be felt. Its vein, which lies superficial, and rather external to it, must be cautiously separated and drawn outwards, and the needle be passed between them.

XVI. Posterior Tibial Artery.—The operation usually recommended for tying this artery in the upper part of the leg is performed thus. The limb being placed on its outer side, with the knee bent and the foot extended, an incision four inches in length must be made through the skin and fascia over the inner margin of the tibia, avoiding the saphena vein. The edge of the gastrocnemius thus exposed is to be turned back. A director must then be insinuated beneath the inner head of the solæus, and this muscle must be divided from its attachment to the tibia. The strong and tense fascia beneath it must next be divided in the same manner. Then the muscles being relaxed as much as possible by bending the knee and extending the foot, the artery may be felt about an inch from the edge of the tibia. The veins are to be separated from it, and an aneurism-needle passed round it from without, inwards, so as to avoid the nerve. The incision for this operation is shown in the following figure.

This operation, however, is considered by Mr. Guthrie to be so " painful, difficult, bloody, tedious, and dangerous," that he proposes to reach the artery by making a perpendicular incision six or seven inches in length, at the back of the leg, through the skin, gastrocnemius, plantaris, and solæus—then the fascia will be exposed with the artery beneath it, and the nerve to the outer side.

The Posterior tibial artery may be easily exposed, in the lower third of the leg, by cutting parallel to the tendo Achillis, and on its inner side, for the extent of two or three inches, through the skin and two layers of fascia. The cellular tissue and sheath of the vessel must next be cautiously divided, and the venæ comites having been separated from it, the needle must be passed round the vessel from the outer side.

This artery may also be tied behind the inner ankle. A semilunar incision, two or three inches long, is made in the hollow between the heel and the ankle, but rather nearer to the latter. The integuments, the superficial fascia, and a very strong tendinous aponeurosis, continuous with the deep fascia of the leg, must be successively divided to the same extent. The sheath of the vessels which will be thus exposed, must be

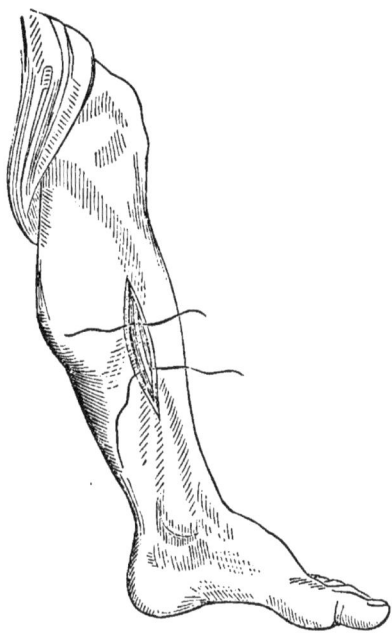

opened—the venæ comites separated, and the needle passed from the heel towards the ankle in order to avoid the nerve, which lies a little nearer to the heel.

XVIII. THE PERONÆAL artery may be exposed in the upper part of the leg by an incision similar to that which Mr. Guthrie proposes for the ligature of the posterior tibial, only rather more external. For the first few inches of its course, this vessel lies underneath the deep fascia—afterwards it lies concealed under the inner edge of the flexor longus pollicis, which must be turned aside to expose it.

XIX. THE ANTERIOR TIBIAL artery in the first third of its course, where it is covered by the extensor muscles, is very difficult to reach. If, however, it is expedient to place a ligature on it, an incision four or five inches in length must be made down to the fascia, in the direction of a line drawn from the head of the fibula to the base of the great toe. The intermuscular septum, between the tibialis anticus and extensor digitorum muscles must then be cut into, and the muscles be separated down to the interosseous ligament, where the artery will be found. The foot should be moved backwards and forwards at the ankle, in order to ascertain with exactness the junction of those muscles.

Below the middle of the leg, at any point to the termination of its course, this artery may be found on the fibular side of the extensor proprius pollicis tendon, which must be the guide for the incision. The coverings must be divided with the usual precautions, and neither the

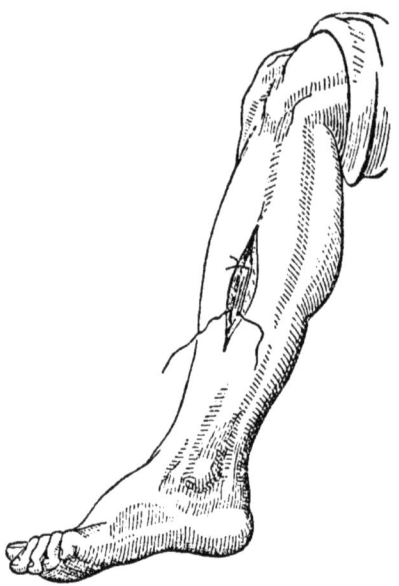

peronæal nerve nor the venæ comites should be wounded with the knife, or be included in the ligature.

In wounds of the arteries in the sole of the foot, (except perhaps of the external plantar, opposite the base of the little toe,) it is scarcely judicious to enlarge the wound with the view of securing the bleeding point. But methodical pressure should be applied after the manner recommended at page 288; and if that fails, the posterior tibial artery should be tied behind the inner ankle—and the anterior tibial on the dorsum of the foot likewise, if necessary.

# APPENDIX OF FORMULÆ.

---

### F. 1. *Tonic Draught.*

℞. Acidi sulphurici diluti ♏ v.—xv.; syrupi aurantii f3j.; infusi cascarillæ, (*vel* decocti cinchonæ,) f℥x. Misce, fiat haustus, ter vel quater die sumendus.

### 2. *Quinine draught.*

℞. Quinæ disulphatis gr. ii.—v.; tincturæ opii ♏. ii.—v.; spiritûs ætheris compositi, spiritûs ammoniæ aromatici, aa f℥ß.; decocti cinchonæ f℥x. Misce, fiat haustus, ter vel quater die sumendus.

### 3. *Quinine Draught.*

℞. Quinæ disulphatis gr. ii.—v.; Acidi hydrochlorici ♏ x.—xv.; camphoræ gr. ii.; spiritus ætheris nitrici f3j.; tincturæ cardamomi compositæ f3j.; aquæ menthæ viridis f℥x. Misce, fiat haustus, sextâ quâque horâ sumendus.

### 4. *Black Draught.*

℞ Sennæ foliorum ℨvj.; zinziberis concisi ℨß.; extracti glycyrrhizæ ℨii.; aquæ ferventis f℥ix. Post horas tres cola, et adde spiritus ammoniæ aromatici f℥ii.; tincturæ sennæ, tincturæ cardamomi compositæ aa f℥ß. Dosis f℥ißß.

### 5. *Saline Draught.*

℞. Potassæ nitratis Əij.; sodæ sesquicarbonatis Əß; vini antimonii f℥ii.; syrupi croci, spiritus ætheris nitrici, aa f℥ii.; aquæ f℥v. Misce. Dosis f℥ißß, quartâ quâque horâ.

65

### 6. *Calomel Pill.*

R. Calomelanos gr. i.—iii.; antimonii potassio-tartratis gr. ⅛—¼; extracti hyoscyami (*vel* conii) gr. iii. (*vel* pulveris opii gr. ½.) Misce, fiat pilula tertiâ—sextâ quâque horâ sumenda.

### 7. *Alterative Pill.*

R. Pilulæ hydrargyri gr. iii.; extracti hyoscyami (*vel* pulveris Doveri) gr. iii.; pulveris ipecacuanhæ gr. j. Misce, fiant pilulæ duæ omni nocti sumendæ.

### 8. *Cordial Aperient Draught.*

R. Pulveris rhei, potassæ sulphatis aa ɔj.; decocti aloes compositi, aquæ menthæ viridis aa fȝvj.; spiritus ammoniæ compositi fȝß. Misce, fiat haustus.

### 9. *Aperient Draught.*

R. Sodæ potassio-tartratis ȝiv.; tincturæ sennæ fȝiii.; spiritus myristicæ fȝß.; aquæ fȝiß. Misce, fiat haustus.

### 10. *Alterative Powder.*

R. Hydrargyri cum creta gr. iii —vi.; pulveris Doveri gr. i.—v. Misce, fiat pulvis omni nocte sumendus.

### 11. *Lead Lotion.*

R. Liquoris plumbi diacetatis fȝj.; acidi acetici diluti, spiritus rectificati aa fȝß.; aquæ fȝix. Misce, fiat lotio.

### 12. *Frigorific Mixture.*

R. Sodii chloridi, potassæ nitratis, ammoniæ hydrochloratis, partes æquales; aquæ quantum satis sit ad solvendas.

### 13. *Spirit Lotion.*

R. Spiritus vini rectificati fȝj.; aquæ fȝxv. Misce fiat lotio.

### 14. *Stimulating Liniment.*

R. Liquoris ammoniæ fȝii.; linimenti saponis (*vel* linimenti camphoræ compositi) fȝj. Misce, fiat linimentum.

### 15. *Zinc Lotion.*

R. Zinei sulphatis ȝj.; aquæ octarium. Misce, fiat lotio.

## 16. *Discutient Lotion.*

R. Ammoniæ hydrochloratis ℥ß.; acidi acetici diluti, spiritus rectificati aa f ℥ß.; misturæ camphoræ f℥xv. Misce, fiat lotio.

## 17. *Nitric Acid Lotion.*

R. Rosæ petalorum ℈j.; aquæ ferventis f℥viij.; acidi nitrici diluti f℥iiß. Misce, et cola post horam, ut fiat lotio.

## 18. *Castor Oil and Turpentine Draught.*

R. Olei terebinthinæ, olei ricini aa f℥vj.; tincturæ sennæ f℥ij.; mucilaginis acaciæ f℥ii,; acquæ menthæ quantum satis sit, ut fiat haustus.

## 19. *Demulcent Mixture for Gonorrhœa.*

R. Potassæ nitratis ℈ß.; sodæ sesquicarbonatis ℈ß.; (*vel* liquoris potassæ f℥ij.;) tincturæ hyoscyami, spiritus ætheris nitrici aa f℥ij; liquoris opii sedativi ℳ xx.—xxx.; misturæ amygdalæ f℥viiß. Misce, sumantur cochlearia tria ampla quartâ quâque horâ.

## 20. *Copaiba Mixture.*

R. Copaibæ f℥ii.—iv.; mucilaginis acaciæ f℥iv.; spiritus ætheris nitrici, spiritus lavandulæ aa f ℥ii.; olei cinnamomi guttas vi.; aquæ f℥v. Misce. Dosis f℥j. ter die.

## 21. *Acetate of Zinc Injection.*

R. Zinci sulphatis gr. v.; liquoris plumbi diacetatis f℈ß.; aquæ rosæ f℥iv. Misce, fiat injectio.

## 22. *Acetate of Copper Injection.*

R. Cupri sulphatis gr. v.; liquoris plumbi diacetatis f℈ß.; aquæ rosæ f℥iv. Misce, fiat injectio.

## 23. *Ammoniaret of Copper Injection.*

R. Liquoris cupri ammonia-sulphatis ℳ xx.; aquæ rosæ f℥iv. Misce, fiat lotio.

## 24. *Pearson's Liniment.*

R. Olei olivæ f℥iß.; olei terebinthinæ f ℥ß.; acidi sulphurici fortissimi f ℥iß. Misce grandatim.

### 25. *Scott's Ointment.*

R. Unguenti hydrargyri fortioris, cerati saponis aa ℥j. camphoræ pulverizatæ ʒj. Misce. (*Vide* p. 264.*)

### 26. *Battley's Liquor Cinchonæ.*†

R. Liquoris Cinchonæ flavæ ℳxx.; aquæ pimentæ f℥j. Misce, fiat haustus quater die sumendus.

### 27. *Antacid Mixture for Children.*

R. Magnesiæ ustæ ℈j.; spiritus ammoniæ aromatici fʒß.; syrupi aurautii fʒiii.; aquæ calcis, aquæ destillatæ aa f℥iij. Misce, sumantur cochlearia duo magna ter die.·

### 28. *Steel and Aloes Mixture.*

R. Ferri sulphatis ℈j.; sodæ subcarbonatis gr. xxv.: ammoniæ sesquicarbonatis ℈j.: vini aloes fʒß.; spiritus myristicæ fʒiii.; aquæ destillatæ f℥vij. Misce. Dosis fʒß. ter die.

### 29. *Sarsaparilla and Nitric Acid.*

R. Decocti sarsæ compositi f℥iv.; acidi nitrici diluti ℳ xx.—lx.; tincturæ hyoscyami fʒß. Misce, fiat haustus ter die sumendus.

### 30. *Corrosive Sublimate Pills.*

R. Hydrargyri sublimati corrosivi, ammoniæ hydrochloratis aa gr. i.—ii.; aquæ destillatæ guttam; micæ panis quantum satis est, ut fiant pilulæ xii., quarum sumatur una ter die.

### 31. *Bark and Guaiacum.*

R. Tincturæ guaiaci ammoniatæ tincturæ humuli aa fʒß.; decocti cinchonæ lancifoliæ f℥ii. Misce, fiat haustus, ter die sumendus.

### 32. *Eye Snuff.*

R. Pulveris asari partes tres, pulveris florum lavandula partes duas. Misce. *Vel.* R. Pulveris euphorbii partem unam, pulveris amyli partes septem. Misce.

---

* This ointment may easily be combined with pulv. opii, or ext. belladonnæ.
† One fluid drachm of this solution is equal to an ounce of the finest bark.

### 33. *Mercurial Eye Snuff.*

℞. Hydrargyri sub-sulphatis fiavi ʒß.; pulveris glycyrrhizæ ʒii. M'isceintime.

### 34. *Schmucker's Pills.*

℞. Sagapeni, galbani, saponis aa ʒj.; rhei ʒiß.; antimonii potassic-tartratis gr. xv.; succi glycyrrhizæ ʒj. Misce. Dosis gr. xv. bis die.

### 35. *Richter's Pills.*

℞. Ammoniaci, assafœtidæ, saponis, valerianæ, arnicæ, aa ʒii.; antimonii potassio-tartratis gr. xviii.; syrupi quantum satis est, ut fiat massa. Dosis gr. xx.—xxx. ter die.

### 36. *Collyria.*

℞. Zinci sulphatis gr. i.—iv.; *vel* aluminis gr. i.—iv.; *vel* cupri sulphatis gr. ½—ii.; *vel* argenti nitratis gr. i.—iv.; *vel* zinci acetatis gr. i.—vi.; *vel* liq. plumbi diacetatis ℳ x.; aquæ destillatæ f ʒj. Misce.

### 37. *Corrosive Sublimate Collyrium.*

℞. Hydrargyri sublimati corrosivi gr. j.; aquæ destillatæ f ʒviij. Misce. (*Mackenzie.*)

### 38. *Tartar Emetic Ointment.*

℞. Antimouii potassio-tartratis ʒj.; adipis ʒj. Misee.

### 39. *Detergent Gargle.*

℞. Liquoris calcis chlorinatæ f ʒiv.; mellis ʒj.; aquæ destillatæ f ʒiii. Misce. *A tablespoonful to be mixed with a glass of warm brandy and water, and to be used as a gargle.*

### 40. *Cooling Gargle.*

℞. Mellis confectionis rosæ caninæ aa ʒii.; aceti destillati f ʒß,; acidi hydrochlorici ℳ xx.; aquæ rosæ f ʒj.; aquæ puræ f ʒvj. Misce.

### 41. *Astringent Gargle.*

℞. Aluminis ʒj.; acidi sulphurici diluti ℳ xx.; tincturæ myrrhæ f ʒii.; decocti cinchonæ, f ʒvi. Misce.

### 42. *Aperient Electuaries.*

℞. Pulveris potassæ supertartratis, ʒß.; sulphuris præcipitati, ʒii—iv.; confectionis sennæ, ʒj.; syrupi zinziberis, quantum satis sit.

℞. Magnesiæ ustæ, potassæ supertartratis, florum sulphuris, pulveris rhei, aa. ʒj.; pulveris zinziberis, ʒß.; theriacæ, quantum satis sit.

℞. Mannæ, confectionis sennæ, aa. ʒj; sulphuris ʒiij., syrupi quantum satis sit; dosis, ʒi—ʒiv., omni nocte horâ somni.

### 43. *Ointment for Piles.*

℞. Pulverisgallæ ʒj.; liquoris plumbi diacetatis ♏xv.; adipis ʒj. Misce.

### 44. *Mustard Poultice.*

℞. Lini seminum, sinapis singulorum contritorum libram dimidiam; aceti fervefacti, quantum satis sit; ut fiat cataplasmatis crassitudo. Misce. (Pharm. Lond.)

### 45. *Linseed Meal Poultice.*

The highest authority on poultices was Mr. Abernethy, who seemed to revel in the idea of them. "Scald your basin," he says, "by pouring a little hot water into it, then put a small quantity of finely-ground linseed meal into the basin, pour a little hot water on it and stir it round briskly until you have well incorporated them; add a little more meal and a little more water, then stir it again. Do not let any lumps remain in the basin, but stir the poultice well, and do not be sparing of your trouble. If properly made, it is so well worked together that you might throw it up to the ceiling, and it would come down again without falling in pieces; it is in fact like a pancake. What you do next, is to take as much of it out of the basin as you may require, lay it on a piece of soft linen, let it be about a quarter of an inch thick, and so wide that it may cover the whole of the inflamed part"

### 46. *Yeast Poultice.*

℞. Farinæ ℔. i ; cerevisiæ fermenti f ʒ i. Misce, et calorem lenem adhibe donec intumescant. (Pharm. Lond.)

### 47. *Bread Poultice.*

"I shall now speak," says Mr. Abernethy, "of the bread and water poultice. The way in which I direct it to be made is the following:— Put half a pint of hot water into a pint basin, add to this as much of the crumb of bread as the water will cover; then place a plate over the basin and let it remain about ten minutes; stir the bread about in the water, or, if necessary, chop it a little with the edge of the knife, and drain off the water by holding the knife on the top of the basin, but do not press the bread, as is usually done; then take it out lightly, and spread it about one-third of an inch thick on some soft linen, and lay it upon the part."

A very admirable soft poultice for parts that are excoriated, or that threaten to slough from pressure, during long illnesses, may be made by mixing together equal parts of bread crumbs and of mutton suet grated very fine, with a little boiling water, and stirring them into a saucepan over the fire till they are well incorporated.

### 48. *Opiate Enema.*

℞. Decocti amyli f ℥iv.; tincturæ opii f℥ß—ʒj. Misce. (Pharm. Lond.)

### *Opiate Suppository.*

℞. Pulveris opii gr. i.—iv; saponis gr. x.; contunde simul.

### 49. *Turpentine Enema.*

℞. Olei terebinthinæ f ℥j.; vitelli ovi, (vel mucilaginis acaciæ,) quan-tum satis sit; tere simul et adde, decocti hordei, *vel* decocti avenæ f ℥xix.

### 50. *Tobacco Enema.*

℞. Tabaci foliorum ʒß.; aquæ octarium dimidium; macera per horæ quartam partem, et cola.

### 51. *Castor Oil Enema.*

℞. Olei ricini f ℥iii.; potassæ carbonatis gr. xv.; saponis ʒj.; aquæ ferventis octarium; tere simul donec bene misceantur.

### 52. *Alterative Powder.*

℞. Hydrargyri cum creta gr. ii.; pulveris rhei gr. v. Misce, fiat pulvis, omni nocte sumendus.

### 53. *Zinc Mixture.*

℞. Zinci sulphatis gr. vj.; acidi sulphurici diluti ♍ xxx; syrupi aurantii f ʒß.; infusi aurantii f ʒvß. Misce, sumantur cochlearia duo ter die.

### 54. *Antacid Mixture.*

℞. Sodæ susquicarbonatis ʒß.; spiritus ammoniæ aromatici f ʒiii; syrupi zinziberis f ʒß.; tincturæ cardamomi compositæ f ʒ ß. aquæ cin-namomi f ʒv. Misce, sumantur cochlearia duo ter die, (*after meals.*)

### 55. *Rheubarb and Magnesia.*

℞ Pulveris rhei gr. x.; magnesiæ ustæ gr. v.; pulveris zinziberis gr. ii. Misce, fiat pulvis, omni mane sumendus.

### 56. *Alkaline Infusion of Sarsaparilla.*

R. Sarsaparillæ Jamaicensis radicis, concisæ et contusæ ℥ii.; radicis glycyrrhizæ concisæ Ʒii.; liquoris potassaæ ℳ xl.—lx.; aquæ destillatæ ferventis f℥x.; tincturæ cardamomi compositæ fℨiii. Macera per horas viginti quatuor et, cola. Sumatur totum quotidie.

### 57. *Sarsaparilla and Lime Water.*

R. Sarsaparillæ ℥ii.; glycyrrhizæ Ʒii.; liquoris calcis f℥x. Macera per horas viginti quatuor et cola. Sumatur totum indies.*

### 58. *Corrosive Sublimate and Bark for Children.*

R. Hydrargyri sublimati corrosivi gr. j.; tincturæ cinchonæ (*vel* tincturæ rhei) ℥ii.; solve. Dosis fℨj.; ter die ex aquâ.†

### 59. *Epsom Salts and Tartar Emetic.*

R. Magnesiæ sulphatis ℥j.; antimonii tartarizati gr. j.; sp. ætheris nitrici Ʒii.; aquæ menthæ f℥x. Misce, sumantur cochlearia magna tria, quartâ quâque horâ.

### 60. *Lead Pills.*

R. Plumbi acetatis gr. iii.; pulveris opii gr. jß.; micæ panis Ʒß. Misce; fiant pilulæ sex; quarum summatur una, quartâ quâque horâ, cum haustu sequente.

### 61. *Vinegar Draught.*

R. Aceti destillati fℨiii.; syrupi papaveris fℨj.; aquæ f℥j. Misce.

### 62. *Ammoniated Iron.*

R. Ferri ammonio-chloridi gr. xii—xx.; sodæ sesquicarbonatis gr. xii.; ammoniæ sesquicarbonatis Ʒj.; syrupi f℥ß.; aquæ destillatæ f℥vß. Misce. Dosis fℨj. ter die.

### 63. *Chalybeate Mixtures.*

R. Tincturæ ferri sesquichloridi fℨii.; spiritus ætheris nitrici, syrupi

---

* 56, 57. It is far better to give sarsaparilla in a concentrated form, than to flood the stomach with a pint of it. Besides, private patients will not drink a whole pint; it makes them cold, windy, and comfortless.

† 58. This, as well as arsenic, iodine, and other irritating medicines, should be taken after meals.

croci āā f℈iii.; misturæ camphoræ f℥v. Misce. Sumantur cochlearia duo magna ter die.

℞. Vini ferri f℥vi.; tincturæ ferri sesquichloridi ℳ xx. ; aquæ destillatæ f℥vj. Misce. Sumantur cochlearia duo ter die.

### 64. *Opiate Lotion.*

℞. Pulveris opii ℈ß.; aquæ destillatæ ferventis f℥viii.; macera per horas duas, et cola.

### 65. *Opiate Poultice.*

℞. Micæ panis, et *lotionis opiatæ* suprapræscriptæ, singulorum, quantum satis sit.

### 66. *Conium Lotion.*

℞. Extracti conii ℨj.; aquæ destillatæ f℥iii. ; tere simul, et macera per horas duas; dein cola.

### 67. *Conium Poultice.*

℞. Cataplasmatis panis (F. 47) quantum satis sit; extracti conii ℈j. Misce.

### 68. *Arsenical Lotion.*

℞. Liquoris arsenicalis f℈i—ii.; aquæ destillatæ f℥j. Misce.

### 69. *Steel and Acid Mixture.*

℞. Ferri sulphatis gr. xii.; acidi sulphurici diluti f℈j.; tincturæ cardamomi compositæ f℥ß.; infusi rosæ compositi f ℥vß. Misce; sumantur cochlearia duo magna ter die.

### 70. *Black Wash.*

℞. Calomelanos ℨj.; mucilaginis acaciæ f℥ß; liquoris calcis f℥vß. Misce.

### 71. *Yellow Wash.*

℞. Hydrargyri sublimati corrosivi gr. vi.—℈j.; liquoris calcis f℥vj. Misce.

### 72. *Peruvian Balsam Ointment.*

℞. Balsami Peruviani ℨj.; unguenti cetacei ℨj. Misce.

### 73. *Diluted Citrine Ointment.*

℞. Unguenti hydrargyri nitratis ℨß.; olei amygdalæ f℥ß. Solve leni calore.

66

### 74. *Iodine Mixture.*\*

℞. Iodinii gr. ¼; potassii iodidi gr. j.; aquæ destillatæ f ℥vj.

*Vel.* ℞. Tincturæ iodinii compositi (p. l.) ℳ xx.; aquæ destillatæ f ℥vj.

*Vel.* ℞. Liquoris potassii compositi (p. l.) f ℨ ß.; aquæ destillatæ f ℥vß. Misce. Sumatur totum indies divisis dosibus.

### 75. *Iodine Ointment.*

℞. Iodinii gr. vj.; potassii iodidi ϶ii.; adipis ℥j. Misce.

### 76. *Iodine Lotion.*

℞. Liquoris potassii iodidi compositi f ℨj.; aquæ destillatæ f ℥x. Misce. *For scrofulous ulcers, fistulæ, ophthalmia, &c.*

### 77. *Rubefacient Solution of Iodine.*

℞. Iodinii ℨiv.; potassii iodidi ℨj.; aquæ destillatæ f ℨvj. Misce. *'To touch very indolent sores; the edges of the eyelids, ozena, &c.*

### 78. *Caustic Solution of Iodine.*

℞. Iodinii, potassii iodidi āā ℨj.; aquæ destillatæ f ℨii. Misce. *To destroy weak granulations, ragged edges of sores, &c.*

### 79. *Iodine Bath.*

Should contain, for children, half a grain of iodine to cach quart of warm water;—and for adults, one drachm to twenty-five gallons. The body may be immersed ten minutes.†

### 80. *Tonic Aperient and Antacid Powder.*

℞. Sodæ carbonatis exsiccatæ gr. v.; pulveris calumbæ gr. x.; pulveris rhei gr. ii. Misce; fiat pulvis quotidie, ante prandium sumendus.

### 81. *Strong Camphor Mixture.*

℞. Camphoræ gr. xxv.; amygdalas dulces decorticatas sex; sacchari purificati ℨiii.; optime contere, dein adde gradatim, aquæ menthæ viridis

---

\* These three formulæ are of the same strength. The dose of iodine may be gradully increased to gr. 4·5ths, or gr. i. daily.

† Vide Essays on the Effects of Iodine in scrofulous diseases, by Lugol; translated by O'Shaughnessy; London, 1831.

f ℥viiß. ut fiat mistura, cujus sumantur cochlearia tria magna, quartâ quâque horâ. (*Hooper.*)

### 82. *Steel, Soda, and Rhubarb.*

℞. Ferri sesquioxydi Əj.; sodæ sesquicarbonatis gr. iii.; pulveris rhei gr. iii. Misce. Fiat pulvis, ter die sumendus.

### 83. *Demulcent Mixture for Gonorrhœa.*

℞. Liquoris potassæ f℈ii.; liquoris opii sedativi f℈ß.; misturæ amygdalæ f ℥vj. Misce. Sumantur cochlearia duo quartâ quaque horâ.

### 84. *Copaiba and Oil of Cubebs.*

℞. Copaibæ f℈iii.; olei cubebæ ♏ xx.; liquoris potassæ f℈ii.; sp. myristicæ f℈iii.; misturæ camphoræ f ℥vii. Misce. Sumantur cochlearia tria magna ter die.

### 85. *Cubebs and Soda.*

℞. Pulveris cubebæ Əii.; sodæ sesquicarbonatis, potassæ bitartratis āā Əß. Misce; fiat pulvis, ter die sumendus.

### 86. *Copaiba and Kino.*

℞. Copaibæ f ℥ß; pulveris kino ℈j.; mucilaginis acaciæ f℈iii.; spiritus lavandulæ compositi f℈iii.; aquæ f ℥v. Misce. Sumantur cochlearia duo magna ter die.

### 87. *Copaiba and Catechu.*

℞. Copaibæ f ℥ß.; tincturæ catechu f℈vj.; olei juniperi guttas duas; mucilaginis f℈iii.; aquæ f ℥v. Misce.

### 88. *Cantharides and Zinc.*

℞. Zinci sulphatis gr. xxiv.; pulveris cantharidis gr. vj.; pulveris rhei ℈j.; terebinthinæ venetiensis quantum satis sit, ut fiant pilulæ viginti qûatuor, quarum sumantur duo ter die.

### 89. *Cantharides and Steel.*

℞. Tincturæ ferri sesquichloridi, tincturæ cantharidis, āā f℈ii.; tincturæ capsici f℈i.; syrupi croci f℈iii.; aquæ pimentæ f ℥vj. Misce; sumantur cochlearia duo ter die.

### 90. *Turpentine and Copaiba.*

℞. Olei terebinthinæ f℈ii.; copaibæ f℈vj. Misce; sumantur guttæ quadraginta ter die, ex cyatho aquæ.

### 91. *Buchu and Uva Ursi.*

℞. Foliorum buchu, et uvæ ursi, āā ℨii.; aquæ ferventis f℥vj. Macera per horas duas; dein cola, et adde liquoris potassæ fℨj.; tincturæ cinnamoni, tincturæ hyoscyami āā f℥iii. Misce; sumantur cochlearia duo ter die.*

### 92. *Tannin Gargle.*

℞. *Tannin†* ℈j.; *Brandy* f℥ß; misturæ camphoræ f℥vß. Misce. *For salivation, spongy gums; relaxed throat, &c.*

### 93. *Iodide of Potassium.*

℞. Potassii iodidi, extracti conii āā ℨß. Misce; fiant pilulæ xij.; quarum sumatur una, ter die.

### 94. *Warm Emetic.*

℞. Pulveris ipecacuanhæ, ammoniæ sesquicarbonatis aa ℈ß.; spiritus lavandulæ compositi ♏x.; aquæ f℥j. Misce; fiat haustus. Bibat æger posteà infusi anthemidis tepidi octarium.

### 95. *Colchicum and Magnesia.*

℞. Vini colchici f℥ii.; solutionis magnesiæ‡ f℥iß.; syrupi croci f℥ii.; misturæ camphoræ f℥ivß. Misce; sumantur cochlearia duo quartâ quâque horâ.

### 96. *Steel and Bitters.*

℞. Infus. quassiæ f℥ß.; tincturæ ferri ammoniati f℥ß.; ammoniæ sesquicarbonatis gr. vj.; syrupi aurantii f℥j.; aquæ destillatæ f℥vii. Misce; fiat haustus, bis vel ter quotidie sumendus. *For hysterical women. (Brodie.)*

### 97. *Opiate Collyrium.*

℞. Zinci sulphatis gr. xii.; (*vel* liquoris plumbi diacetatis f℥ß.) tincturæ opii f℥ii.; aquæ destillatæ f℥vj. Misce.

### 98. *Anti-Phosphatic Mixture.*

℞. Acidi nitrici diluti; acidi muriatici diluti aa f℥ii.ß.; syrupi aurantii f℥i.; aquæ florum aurantii f℥j.; aquæ destillatæ f℥xiiiß. Misce; sumatur cyathus vinarius, ter vel quater die. (*Brodie.*)

---

* The alkali to be omitted, if the urine tends to be alkaline.
† To be had at Morson's, Southamptom Row.
‡ Made by Murray, or Dinneford. This is the best application of this much-advertised nostrum.

### 99. *Anti-Lithic Pill.*

R. Extracti colchici acetici, pilulæ hydrargyri aa gr. j.; extracti colocynthidis compositi gr. ii. Misce; fiat pilula omni nocte sumenda.

### 100. *Corrosive Sublimate Gargle.*

R. Hydrargyri sublimati corrosivi gr. ii.; acidi hydrochlorici ℳ xx.; mellis ʒj.; aquæ destillatæ f ʒvii. Misce.

### 101. *Sulphuric Acid, and Æther.*

R. Acidi Sulphurici diluti ℳ xl.; spiritus ætheris sulphurici compositi f ʒii.; sacchari albi ʒss.; aquæ menthæ viridis f ʒvj. Misce. Sumatur pars quarta, quater die. (*An admirable restorative after illness.*)

### 102. *Chalk Ointment.*

R. Cretæ, subtilissimi pulverizatæ ʒj.; olei olivæ ʒii.; adipis ʒss. Misce. (*For burns, excoriations with acrid discharge, &c.*)

# INDEX.

LEA & BLANCHARD HAVE JUST PUBLISHED:

# MIDWIFERY ILLUSTRATED,

## BY FRANCIS H. RAMSBOTHAM, M. D.

*Physician to the Royal Maternity Charity, and Lecturer on Midwifery at the London Hospital, &c.*

The Principles and Practice of Obstetric Medicine and Surgery, in Reference to the Process of Parturition. Illustrated by One Hundred and Forty-Two Figures. First American Edition, Revised. In One large Octavo Volume.

From among numerous commendations of this work of Dr. Ramsbotham the American publishers append a few, and would particularly call the attention of the medical public to the execution of the numerous plates which form a most important feature in the volume. The great expense they have incurred in its production calls for an extended sale, which they trust the merits of the work will command.

" It is a good and thoroughly practical treatise; the different subjects are laid down in a clear and perspicuous form, and whatever is of importance is illustrated by first rate engravings. As a work conveying good, sound, practical precepts, and clearly demonstrating the doctrines of obstetrical science, we can confidently recommend it either to the student or practitioner."—*Edinburgh Journal of Medical Sciences.*

" It is *the* book on Midwifery for students : clear, but not too minute in its details, and sound in its practical instructions. It is so completely illustrated by plates (admirably chosen and executed) that the student must be stupid indeed who does not understand the details of this branch of the science, so far at least as description can make them intelligible."—*Dublin Journal of Medical Science.*

" We strongly recommend the work of Dr. Ramsbotham to all our obstetrical readers, especially to those who are entering upon practice. It is not only one of the cheapest, but one of the most beautiful works in Midwifery."—*British and Foreign Medical Review.*

" We feel much pleasure in recommending to the notice of the profession one of the cheapest and most elegant productions of the medical press of the present day. The text is written in a clear, concise, and simple style. We offer our most sincere wishes that the undertaking may enjoy all the success which it so well merits."—*Dublin Medical Press.*

" We most earnestly recommend this work to the student, who wishes to acquire knowledge, and to the practitioner who wishes to refresh his memory, as a most faithful picture of practical Midwifery ; and we can with justice say, that altogether it is one of the best books we have read on the subject of obstetrical medicine and surgery."—*Medico Chirurgical Review.*

" It is intended expressly for students and junior practitioners in Midwifery ; it is therefore as it ought to be, elementary, and will not, consequently, admit of an elaborate and extended review. Our chief object now is to state our decided opinion, that this work is by far the best that has appeared in this country, for those who seek practical information upon Midwifery, conveyed in a clear and concise style. The value of the work, too, is strongly enhanced by the numerous and beautiful drawings, by Bagg, which are in the first style of excellence. Every point of practical importance is illustrated, that requires the aid of the engraver to fix it upon the mind, and to render it clear to the comprehension of the student."—*London Medical Gazette.*

" Among the many literary undertakings with which the Medical press at present teems, there are few that deserve a warmer recommendation at our hands than the work—we might almost say the *obstetrical library*, comprised in a single volume—which is now before us. Few works surpass Dr. Ramsbotham's in beauty and elegance of getting up, and in the abundant and excellent engravings with which it is illustrated. We heartily wish the volume the success which it merits, and we have no doubt that before long it will occupy a place in every medical library in the kingdom. The illustrations are admirable; they are the joint production of Bagg and Adlard; and comprise, within the series, the best obstetrical plates of our best obstetrical authors, ancient and modern. Many of the engravings are calculated to fix the eye as much by their excellence of execution, and their beauty as works of art, as by their fidelity to nature and anatomical accuracy."—*The Lancet.*

# DUNGLISON'S PRACTICE OF MEDICINE,

## OR

## A TREATISE ON SPECIAL PATHOLOGY AND THERAPEUTICS.

### BY ROBLEY DUNGLISON, M. D.,

*Professor of the Institutes of Medicine, &c., in the Jefferson Medical College, Phila-
delphia; Lecturer on Clinical Medicine, and attending Physician at the Philadelphia Hospital &c. &c.*

CONTAINING

| | |
|---|---|
| The Diseases of the Alimentary Canal, | Diseases of the Respiratory Organs, |
| "    Circulatory Apparatus, | "    Glandiform Ganglions, |
| "    Glandular Organs, | "    Nervous System, |
| "    Organs of the Senses, | "    Organs of Reproduction, |

Diseases involving Various Organs, &c. &c.

### IN TWO VOLUMES OCTAVO.

" Enough, perhaps, has been said to convey to the reader a pretty just conception of the general plan and mode of execution of the work before us. Our examination of it has necessarily been hasty, and we are confident that we are very far from having done it all the justice which it deserves. Its author has not only given evidence of the most extensive research, but of much judgment in the choice and arrangement of his materials, and whilst he carefully recounts the various opinions of medical men upon numerous points, he equally avoids the admission of any thing like confusion into his descriptions. In the midst of conflicting opinions, the expression of his own views is marked by much clearness of conception and justness of conclusion. The whole character of the work is eminently practical. It has no tendency to lead the reader to the adoption of exclusive views; but, on the contrary, presents him with a remarkably just estimate of the state of opinion on most points. With these and other features previously noticed, of the work before us, we have been highly gratified, and we have little doubt that our readers, when they shall have an opportunity of forming their own opinions by a perusal of it, will agree with us that it contains a vastly more complete digest of the state of our knowledge in reference to Pathology and Therapeutics than any previous treatise of a similar character."—*American Medical Journal.*

" We have endeavoured to convey a general idea of the scheme of this important work, that physicians may have some data to go upon in deciding upon its character Dr. Dunglison appears to have collected every essential fact within the compass of an extensive field of observation, and has so arranged the whole mass of materials, that there is not even an opportunity for finding fault."—*Boston Medical and Surgical Journal.*

" The science of Medicine and the art of Medicine are both very well posted up, not up to the beginning of the century or to the close of the late war—or to the first year when the Professor began to lecture (as would be the case were some learned professors to print their lectures) but up to the present time, up to 1842. The student will here find a clear distinct digest of medical science—the practitioner will here see at a glance all that has been done, on any important point in practical medicine upon which he may need information. We wanted something of the kind very much, and this supplies the want The text books which teachers have been obliged to place in the hands of their students, "*faute de mieux*," are all extremely defective Those of Eberle and Dewees are evidently not the productions of medical scholars; that of Mackintosh, though full of practical sagacity, is exceedingly defective, and besides abounds in whims and notions; that of Gregory, though perhaps upon the whole the best, though full enough upon the art of medicine is lamentably deficient in the science of disease. The work of Professor Dunglison is superior to either, and will, we 'hope, soon supercede them. Most assuredly it shall with those over whose medical studies we may have control."—*New York Medical Gazette, March 2, 1842.*

" Considering the task which the learned author has undertaken to perform, and the manner in which it has been executed, we without hesitation recommend it to our readers as the best exposition of the present state of practical medicine, that has been written in the United States. In the work before us, the student will not find out what was the state of Medicine some ten or twenty years ago, but what it is at the present period In it will be found an account of all the latest pathological improvements and therapeutical changes that have been made, and to no work can he refer in which he will meet, in a small compass, with so large an amount of information that will be useful to him in actual practice."—*Western and Southern Medical Recorder, April, 1842.*

" This work supplies a want which has been long felt—an elementary treatise for students which includes the recent additions which have been made to medicine The older works, not excepting those published some ten or fifteen years since, are all deficient in this respect, and we have no doubt, that this new one will be received in a manner which will be highly gratifying to the author.

" The references in the work, as well as the formulæ, which are numerous, are included in the body of the text, and the author, with feelings of honourable justice towards his professional brethren, has mentioned the different writers whose opinions he cites. To the practitioner it will prove interesting, while it will furnish to the student—for whom it seems to be principally designed—a vast amount of useful, and, to the larger number novel, information. We are obliged to content ourselves with expressing the gratification the work has afforded us, and the belief that it will prove generally useful and acceptable."—*Philadelphia Medical Examiner, March 5, 1842.*

# LEA & BLANCHARD,

## Philadelphia,

HAVE RECENTLY PUBLISHED,

# MIDWIFERY ILLUSTRATED,

## BY FRANCIS H. RAMSBOTHAM, M.D.,

PHYSICIAN TO THE ROYAL MATERNITY CHARITY, AND LECTURER ON MIDWIFERY AT THE
LONDON HOSPITAL, ETC.

———

## THE PRINCIPLES AND PRACTICE

OF

# OBSTETRIC MEDICINE AND SURGERY,

IN REFERENCE TO THE

## Process of Parturition,

### ILLUSTRATED BY ONE HUNDRED AND FORTY-TWO FIGURES.

#### FIRST AMERICAN EDITION, REVISED.

In one large octavo volume.

From among numerous commendations of this work of Dr. Ramsbotham, the American publishers append a few, and would particularly call the attention of the medical public to the execution of the numerous plates, which form a most important feature in the volume. The great expense they have incurred in its production calls for an extended sale, which they trust the merits of the work will command.

"It is a good and thoroughly practical treatise; the different subjects are laid down in a clear and perspicuous form, and whatever is of importance is illustrated by first rate engravings. As a work conveying good, sound, practical precepts, and clearly demonstrating the doctrines of obstetrical science, we can confidently recommend it either to the student or practitioner."—*Edinburgh Journal of Medical Science.*

"It is *the* book on Midwifery for students: clear, but not too minute in its details, and sound in its practical instructions. It is so completely illustrated by plates (admirably chosen and executed) that the student must be stupid indeed who does not understand the details of this branch of the science, so far at least as description can make them intelligible."—*Dublin Journal of Medical Science.*

"There is so much in the practice of Midwifery which cannot be understood without pictorial illustrations, that they become almost essential to the student; but hitherto the expense has proved an impediment to their being employed so much as desirable. The work has only to be known to make the demand for it very extensive."—*Medical Gazette.*

"We strongly recommend the work of Dr Ramsbotham to all our obstetrical readers, especially to those who are entering upon practice. It is not only one of the cheapest, but one of the most beautiful works in Midwifery."—*British and Foreign Medical Review.*

"We feel much pleasure in recommending to the notice of the profession one of the cheapest and most elegant productions of the medical press of the present day. The text is written in a clear, concise, and simple style. We offer our most sincere wishes that the undertaking may enjoy all the success which it so well merits."—*Dublin Medical Press.*

"We most earnestly recommend this work to the student, who wishes to acquire knowledge, and to the practitioner who wishes to refresh his memory, as a most faithful picture of practical Midwifery; and we can with justice say, that altogether it is one of the best books we have read on the subject of obstetrical medicine and surgery."—*Medico-Chirurgical Review.*

"It is intended expressly for students and junior practitioners in Midwifery; it is therefore, as it ought to be, elementary, and will not, consequently, admit of an elaborate and extended review. Our chief object now is to state our decided opinion, that this work is by far the best that has appeared in this country, for those who seek practical information upon Midwifery, conveyed in a clear and concise style. The value of the work, too, is strongly enhanced by the numerous and beautiful drawings, by Bagg, which are in the first style of excellence. Every point of practical importance is illustrated, that requires the aid of the engraver to fix it upon the mind, and to render it clear to the comprehension of the student."—*London Medical Gazette.*

"Among the many literary undertakings with which the Medical press at present teems, there are few that deserve a warmer recommendation at our hands than the work—we might almost say the *obstetrical library*, comprised in a single volume—which is now before us. Few works surpass Dr Ramsbotham's in beauty and elegance of getting up, and in the abundant and excellent engravings with which it is illustrated. We heartily wish the volume the success which it merits, and we have no doubt that before long it will occupy a place in every medical library in the kingdom. The illustrations are admirable; they are the joint production of Bagg and Adlard; and comprise, within the series, the best obstetrical plates of our best obstetrical authors, ancient and modern. Many of the engravings are calculated to fix the eye as much by their excellence of execution and their beauty as works of art, as by their fidelity to nature and anatomical accuracy."—*The Lancet.*

# THE PRACTICE OF MEDICINE,

OR A

## TREATISE ON SPECIAL PATHOLOGY AND THERAPEUTICS.

### BY ROBLEY DUNGLISON, M. D.,

PROFESSOR OF THE INSTITUTES OF MEDICINE, ETC. IN THE JEFFERSON MEDICAL COLLEGE,
PHILADELPHIA, LECTURER ON CLINICAL MEDICINE, AND ATTENDING
PHYSICIAN AT THE PHILADELPHIA HOSPITAL, ETC.

CONTAINING

THE DISEASES OF THE ALIMENTARY CANAL,
THE DISEASES OF THE CIRCULATORY APPARATUS,
DISEASES OF THE GLANDULAR ORGANS,
DISEASES OF THE ORGANS OF THE SENSES,
DISEASES OF THE RESPIRATORY ORGANS,
DISEASES OF THE GLANDIFORM GANGLIONS,
DISEASES OF THE NERVOUS SYSTEM,
DISEASES OF THE ORGANS OF REPRODUCTION,
DISEASES INVOLVING VARIOUS ORGANS,
&c. &c.

## In Two Volumes Octavo.

"This new work, from the press of Lea and Blanchard, forms a valuable addition to our Medical Literature, and fills up a void in our libraries, which the numerous improvements in medical science had long since created; and we congratulate the profession in being put in possession of a work on the practice of medicine, in which not only are found the latest and most approved views of Pathology, united with the soundest practical deductions, but which is here interspersed throughout with the most valuable recipes for administering the various medicines suggested.

"The object of the author has been, as he states, to incorporate the improvements and modifications incessantly taking place in the departments of Pathology and Therapeutics, so as to furnish those to whom the different general treatises, monographs and periodicals are not accessible, with the means of appreciating their existing condition. The examination we have made of the work satisfies us that in this aim he has been eminently successful, and that he has presented to the profession the most complete work on the Practice of Medicine to be found in any language—for we know of no similar work in which is embodied such an amount of scientific and practical information. No one, therefore, who desires to keep himself au nouveau du siecle, will fail to include in his collection a work which thus brings before him the latest views of subjects, in which scientific investigations have lately wrought so many changes.

"This is not the place of course, to speak in detail of the merits of such a work. We may therefore say that the two volumes before us give evidence throughout of extensive research, deep reflection, and abilities for which, indeed, the author's name is always a guarantee; and that we can confidently recommend them to all who desire to keep pace with the progress of medical science."— Balt. Pat.

"We hail the appearance of this work, which has just been issued from the prolific press of Messrs. Lea & Blanchard, of Philadelphia, with no ordinary degree of pleasure. Comprised in two large and closely printed volumes, it exhibits a more full, accurate, and comprehensive digest of the existing state of medicine than any other treatise with which we are acquainted in the English language. It discusses many topics—some of them of great practical importance, which are entirely omitted in the writings of Eberle, Dewees, Hosack, Graves, Stokes, McIntosh, and Gregory; and it cannot fail, therefore, to be of great value, not only to the student, but to the practitioner, as it affords him ready access to information of which he stands in daily need in the exercise of his profession, It has been the desire of the author, well-known as one of the most abundant writers of the age, to render his work strictly practical; and to this end he has been induced, whenever opportunity offered, to incorporate the results of his own experience with that of his scientific brethren in America and Europe. To the former, ample justice seems to have been done throughout. We believe this constitutes the seventh work which Professor Dunglison has published within the last ten years; and, when we reflect upon the large amount of labour and reflection which must have been necessary in their preparation, it is amazing how he could have accomplished so much in so short a time."—Louisville Journal

"As a system of Practical Medicine, this work will meet a cordial welcome from all who know the untiring assiduity and laborious habits in the pursuit of knowledge, of the author, who has already presented the public with numerous excellent works, bearing the stamp of originality as well as of profound research.

"The object of Professor Dunglison is to present, in as compact a form as was consistent with accuracy and perspicuity, a history of all the affections which properly come under the care of the physician, with all the improvements and modifications which have taken place latterly in Pathology and Therapeutics, so as to enable the student and practitioner 'to appreciate their present condition,' and to avail themselves of knowledge scattered about in various journals and monographs.

"This task has been faithfully executed, and the work may be recommended as a good class-book, in which the soundness of the author's views and his freedom from exclusive opinions have enabled him to select from the experience of others those facts and views, which, together with his own experience, were to furnish the proper data for correct descriptions and for sound practical deductions."—New York American,

# LEA AND BLANCHARD

HAVE JUST PUBLISHED

A NEW AND CHEAPER EDITION

OF

# THE LIBRARY

OF

# PRACTICAL MEDICINE:

CONDUCTED BY

## ALEXANDER TWEEDIE, M.D., F.R.S.

PHYSICIAN TO THE LONDON FEVER HOSPITAL, AND TO THE FOUNDLING HOSPITAL ; EDITOR OF THE
CYCLOPEDIA OF PRACTICAL MEDICINE, ETC.

## WITH THE ASSISTANCE OF NUMEROUS CONTRIBUTORS.

THE WHOLE REVISED, WITH NOTES AND ADDITIONS,

BY

## W. W. GERHARD, M.D.,

LECTURER ON CLINICAL MEDICINE TO THE UNIVERSITY OF PENNSYLVANIA, PHYSICIAN TO
THE PHILADELPHIA HOSPITAL, BLOCKLEY, ETC.

*The whole Five Volumes of the former edition, now complete in Three large*
*Volumes,*

AND FOR SALE BY ALL BOOKSELLERS.

The design of this work is to supply the want, generally admitted to exist in the medical
literature of Great Britain, of a comprehensive System of Medicine, embodying a condensed,
yet ample, view of the present state of the science. The desideratum is more especially felt by
the Medical Student, and by many Members of the Profession, who, from their avocations and
other circumstances, have not the opportunity of keeping pace with the more recent improvements in the most interesting and useful branch of human knowledge. To supply this deficiency, is the object of THE LIBRARY OF MEDICINE; and the Editor expresses the hope, that
with the assistance with which he has been favoured by Contributors, (many of great eminence,
and all favourably known to the Public,) he has been able to produce a work, which will form
a Library of General Reference on Theoretical and Practical Medicine, as well as a Series of
Text Books for the Medical Student.

It is intended to treat of each Department, or Division of Medicine, each SERIES forming a
complete Work on the subject treated of, which may be *purchased separately* at a very moderate price, or it will constitute a part of THE LIBRARY OF MEDICINE. This arrangement is
made with the view of giving those persons who may wish to possess ONE OR MORE OF THE
SERIES, the opportunity of purchasing such Volumes only, and thus avoid the inconvenience
of making a larger addition to their stock of Books than their wants or circumstances may
require.

Each treatise is authenticated by the Name of the Author ; and from the care bestowed in
the arrangements, it is confidently hoped that the want of uniformity noticed in works of a
similar kind, has been obviated, at least, as far as is compatible with the execution of the work
by a numerous body of united Authors.

# THE AMERICAN PUBLISHERS TO THEIR NEW EDITION
## IN THREE VOLUMES.

The matter embraced in the Three Volumes now presented, was published in London in five separate volumes, and at intervals republished in this country. The rapid sale of these volumes, embracing as they do a History of Practical Medicine, is the best evidence of the favour with which it has been received by the physicians of the United States. Embodying as it does the most recent information on nearly every disease, and written by men who have specially devoted themselves to the study of the disorders which form the subject o their articles, the work is the most valuable for reference within the reach of a practitioner The arrangement of the Library into classes of diseases, grouped according to the cavities o the body, is much more agreeable to the reader than the alphabetical order, and nearly as convenient for reference.

The reader will not fail to perceive some inequality in the articles, even of the same authors; the subjects with which an author is most familiar, and upon which he had pre-viously written, are usually the best treated and most elaborate. Among the most finished treatises are those of Dr. Christison on the urinary organs, and of Williams and Joy on the thoracic viscera; several other essays are excellent monographs, and very few fall much below the average standard of the series.

The object of the publishers in compressing the five volumes of the former edition into three is to place the work at such a price as to be within the reach of every reader. There is no abridgement or alteration whatever of the text of the former edition, and the general ap-pearance of the volumes is scarcely inferior. The notes added to the last four volumes have been revised, and some additions made to them. New notes have also been added to the first volume, which was not revised in the former edition. For the note on Remittent Fever, the American Editor is indebted to Dr. Stewardson, for those on Ophthalmia to Dr. W. P. Johnston. The principal notes are one on Typhoid Fever, another on Remittent, one on Tuberculous Meningitis, and a fourth on Delirium Tremens. It was neither intended nor wished to over-load the work with annotations; the notes refer either to some trivial errors which have crept into the text, or to subjects which were treated less completely than they deserved to be; they are, therefore, comparatively few in number. Several diseases are, from the difference of cli mate, more frequent and severe in the United States than in Great Britain, and the article which relate to them required some additional matter.

The notes which appeared in the London edition are designated by the word Author. Thos of the American Editor are indicated by the letter G.

The Editor of this edition did not feel himself at liberty to make any change in the for mulæ of the prescriptions, which are published towards the end of the last volume, believing as he does, that very strong reasons alone can justify such use of a scientific work. On alteration, which adapts them to the custom of this country, was, however, made;—that is, th translation of the directions for the doses and administration of the prescriptions from Lati into English: there is an obvious convenience in this change.

The Three Volumes now presented contain the first series, that on *Practical Medicine*, of Library of Medicine, edited by Dr. Tweedie, and now in course of publication, and are com piete in themselves. The series will be continued in London, embracing works on Midwifery, Surgery, Anatomy, and the other Departments of Medical Science. Such of them as may b deemed worthy of republication will be issued here with notes and additions, each work unde its particular title, but in a style and manner to match this work.

---

\* The work on Midwifery, by Edward Rigby, with numerous wood cuts, has lately been issued by the pul lishers of these volumes.

# LEA & BLANCHARD,

## PHILADELPHIA,

### HAVE RECENTLY PUBLISHED

#### A NEW SERIES OF

##### THE

#### AMERICAN

# JOURNAL OF THE MEDICAL SCIENCES,

##### EDITED BY

## ISAAC HAYS, M. D.

##### COMMENCED ON THE 1st OF JANUARY, 1841.

#### TERMS.

Each number contains 260 pages, or upwards, and is frequently illustrated by coloured engravings. It is published on the first of January, April, July, and October. Price Five Dollars per annum, payable in advance.

Orders, enclosing the amount of one year's subscription, addressed to the publishers, or any of the agents, will receive prompt attention. The year of this work commences with the January number.

Persons sending Twenty Dollars will be entitled to five copies of the work, to be forwarded as they may direct. All persons desirous of advancing the interest of medical science, are requested to use their efforts to increase its circulation.

The postage per number is, within 100 miles, about 16 cents; over 100 miles, about 28 cents.

A few complete sets of the old series may be had at a large discount from the subscription price. Odd numbers can be furnished to complete sets.

---

##### PRACTICAL

# GEOLOGY AND MINERALOGY,

##### WITH INSTRUCTIONS FOR

## THE QUALITATIVE

## ANALYSIS OF MINERALS.

##### BY JOSHUA TRIMMER, F.G.S.

### WITH 212 WOOD CUTS.

*A handsome Octavo Volume bound in Embossed cloth.*

This is a systematic introduction to Mineralogy and Geology, and admirably calculated to instruct the student in those sciences. The organic remains of the various formations are well illustrated by numerous figures which are drawn with great accuracy.

EMBRACING,

I. The Adaptation of External Nature to the Moral and Intellectual Constitution of Man. By the Rev. Thomas Chalmers.

II. The Adaptation of External Nature to the Physical Condition of Man. By John Kidd, M. D., F. R. S.

III. Astronomy and General Physics, considered with Reference to Natural Theology. By the Rev. William Whewell.

IV. The Hand: Its Mechanism and Vital Endowments as Evincing Design. By Sir Charles Bell, K. H., F. R. S. With numerous wood cuts.

V. Chemistry, Meteorology, and the Function of Digestion. By Wm. Prout, M. D., F. R. S.

VI. The History, Habits, and Instincts of Animals. By the Rev. William Kirby, M. A., F. R. S. Illustrated by numerous engravings on copper.

VII. Animal and Vegetable Physiology, considered with Reference to Natural Theology. By Peter Mark Roget, M. D. Illustrated with nearly Five Hundred Wood Cuts.

VIII. Geology and Mineralogy, considered with Reference to Natural Theology. By the Rev. William Buckland, D. D. With numerous engravings on copper, and a large coloured Map.

☞ The work of BUCKLAND, KIRBY and ROGET, may be had separate.

---

## THIRD EDITION BROUGHT UP TO 1841,

OF

# NEW REMEDIES.

## THE METHOD OF PREPARING AND ADMINISTERING THEM;

### THEIR EFFECTS

UPON THE

## HEALTHY AND DISEASED ECONOMY, &c. &c.

### BY ROBLEY DUNGLISON, M. D.

*Professor of the Institutes of Medicine and Materia Medica in Jefferson Medical College of Philadelphia; Attending Physician to the Philadelphia Hospital, &c.*

### IN ONE VOLUME, OCTAVO.

[Extract from the Preface to the Third Edition.]

" This edition has been subjected to an entire revision, and the author has modified in certain respects the arrangement, and altered the nomenclature so as to cause it to correspond more nearly to that adopted in the Pharmacopœia of the United States."

---

## THIRD EDITION BROUGHT UP TO 1842,

OF

# DUNGLISON'S DICTIONARY

OF

# MEDICAL SCIENCE AND LITERATURE:

CONTAINING

*A concise account of the various Subjects and Terms, and Formulæ for various officinal and empirical preparations, &c.*

### IN ONE ROYAL OCTAVO VOLUME.

This new Edition includes in the body of the work, The Index, or Vocabulary of Synonymes that was in the former Editions printed at the end of the Volume, and embraces many corrections, with the additions of many new words.

FOURTH EDITION, IMPROVED WITH ADDITIONS UP TO 1842,

OF

# DUNGLISON'S HUMAN PHYSIOLOGY:

### ILLUSTRATED WITH NUMEROUS ENGRAVINGS.

### IN TWO VOLUMES OCTAVO.

---

# THE MEDICAL STUDENT;

## OR, AIDS TO THE STUDY OF MEDICINE.

Including a Glossary of the Terms of the Science, and of the mode of Prescribing; Biblio-
graphical Notices of Medical Works; the Regulations of the Different
Medical Colleges of the Union, &c.

### BY ROBLEY DUNGLISON, M. D., &c. &c.

*In One Volume, Octavo.*

---

## THE FIRST PRINCIPLES OF MEDICINE.

### BY ARCHIBALD BILLING, M. D. A. M.

*Member of the Senate of the University of London, Fellow of the Royal College of Physicians,
&c. &c.*

In One Volume, 8vo. First American from the Fourth London Edition.

" We know of no book which contains within the same space so much valuable information, the result not of fanciful theory, nor of idle hypothesis, but of close persevering clinical
observation, accompanied with much soundness of judgment, and extraordinary clinical
tact."—*Medico-Chirurgical Review.*

---

### A NEW EDITION (THE SIXTH) OF

# THE MEDICAL FORMULARY OF DR. ELLIS,

This edition is completely revised, with many additions and modifications, and brought up to
the present improved state of the Science,

### BY SAMUEL GEORGE MORTON, M. D.

*Professor in the Pennsylvania College of Medicine, &c. &c.*

---

## A PRACTICAL TREATISE ON THE HUMAN TEETH,

Showing the causes of their destruction and the means of their preservation. By Wm.
Robertson. With plates. First American, from the second London
edition. In One Volume.

---

### OUTLINES OF A

## COURSE OF LECTURES ON MEDICAL JURISPRUDENCE.

### BY THOMAS STEWART TRAILL, M. D.

*From the Second Edinburgh Edition, with American Notes and Additions.*

---

## ARNOTT'S ELEMENTS OF PHYSICS.

*Complete in One Volume.*

A New Edition of Elements of Physics, or Natural Philosophy, general and medical, written for universal use, in plain or non-technical language, and containing New Disquisitions
and Practical Suggestions, comprised in five parts:—1st. Somatology, Statics and Dynamics.
2d. Mechanics. 3d. Pneumatics, Hydraulics and Acoustics. 4th. Heat and Light. 5th.
Animal and Medical Physics. Complete in one volume, by Neil Arnott, M. D., of the Royal
College of Physicians. A new edition, revised and corrected from the last English edition,
with additions, by Isaac Hays, M. D.

---

## A PRACTICE OF PHYSIC.

Comprising most of the diseases not treated of in Diseases of Females and Diseases of
Children, second edition. By W. P. Dewees, M. D., formerly adjunct professor in the University of Pennsylvania. In one volume, octavo.

# A COMPENDIOUS SYSTEM OF MIDWIFERY.

### BY DR DEWEES.

Chiefly designed to facilitate the Inquiries of those who may be pursuing this branch of study. Illustrated by occasional cases and with many plates. The ninth edition, with additions and improvements. In one vol. 8vo.

## DEWEES ON THE DISEASES OF FEMALES.

The seventh Edition, Revised and Corrected. With Additions and Numerous Plates. In One Vol., 8vo.

## DEWEES ON THE PHYSICAL AND MEDICAL TREATMENT OF CHILDREN

With Corrections and Improvements. The seventh edition. In one volume, 8vo.

## A FLORA OF NORTH AMERICA.

With 108 Coloured Plates. By W. P. C. Barton, M. D. In three volumes, quarto.

A Treatise on Special and General Anatomy. By W. E. Horner, M. D., Professor of Anatomy in the University of Pennsylvania, &c., &c. Fifth edition, Revised, and much improved. In two volumes, 8vo.
This work is extensively used as a Text Book.

A System of Midwifery, with numerous wood cuts, by Edward Rigby, M. D., Physician to the General Lying-in Hospital, Lecturer on Midwifery at St. Bartholomew's Hospital, &c., with notes and additional illustrations by an American Practitioner. In One Volume.

*Extract from the Editor's Preface.*—"This System of Midwifery, complete in itself, was published in London, as part of Dr. Tweedle's ' Library of Medicine.' The first series of the Library, that on ' Practical Medicine,' recently completed, has been received with extraordinary favour on both sides of the Atlantic, and the character of the publication is fully sustained in the present contribution by Dr. Rigby, and will secure for it additional patronage.

"The late Professor Dewees, into whose hand this volume was placed, a few weeks before his death, in returning it expressed the most favourable opinion of its merits, and the judgment of such high authority renders it supererogatory to add a word farther of commendation."

A Treatise on Pulmonary Consumption, comprehending an inquiry into the Nature, Causes, Prevention, and Treatment of Tuberculous and Scrofulous Diseases in General. By James Clark, M. D., F. R. S.

*Essays on ASTHMA, APHTHÆ, ASPHYXIA, APOPLEXY, ARSENIC, ATROPA, AIR, ABORTION, ANGINA-PECTORIS, and other subjects Embraced in the Articles from A to Azote, prepared for the Cyclopædia of Practical Medicine.* By Dr. Chapman and others.
Each article is complete within itself, and embraces the practical experience of its author, and as they are only to be had in this collection will be found of great value to the profession.
*⁎⁎⁎* The two volumes are now offered at a price so low, as to place them within the reach of every practitioner and student.

A Practical Treatise on Medical Jurisprudence, with so much of Anatomy, Physiology, Pathology, and the Practice of Medicine and Surgery, as are essential to be known by Members of the Bar and Private Gentlemen ; and all the laws relating to Medical Practitioners, with explanatory plates. By J. Chitty, Esq. Second American edition : with Notes and Additions, adapted to American works and Judicial Decisions, 8vo.

Abercrombie's Pathological and Practical Researches on Diseases of the Stomach, the Intestinal Canal, the Liver, and other Viscera of the Abdomen. Third American, from the second London edition, enlarged. In 1 vol. 8vo.

A Treatise on Fever. By Southwood Smith, M. D., Physician to the London Fever Hospital. Fourth American edition. In 1 volume, 8vo.

The Anatomy, Physiology, and Diseases of the Teeth. By Thomas Bell, F. R. S., F. L. S.,

Lightning Source UK Ltd.
Milton Keynes UK
UKHW022215140219
337291UK00006B/458/P